Nursing
Leadership
and Management
in Canada

Nursing
Leadership
and Management
in Canada

THIRD EDITION

Judith M. Hibberd
Donna Lynn Smith

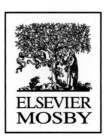

ELSEVIER
MOSBY

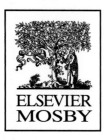

NOTICE

Pharmacology is an ever-changing field. Standard safety precautions must be followed, but as new research and clinical experience broaden our knowledge, changes in treatment and drug therapy may become necessary or appropriate. Readers are advised to check the most current product information provided by the manufacturer of each drug to be administered to verify the recommended dose, the method and duration of administration, and contraindications. It is the responsibility of the licensed prescriber, relying on experience and knowledge of the patient, to determine dosages and the best treatment for each individual patient. Neither the Publisher nor the editor assume any liability for any injury and/or damage to persons or property arising from this publication.

Library and Archives Canada Cataloguing in Publication

Hibberd, Judith M. (Judith Mary). 1934-
Nursing leadership and management in Canada/Judith M. Hibberd, Donna Lynn Smith. –3rd ed.
Includes index.
First 2 eds. had title: Nursing management in Canada.
ISBN-13: 978-0-9205-1389-7   ISBN-10: 0-9205-1389-1

I. Nursing services–Canada–administration. I. Smith, Donna Lynn, 1945-
II. Title. III. Title: Nursing management in Canada.

RT89.H53 2004   362.17'3'068   C2004-905989-0

Publisher: Ann Millar
Managing Developmental Editor: Martina van de Velde
Project Manager: Liz Radojkovic
Copy Editor: Kelly Davis
Proofreader: Rachelle Redford
Typesetting and Assembly: Judith Campbell
Printing and Binding: R.R. Donnelley

Elsevier Canada
1 Goldthorne Ave., Toronto, ON, Canada M8Z 5S7
Phone: 1-866-896-3331
Fax: 1-866-359-9534

Printed in the United States of America.

2 3 4 5   10 09 08 07 06 05

Dedication

In this dedication we honour all those uncelebrated nursing leaders in Canada whose professional competence, intellectual curiosity, and sense of adventure have enriched the quality of health and life of the people in their communities. Elizabeth Crockett Davidson was one such person. Born in 1903, she was a graduate of Royal Alexandra Hospital School of Nursing in Edmonton. She became Matron of the Calgary Red Cross Children's Hospital (c. 1929), and in the early 1930s she worked with one of the travelling medical clinics established by the government of Alberta to serve economically depressed areas of the province. Between 1932 and 1934 she was the second District Nurse at Worsely, Alberta. She married and gave birth to four children in an isolated farm home with the assistance of another district nurse. After moving to Ontario with her family in 1943, she provided informal health teaching and consultation to other women in her community. She died in 1951.

Preface

Authors and editors of any textbook face inevitable challenges and choices. They must clarify their general view as to the purpose of the textbook and give thought to the audience to be addressed. They must make a critical decision about what to include in the book and what to leave out. In doing this, they expose and express their values. In this preface we explain our approach to designing this book in the hope that this will help all readers use it to best advantage for their immediate and reference purposes.

Who Should Read this Book and Why?

As this book goes to press, it continues to be the only Canadian book with a specific focus on nursing leadership and management. Previous editions have been used as textbooks in both undergraduate and graduate courses on nursing leadership and administration, or in courses about nursing issues. The book is also widely used by nurses who are leaders at various levels in different types of health service organizations. It is sometimes consulted as a reference source by people from outside the nursing discipline who want to know what nurses are taught about leadership and management, or what to expect of nurses who hold leadership positions. As authors and editors we have endeavoured to design this third edition with the needs of all these audiences in mind. This helps to explain the purpose, structure, length, and scope of the book.

The Purpose and Objectives of this Book

In the *Concise Oxford Dictionary,* a textbook is defined as a manual of instruction and as a standard book in a branch of study. Textbooks therefore have a practical purpose: to acquaint readers with established knowledge so that they can use it as a basis for further study in the discipline, or apply it to professional practice. As in any scientific field, knowledge in the health care field is expanding. New discoveries and research findings have to be evaluated for their potential to become useful knowledge for inclusion in a textbook on nursing leadership and management.

Our objective in this book is to transmit established knowledge in the domain of nursing leadership and management and to encourage the excellence in practice, teaching, scholarship, and research that is needed to develop and refine knowledge in this domain. More specifically, our objectives as authors and editors are to:

- transmit the body of established knowledge in a fashion that facilitates learning by undergraduate students and beginning nursing leaders;
- challenge outstanding undergraduate students to pursue further study and careers in the field of nursing leadership and management;
- assist faculty colleagues at universities and colleges in their teaching and scholarship in this field of study;
- address the needs of students and faculty in graduate programs for nursing leadership by examining practical leadership problems within a scholarly framework of theory and research; and
- provide evidence and support for policy and evidence-based practice by nurse leaders and other leaders and policy-makers who make decisions about the organizational arrangements, resources, and management practices affecting nurses and the nursing discipline.

Identifying Established Knowledge in a Rapidly Changing Context

Nursing and nursing administration emerged as a professional discipline and field of study at about the same time as management theories began to be developed. This occurred long before the field of health services administration and business administration were recognized as formal fields of study. As a mature, self-regulated profession, nursing is comparable only to medicine in terms of the length of its history and published literature, and the extent of its societal impact and influence.

The field of nursing leadership and administration is, itself, an area in which there is established knowledge that has been formally transmitted for over a century through textbooks and an ever-expanding periodical literature. Nursing leadership and administration were among the first areas of nursing practice to be the focus of graduate education programs in universities, and they continue to be the focus of specialized graduate study at the master's and doctoral level in universities in many western countries, including Canada.

As Dr. Heather Spence Laschinger has explained in her chapter *Nursing Administration Research*, knowledge is not generated from single studies, but rather from programs of reproducible research that have as their ultimate goal the development or testing of theories to guide practice. Claims and assertions about the content and credibility of established knowledge need to be appraised and evaluated in terms of the type of evidence used to substantiate them. Evidence and knowledge are not the same thing. Single elements and sources of evidence must be confirmed by similar methods, reconfirmed through multiple approaches and methods, reproduced under controlled conditions, and applied to achieve anticipated results before claims of knowledge can be made.

In planning, writing, and editing this book, we have been conscious of our professional and scholarly responsibilities to evaluate and present evidence of various kinds. The references cited in each chapter provide readers with insights into the type of evidence upon which particular claims or arguments are based. We take the position that recency of publication, even in the most prestigious of peer-reviewed journals, is not in itself a criterion for the relevance or applicability of specific evidence to practical problems of decision-making and leadership in nursing or any other field.

We believe there is value in publishing single anecdotal or case reports for illustrative or analytical purposes, but neither a single case nor a single report of a rigorous study can be assumed to be established knowledge. Rather it is to be hoped that cumulative research in a particular area will reveal how data have been collected, analyzed, and described in a disciplined and systematic fashion, so that knowledgeable readers will be able to evaluate the evidence being presented. More importantly, for the benefit of novice readers in a subject area, it is critical that claims for the relevance, significance, and credibility of evidence from any single publication not be exaggerated. We believe that learning to read critically and assess evidence in a domain of study is one of the most important objectives of post-secondary education.

In this book, bibliographic citations for each chapter include references to original studies, historical documents, classic titles, and basic textbooks in relevant fields. Writings of professional experts and reports of peer-reviewed research have been included to enable readers to trace the evolution of ideas, concepts, and theories and to present evidence from a variety of different sources. The types of evidence presented in this text include statistics, the opinions and experiential knowledge of experts, as well as real life and hypothetical examples. The narrative text and pedagogical features such as case studies, case examples, learning exercises, and learning resources are intended to facilitate objective analysis and critical appraisal of information and ideas presented.

The Relative Importance of Leadership and Management

In the preface to the second edition of this book, we challenged the tendency in many textbooks and some periodical literature to make a dichotomous distinction between leadership and management. We reiterate our belief that leaders who lack management skills are as much of a liability to modern organizations and the communities they serve as are managers who lack the vision of leadership. In 2005, we re-affirm this position, pointing out that many so-called "visionary" changes to the health system and the structure and management practices of health agencies over the past decade have been poorly chosen, planned, and implemented. For these and other reasons (including the possibility that they were faddish or foolish with no basis in evidence or expert knowledge), health organizations and professionals now are experiencing change fatigue.

Financial savings and quality outcomes predicted and promised by the proponents of many faddish changes have not materialized. It is now highly instructive to re-evaluate these initiatives in light of the evidence, if any, that was available for decision-making at the time these management strategies were advocated and hastily implemented. In many instances, the ethical precept "first, do no harm" can be seen to have been violated. The direct costs of implementing administrative "quick-fixes" in the health system have often been significant. However, these are now recognized as inconsequential in relation to a more profound loss of capacity and confidence that has resulted in cynicism and attrition among health professionals. As readers of this text will discover, the nursing discipline and nursing leaders at all levels have been disproportionately affected by this problem in recent years.

Two major issues currently dominate public and professional discourse of health policy and health services administration. These are the related concerns about patient safety and leadership accountability for the "blunt end" conditions that undermine safety and quality in the health system. These pervasive themes are reflected in the programs of conferences for health system leaders and in the health services administration literature. Appropriate knowledge appraisal and the application of best practices from established knowledge in the field of management might have prevented the problems that have resulted from importing so-called "visionary" ideas and practices from less complex business and industrial contexts. Best leadership and management practice now is needed to correct these problems and to select innovations that have the greatest potential to improve the delivery and outcomes of health services.

Is this Book Practical or Theoretical?

As authors and editors, we have occasionally been asked why we chose to include certain chapters in the book — particularly those that are theoretical and do not seem to have a direct or immediate application to basic nursing or nursing leadership practice. Our answer to this question is that nursing leadership and management occur in complex political and organizational contexts and also in a context of changing values and ideas about what the health system is and what its goals and policies should be. There are some uniquely Canadian perspectives on the values, goals, and priorities of the health system. Some of these are highlighted in Section I of the book titled *The Context for Health Services in Canada*. Readers will find the material in this section to be more discursive than prescriptive and with an intentionally forward looking and sometimes theoretical focus. There are two entirely new chapters in this section, Chapter 3, *A Population Health Approach to Planning*, and Chapter 6, *The Nursing Workforce in Canada*.

In Section II, *Structure and Organization*, readers will find historical and current information about how the health system, health organizations, and nurses' work are structured. Understanding the history of knowledge on a topic is a basic requirement for conducting research or for evaluating current evidence and debate on the subject. Therefore, some material in this section is basic and factual, intended to enable readers to understand the organizational arrangements they directly observe and experience, and to explain how these have come to be. Other material is intended to introduce the reader to the evolution of theoretical ideas and research about organizational variables and is of relevance not only to nurses and nursing leaders, but to all policy- and decision-makers in the health system. The final chapter in this section intentionally illustrates the use of a critical perspective and will be of particular interest to graduate students and researchers.

In Section III, *Standards and Accountability*, information about the legal framework for health services and agencies provides a background for understanding existing standards and approaches to quality management and emerging issues about safety and accountability in the health system. The material in this section has undergone major revision and in Chapters 12 (*Standards and Quality in the Canadian Health System*) and 13 (*Accountability in the Canadian Health System*), the intention has been to supplement expository material with theoretical and critical analysis.

Section IV, *Professional Leadership*, deals with leadership issues that are particularly relevant to nurses and the nursing discipline. Readers prepared in other disciplines will find that these issues can be extrapolated to the more general but pressing problem of how to structure health service organizations so that the development and application of disciplinary knowledge is encouraged and optimized. There are three entirely new chapters in this section. Chapter 14, *Leadership and Leaders*, is intended to inform and inspire through a discussion of leadership theories and by presenting profiles of registered nurses who have achieved positions of senior leadership in various parts of Canada. The challenging material in the new Chapters 18 (*Nursing Information and Outcomes*) and 19 (*Nursing Administration Research*) will be of particular interest to graduate students and senior leaders who are concerned about improving and speeding up the process of knowledge transfer that has now become a public policy priority.

Section V, *Leadership and Management Skills*, is entirely practical, and readers will see in this section the type of material that is most frequently the focus of traditional textbooks on management. The content of Chapters 21 through 30 is typically covered in courses focused on the role of the front-line or middle managers and is generally applicable to all disciplines. The material in Chapter 31, *Policy Analysis: From Issues to Action*, is intentionally more difficult and has been added for the benefit of graduate students, researchers, and senior leaders.

Another new feature of this book is that each section is preceded by an introduction explaining the relevance of each chapter to the study of nursing leadership and management.

How Should Readers Approach This Book?

We hope that all readers will approach this book with discipline and concentration. If you are an undergraduate student or a beginning front-line manager, you will begin by reading for information and basic understanding. The organization of the book and of each chapter is intended to help you do this. The objectives, headings, and summaries are designed to highlight key points.

Once you have grasped the terminology and concepts in a chapter, you should be able to apply these to practical situations. The case examples, case studies, and learning exercises are designed to assist you. Learning Resources and Further Readings at the end of the chapters offer more detailed discussions of particular topics. We have been highly selective in the Internet Resources listed at the end of chapters, choosing those that are informative and likely to be maintained.

We are firm in our resolve to challenge and not patronize all readers of this book. We are optimistic that all readers, but particularly advanced students, senior leaders, and decision-makers, will approach the material critically and analytically. Ultimately, the evaluation of the evidence and knowledge presented in this book will require that readers be more disciplined, discerning, and knowledgeable than the original writers. If or when this is the case, we will have achieved our most important objective as teachers and scholars.

Judith M. Hibberd and Donna Lynn Smith
January 2005

Acknowledgments

This book is a collaborative venture and has been completed with the assistance of a virtual team. Its depth, breadth, and scholarship has been enriched by professional colleagues from all regions of Canada and from teachers and practitioners of nursing leadership and management. We thank all contributing authors for their support, diligence, and intellectual contributions.

As faculty members, we acknowledge our debt to the students whom we have taught in leadership and management courses and whose research we have supervised. Several past or present students are among the co-authors and contributors to this edition. Material that is new to this edition and revisions or additions to previously published material is, in many cases, a response to these students' needs and questions. The pedagogical features of this third edition have been designed to facilitate teaching and learning, and they have benefited from the opinions of our students and faculty colleagues.

Reviewers have played an important role in the development of this third edition. Reviews of the second edition provided a basis for identifying its strengths and for confirming that the book was serving, and should continue to serve, a number of different audiences. As previous chapters were revised and updated and new chapters written, each was anonymously reviewed by four colleagues teaching in this field. We thank all reviewers for their detailed comments and hope that each will find our responses to the issues they raised.

As authors and editors, our own work has been facilitated by colleagues who have assisted in bibliographic search. We particularly thank the following people for their assistance in these areas: Taranjeet Birdi, BA, MPH; Jane E. Smith, RN, MN; and Vickie Boechler, RN, MN.

We also thank the following colleagues who provided consultation, advice, or reviews of specific chapters: Greta Cummings, Assistant Professor, Faculty of Nursing, University of Alberta; Susan Wagner, Professor, College of Nursing, University of Saskatchewan; Richard Fraser, QC, Edmonton; Kathleen E. Oliver, Director of Clinical Informatics, Chinook Health Region; Barbara Rocchio, President, Innovative Health Care Consulting, Inc.; and Linda D. MacKay, Nursing Instructor, Red Deer College. We express our appreciation to Llyn Madsen who has assisted us with bibliographic search, communications, and instructional design.

Finally, we thank Ann Millar, Publisher, and her colleagues at Elsevier Canada for their belief in the importance of this book, their patience with our idiosyncrasies, and their professional advice and skills.

JMH & DLS

Contents

Contents

Governing boards and senior leaders bear the main responsibility for monitoring and interacting with forces in the complex external environment of health agencies. Factors and trends in the political, social, and economic context of the health system may seem distant from the daily activities of clinical professionals and first-line or middle managers; however, a basic understanding of these factors can help clinical care providers and leaders at all levels understand and influence the context of their work. Section I provides a broad view of the Canadian health system and identifies issues of key importance to nurses and nursing leaders.

In Chapter 1, *Political, Social, and Economic Forces Shaping the Health Care System*, key characteristics and developmental milestones in the evolution of the Canadian health system are described. The authors are distinguished scholars who have observed and studied the development of the Canadian health system and who have made major contributions to the education of health system leaders in Canada. For most readers, the details of this chapter will be less important than the broad overview it provides; however, this chapter will also be a helpful reference for readers who need to confirm specific principles or facts about the health system that is so prized by Canadians and admired around the world.

Although health economics is a specialized field, many issues in this area of scholarship are now presented in daily newspapers as well as in research reports and government policy documents. In Chapter 2, *Health Economics and Health System Reform,* a prominent Canadian health economist introduces readers to basic concepts and information in this field of growing importance. An understanding of the way health services are funded and how financial incentives have developed and changed is now relevant to both clinical and leadership practice.

Canada has led the world in the development and application of *A Population Health Approach to Planning,* described and discussed in Chapter 3 by a team of experts. Although the concepts and principles of this approach were originally associated exclusively with the field of public health, they are now recognized as essential to setting goals and measuring outcomes in all sectors of the health system. When there is competition for resources, it is important to be able to assess whether expenditures are resulting in demonstrable improvements to the health of individuals and groups. Therefore, there has been growing recognition of the need to apply population health principles in the planning and evaluation of services provided in hospitals and all other care settings.

In Canada, community health centres have developed as an organizational model for implementing primary health services, and it can be expected that they will increase in number and variety in the years to come. Chapter 4, *Implementing Primary Health Care through Community Health Centres*, describes how community health centres have developed and how they are operated. Many readers will find this information useful as they will have opportunities to participate in these agencies as clinicians, nurse practitioners, or leaders. The authors of this chapter are particularly well equipped to address this topic—one has conducted research on community health centres for over a decade, and the other is directly involved as a nurse practitioner in an innovative community health centre. Although it began with charitable services to disadvantaged or marginalized groups, primary health care is now recognized as being critical to the improvement of health for the entire population.

In Chapter 5, readers are introduced to contemporary conceptualizations and current and emerging issues in *Continuity of Care, Service Integration, and Case Management* by a team of authors directly involved in research, education, and practice in this area. The need to integrate services and provide continuity of health care has been recognized in the professional literature since the 1960s; however, the number of health disciplines and the settings for delivery of health services has dramatically increased since that time. Specialized fields of knowledge and practice, fragmented health services, and problems in crossing boundaries between health and other human services now present bewildering complexities, costs, and inconveniences to citizens who must seek services or manage ongoing health concerns. Improving the integration of services and achieving improved continuity of care have become explicit goals of health reform initiatives in Western countries and are factors in the restructuring of the Canadian health system. Case management is an intervention that has proven to be effective in achieving and improving continuity of care, and many readers of this chapter will be familiar with one or more case management models and the requirements for this professional role. Structural changes to create regional systems and services have improved continuity for some populations or in some programs, but have also created new sources of discontinuity. Therefore, the integration of services and the achievement of continuity of care through case management services, and other means, will remain high-level policy and administrative priorities for federal and provincial governments and individual health organizations.

The ability to maintain quality in traditional health services and to implement initiatives to improve population health, primary health care, and continuity of care is highly dependent upon the professional nursing workforce. This important health policy and planning issue is discussed in Chapter 6, *The Nursing Workforce in Canada*. Registered nurses (RNs) provide essential health services and are uniquely prepared with the knowledge required to assure quality and to advance needed reforms in the health system. Ironically, as a professional group, they have been subject to conflicting political and organizational policies and funding cycles that, in turn, have created fluctuations in the number of nurses available. Many readers of this book will have direct experience of the effects of these cycles and will be aware of factors in the work environment that affect the retention and, therefore, the supply of RNs. The authors of this chapter are members of a research team who are making a contribution of knowledge and policy recommendations to this area of health workforce planning, which is a concern to all practicing nurses and health system leaders.

POLITICAL, SOCIAL, AND ECONOMIC FORCES SHAPING THE HEALTH CARE SYSTEM

Janet L. Storch and Carl A. Meilicke

Learning Objectives

In this chapter, you will learn:

- Major forces and events that shaped the health care system from before Confederation in 1867 until the early days of the 21st century

- The division of power between federal and provincial governments in relation to health care services

- The act of parliament that originally established and continues to influence jurisdiction for health services in Canada

- The five principles upon which the Canadian health care system is founded

- About influential reports that affected development of health and social welfare programs in Canada, and their significance for social policy

- Legislation that has had major impacts on development of the health care system

- The main reasons provincial and federal governments continue to debate how to reform the health care system

This chapter briefly describes the Canadian health care system, with attention to the political, social, and economic forces that have shaped it. A historical-analytical approach has been adopted to trace the causes and consequences of the development of the Canadian health care system, beginning with the period predating Confederation and ending with the 21st century. The chapter concludes with a discussion of current issues and trends and future policy implications relative to the Canadian health care system.

General Structure of the Canadian Health Care System

Knowing the general types of health care systems that exist across the industrialized nations helps to place the Canadian health care system in context. Four general types ("ideal types") of health care systems are apparent, ranging from those in which governments play a residual role in a system governed by a market orientation (private health insurance systems), to the opposite extreme in which governments define health care as an essential service (socialized health care systems) (Najman & Western, 1984; Storch, 2003). In private health insurance systems, preservation of the autonomy of physicians, health institutions, and clients take priority. The fact that a substantial minority of people might be without health care in such a system is viewed as unfortunate but unavoidable. In socialized health care systems, minimal autonomy of the health provider and patient is accepted since the goal is to preserve the collective good by ensuring optimal productivity of citizens.

Between these opposite types of health care systems are two other approaches to the delivery of health care. In one of these, the role of government in health services is viewed as a necessary vehicle for reasonable social distribution of resources (national health service). Health services are seen to be a natural resource that should be available to all based on need, not ability to pay. Physician, institution, and patient autonomy are secondary to public need. In the final general type of health care system, government attempts to balance autonomy with the collective good through public insurance programs (national health insurance). In this type of system, physician, institution, and patient autonomy are preserved, but within a context of equitable access to health services for all citizens.

If the private health insurance system is typified by the general approach to delivering health care in the United States, and the national health service system is typified by the approach initially taken by the United Kingdom, then the Canadian health care system (the national health insurance system) falls somewhere in between these ideal types (i.e., the American and British approaches). By encouraging autonomy of health professionals and health agencies while ensuring relatively equal access to health care by all individuals regardless of their ability to pay, two important values in Canadian society are protected.

Principles of Canadian Health Care

In attempting to protect and preserve autonomy and equity, the Canadian health care system has been built upon five main principles: universality, accessibility, comprehensiveness, portability, and public administration. Provincial tax revenues and, to a declining degree, federal tax revenues fund medical and hospital service delivery in all provinces as long as the five essential principles are honoured.

Only three provinces (Alberta, British Columbia, and Ontario) levy premiums to assist with costs of health services. However, for the most part, there are no user fees or extra billing for services considered medically necessary because such fees are seen to violate the principle of accessibility. Thus, coverage of basic hospital care (e.g., X-rays, medications, diagnostic testing) and physician care is provided "free" to all Canadian citizens. Private health insurance (e.g., Blue Cross) covers only supplemental benefits, such as private accommodation, ambulance services, out-of-country costs not covered under the public plan, and other health benefits.

Although publicly funded health insurance remains the dominant coverage, it must be acknowledged that during the 1990s and into the 21st century, there has been a steady erosion of what is defined as "medically necessary service." Each province has the authority to determine this definition. For example, many provinces once included chiropractic, optometry, physiotherapy, and other services as medically necessary. By 2003, many of these services had been largely withdrawn. (These changes will be discussed in further detail in the final sections of this chapter.)

The Canadian health care system is part of a broader network of social security programs that have developed over time. This network of programs, made accessible to all, is a remarkable achievement for a relatively young nation. Although the phrase "Canadian health care system" is commonly used, it is important to remember that Canada does not have a federal health care system—it has ten provincial plus three territorial health care systems. The federal government has provided principle-based leadership and monetary support (since 1968) through various means over the years. It also plays a more direct role in care in the three territories, although they have moved toward greater autonomy in the last few years.

The range of social programs reflects basic values that have evolved over more than 200 years. Some of the most notable commitments developed in the early part of the 20th century, particularly in Saskatchewan, where a number of innovative approaches to health care occurred. These innovations became part of the background for establishing a national blueprint of Canadian social security in the mid-1940s. The values underlying these innovations continued to shape health care policy and programs in the 1990s. As Deber and Vayda (1992) noted, "Historically, Canadians have accepted government intervention in social programs and have welcomed sponsorship of health care" (p. 3).

Understanding how this network of programs took shape is critical to understanding the strengths and challenges of the system in the 21st century. Therefore, the historical perspective presented below outlines seven main eras of health policy and program development and highlights the nature and dynamics of the changes that shaped their evolution. Each era is characterized by distinctive concerns and activities. The following eras are considered: (a) the days of the earliest settlements until Confederation in 1867, (b) Confederation to the mid-1940s,

(c) the mid-1940s to the mid-1960s, (d) the mid-1960s to the mid-1970s, (e) the mid-1970s to 1989, (f) the 1990s, and (g) 2000 onward. These time periods are approximate, of course, because multidimensional historical dynamics defy precise categorization into unidimensional time periods.

Era One: Pre-Confederation and Ad Hoc Arrangements for Health Care

In the young and developing Canadian nation predating Confederation, self-reliance was necessary and valued. Self-reliance involved providing for the necessities of life, looking after one's family, and providing health care. The natural outcome of this focus on self-reliance was the belief that there should be limited government involvement in social security, other than a modicum of services for the sick, mentally ill, and delinquents (Cassidy, 1947; Splane, 1965). Typical examples of the limited legislation and programs were acts (dating from the early 1700s) to control the sale of meat, establish quarantine stations, deal with foundlings, and make provision for sick and disabled seamen (Gelber, 1973; Gregoire, 1962; Heagerty, 1934). Buildings were provided for the insane (lunatic asylums), provisions were made for the care of lepers, and procedures were implemented to handle epidemics of cholera, smallpox, and typhus. The procedures for dealing with epidemics were ad hoc measures, with no permanent boards of health. This ad hoc approach was typical—governments chose not to develop proactive policies because these might be viewed as interfering with self-reliance. Instead, they reacted only to the major crises of the day. As Wallace (1950) noted, Canada's population was primarily rural, and problems that might now be defined as social problems were then viewed as problems to be addressed by families, local communities, or the Church, rather than the state.

These were among the reasons the *British North America (BNA) Act (1867)*, one of the constituting acts of Canada, made provision only for residual needs; the authors assumed that the family, community, or Church was capable of handling the major concerns. Thus, Section 91 of the *BNA Act* outlines federal responsibilities as raising money by a mode or system of taxation, providing for census and statistics, providing for quarantine, establishing and maintaining marine hospitals, and being responsible for Indians and their reserved lands.

The only items relevant to health care are in Section 92, which outlines provincial responsibilities. Provinces were responsible for the "establishment, maintenance, and management of hospitals, Asylums, charities, and eleemosynary institutions in and for the province, other than marine hospitals" and for "generally all matters of a merely local or private Nature in the Province" (*BNA Act*, 1867, as cited in Van Loon & Whittington, 1976, p. 483). This short-sighted delineation of legal responsibilities left virtually all health service provision in the hands of the provinces, which had insufficient tax bases to support such extensive services to meet the needs of the Canadian public. "The fathers of Confederation proved to be poor prophets. The resulting imbalance between fiscal resources and constitutional responsibilities has made federal-provincial relations the primary concern of Canadian politics" (Deber & Vayda, 1992, p. 3).

Since the *BNA Act* contained such limited provisions for determining federal and provincial responsibilities in matters of health and welfare, and with the lion's share of responsibility resting with the provinces, only three options were open to federal and provincial governments to deal with this anomaly: (a) they could go ahead on their own, (b) they could push for a constitutional amendment, or (c) they could enter into cost-shared programs (Taylor, 1987). All these strategies are evident in the system that unfolded during the ensuing years.

It is important to remember that the division of power and the use of these strategies are not only historically interesting, but are also important in understanding the Canadian health care system of today. These same provisions still prevail because the *BNA Act* became part of the constitutional package under the *Constitution Act (1982)*, part of the process that created the *Canadian Charter of Rights and Freedoms* and a constitutional amending formula.

Era Two: Confederation to the Mid-1940s— The Creation of a Blueprint for Health Care

The second era was characterized by growing awareness that organized action was necessary to deal with the social security needs of an increasingly urbanized and industrialized nation. This awareness led to extensive developments in government and voluntary programs and, eventually, to a profoundly important clarification of federal versus provincial authority in matters relating to social security. This era is characterized by increasing government involvement and a slow but steady progression from reactive ad hoc programming to beginning efforts to effect planned change.

Between Confederation in 1867 and 1920, municipal and provincial programs in health and social security were expanded considerably, and many important voluntary organizations were formed. For example, organizations now known as the Toronto Children's Aid Society (1891), the Red Cross (1896), the Victorian Order of Nurses (1897), the Canadian Mental Health Association (1918), the Canadian Institute for the Blind (1918), and the Canadian Council of Social Development (1920) were organized during this time (Armitage, 1975).

Growth in municipal and provincial government activities during this period occurred because the *BNA Act* was silent on matters of health and welfare services, reflecting the conviction that these matters, insofar as they were the responsibility of government, were of proper concern only to local and provincial authorities (Splane, 1965; Wallace, 1950). Representative of such activities was the substantial expansion of welfare services in Ontario, the implementation of municipal doctor plans and union hospitals in Saskatchewan, an income support plan for widowed mothers in Manitoba, and municipal hospital plans in Manitoba and Alberta (Gelber, 1966; Morgan, 1961; Rorem, 1931; Splane, 1965; Taylor, 1949).

These municipal and provincial developments proceeded apace through to the 1940s. At that time, the federal government—in response to growing public demand for social services and to the social disruptions caused by World War I (1914–1918) and the Great Depression (1930s)— began to consolidate its health responsibilities and respond to needs newly deemed to require federal assistance. These initiatives were largely reactive rather than planned (e.g., grants-in-aid scheme for venereal disease control, *Soldiers' Settlement Act* of 1920), and relatively few programs were actually established. However, one program, the *Old Age Pensions Act (1927)*, was significant in being Canada's first nationwide income support plan and the first major continuing federal-provincial cost-shared social security program (Bryden, 1974; Cameron, 1962; Morgan, 1961). Various ad hoc unemployment measures also were undertaken by the federal government during the Depression because thousands of individuals were no longer self-reliant, and neither municipal nor provincial governments were capable of financing the relief programs required (Bellamy, 1965; Gelber, 1973).

The problems inherent in an ad hoc approach were dramatized in 1937 when the *Employment and Social Insurance Act (1935)*, designed to provide an extensive federal program for dealing with the economic and social problems created by unemployment, was declared unconstitutional because the federal government did not have the power to levy direct premiums on provincial residents for health and welfare programs (Taylor, 1987). A commission was established to deal with this first major federal-provincial controversy and was charged with determining areas of federal-provincial jurisdiction in a wide variety of fields, including social security. In this case, the strategy of pressing for a constitutional amendment was employed but was not effective until 1940 when federal responsibility for unemployment insurance was added to Section 91 of the *BNA Act*.

The end of this era was dominated by the federal government's efforts to evolve a planned approach to long-range policy and program development based on a careful definition of national needs. Ultimately, these efforts floundered because of the problem of federal versus provincial authority. Passage of the *Unemployment Insurance Act* in 1940 permitted the federal government to implement a compulsory contributory insurance program at the national level. A variety of pressures further stimulated federal government action. These included serious concerns about social and economic dislocations caused by the Depression and World War II (1939–1945) and a commitment to the *Atlantic Charter* of 1941, which stressed the concept of individual freedoms and rights. The federal government undertook two major reports during this period, commonly known as the Marsh Report and the Heagerty Report (Collins, 1976; Heagerty, 1943; Marsh, 1975; Storch, 2003).

The Marsh Report, prepared in 1943, has been cited as the "single most important document in the development of the post-war social security system in Canada" (Collins, 1976, p. 5). It took a long-range perspective and outlined a comprehensive national plan for social security in Canada. It recommended social insurance for interruptions of earning capacity (e.g., job loss), for occasions requiring special expenditure (e.g., major accidents or illness), and for chronic poverty. Marsh also emphasized the need for integration of social security programs.

The Heagerty Report was more limited in scope than the Marsh Report but more specific in its proposals. Heagerty considered it essential that everyone in Canada be provided with health insurance but that no compulsion should be placed on the provinces other than all indigents be included in the plan. Health program benefits were to be broad in scope, including medical, dental, and pharmaceutical benefits. Additional program grants to the provinces also were proposed, including grants for tuberculosis, mental health, and professional training. Heagerty stressed integration of public health and medical care, with the goal of "raising and maintaining the standard of health care of the Canadian people" (Heagerty, 1943, p. 5).

The only apparent immediate result of these remarkably prescient reports, however, was the passage of the *Family Allowance Act* in 1944. It provided for payment by the federal government of monthly allowances for every child less than 16 years of age. The prime reason this program went forward was the perceived urgent need for its expected economic stabilization effects through income redistribution (Bellamy, 1965; Lindenfield, 1959). The challenges inherent in federal versus provincial responsibilities meant that it would be many years before the Marsh and Heagerty concepts could be realized. Ultimately, a great deal of the leadership came from the provinces rather than from the federal government.

The Marsh and Heagerty Reports formed the basis for a major document considered at the Dominion-Provincial Conference on Reconstruction in 1945. Proposals in the document stressed the need for cooperation among all levels of government and groups in the country to attain high levels of employment, increased welfare, and security. The proposals also outlined strategies to address three main gaps in the present system: health insurance, national old age pensions, and unemployment assistance (Dominion-Provincial Conference on Reconstruction, 1945).

Because the social security proposals were part of larger proposals relating to financial matters upon which there was no provincial consensus, the innovative concept of comprehensive, integrated, coordinated, national programming for social security was eventually abandoned. This unfortunate outcome impelled the federal and provincial governments to independently seek ways to influence health policies. However, the extensive investigations and discussions associated with the conference had established political and social pressures for action that were not to be denied (Taylor, 1987). This pressure toward integrating health and welfare services led to amalgamation of health and welfare under one common federal department in 1944. The minister of the new Department of Health and Welfare now had responsibility for "all matters relating to the promotion or preservation of the health, social security, and social welfare of the people of Canada over which the Parliament of Canada has jurisdiction" (Cameron, 1962, p. 1).

Era Three: Mid-1940s to Mid-1960s— Disjointed Incrementalism

The third major era in the development of social security policy and programs in Canada was marked by consolidation of a dominant government role in social security and by remarkable progress (at both the federal and provincial levels) in establishing a range of new programs and improving those that already existed (Taylor, 1956). It was a period of what is termed "disjointed incrementalism" because the order in which new programs were implemented and the relationship between them were not guided by a formal rational plan as had been conceived by Marsh and Heagerty.

The one exception to this disjointed approach was in Saskatchewan, which was to lead health care planning and programming for all of Canada during the next 20 years. In 1944, the Co-operative Commonwealth Federation (CCF) party came to power. This democratic-socialist agrarian protest movement put forth a platform promising a "complete system of socialized health services" (Sigerist, 1944, p. 3). Dr. Henry Sigerist of Johns Hopkins University was engaged to develop the plan that would guide health policy and program development in Saskatchewan.

The most dramatic immediate action of the Saskatchewan government was the establishment of a Hospital Services Plan on January 1, 1947. This was the first compulsory and comprehensive hospital insurance plan in North America. During the next three years, provincial plans were also implemented in Alberta, British Columbia, and Newfoundland (Taylor, 1987). As a result of these developments, the provinces requested that health insurance be placed on the agenda of the 1955 federal-provincial conference. Subsequent federal-provincial negotiations resulted in federal proposals to pay approximately 50% of the costs of insured hospital services, based on a cost-sharing formula (Taylor, 1973). By 1958, the federal *Hospital Insurance and Diagnostic Services Act* was implemented in five provinces; the remaining provinces joined the plan by 1961.

Several other important federal programs also were developed during this time. In 1948, national health grants were introduced. These grants had been part of the Proposals on Reconstruction and were designed to enable the provinces to establish the foundations for comprehensive health insurance. This grants-in-aid program targeted public health, tuberculosis control, mental health care, venereal disease control, crippled children's diseases, cancer, professional training, public health research, hospital construction, and health survey capability (Martin, 1948). A number of positive modifications also were made to income security programs during this era.

In 1962, Saskatchewan again took the lead in health care when it introduced a medical insurance plan. The plan faced adamant opposition from the medical profession, opposition that resulted in the famous "doctors' strike" (Badgely & Wolfe, 1967; Meilicke, 1967; Tollefson, 1964). The fact that public opinion moved against the striking doctors ensured that medical insurance plans could be introduced in other provinces and, eventually, at the federal level. In 1964, the federal Royal Commission on Health Services, headed by Chief Justice Emmett Hall (the first "Hall Commission"), released its report. It recommended that the federal government enter into agreements with the provinces to assist them in introducing and operating a "comprehensive, universal, provincial program of personal health services" (Royal Commission, 1964, p. 19). This led, in 1966, to the passing of the federal *Medical Care Act* that took effect in 1968. This act provided for federal sharing of approximately 50% of the costs of provincial medical insurance if it incorporated comprehensive medical coverage, a universally available plan, portable benefit coverage, and public authority administration. This covered four of the five principles of medicare, that is, Canadian health care. The fifth principle, accessibility, was added in the *Canada Health Act* of 1984.

Several other federal programs began in the 1960s:

- National Welfare Grants in 1962;

- Youth Allowance Program in 1964;

- Canada Pension Plan in 1965 (an extension to the *Old Age Pensions Act* of 1927);
- Canada Assistance Program in 1966 (a comprehensive program for federal sharing of provincial expenditures for public assistance and for welfare services on a conditional cost-sharing basis similar to that in health); and the
- *Health Resources Act* (federal payments over a 15-year period for construction, acquisition, and renovation of facilities for training health care workers and for research in health fields) (Hacon, 1967).

In only 20 years, Canada had moved from what has been described as a "backward position in welfare state development by international standards" (Collins, 1976, p. 6) to a point where at least the major social security programs necessary for a modern industrial nation were in place. The speed of progress and the scope and range of the programs generated a vast array of new problems; these problems were to become the focus of the next era.

Era Four: Mid-1960s to Mid-1970s— Extensive Reappraisal

The 10-year period from the mid-1960s to the mid-1970s was characterized by the commissioning of special inquiries and reports. These examined the numerous and complex social security programs established in the previous 20 years, reassessed needs, and made recommendations for improvements in services, organization, financing, and cost control. One of the most ambitious investigations began in Quebec in 1966 with establishment of the Commission of Inquiry on Health and Social Welfare (the Castonguay-Nepveu Commission). Ontario established the Committee on the Healing Arts and the Ontario Council of Health in that same year. In the years following, almost every province instituted one or more mechanisms of inquiry into general or specific aspects of their respective social security services. For an extensive listing of these and other reports, see Storch and Meilicke (1979), and for a summary and comparison of six of the most significant provincial and federal government sponsored reports during this 10-year period, see Browne (1980).

At the federal level, several inquiries were established:
- The Report of the Task Force on the Cost of Health Services (National Health & Welfare Canada, 1969) suggested ways to restrain health care costs;
- The report of the Special Senate Committee on Poverty in Canada (1971) highlighted that poverty is reflective of a social attitude translated into economic and political policies;
- The report of the Community Health Centre Project (Hastings, 1972) suggested establishing people-centred primary care centres.

The community health centre project was significant because it was the first attempt to shift the pattern of service delivery away from the institutional focus introduced by the *Hospital Insurance and Diagnostic Services Act (1957)*, a shift that continued to defy the most brilliant of strategies. The principles of the project were simple, but implementing the ideas would have required a serious realignment of power within health care. It was a concept ahead of its time, but the principles were valid and continue to be valid today; they have been incorporated into virtually all of the subsequent major reports to date. Table 1.1 presents a comparison of community health centre and primary health care concepts.

In 1974, Federal Health Minister Marc Lalonde issued a report on the determinants of health, titled *A New Perspective on the Health of Canadians* (Lalonde, 1974). This report maintained that a new emphasis on human biology, environment, and lifestyle, equal to the traditional emphasis on health care delivery, was necessary to improve the health of Canadians. He also issued a *Working Paper on Social Security* (Lalonde, 1973), which upheld proposals similar to those of the Marsh Report of 1943 (i.e., the need for an employment strategy, a social insurance strategy, an income supplementation strategy, a social and employment services strategy, and a federal-provincial strategy).

Table 1.1 Comparison of Community Health Centre Concepts (1972) and Primary Health Care Concepts (2002)

1972: Community Health Centre Concepts (Hastings, 1972)	2002: Primary Health Care Concepts (Fooks & Lewis, 2002)
For individual and family access to obtain initial and continuing care	For continuity of services 24 hours a day, 7 days per week in person or by phone
Care provided through a team of health professionals working in an accessible and well-managed setting	Genuinely interdisciplinary teams of health professionals going beyond the family physician and a nurse
The community health centre must form a responsive and accountable health services system	Funding would be mixture of capitation, fee for service for specialized services, and program funding
Health services closely coordinated with social and related services to help individuals, families, and communities deal with the many-sided problems of living	A focus on wellness and health promotion activities
	Ability of patients to choose their primary care provider(s), and, in some cases, the expectation they will sign up (roster) with their choice for a minimum period of time

Source: Adapted from *The Community Health Centre in Canada: Report of the Community Health Centre Project to the Health Ministers (Vol 1)*, by J.E.F. Hastings, 1972, Ottawa: Information Canada; *Ramanow and Beyond: A Primer on Health Reform Issues in Canada*, by C. Fooks and S. Lewis, November 2002, discussion paper No. H/05 Health Network, Ottawa: Canadian Public Policy Research Networks Inc.

An important reappraisal process began in December 1970, when the federal government initiated discussions regarding new federal-provincial cost-sharing formulas. Dialogue between the federal and provincial governments continued sporadically, and in 1975, the federal government served notice of its intent to terminate the existing formula for hospital cost sharing. After drawn-out negotiations with the provinces, the *Established Programs Financing Act* was created in 1977, whereby federal cost sharing for both hospital and medical insurance was changed from a conditional grant to a modified block grant system. The intent of this change was to provide greater provincial flexibility and facilitate the containment of costs to the federal treasury (Van Loon, 1978).

Thus, the fourth era in the development of the Canadian social security program was a time of extensive reappraisal. Although few definitive solutions were found, many problems and issues were more clearly identified, and a rich variety of ideas and proposals were generated. Among the themes most frequently heard were the need for a comprehensive and integrated approach to planning, organizing, administering, and evaluating social security; the need to control costs; and the need to define and control quality better.

Era Five: 1977 to 1989—Renewed Federal Leadership

The fifth era was characterized by federal government attempts to uphold the principles of health care while reducing its cost commitments to the health enterprise. Still operating within the context of the provisions in the *BNA Act,* the federal government's only real enforcement mechanism to maintain the principles of accessibility, universality, comprehensiveness, portability, and non-profit administration was the power to withhold grant monies to coerce conformity. With the change in funding involving block grants and tax point transfers, the financial transfer to the provinces became less valuable than that realized during the period of conditional cost sharing. Thus, even the threat of withholding a portion of the block grant was not as serious as it might have been.

In 1984, the federal government introduced the *Canada Health Act*; this was intended to re-establish the five principles of Canadian health care and replace the *Hospital Insurance and Diagnostic Services Act* and the *Medical Care Act.* The provinces and organized medicine bitterly opposed the *Canada Health Act*—the provinces resented intrusion into what they considered their constitutional domain, so, too, did organized medicine. Provinces could be penalized for not adhering to the Act; for example, if a province allowed extra-billing practices (i.e., user fees and so-called "balance billing"), the federal government could withhold funds from the block grant transfer on the basis of one dollar for every dollar collected by extra billing. Organized medicine opposed these constraints, contending that user fees and balance billing represented a means for raising health revenues and for exercising physicians' unencumbered professional freedom, which it considered to be an inalienable right of the profession (Taylor, 1987). There were numerous challenges to this Act, most notably from within Ontario in the form of a physicians' strike in 1986. Once again, public opinion moved against the doctors in this strike, and the medical profession failed to sustain a united front. Ontario banned extra billing, and the last province holding out (Alberta) banned the practice five weeks later.

During this era, numerous government commissions and inquiries examined ways in which health care might be delivered in a more cost-effective manner (for a synopsis of these reports, see Angus, 1991). The growing cost constraint brought about by a downturn in the economy forced the provinces to reconsider the structure of the health care system and confirm that major reforms were needed to create an affordable system. The *Rainbow Report* from Alberta and the *Closer to Home Report* from British Columbia are only two of numerous reports produced during this time that called for fundamental changes in the delivery of health care, stronger emphasis on health promotion and primary care, and care delivered outside institutions.

Era Six: The 1990s—Economic Downturn, Downsizing, and Reform

By the early 1990s, a dramatic change had occurred in the way health services were planned and financed. The federal government basically restricted its role to maintenance of the five principles of health care, and the provincial governments were left with the main responsibility for funding. In the face of growing budget deficits, this placed pressure on provincial and territorial governments to economize on health expenditures. In turn, this created a climate for change in the organization and management of health services that transcended all others since the current system was founded more than 25 years earlier.

Changes evident throughout the system included mergers, amalgamations, and regional planning. There was growing activity to refine the operational mission and role of health care organizations and to minimize costs associated with inappropriate or unnecessary distribution and utilization of resources. Provincial and territorial funding agencies began funding systems that more directly encouraged efficient management of resources, such as providing funding to hospitals based on severity of illness measures (Meilicke, 1990). As noted earlier in this chapter, there also were modifications made to narrow the definition of basic health services ("medically necessary services") mentioned in the *Canada Health Act*.

Along with these activities were efforts to improve hospital information systems and rationalize technology assessment and distribution. This was considered essential to allow more precise definitions of intra-institutional responsibility, to improve the appropriateness of patient placement relative to care alternatives, and to develop guidelines for clinical decision making in physician practice. To some extent, health promotion and disease prevention activities were also expanded, although the investment of funding to elevate the status of these activities was still modest. Changes in delivery systems were beginning, with the intent of focusing on community-based services.

Different patterns of governance, such as regional planning agencies and area health authorities, were discussed, planned, and implemented in most provinces. In Saskatchewan, for example, plans were underway to replace the existing 400 separate boards with 30 autonomous health district boards to administer the province's health care budget. Such planning for health districts was reminiscent of the work of the Sigerist Commission in the mid-1940s (Sigerist, 1944).

Accepting their fundamental responsibility for health, the provincial ministers of health and their deputies began meeting to share their approaches to health care reform and to unite in their common struggle for cost containment. The intensity of these deliberations was similar to meetings preceding the Dominion-Provincial Conference on Reconstruction in 1945. The agenda had changed, however, from one requesting federal government assistance in funding health care to one that assumed greater provincial responsibility. The meetings were designed to provide mutual support and consultation to effect health care reform. The common fundamentals of government reform articulated for this era were

- to improve the health status of all Canadians;
- to reaffirm the five principles of the Canada Health Act;
- to ensure a more cost-effective system; and
- to provide a continuum of services characterized by a shift from institution-based to community-based services, by healthy public policy, and by an emphasis on health promotion (Background paper, 1992).

A prime example of unity across the provinces and territories was evident in the commissioning of a study on physician resources in Canada (Barer & Stoddart, 1991). Not only were the provinces instrumental in examining the numbers of physicians in the system and entering the system, they also took action to deal with several recommendations of the report, such as implementing reductions in medical school enrolment.

By 1993, there were clear signals that health care restructuring with a view to health care reform was more than rhetoric and that virtually all policies and services were vulnerable to change. As the provinces accepted increasing responsibility for health care, they began to reconsider consumers' needs in a more orderly manner—needs for first access care, continuity of care, emergency care, community care, and social welfare. In many respects, a return to some of the ideals promoted in the Marsh and Heagerty Reports, and reiterated in the plethora of reports issued during the fourth era, was becoming evident.

In late 1994, shortly after a Liberal government was returned to power, Prime Minister Jean Chrétien established the National Health Forum to involve and inform Canadians and to advise the federal government on innovative ways to improve the health care system and the health of Canadians (National Health Forum, 1997). The Forum focused attention in four key areas:

1. Values (exploring core values Canadians connect to the health care system)
2. Striking a Balance (examining health resource allocation)
3. Determinants of Health (identifying actions to address population health and non-medical aspects of health)
4. Evidence-Based Decision Making (considering how policy makers, practitioners, and individuals can have the best access to and use of evidence upon which to base their decisions)

The Final Report of the National Health Forum, released in early 1997, concluded that Canadians had inherited an excellent health care system, which had been developed over four decades and that continued to enjoy strong support from the people of Canada. It was deemed essential to protect that legacy by preserving what had been acquired and by developing more integrated systems of care and broader approaches to promoting health.

Also released in 1997 was *A Renewed Vision for Canada's Health System* (Provincial/Territorial Ministers of Health, 1997) from the Conference of Provincial/Territorial Ministers of Health, which represented a consensus of all provinces and territories except Quebec. This report recommended a new administrative mechanism to secure the future of the *Canada Health Act*. An expert advisory panel was to serve as a reference body to make recommendations on disputes and issues referred by the federal government, provinces, or territories. This panel's duties would include clarifying and interpreting the Act and its five principles and reviewing provincial and territorial application and adherence to the principles. With the return of the Liberal government to a second term in June 1997, the potential for preserving the values of the current system seemed promising.

Meanwhile, most provinces were devolving authority relative to health and social services to regional levels, with the intent to control costs, increase responsiveness and flexibility, better integrate services, and improve health outcomes. Five provinces led the way in these initiatives: Quebec, New Brunswick, Saskatchewan, Prince Edward Island, and Alberta (all of which commenced implementation prior to 1994). Alberta implemented regional health authorities so rapidly that it came to be regarded as a leader in health care restructuring (Lomas, Woods, & Veenstra, 1997a).

In Alberta, the severity and rapidity of reduction and restructuring, with closure of several major urban hospitals, led to serious questioning of government motives by many citizens and health providers. Critics claimed that reduction and restructuring were informed more by political ideology than by rational planning. At least two commentators suggested that the rapid changes, based upon the argument that health care costs were out of control, could not be justified. They claimed that this argument was a clever ruse for those attempting to privatize Canada's health care system and was a mask for the real cause of provincial deficits, namely, massive subsidies to the private sector, not public expenditure on health (Nelson, 1995; Taft, 1997).

Toward the turn of the century, tensions characterizing regionalization efforts were common in almost every province. These included tensions between provincial and regional roles (particularly in regard to budgetary control), between regional authorities and health care professionals and providers, and between regional authorities and the public they were intended to serve (Lomas, Woods, & Veenstra, 1997b). At the core of these tensions was a fundamental questioning of whether devolution of health care was a good thing for Canadian health care and for the health status of Canadians. With the Ontario government proceeding with major restructuring of health and welfare, the distribution of financial responsibility for health and welfare that was characteristic of the 1940s loomed as a distinct possibility for the future. In 1940, for example, municipalities paid 22.3% of public health and welfare costs, the province paid 41.5%, and the federal government contributed 36.2% (Cassidy, 1945).

Such redistribution of fiscal and moral responsibility threatened the concept of a national health care (and social service) system. Further, as Stingl (1996) noted, "The current health reform debate in Canada is not just about the kind of health system we want for ourselves and our family members. At a deeper and more far-reaching level, it is about the kind of society we want to live in, one that feels an obligation to care for its sick and injured or one that does not" (p. 17).

Era Seven: Entering the 21st Century—At a Crossroads

Given the advances in society and medical science in the last 150 years, it may seem irreverent to suggest that there are parallels in the health care problems and issues of pre-Confederation and those of the 21st century. Nevertheless, there are uncanny similarities that should be noted.

First, communicable diseases, once thought to be largely conquered and a part of our past, have returned to challenge us in numerous ways. Many of these diseases are relatively new, poorly understood, and difficult to treat (e.g., AIDS, SARS, Mad Cow Disease, West Nile Virus). Also, our ability to detect and quarantine infected people in a time of widespread travel has proven not to be as easy as putting a sailing ship or two into isolation. Our governments and senior health officials often seem slow to respond to the new challenges and are back to reactive rather than proactive measures in managing these problems of the 21st century.

Second, and related to communicable disease control, is that we can no longer take our air and water supply for granted. Water quality, for example, has become a major issue for numerous communities across Canada. Serious disease outbreaks (e.g., the Walkerton, Ontario, *Escherichia coli* outbreak of 2001) threaten many communities as a result of an inattention to sanitary measures that is not too dissimilar from conditions of pre-Confederation.

Third, in attempting to deal with these serious public health problems, we are confronted with boards of health that have been seriously weakened through financial cutbacks over the years and with a comparable reduction in knowledgeable health scientists at all levels of government (once again, due to serious and short-sighted cutbacks to basic health-related technical services).

Fourth, the terrorist attacks on the World Trade Center in New York on September 11, 2001, exposed our vulnerability to worldwide terrorism and forced international actions that have diverted funds to national and international defense. This, too, is not dissimilar from war efforts in earlier eras when money and political commitment were diverted from health issues.

Against this backdrop, the beginning of the 21st century is characterized by continued, sometimes contradictory, and often perverse reform efforts of governments, by continued federal-provincial wrangling, by yet another round of major provincial and federal reports, and by dissonance in regards to which values should inform health care policy and program delivery. This confusion is largely driven by a clear and steady attempt on the part of some to move greater responsibility back to individuals, families, communities, and municipalities—a return to a structure not unlike the one existing around the time of Confederation.

As attempts at reform continue, the Canadian public continues to receive dubious messages about a "crisis in health care." As a critical carry-over from the 1990s, the public is bombarded with messages of fiscal crises while enduring extensive cutbacks to health services. As the system seems unable to respond to real and perceived health needs, some citizens choose to purchase MRIs, CAT scans, and cataract and other available surgeries to shorten their waiting periods for diagnosis and treatment. With only one option offered to offset the problem (i.e., privatization), citizens' actions become a self-fulfilling prophecy. At the same time, countless reports and analyses point out that it is not the spending on public health or public health insurance that reduces the monies available, but rather private industry subsidies or concessions (such as the concessions given to private clinics and multinational pharmaceutical companies).

There are many other similar problems in health care today. One is the lack of progress toward evidence-based assessment of care and patient safety; another is the lack of political will to address issues of health human resource planning and teamwork. It is noteworthy, for example, that all levels of government promote the use of best evidence to support practices, while at the same time those governments routinely ignore the evidence supplied by well-reputed research foundations, such as the Canadian Health Services Research Foundation (CHSRF). (See, for example, CHSRF's Mythbuster series in the Internet Resources at the end of this chapter.) Another critical problem is the absence of adequate funding for staffing resources when numbers of nurses and many other health professionals are at an all-time low in many parts of the country. One particularly unfortunate consequence of this is the necessity for family and friends to provide informal home care for loved ones, with few supports available to them, the justification being that this is a return to placing greater responsibility on individuals and families (Peter, 2004; MacAdam, 2000). The fact is that it is a Third World solution by a First World country.

There is little question that the seemingly endless debate about which level of government is in charge of health care further obscures attention to the real issues and allows for continued erosion of health care through inaction or poorly conceived action.

Provincial Reports of the Early 21st Century

Several significant reports have been released in the early years of the 21st century. Among these were four provincial reports out of Quebec, Saskatchewan, Alberta, and British Columbia. The substance of these reports will be summarized briefly, noting their similarities and differences while outlining the choices that have been mapped out for Canadians.

As with the Castonquay Report of 1968, Quebec once again led the way with a report released in December 2000 that addressed issues facing the health and social services system. The recommendations of this report were in keeping with objectives established by the World Health Organization (2000), namely, to improve health by reducing disparities in health and welfare, to respond to legitimate expectations of individuals and groups without discrimination, and to ensure fairness in financing (Commission d'étude, 2001). Such fairness was seen to include a wide range of resources, a high level of prepayment, and good stewardship to improve the performance of the system, including making conscious choices about what services will have priority.

In Saskatchewan, Ken Fyke was appointed as a one-man commission (Commission on Medicare, 2001) with a mandate to identify key challenges and to recommend action that would be sustainable, embody the core values of medicare, and preserve long-term stewardship of a publicly administered system. His report focused on sustaining a quality system with attention to patient safety (reduction and elimination of error) and performance measurement. A significant contribution of the Fyke Report was its emphasis on "everyday service," in short, a strong focus on primary health care services involving teamwork.

Alberta's 2001 *Report of the Premier's Advisory Council on Health*, also known as the Mazankowski Report, contained several novel recommendations, such as health education as a way to stay healthy; a 90-day "guarantee" of access to care; a need to redefine comprehensive care; more choice in health care, including more competition; and diversifying revenue streams (Premier's Advisory Council, 2001).

Finally, British Columbia's Select Standing Committee on Health (2002) recommended moving the province from 52 health authorities to five health regions, closing or transforming small hospitals, utilizing fact-based information, enacting clean water protection, and establishing needs-based access to long-term care. Little explicit mention was made of BC's intent to stimulate competition, develop public-private partnerships, and diversify revenue; nevertheless, silent but steady movement towards privatization is underway in that province.

Federal Reports of the Early 21st Century

Two significant federal reports were released in the fall of 2002, namely, the Romanow Report and the Kirby Report. The Romanow Commission was appointed to "inquire into and undertake dialogue with Canadians on the future of Canada's public health care system, and to recommend policies and measures… required to ensure long term… sustainability" (Commission on the Future, 2002, p. iii). The Kirby Report was authorized by the Senate to examine the fundamental principles on which Canada's publicly funded system is based, its historical development, the pressures and constraints on the system, and the role of the federal government in Canada's health care system. In the process of review, Romanow heard from about 40,000 Canadians after soliciting an exemplary range and variety of input, while Kirby involved a total of 400 witnesses, individuals, and organizations (Commission on the Future, 2002; Standing Senate Committee, 2002; Roberge, 2003). Both recommended that more public money be put into health care, but their priorities for use of such funds differed in both priority and amount.

Romanow took as top priorities creating a Canada Health Covenant, modernizing the *Canada Health Act*, providing funds for rural and remote access, creating a new diagnostic services fund, improving primary health care, strengthening home care, and offering a catastrophic drug transfer. The Kirby Report did not address the core values underpinning the system; recommended no change to the *Canada Health Act*; and took as priority the need for service-based funding for hospitals, granting greater responsibility to regional health authorities for delivering and/or contracting out publicly insured health services, reforming primary health care, offering a health care guarantee, providing coverage of catastrophic prescription costs, and improving home care. Both reports stressed accountability for funding and services provided, with the Romanow Report recommending the establishment of accountability as the sixth principle under the *Canada Health Act* and promoting the concept of a National Health Council with wide responsibility for indicators, benchmarks, and performance measurement (reminiscent of the establishment of the Dominion Council of Health in 1919). Kirby suggested a more bureaucratically appointed council of fewer members with limited advisory functions.

Kirby presented a profoundly significant position when he supported a single payer system but also left the door open to private sector involvement. As Roberge (2003) observed,

One of the ironies of the current crisis and the nature of the debate is that it was the desire to ensure access that led to the creation of public health insurance in Canada in the first place. Now it appears that a desire to ensure access is being used as an argument to move away from a public system. Public health insurance was designed to shift the burden from the individual to the collective through government funding. Now the fiscal burden of health care on governments has led to reduced access and there is pressure to shift the burden, at least, in part, back to the individual (p. 39).

First Ministers' Health Policy Discussions

By February 2003, the provincial premiers at their First Ministers' Conference passed the Health Care Renewal Accord (2003), which was based upon agreements they had struck in September 2000 for health system renewal. Reaffirming their commitment to the five principles of health care, they specified the purpose of their accord was to ensure that Canadians

- have access to a health provider 24 hours a day, 7 days a week;
- have timely access to diagnostic procedures and treatments;
- do not have to repeat their health histories or undergo the same tests for every provider they see;
- have access to quality home care and community care services;
- are able to access quality care no matter where they live; and
- see their health care system as efficient, responsive, and adapting to their changing needs and those of their families and communities now and in the future (Health Care Renewal Accord, 2003).

To achieve these goals, the Government of Canada agreed to establish a long-term Canada Health Transfer (CHT) by March 31, 2004, and to include a portion of the current cash and tax points corresponding to provincial expenditures and with predictable annual increases. By July 2003, however, the political climate had changed, and a group of premiers chose to delay formation of the National Health Council, declared health care to be a "provincial responsibility," and proposed to establish a Council of the Federation as a common forum for premiers to discuss common positions on issues. Meanwhile, the silence of the federal government was both puzzling and worrisome. If Prime Minister Chrétien, who retired in December 2003, hoped to leave a legacy of a renewed health care system (as many believed he had intended to do), time was slipping away as the erosion of health care continued.

Perhaps Canadians are at a true crossroads in health care renewal, a crossroads involving a change in values. Some have questioned whether the federal government has lost the moral authority to lead (Kenny, 2002; Roberge, 2003). Since the Romanow and Kirby Reports took a different approach to values in health care, the view of the Canadian public is uncertain. Can Romanow and 40,000 Canadians be wrong? Or, as some have suggested, do the efforts to accomplish a shift in values reflect only the view of the most powerful in society whose personal interests are better served by ignoring the call for upholding the traditional Canadian values of health care (Williams, Deber, Baranek, & Gildiner, 2001; Armstrong & Armstrong, 2003)?

Romanow proposed a Health Covenant for Canadians to restore their confidence in their health care system (Commission on the Future, 2002). Reminiscent of the Health Charter for Canadians prominent in the Royal Commission on Health Services (Vol. I) (Royal Commission, 1964), the Covenant was offered as an essential step in "re-affirming our collective commitment to medicare" (Commission on the Future, 2002, p. 52). This was greeted favourably by many and scorned by some. The tensions inherent in a value-based system of health care versus a market ideology resurfaced in many of the public debates following release of these two federal reports (Pauly, 2004; Williams et al., 2001). Some of the rhetoric was not dissimilar to the debates surrounding the introduction of Canada's first social security program in 1927, the Old Age Pension Plan (Bryden, 1974).

Despite the evidence that health markets "are not like other markets and single payer, publicly administered health care systems are optimal both on efficiency and equity grounds" (Williams et al., 2001, p. 8), medicare faces continuing political assaults. Because it is a public program in an era when neo-conservatives consider governments to be sources of waste, inefficiency, and abuse, the fascination with competitive global markets dominates the agenda of many of the more powerful people in Canadian society. This leaves unattended the basic causes of poor health—poor sanitation, environmental pollution, poverty, unemployment, poor housing, lack of education, and so on—none of which can be solved and most of which will be exacerbated by transforming health care into a free market model.

These realities highlight the importance of comments by ethicists such as Nuala Kenny, a prominent Canadian health ethicist and physician who argues strongly that health policy discussions are moral discussions and that values should be considered as outcomes. She identifies key values in health reform as solidarity (or collective responsibility), equity (fairness), compassion (recognizing the needs of the most vulnerable), efficiency (of public administration of a public good), and civility (the capacity to discuss and decide as citizens) (Kenny, 2002).

There is no doubt that in the 21st century governments and the Canadian public will have to choose their course of action. While it is clear that the Canadian health care system faces concerns similar to other health care systems, the strengths of the Canadian system should not be abandoned without a great deal of consideration. Reflecting the words of former Prime Minister Joe Clark (1994), who said in his book that we have a country too good to lose, one might well add that we have a health care system too good to lose.

Leadership Implications

Although history rarely repeats itself exactly, it is clear that similar problems in health care delivery emerge in different contexts across the years. Knowledge of the past, therefore, allows a respect for history and can contribute a useful degree of wisdom in the creative search for new solutions while reducing the likelihood of repeating past mistakes. Knowledge of the development of Canadian health care delivery is critical to understanding the social, political, and economic forces that have shaped the system and that will continue to influence future changes within it.

Health care professionals traditionally have taken a keen interest in the evolution of the health care system. National and provincial associations for health professionals and organizations, including nursing associations, have provided leadership in advising both levels of government on health care policy issues. They also serve as monitors, advocates, and critics of the ongoing health care system debates between federal, provincial, and territorial governments, and they are unlikely to relinquish these roles in the future.

Summary

- The division of power relative to health care between the federal and provincial governments (under the *British North America Act*) has been a major factor shaping the Canadian health care system.
- Current health care restructuring programs to control costs, increase responsiveness and flexibility, better integrate services, and improve health outcomes have their roots in past reports and commissions.
- Canadians generally support the five principles upon which the Canadian health care system is founded.
- Although significant restructuring is in progress, there is, as yet, limited evidence of reform.

Applying the Knowledge in this Chapter

Exercise

Select and read one or more of the Mythbuster essays available from the Canadian Health Services Research Foundation. See Internet Resources for the CHSRF Web site and a list of myths.

Discuss this question: If we accept the fact that the information provided by the CHSRF is valid, how might we explain or account for the fact that many politicians, health care leaders, and policy makers choose to ignore this information?

Resources

evolve Internet Resources

Canadian Centre for Policy Alternative:

http://policyalternatives.ca/index.html

This is a good site for background reports on health care and other issues affecting health status.

Canadian Health Services Research Foundation, Mythbusters:

www.chsrf.ca/mythbusters/index_e.php

Myth: A parallel private system would reduce waiting times in the public system

Myth: User fees would stop waste and ensure better use of the health care system

Myth: For-profit ownership of facilities would lead to a more efficient health care system

Myth: Seeing a nurse practitioner instead of a physician is second-class care

Myth: The cost of dying is an increasing strain on the health care system

Myth: An ounce of prevention buys a pound of cure

Romanow Commission background reports:

http://hc-sc.gc.ca/english/care/romanow/index.html

Further Reading

Meilicke, C.A., & Storch, J.L. (Eds.). (1980). *Perspectives on Canadian health and social services policy: History and emerging trends*. Ann Arbor, MI: Health Administration Press.

This book of previously published articles is a collection of historical perspectives on the development of Canadian health and social services policy. Perspectives include those of government bureaucrats, journalists, academics, and agency personnel who collectively provide a rich review of policy and practice in health care and social welfare. Integration of the numerous articles is provided through an introduction and brief commentaries on each section.

Taylor, M.G. (1987). *Health insurance and Canadian public policy: The seven decisions that created the Canadian health insurance system and their outcomes* (2nd ed.). Montreal, QC: McGill-Queen's University Press.

This book contains an interesting and brilliant analysis of the critical steps in development of Canada's health insurance system and of policy making at federal and provincial levels of government. Featuring three federal and four provincial key decisions, Taylor describes the inputs to those decisions as well as immediate and long-term outcomes.

References

Angus, D.E. (1991). Review of significant health care commissions and task forces in Canada since 1983–84. Ottawa, ON: Canadian Hospital Association.

Armitage, A. (1975). Social welfare in Canada: Ideals and realities. Toronto, ON: McClelland & Stewart.

Armstrong, P., & Armstrong, H. (2003). *Wasting away: The undermining of Canadian health care* (2nd ed.). Don Mills, ON: Oxford University Press.

Background paper on health care reform initiatives. (1992). Health reform paper for provincial health ministers meeting in Newfoundland. Regina, SK: Saskatchewan Health Planning and Policy Development Branch.

Badgely, R.F., & Wolfe, S. (1967). *Doctors' strike: Medical care and conflict in Saskatchewan.* Toronto, ON: Macmillan of Canada.

Barer, M.L., & Stoddart, G.L. (1991). *Toward integrated medical resource policies in Canada.* Winnipeg, MB: Manitoba Health.

Bellamy, D. (1965). Social welfare in Canada. In *Encyclopedia of Social Work* (15th ed.). New York: National Association of Social Workers.

Browne, J. (1980). Summary of recent major studies of health care in Canada. In C.A. Meilicke & J.L. Storch (Eds.), *Perspectives on Canadian health and social service policy: History and emerging trends* (pp. 293–305). Ann Arbor, MI: Health Administration Press.

Bryden, K. (1974). *Old age pensions and policy-making in Canada.* Montreal, QC: McGill-Queen's University Press.

Cameron, G.D.W. (1962). The department of national health and welfare. In R.D. Defries (Ed.), *The federal and provincial health services in Canada* (2nd ed., pp. 1–17). Toronto, ON: Canadian Public Health Association.

Cassidy, H.M. (1945). *Public health and welfare reorganization: The post-war problem in the Canadian provinces.* Toronto, ON: Ryerson Press.

Cassidy, H.M. (1947). The Canadian social services. *Annals of the Academy of Political and Social Science, 253,* 191–198.

Clark, J. (1994). *A nation too good to lose: Renewing the purpose of Canada.* Toronto, ON: Key Porter Books Limited.

Collins, K. (1976, January-February). Three decades of social security in Canada. *Canadian Welfare, 51,* 5–7.

Commission d'étude sur les services de santé et les services sociaux. (2001). *Emerging solutions: Report and recommendations.* Chair: M. Clair. Quebec City, QC: Ministry of Health and Social Services.

Commission on the Future of Health Care in Canada. (2002, November). *Building on values: The future of healthcare in Canada* – Final report. Commissioner: R. Romanow. Ottawa, ON: Parliament of Canada.

Commission on Medicare. (2001). *Caring for medicare: Sustaining a quality system.* Commissioner: K. Fyke. Regina, SK: Government of Saskatchewan.

Deber, R., & Vayda, E. (1992). The political and health care systems of Canada and Ontario. In R. Deber (Ed.), *Case studies in Canadian health policy and management Vol. 1* (pp. 1–16). Ottawa, ON: Canadian Hospital Association Press.

Dominion-Provincial Conference on Reconstruction. (1945). *Proposals of the Government of Canada.* Paper presented at the meeting of the Dominion-Provincial Conference on Reconstruction. Ottawa, ON: Queen's Printer.

Fooks, C., & Lewis, S. (2002, November). *Romanow and beyond: A primer on health reform issues in Canada* (Discussion paper No. H/05 Health Network). Ottawa, ON: Canadian Public Policy Research Networks Inc.

Gelber, S.M. (1966, June). The path to health insurance. *Canadian Public Administration, 9,* 211–220.

Gelber, S.M. (1973). *Personal health services in Canada: The early years.* Address to the Association of University Programs in Hospital Administration, Faculty Institute, Ottawa, Ontario.

Gregoire, J. (1962). The ministry of health of the province of Quebec. In R.D. Defries (Ed.), *The federal and provincial health services in Canada* (2nd ed.). Toronto, ON: Canadian Public Health Association.

Hacon, W.S. (1967, October 28). Improving Canada's health manpower resources. *Canadian Medical Association Journal, 97,* 1104–1108.

Hastings, J.E.F. (1972). *The community health centre in Canada: Report of the community health centre project to the health ministers Vol. 1.* Ottawa, ON: Information Canada.

Heagerty, J.J. (1934). The development of public health in Canada. *Canadian Journal of Public Health, 25* (February), 54–56.

Heagerty, J.J. (1943). *Report of the advisory committee on health insurance.* Ottawa, ON: Queen's Printer.

Health Care Renewal Accord. (2003). *First ministers' health accord.* Retrieved August 20, 2003, from http:// www.hc-sc.gc.ca

Kenny, N.P. (2002). *What 'good' is health care? Reflections on the Canadian experience.* Ottawa, ON: Canadian Healthcare Association Press.

Lalonde, M. (1973). *Working paper on social security.* Ottawa, ON: Government of Canada.

Lalonde, M. (1974). *A new perspective on the health of Canadians: A working document.* Ottawa, ON: Government of Canada.

Lindenfield, R. (1959). Hospital insurance in Canada. *Social Service Review, 33,* 149.

Lomas, J., Woods, J., & Veenstra, G. (1997a). Devolving authority for health care in Canada's provinces: 1. An introduction to the issues. *Canadian Medical Association Journal, 156*(3), 371–377.

Lomas, J., Woods, J., & Veenstra, G. (1997b). Devolving authority for health care in Canada's provinces: 3. Motivations, attitudes and approaches of board members. *Canadian Medical Association Journal, 156*(5), 669–676.

MacAdam, M. (2000). Home care: It's time for a Canadian model. *Healthcare Papers, 1*(4), 9–36. Retrieved August 15, 2003, from http://www.longwoods.com/hp/fall00/lead.html

Marsh, L. (1975). *Report on social security for Canada: 1943.* Toronto, ON: University of Toronto Press.

Martin, P. (1948). A national health program for Canada. *Canadian Journal of Public Health, 39,* 220–223.

Meilicke, C.A. (1967). *The Saskatchewan medical care dispute of 1962: An analytical social history.* Unpublished doctoral dissertation, University of Minnesota.

Meilicke, C.A. (1990). International perspectives on healthcare: Canada. *Healthcare Executive, 5*(4), 25–26.

Morgan, J.S. (1961). Social welfare services in Canada. In M. Oliver (Ed.), *Social purpose for Canada.* Toronto, ON: University of Toronto Press.

Najman, J.M., & Western, J.S. (1984). A comparative analysis of Australian health policy in the 1970's. *Social Science and Medicine, 18*(1), 949–958.

National Health Forum. (1997). *Canada health action: Building on the legacy.* Final report of the National Health Forum (Vols. I and II). Ottawa, ON: Minister of Public Works and Government Services.

National Health & Welfare Canada. (1969). *Report of the task force on the cost of health services in Canada: Summary* (Vol. 1). Ottawa, ON: National Health & Welfare.

Nelson, J. (1995, January-February). Dr. Rockefeller will see you now: The hidden players privatizing Canada's health care system. *Canadian Forum, 73,* 7–12.

Pauly, B. (2004). Shifting the balance in funding and delivery of health care in Canada. In J. Storch, P. Rodney, & R. Starzomski (Eds.), *Toward a moral horizon: Nursing ethics for leadership and practice* (pp. 181–208). Don Mills, ON: Pearson Prentice Hall.

Peter, E. (2004). Home health care and ethics. In J. Storch, P. Rodney, & R. Starzomski (Eds.), *Toward a moral horizon: Nursing ethics for leadership and practice* (pp. 248–261). Don Mills, ON: Pearson Prentice Hall.

Premier's Advisory Council on Health. (2001). *A framework for reform.* Report of the Premier's Advisory Council on Health. Chair: D. Mazankowski. Edmonton, AB: Government of Alberta.

Provincial/Territorial Ministers of Health. (1997). *A renewed vision for Canada's health system: A report of the Conference of Provincial/Territorial Ministers of Health.* Ottawa, ON: Health Canada.

Roberge, G. (2003). *A four part paper on health policy and management implications of the Romanow and Kirby reports.* Unpublished paper, Faculty of Human and Social Development, University of Victoria, British Columbia, Canada.

Rorem, R.C. (1931). *The municipal doctor system in rural Saskatchewan.* Chicago: University of Chicago Press.

Royal Commission on Health Services. (1964). *Report: Royal Commission on health services* (Vol. 1). Ottawa, ON: Queen's Printer.

Select Standing Committee on Health Report. (2002). *Patients first 2002: The path to reform.* Victoria, BC: Legislative Assembly.

Sigerist, H.E. (1944). *Saskatchewan Health Services Commission: Report of the Commissioner.* Regina, SK: King's Printer.

Special Senate Committee on Poverty. (1971). *Poverty in Canada: Report of the Special Senate Committee on Poverty.* Ottawa, ON: Information Canada.

Splane, R.B. (1965). *Social welfare in Ontario: A study of public welfare administration*. Toronto, ON: University of Toronto Press.

Standing Senate Committee on Social Affairs, Science and Technology. (2002). *The health of Canadians – The federal role*. Final report on the state of the health care system in Canada. Volume 6, Recommendations for reform. Chair: The Honourable M.J.L. Kirby. Ottawa, ON: Parliament of Canada.

Stingl, M.S. (1996). Equality and efficiency as basic social values. In M. Stingl & D. Wilson (Eds.), *Efficiency and equality: Health reform in Canada*. Halifax, NS: Fernwood Publishing.

Storch, J.L. (2003). The Canadian health care system and Canadian nurses. In M. McIntyre & E. Thomlinson (Eds.), *Realities of Canadian nursing: Professional, practice, and power issues* (pp. 34–59). Philadelphia, PA: Lippincott, Williams & Wilkins.

Storch, J.L., & Meilicke, C.A. (1979). *Health and social services administration: An annotated bibliography*. Ottawa, ON: Canadian College of Health Service Executives.

Taft, K. (1997). *Shredding the public interest*. Edmonton, AB: University of Alberta Press.

Taylor, M.G. (1949). *The Saskatchewan hospital services plan*. Unpublished doctoral dissertation, University of California, Berkeley.

Taylor, M.G. (1956). *The administration of health insurance in Canada*. Toronto, ON: Oxford University Press.

Taylor, M.G. (1973, January-February). The Canadian health insurance program. *Public Administration Review, 33*, 35.

Taylor, M.G. (1987). *Health insurance and Canadian public policy: The seven decisions that created the Canadian health insurance system* (2nd ed.). Montreal, QC: McGill-Queen's University Press.

Tollefson, E.A. (1964). *Bitter medicine: The Saskatchewan medical care dispute*. Saskatoon, SK: Modern Press.

Van Loon, R.J. (1978, Winter). From shared cost to block funding and beyond. *Journal of Health Politics, Policy and Law, 2*, 460.

Van Loon, R.J., & Whittington, M.S. (1976). *The Canadian political system: Environment, structure and process* (2nd ed.). Toronto, ON: McGraw-Hill Ryerson.

Wallace, E. (1950). The origin of the social welfare state in Canada, 1867-1900. *Canadian Journal of Economics and Political Science, 16*, 384.

Williams, A.P., Deber, R., Baranek, P., & Gildiner, A. (2001). From medicare to home care: Globalization, state retrenchment, and the profitization of Canada's health care system. In P. Armstrong, H. Armstrong, & D. Coburn (Eds.), *Unhealthy times: Political economy perspectives on health and health care in Canada* (pp. 7–30). Toronto, ON: Oxford University Press.

World Health Organization. (2000). *World health report 2000 – Health systems: Improving performance*. Geneva, Switzerland: Author.

2

HEALTH ECONOMICS AND HEALTH SYSTEM REFORM

Philip Jacobs

Learning Objectives

In this chapter, you will learn:

- Three functions of a health care system: finance, funding, and delivery

- Traditional ways of funding medical and hospital care in the Canadian health care system, and the effects these funding methods have had on care in recent years

- Relationships between the traditional funding methods and the call for reform in Canada

- Reforms that have been proposed (a) to replace fee-for-service funding of physicians, (b) to develop better links between hospital and community care, and (c) to find new sources of money for the health care system

- Effects such reforms may have

At the beginning of the 1990s, Canada, along with many other countries, was faced with a deep financial problem. Health care expenditures per person were increasing annually at an alarming rate. As shown in Figure 2.1, total per-person expenditures rose from $911 in 1980 to $2,200 in 1990 (Health Canada, 2002). Federal and provincial governments were distressed with this growth because they paid roughly 75% of total health expenditures—government deficits were growing, and health care was one contributing factor. Adding to the alarm was a steadily aging population, which generates more health care expenditures as older people require more health services. Finally, a widespread evidence-based movement was under way; there was a growing feeling that many health care practices (especially aspects of inpatient care) were unproven in terms of how they influenced health status, which is the presumed outcome of health care.

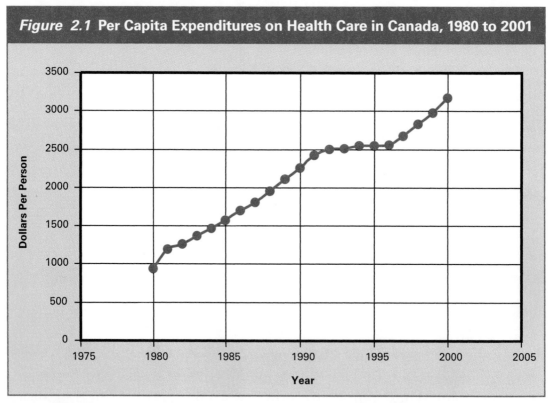

Figure 2.1 **Per Capita Expenditures on Health Care in Canada, 1980 to 2001**

Source: Adapted from *National Health Expenditures in Canada, 1975–1996,* by Health Canada Fact Sheets, Table 1, 2002. Adapted and reproduced with the permission of the Minister of Public Works and Government Services Canada, 2004.

These factors led to calls for health reform in Canada. Governments put the brakes on health care spending during the early 1990s, and these expenditures levelled out (see Figure 2.1). The prior growth in health care expenditures caused governments and analysts to scrutinize the health care system beyond looking merely at the levels of expenditures. Many analysts concluded that, because of the way it was structured, the health care system contained inflationary incentives, and fundamental changes needed to be made. Most provinces began making reforms to their health care systems at varying degrees of speed.

In the late 1990s, the cutbacks of the previous several years led to increasing waiting lists for services in a number of provinces and to projected shortages of many types of personnel, including nurses and physicians. These changes were accompanied by an improved overall economic climate, so federal and provincial governments responded to economic pressures and increased health care spending. As seen in Figure 2.1, per capita health expenses began increasing rather rapidly again after 1996. Both provincial and federal governments then established large-scale studies to again address the issue of health care reform.

In the first several years of the second millennium, a number of federal and provincial reports were issued. There were two federal reports—The Romanow Report (Commission on the Future of Health Care, 2002) and the Kirby Report (Standing Senate Committee, 2002)—and a number of provincial reports, including the Fyke Report (Commission on Medicare, 2001), the Mazankowski Report (Premier's Advisory Council, 2001), and the Clair Report (Commission d'étude, 2001). These reports varied in their recommendations, but they set the policy stage in Canadian health care for years to come. We briefly will return to them later in this chapter; first, however, we introduce the tools that are needed to analyze the policies—those that represent the discipline of economics.

Economics is the science that deals with how scarce means are allocated among competing ends. This is a broad definition, and one can better see what kinds of subjects are tackled by looking at the three general ways that economists conduct studies:

- Economists can *describe* what is happening; providing intelligence is an important component of economics because one needs good data to know what is going on.
- Economists can *explain* what is happening or predict what will happen; this task is important because one needs to know how health care systems will react to incentive changes.
- Economists can *evaluate* interventions that have been implemented; this is important because one needs to be able to rank alternative policies and interventions on a better or worse basis.

Health economics is a branch of economics that deals with the use of resources to achieve health. As a discipline, it can address the subjects of health care reform and health care incentives. Using health economics, one can explain how a health care system works, in effect, by pushing resources in one direction or another. In this chapter, you will be introduced to the science of economics as it is applied to understanding health care resource use. The chapter begins with a description of the traditional health care system, discusses the incentives inherent in that system, and finally examines how health reform is being envisaged to alter the system.

The Traditional Health Care System

Any health care system can be characterized as having three main functions: finance, funding, and delivery. Sometimes these functions are combined.

The *finance function* refers to the manner in which money is transferred from consumers and taxpayers (the ultimate payers) directly to providers or, more usually, to intermediaries (e.g., insurers, regional health authorities) who then pay the providers. Payments can be in the form of taxes (e.g., income taxes, general sales taxes), insurance premiums, or direct out-of-pocket payments.

When the health care system is government-financed, most of the money is raised in the form of taxation. When private health insurance is a major form of finance, the consumers or their employers pay insurance premiums to the insurers. Finally, consumers can pay directly out of pocket to the health care providers. The type of payment has implications in terms of how much different groups pay. Income taxes increase with income, so the average contribution for this form of finance is higher for higher-income families. On the other hand, insurance and health plan premiums do not vary with income, so as incomes increase, the family's average contribution to health care expenditures declines.

Figure 2.2 depicts the financial flows of the traditional Canadian health care system. As can be seen from this diagram, all three forms of finance are used in Canada. Most health care (about 75%) is financed through the government-run health insurance programs. In this program plan, individuals and companies pay taxes to both the federal and provincial governments. The federal government transfers funds to the provincial governments to enable them to operate health care insurance programs that cover medically necessary services for the general population.

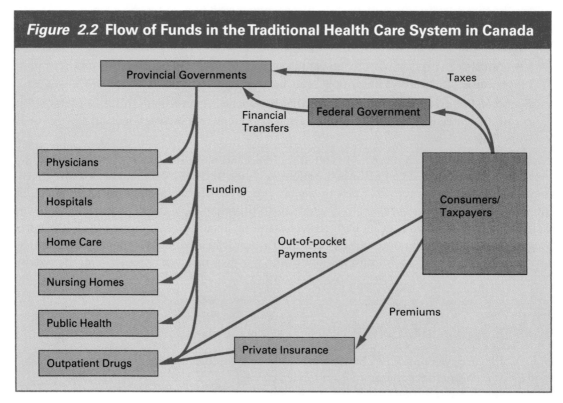

Figure 2.2 Flow of Funds in the Traditional Health Care System in Canada

Medically necessary services include medical (physician) and hospital care. Necessary is a term related to essential, but, in fact, this term has never been clearly defined. Transfers from the federal to the provincial governments cover roughly one-half of the cost of the provincial medicare programs. In addition to hospital and physician care, provincial health programs cover professional home care, long-term (nursing home) care, public health, and some outpatient drugs for welfare recipients and the elderly. Outpatient drugs for the remainder of the population are covered through private insurance (for which individuals or employers pay insurance premiums) or are paid for directly out of pocket. The arrow in Figure 2.2 shows consumers paying co-payments for outpatient drugs only, but in fact, there can also be co-payments for a number of other provincial services.

The *funding function* of the health care system refers to the manner in which provincial health plans pay the providers of care. The prime form of funding for physicians has been fee for service, by which physicians are paid separately for each service provided. Hospitals have been funded on an overall global budget, a lump-sum payment to the hospital adjusted annually on the basis of numbers and types of cases treated or numbers of bed-days. Other providers have been funded by budgets (public health), fee per service (home care), or fee per day (nursing home care).

The *delivery function* refers to the manner in which health care services are provided to the public. Traditionally, each type of care provider has been organized separately. Physicians were organized privately, like businesses. Hospitals were operated by boards of governors; they were organized separately from nursing homes and home care (which had their own governing boards). Institutional providers were, for the most part, not-for-profit; however, a number of for-profit providers have existed in the nursing home sector. Outpatient drugs were prescribed by physicians but funded by private insurance or government plans.

Health Care Incentives

Many aspects of this traditional health care system created an inflationary orientation. Under the *Canada Health Act* of 1984, which consolidated a number of previous government acts, consumers were guaranteed free physician and hospital services (i.e., they paid nothing out of pocket). At a zero out-of-pocket price, there was no incentive for patients to cut back their usage.

Patients will reduce their usage of the health care system when they pay for some of their care out of pocket, at the point of care. The Canadian health care insurance program discourages such payments and therefore creates a tendency toward greater use of services. There are reasons why such incentives have been built into the system. When the insurance programs were established, there was a desire to encourage medical care usage. Recently, however, there has been discussion about trying to discourage usage, especially unnecessary usage. Some out-of-pocket payments will discourage usage, though it is not known for certain whether that usage will be "necessary" or not. Additionally, the poor may be disadvantaged more than the wealthy when out-of-pocket payments are required, and it is largely for this reason that out-of-pocket financing has not been used in Canada.

In addition to consumer or patient incentives, there are provider incentives that may influence the system's economic performance. One of these is the fee-for-service payment of physicians. Each provincial government has set up a medical insurance plan that developed a list of services (e.g., complete physical examination, hysterectomy, complete blood count). For each of these services, there is a fixed fee. Each time a physician provides a service, he or she bills the provincial health insurance plan. This system has been identified as encouraging the provision of services since additional services generate additional revenue for the physician. In response, most provinces have placed a cap on the total fees to be paid annually by the plan: when physicians in the province reach this cap, no physician is funded for additional services. With or without the cap, there is an issue of whether fee-for-service funding might encourage provision of some unnecessary services, though the term *necessary* is difficult to define.

Another provider incentive has been the payment to hospitals on the basis of a fixed global (overall) budget. Provincial governments usually needed to adjust these budgets annually for each hospital. Initially, provinces used the total number of days in which patients were treated; however, this per diem payment system encourages hospitals to keep patients longer because they get more money for doing so, with little extra cost. With average hospitalization costs estimated to be about $700 per day, and the marginal cost of an extra day approximately two-thirds of that amount, this was an expensive practice.

In the early 1990s, several provinces, including Ontario and Alberta, switched to a weighted case-mix system, which was akin to the Diagnosis Related Group (DRG) system developed in the United States a decade earlier. According to these new case-mix funding mechanisms, hospital budgets were adjusted on a per-case basis, with the adjustment amount depending on the average degree of severity or "case mix" of the patients. For example, a hospital would be funded less for a patient admitted for routine medical observation than one admitted for a heart transplant. But in neither case would the hospital get more money for keeping the patient in longer. The case-mix system thus provided hospitals with incentive to reduce length of stays, but it also encouraged admission of more cases. This is because hospitals received additional revenue for treating more cases but no additional revenue for having patients stay longer. This created a major change in incentive for those provinces that instituted case-mix funding, and dramatic reductions in stays were experienced in most provinces with this funding.

In addition to drawing attention to the inflationary incentives inherent in the individual components of the health care system, sweeping worldwide views raised issues about the overall organization of the system. In the US, a new form of health care provision has been developing since the 1950s—the health maintenance organization (HMO). The HMO is responsible for provision of several different types of services, including physician services, hospital services, and outpatient drugs. Incorporation of all of these services into one single organization is very different from the separate unit organization style. It makes it easier for services to be coordinated, with potential reductions in hospitalizations. Since the physicians are responsible for organizing the care that a patient receives, physicians can largely influence patterns of practice. HMOs eventually paved the way for managed care, in which the providing organization can monitor and manage how physicians treat their patients (including how much hospitalization takes place). HMOs are not paid for each service provided; rather, they are paid according to the number of members enrolled. This introduction of a per capita funding system destroyed the automatic link between payment and services provided, offering an incentive to reduce service use per person.

In Canada, coordination of care was also lacking, not only between physicians and hospitals, but also between hospitals and types of care that could substitute for (and perhaps be less costly than) hospital care, notably community care. The disconnected organizational structure hampered coordination between units and created barriers to the substitution of community care for hospital care.

The traditional Canadian system has been criticized on several other grounds. First, it did not address inequities among populations and regions within a province. No mechanism existed (other than a very inadequate political process) to ensure that populations within a province were treated equally. The system, with fees for service and global budgeting, was not designed to address that issue. It was designed to pay for "production" but did not address who in the population received services. Second, the traditional system was focused on treatment of the sick, not on prevention of illness. Providers were paid when individuals became sick; therefore, there was little incentive in the system to prevent sickness and poor health from occurring.

It should be stressed that the lack of incentives should not be equated with a lack of concern among providers for good health. Providers were interested in treating patients to help them get healthy, but the system encouraged them to do this by addressing existing illnesses instead of preventing them. As a result, an enormous industry arose that was geared to the diagnosis and treatment of illness, rather than to its prevention.

Health Reform

There is no one single idea of health reform. A number of different groups have embraced the term and have promoted their own changes as "reform." As a result, the term can mean almost anything connected with change. To look at the idea of reform in an orderly manner, it is necessary to return to the initial three functions of the health care system—finance, funding, and delivery—and analyze the concept of reform for each of these categories.

The reform of finance can mean several things. First, it can mean privatizing care—making patients pay more of the total cost of care directly rather than through taxation. This would mean decreasing the government's share of the pie to less than its mid-1990s level of 75%. Some groups have proposed that this be done, largely through de-insuring (a nasty word in some circles) certain "less-than-necessary" services currently covered by the health care insurance plans. A lack of agreement about what constitutes necessary services has hampered the spread of this notion, although some services (e.g., routine eye exams for non-retired adults) have been de-insured in some provinces. As well, there is considerable interprovincial variation in terms of service coverage; for example, chiropractic care is covered in Western provinces, but less so in the eastern regions of Canada.

Second, the reform of finance also can mean changing how the federal government transfers money to the provinces for insured health care. Indeed, the means of transferring funds has changed considerably since Canadian parliament instituted medical and hospital insurance plans, which began in the early 1960s. Initially, provinces were paid roughly half of whatever they spent. Through the years, the federal government, recognizing that this encouraged provinces to spend more, moved to a form of finance with a fixed payment per resident, much akin to the capitation payment discussed below. There is a great deal of discussion as to what form this contribution should take.

A third aspect of finance reform can be found in Alberta's Mazankowski Report. The authors of this report have proposed a number of new forms of finance, including medical savings accounts, direct pay, and taxable benefits. One of the proposals was to make health care services taxable benefits: as one receives services, the government would record the cost of the services as a benefit. Patients then would have to pay taxes on the cost of benefits received. This form of financing would discourage people from using services. Although simply presented, the implementation of such a plan would be very complex because some people with chronic conditions would probably have to be exempt, and it would be very difficult and controversial to develop and enforce such exemptions.

The reform of funding also has a number of different meanings and, in some instances, cannot be separated from the reform of delivery. Many critics call for the reform of fee-for-service payment to physicians. Because the fee-for-service approach encourages the generation of more services (useful or not), many commentators have been looking for another type of payment method and have been inspired by per capitation funding models. Per capitation funding, used by HMOs in the US, is a fixed sum of money paid to providers per individual resident, per year. The provider, then, is responsible for providing all the defined care to the individual during that year. If the provider is an HMO, which includes physician, hospital, and drug care, this can create a powerful incentive to reduce hospitalization (again, whether the health care is useful or not), especially if the HMO can earn a profit on reduced costs.

In Canada, discussion on capitation funding largely has involved the payment to primary care providers of a fixed sum per person, per year, to provide all primary care services. Under such a system, each primary care provider would have a roster of patients and would be required to provide all primary care services for those patients. We should note that, in the view of some writers, primary care can be provided by multidisciplinary teams, so the primary care clinic may not be synonymous with a "doctor's office." Because the budget per patient would be fixed for the year (which is the meaning of capitation), there would be an incentive to minimize services provided to each patient and to recruit patients who are likely to use fewer services. This is a very different set of incentives from fee-for-service or case-mix funding, which encourage the expansion of services.

Introduction of capitation to primary care practitioners would require a clear definition of primary care; specifically, practitioners would need to know what services are to be included in the capitation payment. If primary care practitioners were not responsible for hospital expenses, for example, then they would have an incentive to refer sicker patients to hospitals rather than continually see them at their offices (which increases office costs). A lack of clearly specified covered services also might allow primary care practitioners to refer sicker patients to specialists, who would not be subject to the capitation fees. Although it would be a matter of judgment as to when a patient could legitimately be referred to a specialist, such referral would be encouraged under a capitation system because it would reduce the primary care provider's expenses. Such cost shifting would be a major difficulty; indeed, in countries where capitation systems are in place, such as the US, cost shifting poses a major problem.

Reform of primary care has been an important issue in the US, where 75% of all physicians are specialists. In Canada, specialists represent only about 50% of physicians, and care from family physicians, at least for the general population, is more readily available. Nevertheless, primary care reform has had some attention in Canada; one probable reason for this is an aversion on the part of some analysts to fee-for-service medicine. In Canada, the concept of primary care reform refers to the development of clinics that provide a variety of services by family doctors, nurses (including nurse practitioners), and other professionals and para-professionals, such as nurse assistants. These clinics would not normally be funded on a fee-for-service basis; rather, they might be paid on a capitation payment or a straight budget. Most of the recent reports, including the Romanow, Mazankowski, and Kirby Reports, incorporate proposals for the expansion of primary care.

Reform of fee-for-service medicine has had its proponents for specialized care as well. In the late 1990s, Queen's University changed its funding mechanism from fee for service to a global budget for its entire medical faculty. The faculty was responsible for dividing up the total budget among its individual clinical practitioners, many of whom were specialists. One concern with such reforms is that the incentive to generate services would be reduced under a pure global budget, and therefore availability of specialized services might be reduced.

Several Western and Atlantic provinces have engaged in funding and delivery reform of institutional services. Saskatchewan was the first to do so; in 1993, Saskatchewan eliminated all hospital, nursing home, and public health boards and placed these institutions under the control of regional health authorities (RHAs). Thirty regions were created, and each had an RHA that was jointly responsible for hospital care, home care, nursing home care, and public health services. These regional organizations, as can be seen in Figure 2.3, are akin to HMOs in that they combine several different forms of delivery inside one single organization (drawn inside the dashed lines). This allows RHAs to address the lack of connection between acute care and post-acute care services, as mentioned above. However, Saskatchewan's RHAs do not include physicians and so are not the same as HMOs. Physicians remain as separate funding entities, being paid on a fee-for-service basis.

Funding to RHAs was set according to a needs-based, per capita payment. Each region receives a set fee for each resident based on the provincial average cost of services used by individuals in given age and gender groups. Needs-based funding addresses the inequity issue as individuals in each age group get the same funding regardless of the region in which they live. Each region is responsible for providing care to all individual residents within the region and is required to provide for this care out of capitation funding from the province. Obviously, some people in each age and gender group are healthier than others; therefore, the "needs" among individuals of the same age and gender will differ. To address this point, Saskatchewan (following British practice) introduced an additional needs-based supplement by which regions with less healthy populations receive a needs-based adjustment in addition to the age-based and gender-based capitation payments. Among the bases for making these adjustments were the mortality rate, the number of older adults who live alone, and the premature birth rate for the region. All such factors increase the need for care, and regions with greater need receive needs-based bonuses.

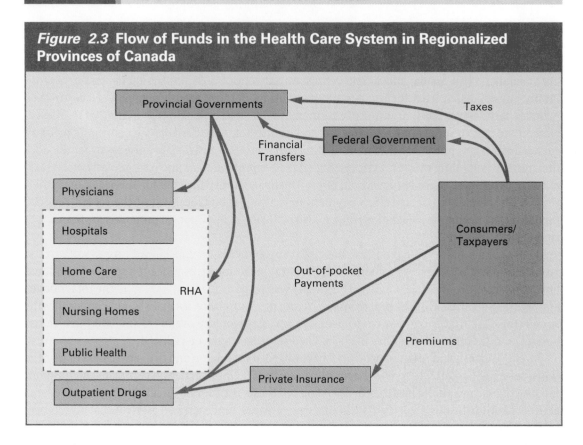

Figure 2.3 Flow of Funds in the Health Care System in Regionalized Provinces of Canada

However, the concept of need is a subjective one. Need may be defined as the minimum amount of health care services that should be provided to bring an individual to a desired level of health. To assess need, therefore, analysts should know what that desired state of health is and what minimum level of services would bring individuals to that level. Further, select target health levels for different groups may differ since it may not be feasible to make everyone completely healthy. In fact, no one yet knows what should go into a needs-based funding formula. A better description of this plan is that it is "equity based."

The regional capitation system itself is not incentive free. The fixed annual payment that is paid to the regions by the provincial governments is based on demographic characteristics and some health status measures, but not on any service characteristics, such as the number of hospitalizations, inpatient length of stay, or emergency room visits. The region cannot generate more money by providing more services. However, there is nothing in this finance mechanism that would encourage more efficient provision of services by the region. If the region is more efficient and produces more services, it will not benefit financially; thus, while this finance mechanism may be fair, it is not efficient. In any payment system, if one obtains one type of benefit or good, one usually ends up sacrificing another. No single payment system will satisfy everyone.

Some people have proposed imposing an out-of-pocket co-payment for medically necessary health services in addition to those for drugs and other provincially provided services like home care and long-term care. This has become a very contentious issue. It would have the impact of choking off demand for services. In all likelihood, the reduced demand would include some services that have an impact on health status, as well as some that have a lesser impact. No one knows for sure how much of each would be affected by a co-payment.

A final type of reform is privatization. In Alberta primarily, but also in other provinces, a number of privately owned clinics and hospitals have been opened or proposed, and these have been encouraged on the basis that the public sector should be able to compete with the private sector, even in health care. Some of these privately operated establishments have been promoted on the basis of their potential export value or the ability of the organizations to market their services to full-paying non-residents. It is felt that perhaps they may even relieve the pressure on the government health insurance systems. However, the ability of physicians to sell services to private and public patients simultaneously raises some concerns. A physician who practices in both sectors has an incentive to build up queues in the public sector so that public patients will move to the physician's private clinic. The Mazankowski Report recommends an increase in the use of private markets in health care (Premier's Advisory Council on Health, 2001) despite the fact that the original federal health care insurance acts prohibited a two-tier system.

Concluding Comments

The Canadian health care system went through considerable changes in the 1990s, and reform continues. Health care reforms are responses to several decades of rising costs; however, they vary in their intent. Some are attacks on fee-for-service medicine, others are attacks on full-service coverage, still others are attacks on government-funded health care.

The incentives created by these reforms are not well understood at this time. It is not clear how much utilization will be reduced as a result, and it is even less clear whether health promotion and disease prevention will increase. Overall, the reforms may reduce costs, but they should not be judged on the basis of cost alone. Changes in outcomes, in terms of health status, must also be assessed. All practices—whether new or existing—should be judged on the basis of solid evidence of their effectiveness.

Leadership Implications

An understanding of how revenues are obtained and administered is an important dimension of administrative competence. It is sometimes assumed that market forces drive the development of health services and the behaviour of citizens who use the health system. However, this simplistic assumption does not take into account the complex mix of service providers and funding incentives within the Canadian health system.

The complex framework of funding incentives reflects the incremental development and implementation of government policy over many decades. Some outdated incentives have remained in place while new incentives have sometimes been added in an attempt to change the behaviour of health service providers or citizens. In some instances, the outcomes of particular interventions, such as the introduction of advanced practice nursing roles, have been studied extensively, but the implementation of these cost-effective interventions has been delayed or prevented by pressure from stakeholder groups who want to maintain current funding incentives. In other instances, new initiatives or policies to change financial incentives have been implemented without evidence that they will improve the quality or lower the cost of service. Many policies and initiatives designed to privatize the delivery of health services fall within this category.

Leaders at all levels of the health system are affected by the framework of funding mechanisms and incentives. In recent decades, as health costs have increased, governments have taken a more interventionist approach to the management of the health system. Health agencies often have had to respond rapidly to changes in funding mechanisms and incentives that arise from the external environment, and which have been implemented without extensive consultation with agency boards or senior leaders. In these circumstances, it often has been impossible to plan for change or to manage it in an orderly fashion. Changes in the external environment of health agencies have, in turn, created instability that can have the effect of increasing both direct and indirect costs.

Not all costs of health services are accounted for within the budgets and accounting systems of health departments. This is particularly true of costs for services that are not covered by the *Canada Health Act*. Changes in the approach to delivering or paying for health services have resulted in the transfer of direct costs to citizens through fees and taxes. The indirect costs of family caregiving, such as time lost from work; costs of medical supplies, equipment, and services; and health problems of caregivers, are not accounted for in health department budgets and represent a rising cost to citizens. Changes in the funding of social services, education, and the justice system also have an impact on the health of the population and the health system.

Summary

- Economics is a science that is used to describe, predict, and evaluate events related to the scarcity of resources. Health economics is the branch of economics that deals with health-related events.
- The health care system has three functions: finance, funding, and delivery. The finance function is the mechanism by which funds are collected from the public via insurance premiums, taxes, and direct charges. The funding function is the means of paying care providers. The delivery function is the means by which health care services are provided to the public.
- In the traditional health care system, physicians were funded by fee for service, and hospitals were funded through global budgets.

- Fee-for-service funding has been perceived as increasing the number of health care services and has therefore been linked to growing health care expenditures.
- Both fee-for-service funding of physicians and global budgeting for hospitals have been perceived as relating to services, rather than to people or needs.
- A number of concepts for health reform have been proposed. These include the privatization of health care, per capita funding for hospitals, and the dismantling of fee-for-service funding for physicians.
- Reforms are being instituted in Canada, including regionalization of health care providers and funding of providers on a per capita basis. These systems are new and should be subject to careful scrutiny. As with their predecessors, they will have drawbacks as well as benefits.

Applying the Knowledge in this Chapter

Exercise

Questions for discussion:

1. What are the three major functions of the health care system?

2. How have these functions traditionally been organized in Canada?

3. Give an example of how each of these functions is proposed to change in reform proposals, and use economic analysis to indicate what the expected change to the health care system will be.

Resources

evolve Internet Resources

Canadian Health Economics Research Association:
   www.chera.ca
   This site contains links to many other Web sites and Canadian studies related to health economics.
Canadian Institute for Health Information (CIHI):
   www.cihi.ca
   The CIHI is one of the primary health data generating agencies in Canada. This Web site contains some series of data and also describes other reports, which must be purchased.

Health Canada:

www.hc-sc.gc.ca

This Web site contains an enormous amount of information about many different aspects of the Canadian health care system and the health status of Canadians.

Institute for Health Economics:

www.ihe.ab.ca

This Web site contains links to studies on a variety of health care issues in Canada.

Statistics Canada:

www.statcan.ca

Statistics Canada is the official federal government data agency. This Web site contains data on demographic and health aspects of the Canadian population.

Further Reading

Commission on the Future of Health Care in Canada. (2002, November). *Building on values: The future of healthcare in Canada – Final report*. Commissioner: R. Romanow. Ottawa, ON: Parliament of Canada. This report contains an extensive set of analyses of the entire health care system and makes a series of recommendations for consideration by the federal government.

Jacobs, P., & Rapoport, J. (2003). *The economics of health and medical care*. (5th ed.). Boston, MA: Jones & Bartlett. This is an elementary level textbook of health economics that focuses on the use of economics to analyze how the health care system works and on the potential impact of policies.

References

Commission d'étude sur les services de santé et les services sociaux. (2001). *Emerging solutions: Report and recommendations*. Chair: M. Clair. Quebec City, QC: Ministry of Health and Social Services.

Commission on Medicare. (2001). *Caring for medicare: Sustaining a quality system*. Commissioner: K. Fyke. Regina, SK: Government of Saskatchewan.

Commission on the Future of Health Care in Canada. (2002, November). *Building on values: The future of healthcare in Canada – Final report*. Commissioner: R. Romanow. Ottawa, ON: Parliament of Canada.

Health Canada. (2002). *National Health expenditures in Canada, 1975–96*. Fact Sheets, Table 1. Ottawa, ON: Author. Retrieved June 5, 2004, from http://www.hc-sc.gc.ca

Premier's Advisory Council on Health. (2001). *A framework for reform. Report of the Premier's Advisory Council on Health*. Chair: D. Mazankowski. Edmonton, AB: Government of Alberta.

Standing Senate Committee on Social Affairs, Science and Technology. (2002). *The health of Canadians – The federal role. Final report on the state of the health care system in Canada. Volume 6, Recommendations for reform*. Chair: The Honourable M. J. L. Kirby. Ottawa, ON: Parliament of Canada.

3

A POPULATION HEALTH APPROACH TO PLANNING

Penelope Lightfoot, Joy Edwards, Nonie Fraser-Lee, Angela Kaida, and Gerald Predy

Learning Objectives

In this chapter, you will learn:

- [ ] What population health is and how it differs from health care

- [ ] The key components of a population health framework

- [ ] Implementation strategies and examples of how to apply a population health approach

Mention the words health or health care and people immediately think of hospitals, surgeries, visits to doctors, pharmaceuticals, or diagnostic tests. However, there is a growing awareness that many of the factors that affect people's health extend well beyond what is traditionally thought of as health care.

Population health takes a broad perspective. It is a way of thinking about health and taking action to improve health not only by treating people when they are ill or injured, but also by addressing the myriad factors that determine the health of large groups of people. These factors include individual characteristics such as biology, personal health practices, and coping skills. Population health also addresses people's access to health services and factors that pertain to the physical, social, and economic environments in which people live. It encompasses the entire range of factors that influence health, going beyond the risk factors for a particular disease or condition.

A population health approach emphasizes understanding the key determinants of health, assessing the health of populations, identifying actions that can be taken by all sectors of society, and evaluating the impact of those actions on improving the health of populations over the long term. Typically, a population health approach focuses on strategies targeted at preventing illness and injury, removing barriers to health, increasing opportunities for people to reach optimal levels of health, and achieving better health outcomes for targeted groups of people as well as the population as a whole.

The following sections provide background information on the development of a population health approach in Canada by describing it, outlining the key components, and providing examples of how this approach can be applied.

The Population Health Approach

The term population health has no widely accepted definition; rather, it continues to evolve amidst considerable discussion. One recent definition proposed by Kindig and Stoddart (2003) defines the term in a comprehensive way that is consistent with the approach adopted in this chapter:

> Population health as a concept of health is defined as the health outcomes of a group of individuals, including the distribution of such outcomes. The field of population health includes health outcomes, patterns of health determinants, and policies and interventions that link these two (p. 380).

For any health issue, there is a spectrum of actions that can be taken to address the problem—from promotion, prevention, and protection strategies to treatment, rehabilitation, and continuing care. The population health approach is distinguished from traditional health care approaches in both its scope and focus. Population health addresses health issues at the population level and focuses on strategies that will achieve greater health for the population as a whole.

The following scenario can be used to illustrate how a population health approach can be applied: An 18-year-old male is brought to an emergency department by ambulance on a Saturday night. He has been in a motor vehicle collision and has a fractured femur and a major head injury. He will require admission to the intensive care unit. Although his life is not in danger, he will require acute care treatment and extensive rehabilitation. Beyond treating the immediate injuries, the health professional considers the individual's relevant living and working conditions. Does he work? Is he in school? Does he have dependents? Does he have family or some support system nearby that will be willing to help? The answers to these questions will not change the immediate treatment, but they may well have implications for ongoing treatment, the rehabilitation plan, and his return home to the community. It is important to consider issues beyond the individual's specific situation and to think of this young man as one of a group of people within the population who have had injuries from motor vehicle accidents. This step involves addressing questions such as the following:

- Who (e.g., age, gender) is having collisions?
- What are the circumstances (e.g., speed, alcohol, environmental factors, time) surrounding the event?
- Is this an isolated event or part of a larger and more common pattern for people with similar circumstances?

The answers to these questions can lead to strategies for preventing further collisions and minimizing injury.

This analysis at a population level emphasizes the importance of understanding the full range of factors that result in high injury rates among young adult males. The physical environment (road and vehicle design) and the social environment (licensing, enforcement, and education) that might contribute to the problem should be explored. Often, policy development and implementation are key strategies used to create change at the population level.

Central to a population health approach is a clear recognition that the health sector does not "own" health problems and cannot address them alone. Public and private sectors (e.g., education, environment, transportation, and industry) collectively share responsibility for the health of a population. However, the health sector is often well placed to take a lead role in identifying issues and coordinating action among sectors to achieve overall improvements in the health of the population. For regions across Canada, a population health approach provides an important way of achieving the goal of "healthy people in healthy communities."

Determinants of Health

A population health approach is based on understanding the range and complex interplay among numerous factors that influence health at individual and population levels. Typically these factors have been called determinants. The lists of determinants and their various categorizations reflect different ideas about how the factors relate to health, how they interact with one another, and their relative importance as a determinant (Hamilton & Bhatti, 1996; US Department of

Health and Human Services, 2000). Despite these different conceptualizations, the lists are quite similar and typically include:

- income and social status;
- social support networks;
- education;
- working conditions;
- physical environments (natural and built);
- biology and genetics;
- personal health practices and coping skills;
- healthy child development; and
- health services (Federal, Provincial and Territorial Advisory Committee, 1994).

The 1994 release of *Why Are Some People Healthy and Others Not? The Determinants of Health of Populations* (Evans, Barer, & Marmor, 1994) stimulated debate about the complex interactions among determinants, applicable research frameworks, and potential policy implications. This discussion also shifted the focus from personal behaviours and the health care system to social and economic factors affecting health. In late 1994, a discussion paper developed by the Federal, Provincial and Territorial Advisory Committee on Population Health was released. It proposed a framework for action that included five categories of health determinants that were supported by

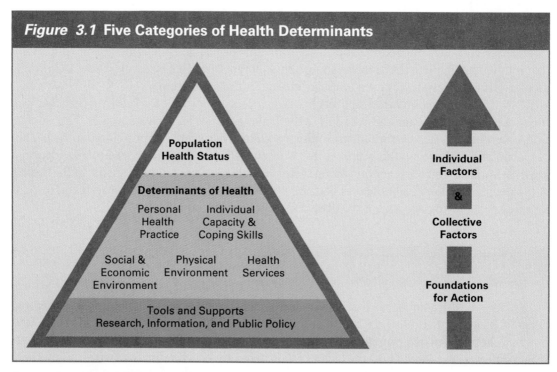

Figure 3.1 Five Categories of Health Determinants

Source: From *Strategies for Population Health: Investing in the Health of Canadians* (p. 30), prepared by the Federal, Provincial and Territorial Advisory Committee on Population Health, 1994, Ottawa, ON: Health Canada.

a foundation of research, information, and public policy (Figure 3.1). The framework is notable for contextualizing the individually oriented behaviours within a collective environment.

Developing a Population Health Approach in Canada

For several decades, Canada has been a leader in developing and implementing a population health approach. Thirty years ago, the Lalonde Report (1974) took the perspective that health is not synonymous with health care but rather is determined by factors beyond health care, namely, human biology, environment, and lifestyle. That perspective was echoed in the Epp Report (1986), which emphasized the importance of reducing inequities between socioeconomic groups by addressing the social determinants of health. It also stressed the need for healthy public policies in all areas of policy development. That same year, the Ottawa Charter (1986) signaled the importance of promoting good health in addition to focusing on treatments for illness and injuries, identified several health challenges, and proposed the following five key strategies:
- Building healthy public policy
- Creating supportive environments
- Strengthening community action
- Developing personal skills
- Reorienting health services.

In 1994, the Federal, Provincial and Territorial Advisory Committee on Population Health developed a discussion paper identifying broad population health strategies that various levels of government could use to work together to improve the health of the Canadian population. The discussion paper argued that there is more to health than health care and that determinants of health included many of the socioeconomic determinants identified in the Ottawa Charter. To address these broader determinants of health, the health sector could not act alone but needed to work together with other sectors, including economic, education, environment, employment, and social services sectors. The paper also emphasized the importance of involvement from various community organizations and the general public (Federal, Provincial and Territorial Advisory Committee, 1994).

At the federal level, recommendations in the National Forum on Health Report (1997) led to the establishment of the Canadian Population Health Initiative (CPHI) in 1997. The CPHI is operated as an integral part of the Canadian Institute for Health Information (CIHI). With financial support from the federal government, the mission of this initiative is to "foster a better understanding of the factors that affect the health of individuals and communities, and to contribute to the development of policies that reduce inequities and improve the health and well-being of Canadians" (CIHI, 2003). CPHI's primary focus is generating knowledge of the determinants of health, developing a national population health information system, synthesizing research evidence and analysis of policy options, and contributing to regular reports to

Canadians on their health and well-being. This work has resulted in the Health Information Roadmap Initiative and the compilation of health indicators for Canadians. In the fall of 2002, a set of comparable health indicators for all provinces and territories was compiled (Health Canada, 2002).

In November 2002, social and health policy experts, community representatives, and health researchers prepared the Toronto Charter after examining the implications of key social determinants on health and discussing policy directions to address some of them (Raphael, 2003). The Toronto Charter recommended that the federal government allocate $1.5 billion towards "two essential determinants of health for children and families: (1) affordable, safe housing, and (2) a universal system of high quality educational childcare" (p. 40). They also recommended that the federal government "establish a social determinants of health task force to consider the findings" (p. 40).

In spite of various reports stressing the importance of taking a population health perspective, Raphael (2003) argues that there is a "policy vacuum on social determinants of health as the costs and delivery of healthcare services have come to dominate the public debate" (p. 35). There is little question that, in recent years, the primary focus of discussion and debate in health care has been centred on rising costs and ensuring the sustainability of the health system over the long term. Several provincial reports—such as the Mazankowski Report in Alberta (2001), the Fyke Commission in Saskatchewan (2001), and the Claire Report in Quebec (2000)—and national reports—such as the Kirby Report (Standing Senate Committee, 2002) and the Romanow Report (Commission, 2002)—have addressed a number of health issues and examined ways of developing an effective and sustainable health system for Canada. While each report takes a different perspective, a consistent message is the need to keep people healthy by preventing illness and injury and promoting good health.

These recent reports have contributed to a growing awareness of the importance of prevention for improving health outcomes and achieving a sustainable health system. A population health approach is consistent with this direction. Policy and decision makers, researchers, health care providers, community agencies, and leaders across sectors can use a population health approach to identify and implement strategies for improving the health of the population.

Implementing a Population Health Framework

The purpose of a population health framework is to (a) achieve a common understanding of the issues at all levels, whether community, municipal, regional, provincial, or national and to (b) provide direction for population health planning and action with appropriate partners. With this type of framework in place, there is a clear understanding of the issues to be addressed, the responsibilities of various players, and the comprehensive range of actions that can be taken together to improve health.

Three key components of a population health framework include the following:
- Principles of population health
- Determinants of health
- Population health process.

Principles of Population Health

The following population health principles, while not unique, guide decision making and action and assist in setting priorities, planning interventions, and evaluating outcomes:

1. *Evidence-based decisions*. Population health decisions are based on evidence of the relationships among health determinants and health, and on evaluations that demonstrate the link between interventions and outcomes.
2. *Multi-level and multi-sectoral responsibility*. Due to the range of skills and knowledge needed to address population health issues, population health takes a multi-level and a multi-sectoral approach. The health sector can often take the lead in identifying issues and coordinating action.
3. *Partnerships*. The population health approach emphasizes individuals, organizations, businesses, service systems, and government working together to achieve common goals.
4. *Shared accountability*. Accountability for population health outcomes extends beyond the health system to all sectors that influence the determinants of health. Each sector is accountable for the outcomes it can affect.
5. *Upstream focus*. Population health focuses upstream, where health problems, disease, and injury start, taking action as early as possible to prevent or reduce future health problems.
6. *Equity*. Population health seeks to reduce inequalities in health status among groups in society and, in so doing, improve the health of everyone.
7. *Holistic view of health*. Population health takes a holistic view of health, addressing the full range of factors that determine health, including (but also going beyond) individual risk factors for disease.

Population Health Process

Implementing a population health process involves four components:
- *Assessing* the health of the population
- *Deciding* on appropriate strategies
- *Taking* action
- *Evaluating* outcomes.

Assessing the Health of the Population

The population health process begins with an assessment of the various determinants of health and the differences in health among subgroups of the population. Using quantitative and qualitative methods, data are analyzed to identify trends and health issues. Key characteristics of the population are examined, including population structure, income and social status, education, employment, social support, health practices and choices, the physical and natural environment, health services, and changes in disease patterns and technology.

Population Structure

Understanding population growth and structure provides important information to help in planning health programs and assessing the current and future health needs of the population. Population data are also necessary to identify, measure, and track trends in rates of certain health and social factors.

The major factors influencing the total population and its age-sex structure are births, deaths, and migration. In simplest terms, the growth or decline of a population depends upon the number of babies born, the number of people who die, and the number of people who move in and out of the population every year. Typically, births outnumber deaths, and the population grows unless a large number of people move away.

Canada's population is growing, but at a very slow pace. In 2001, Canada's population was 30 million, six times as large as it was in 1901 (5.3 million). But from 1996 to 2001, the rate of growth was one of the lowest in our history. There were only two other time periods when the population grew this slowly: during the Depression in the 1930s and between 1981 and 1986 (*Canadian Census Geography,* 2003).

The aging of the baby-boom generation (born between 1946 and 1964) is a key sociodemographic transition occurring across Canada. The boomers' current and projected health status and the implications for the health system are the subject of debate as various scenarios are considered. Will the boomers follow an "older, sicker, increasingly costly care" trajectory? Or will changes in lifestyle and environment mean that older adults will have generally better health status and fewer years of disability than the generation before them? Will society have sufficient economic capacity to absorb the costs associated with an aging population? Anticipating the impact of an aging population is an essential component of future planning for Canada's health care system. Figure 3.2 shows the aging of the population from 1989 to 2007 in an urban health region in Canada.

The growth in the population is not evenly distributed across age groups. The Government of Canada has estimated that the average annual growth of the whole population from 2001 to 2020 will be 0.9%. The average annual growth for people aged 15 to 44 years is estimated to be only 0.1%. In contrast, the growth for people aged 65 years and older is estimated to be 3.0%. At this rate, the percentage of the population aged 65 years and over is expected to grow from 12.7% in 2001 to 17.9% in 2021 (Statistics Canada, 2002).

Growth rates also vary among the provinces. Alberta's population grew 40 fold between 1901 and 2001. In contrast to all other provinces, the population of Alberta increased by 10.3% between 1996 and 2001, almost double its growth in the previous five years. Between 1996 and 2001, there were three provinces and one territory where growth rates were above the national aver-

Figure 3.2 **Population Profile of an Urban Health Region 1989–2007**

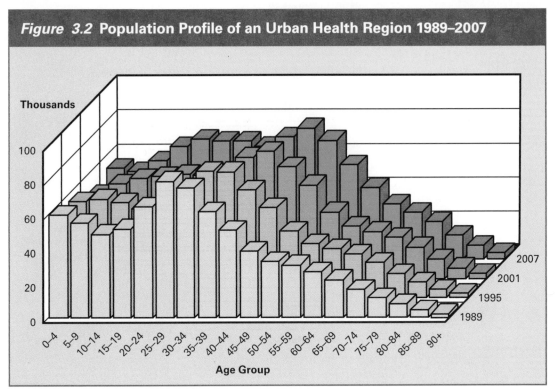

Source: From Capital Health Region Population and Projections (1989–2007), Edmonton, Alberta. The 1989–2001 data are based on the registrants active on the Alberta Health Care Insurance Plan at March 31st of each year. The 2007 population projections were obtained from Alberta Health and Wellness and modified by Capital Health.

age of 4.0%: Alberta had the highest (10.3%), followed by Nunavut (8.1%), Ontario (6.1%), and British Columbia (4.9%). Population movement between provinces was responsible for most of the differences in the growth rates between 1996 and 2001 because the natural increase (births minus deaths) declined in all provinces and immigration remained relatively stable (Statistics Canada, 2003b).

Population pyramids are typically used to show five-year age groupings for males and females by geographic area. The Statistics Canada Web site provides an interesting example of an animated population pyramid that provides a visual picture of Canada's changing population from the early 1900s (Statistics Canada, 2003a). Population pyramids in Figures 3.3 and 3.4 show the age-sex distribution of an area's population, a factor that influences both the health status of the community and the nature and extent of health problems experienced by its members.

Areas with a relatively high proportion of older adults can expect greater numbers of deaths, hospitalizations, visits to physicians, use of home care services, and medication use as a result of chronic diseases (e.g., heart disease, cancer, respiratory conditions). As adults age, their needs also change if they retire, lose a spouse, become more frail, or develop dementia. These changes

Figure 3.3 Example of a Population Pyramid for an Older Population

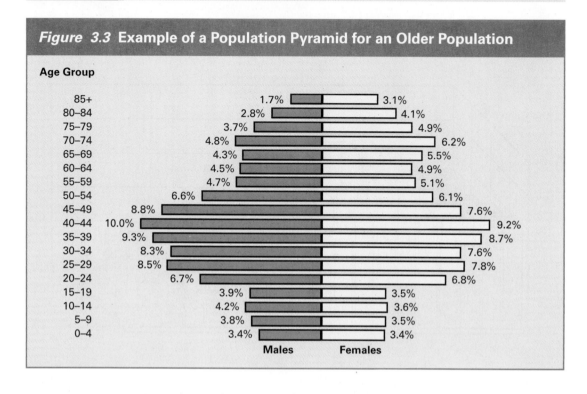

Age Group

	Males	Females
85+	1.7%	3.1%
80–84	2.8%	4.1%
75–79	3.7%	4.9%
70–74	4.8%	6.2%
65–69	4.3%	5.5%
60–64	4.5%	4.9%
55–59	4.7%	5.1%
50–54	6.6%	6.1%
45–49	8.8%	7.6%
40–44	10.0%	9.2%
35–39	9.3%	8.7%
30–34	8.3%	7.6%
25–29	8.5%	7.8%
20–24	6.7%	6.8%
15–19	3.9%	3.5%
10–14	4.2%	3.6%
5–9	3.8%	3.5%
0–4	3.4%	3.4%

Figure 3.4 Example of a Population Pyramid for a Younger Population

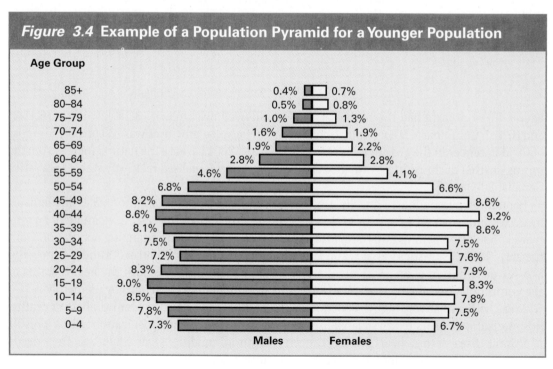

Age Group

	Males	Females
85+	0.4%	0.7%
80–84	0.5%	0.8%
75–79	1.0%	1.3%
70–74	1.6%	1.9%
65–69	1.9%	2.2%
60–64	2.8%	2.8%
55–59	4.6%	4.1%
50–54	6.8%	6.6%
45–49	8.2%	8.6%
40–44	8.6%	9.2%
35–39	8.1%	8.6%
30–34	7.5%	7.5%
25–29	7.2%	7.6%
20–24	8.3%	7.9%
15–19	9.0%	8.3%
10–14	8.5%	7.8%
5–9	7.8%	7.5%
0–4	7.3%	6.7%

could result in the need for specific levels and types of support, care, and health services. Issues such as living independently, adequate housing and transportation, and personal relationships are all important considerations in a population health approach. Despite these challenges, it is important to see the broader picture and the significant contribution older adults make to the community through volunteer activities and support to their families.

In contrast, areas with relatively young populations typically need health services for respiratory illness and injury-related problems. Community issues relate to access to educational and recreational opportunities, day care availability, immunization, and the importance of public policy that supports family values.

Income

Income and the much less studied concept of wealth are known to be both contributors to and consequences of health status. While there are the obvious connections between low income, material deprivation, and health, the most interesting research has pursued a variety of paths. Listed below are some of the research findings that have shaped thinking over the past three decades.

- McKeown's (1979) analysis of declining mortality rates in 19th century England led him to conclude that the increase in the standard of living, not medical care, was responsible for improved health. This generated considerable debate and stimulated new research directions.
- Marmot, Kogevinas, and Elston (1987), after studying 10,000 British civil servants (the Whitehall study), pioneered the idea of a social class gradient in disease rates. The gradient could not be explained by differences in risk factors known to vary among the social classes (e.g., obesity, smoking, higher blood pressure). Poverty could not explain the differences because the gradient applied not only to those at the lowest and highest points on the gradient, but also to those in the middle. Interestingly, those one step removed from the top had rates of disease that were twice as high.
- Evans, Barer, and Marmor (1994) continued to explore the reasons for the gradient and emphasized the importance of social and economic factors over individual behaviour. They focused attention on the persistence of the gradient across disease type, mortality, time periods, occupation, and regions. They brought together research from different fields that hinted at the causal factors (determinants) and their potential physiological pathways.
- Wilkinson (1992) brought to the forefront the importance of income distribution to health status. He compared income distribution and life expectancy for several countries and found a strong link between income inequality and mortality risk, even after controlling for median income variation across countries.
- Ross, Wolfson, and Dunn (2000) challenged the idea that income distribution is linked to the health of a population by analyzing the relationships across Canadian provinces, American states, and metropolitan areas in both countries. The pattern seems to hold in some instances, but not in others. Preliminary explanations for the lack of a relationship are that some areas have an extensive social safety net that buffers the effect of low income.

Understanding the nature of the relationship between income and health remains puzzling. In a recent article by Evans and Stoddart (2003), where the findings of the aforementioned studies are analyzed, the following conclusion is offered: "We think the most plausible view to this point is that the relationship between income and health, or between inequality and health, depends very much on the social and cultural environment in which income differences are experienced" (p. 376).

Education

Education has long been acknowledged as one of the factors that is inextricably linked to socio-economic status and health status. Adults with a lower level of education often have poorer health than those with higher levels of education (Roberge, Berthelot, & Wolfson, 1995). Education increases the opportunity for employment choices, secure income, and job satisfaction. It also helps provide knowledge and skills for all aspects of living. With the rapid changes in society and the growing emphasis on knowledge and ideas, education and lifelong learning are becoming even more important than in the past. Focusing on education is one of the best ways to ensure a healthy population in the long run.

Employment

Employment is a significant determinant of a person's physical, mental, and social health (Federal, Provincial and Territorial Advisory Committee, 1999). Unemployment, underemployment, and stressful or unsafe work are associated with poorer overall health. Evidence suggests that individuals who have more control over their work circumstances and fewer stress-related job demands are healthier and often have a higher life expectancy than those in more stressful or riskier employment.

Employment influences health not only by providing income, but also by offering a sense of identity and purpose, social contacts, and opportunities for personal growth (Federal, Provincial and Territorial Advisory Committee, 1999). Thus, benefits to health through employment are not simply accrued through financial gain, but also through the quality of the job and the workplace environment. The CPRN-Ekos Changing Employment Relationships Survey (a 2000 nationally representative survey of 2500 employees and self-employed individuals) reported that in a job, Canadians value respect, interesting work, good communication, a sense of accomplishment, work-life balance, and opportunities for skill development (Lowe & Schellenberg, 2001). The same survey revealed that Canadians reported work overload and job stress as serious problems. According to Lowe (2002), the gap between employment values and workplace realities is a symptom of unhealthy workplaces, and unhealthy workplaces are associated with poorer health.

Statistics Canada monitors the unemployment rate on a monthly basis. The rates are based on the proportion of people who do not have work but are available and looking for work. This information is important for implementing a population health framework because it allows planners and policy makers to track trends and assess the impact of employment factors on the overall health of the population.

Social Support

As social animals, we rely on a variety of people to provide support when needed. Networks of family, friends, and the larger community are important influences on health. Social support, or the web of social ties that surround people, strongly influence their health-related perceptions and behaviour. While there are many networks that support people, the family, in its myriad forms, is typically the primary source of support. Families are important to consider in relation to the social and economic context within which individuals live and grow. The family provides important socialization, helps interpret influences from the broader community, and is instrumental in encouraging education and social opportunities.

The attributes of the communities that people live in—such as voter turnout, volunteerism, charitable donation rate, crime rate, housing affordability, and commitment to providing public services—are all community-level indicators that are important for a population health assessment (Frankish, Kwan, & Flores, 2002).

Culture and language are also important factors to consider. In communities across the country, there is considerable ethnic diversity in the population, which has a direct impact on health and health-related issues. New Canadians may be more dependent on family support and cultural or religious networks than are other groups who have lived in Canada for many generations.

Health Practices

People are responsible for their behaviour and the lifestyle choices they make, but their choices are strongly influenced by external factors. Behaviour takes place within communities and societies. Family, friends, and the immediate community influence individuals to respond to their environment and its challenges in specific ways. Thus, lifestyle is a combination of choice, chance, and resources. In Table 3.1, three categories illustrate the range of behaviours often considered as components of lifestyle.

Table 3.1 Categories Illustrating the Range of Health Practice Behaviours

Lifestyle Practices	Safety Practices	Health-Related Practices
• Eating habits	• Seatbelt/carseat use	• Immunization
• Physical activity	• Use of safety equipment	• Breast self-examination
• Sleeping patterns	• Use of protective gear	• Pap test
• Leisure activity		• Blood pressure checks
• Sexual behaviour		• Child developmental screen
• Tobacco/alcohol use		• Prostate exam
• Drug use		

Source: From *Dimensions of Health in Edmonton* (p. 80), by P. Macdonald and N. Fraser, 1989, Edmonton, AB: Edmonton Board of Health.

Physical Environment

Both the natural environment and the constructed environment have the potential to critically influence health. Threats to health can exist through air, water and soil quality, the safety of work and recreation sites, and the quality of housing and transportation. In recent years, the public has become more aware of some of the risks in the environment, and their expectations for controlling these risks have increased as a result. Events such as *Escherichia coli* in the Walkerton, Ontario water supply; cryptosporidium in the water in North Battleford, Saskatchewan; and cautions about possible contamination of selected foods have alerted the public to the importance of disease surveillance and prevention strategies. At the same time, people's dependence on the environment encourages protection and enhancement of its health, particularly in relation to the control of solid and toxic wastes and the health of the ecosystem (University of Alberta, 1994).

Health Services

More health care has typically been equated with better health status for individuals and populations. However, over the last two decades, persistent challenges to this idea have been raised. The Black Report from the United Kingdom reported increasing gradients in mortality across social classes despite removal of financial barriers to care (Black, Smith, & Townsend, 1982). Japan continues to have a high ranking on several health indices despite spending relatively less on health care than other developed nations. Examples such as these, and other reports on health care, have reinforced the idea that while health care is no doubt an important contributor to health and well-being, there are socioeconomic factors that exert critically important effects (Frank & Mustard, 1994).

Across the health sector, the importance of being accountable for health outcomes has increased. At a minimum, accountability means knowing that the health system is doing the "right things" and that it is doing the "right things right," namely, providing quality care. Less emphasis has been placed on accountability for achieving the "right outcomes," specifically, improving the health of the population. As a result, there are numerous measures of health system activity, but few assessments of its performance with respect to improving population health. Claims that as much as 30% of medical care is inappropriate have intensified the need to show that resources are being used optimally and that opportunities to spend on other determinants, such as education and social support, are not being missed (Working Group et al., 1995). In recent years, there has been a growing emphasis on accountability for outcomes. Provinces, health regions, and organizations like the CIHI have been measuring outcomes and tracking changes in the health of populations. The CIHI's health indicator framework uses the following eight categories to assess the quality of health care:

- Acceptability
- Accessibility
- Appropriateness
- Competence
- Continuity
- Effectiveness

- Efficiency
- Safety.

Disease Patterns

Changes in disease patterns also have an impact on the overall health of the population and on how health care needs are addressed. During the last century, patterns of disease and types of health problems have changed; for example, in the early 1900s, the primary causes of illness and death were environmental conditions and infectious diseases. Today, the primary causes of illness, disability, and death are chronic diseases. Nevertheless, infectious diseases continue to be of concern as new diseases evolve, necessitating constant vigilance.

Planning for a potential influenza pandemic and the impact of emerging diseases such as the new variant Creutzfeldt-Jakob Disease (CJD), West Nile Virus, and Severe Acute Respiratory Syndrome (SARS) continues in health regions and at provincial, national, and international levels. The outbreak of SARS in 2003 generated worldwide concern and illustrated the ease with which infectious diseases can spread in an era of global travel and trade. Concern has focused on the potentially large health and economic impacts of these diseases. Mandatory surveillance and disease control measures should be priorities for the global community.

Antibiotic resistance is another important concern. Many species of bacteria have developed resistant strains, partly due to the inappropriate use of antibiotics for viral infections and the increasing use of antimicrobial soaps by the general public.

In contrast to the past, chronic diseases such as cancer, cardiovascular disease, diabetes, respiratory disease, and arthritis are now the major causes of illness, disability, and death. These chronic conditions are more frequent among older people; therefore, as our population ages and people live longer, we can anticipate an increase in the number of people affected by chronic conditions and more pressure on the health care system to address and manage these conditions. Health planners are also mindful that the health care expectations of aging baby boomers may be considerably higher than those of their parents.

New Technologies

Ever advancing and changing technology also provides a significant challenge for policy makers and planners in the health care system. Innovative medical imaging techniques, new medications, future gene therapy, and new treatments such as the Edmonton protocol for treating diabetes are being developed on an almost daily basis. New vaccines also continue to be developed; for example, varicella, meningococcal, and pneumococcal vaccines have been recently introduced. These advances in technology require health regions to carefully weigh potential benefits against the costs and to manage public expectations. The public's desire for these innovations increases pressure on decision makers to invest in new treatments and technologies, sometimes at the expense of long-term prevention strategies.

Population Subgroups

Taking a population health approach means not only focusing on assessing the health and health needs of the overall population, but also narrowing the target to look specifically at the needs of various age groups within the population. Clearly, the health needs are very different for infants, children, youths, adults, seniors, males and females, and for special population groups such as

Table 3.2 Health Assessment of Residents by Age Group for an Urban Health Region					
Determinant of Interest	Infants (<1 year)	Children & Youth (1–19 years)	Adults (20–64 years)	Seniors (65+ years)	Special Groups: Aboriginals
Top Causes of Hospital Admissions[1]	Perinatal Conditions	Respiratory Disease Pregnancy & Childbirth Unintentional Injury Digestive Disease Mental Disorders	Pregnancy & Childbirth Digestive Disease Mental Disorders Unintentional Injury	Heart Disease Respiratory Disease Digestive Disease Cancer Musculoskel- etal Disease Unintentional Injury	Not Available
Top Causes of Emergency Department Visits[1]	Respiratory Disease Digestive Disease	Unintentional Injury Respiratory Disease	Unintentional Injury Digestive Disease	Unintentional Injury Heart Disease	Not Available
Top Causes of Death[2]	Perinatal Conditions Congenital Anomalies	Unintentional Injury Intentional Injury Cancer	Cancer Heart Disease Unintentional Injury Intentional Injury	Heart Disease Cancer Respiratory Disease Stroke	Unintentional Injury Intentional Injury Circulatory Diseases Cancer[3]
Health Issues of Concern	Low Birth Weight Preterm Birth	Unintentional Injury Mental Health Teen Pregnancy	Unintentional Injury Suicide Health Practices	Chronic Disease Falls Dementia	Diabetes Unintentional Injury Suicide Premature Death
Social Issues of Concern	Daycare Family Support	Education Family Support Daycare	Employment Poverty Education	Independence Housing Transportation	Poverty Employment Education

Sources:
[1]Capital Health Region, Edmonton, Alberta. Hospital discharge data and emergency department visits for residents of the Capital Health Region for 2001–2003.
[2]Capital Health Region, Edmonton, Alberta. Vital statistics data for residents of the Capital Health Region for 1999–2002.
[3]*A Statistical Profile on the Health of First Nations in Canada*, by Health Canada, 2003, Ottawa, ON: Health Canada. (based on 1999 data)

Aboriginal peoples. One of the key objectives of a population health approach is to identify and reduce inequities in health among various subgroups in the population. Table 3.2 provides examples of the predominant health needs of several population subgroups in an urban health region.

Deciding on Appropriate Strategies

Once the major health issues are identified, the next steps in a population health process are (a) to set priorities, (b) determine what outcomes should be achieved, and (c) decide which strategies are most effective and sustainable in addressing the issues, promoting good health, and reducing the incidence and/or severity of disease.

Deciding on the most effective strategies to implement is different than deciding on treatment and diagnostic services. In the case of treatment and diagnostic services, the costs of the early phases of design and assessment—the initial concept through to piloting, testing, and eventual production—are often borne by suppliers (e.g., pharmaceutical companies). In these situations, health care managers usually deal with the change management associated with implementing a fully tested technology. People working within a population health approach are often directly involved in the design and evaluation of new interventions. Whether a population health intervention has been demonstrated to be successful elsewhere or is being developed from scratch, it must be customized to meet the unique needs of the community where it will be applied. Therefore, the design and evaluation of effective strategies and interventions are critical elements of a population health approach, and the costs typically must be borne by health regions, communities, or provinces.

As noted earlier, one of the key aspects of a population health approach is that decisions on strategies should be based on the best available evidence and, wherever possible, on evaluations that demonstrate the link between interventions and outcomes (i.e., improving health). Strategies should also take into account the resources at different levels in the community and the willingness of various partners to work together to achieve common goals. Decisions about which strategies to adopt for specific health problems should be based on meaningful criteria. For example, the World Health Organization (WHO) suggests health issues be evaluated with respect to

- the degree of impact on population health status (as measured by mortality, morbidity, quality of life, etc.);
- the availability and effectiveness of interventions to address the issue;
- the cost to the community of pertinent health or social conditions and their treatment and prevention; and
- the potential to reduce health inequities (WHO, 1998 as cited in Saskatchewan Health, 1999, p. 20).

Regular assessments of the health of the population guide decisions on setting priorities and taking action to improve the overall health of people in a region and the health of specific groups of individuals. For example, the incidence of low birth weight babies varies across Canada. Although we do not fully understand the complexity of the causes of low birth weight, it is known that alcohol, smoking, and drug use during pregnancy; age of the mother; multiple births; lower socioeconomic status; and inadequate prenatal care all increase the risk of having a low birth weight baby. This information, combined with an understanding of the population profile, helps guide decisions on the most effective strategies for addressing the problem, reducing the rates of low birth weight, and improving the health of newborns.

Taking Action

Once priorities have been set and overall strategies have been determined, the next and often most difficult step is to take action. Because the determinants of health are so broad and far-reaching, it is easy to feel overwhelmed by what needs to be done. Typically, a number of sectors are involved, and sorting out responsibilities and shared accountability can be a challenge. Solutions are often long term, and it may be difficult to see health outcome results in the near future.

The key is to focus on what can be done as part of a coordinated, area-wide effort to take action on identified population health issues. This typically involves a four-step process:

* Determine the entry point for action;
* Identify potential partners and their roles;
* Design and implement appropriate evidence-based actions and strategies;
* Evaluate outcomes and change course as needed.

Determining Entry Points

Determining the most appropriate entry points for population health action includes examining the following:

* Settings – for example, workplaces, schools, and whole communities. Consider factors within the environment or system that affect health.
* Population subgroups – for example, older adults, children, or specific ethnocultural groups. Target actions specifically to those groups.
* Health issues – for example, HIV/AIDS, tobacco use, and chronic diseases. Identify the actions that are most appropriate for addressing those health issues.

Identifying Potential Partners and Their Roles

Potential partners are those who share an interest in the selected entry point and are willing to participate. Potential partners include individuals, families, communities, governments, systems, and sectors in the economy and community. Partners can bring a variety of resources to population health initiatives, including skills, funding, media exposure, added credibility, expertise, and access to settings and population subgroups.

Designing and Implementing Actions and Strategies

Action for population health interventions includes five overlapping strategies. The most effective interventions increase the ability of individuals and the community to take action on issues they identify as important. The interventions are comprehensive, using a combination of strategies and working at different levels. The five types of action strategies include the following:

1. *Develop and implement public policies at an organization and government level.* Healthy public policies that address the broad determinants of health—such as employment,

income, education, and environment—can have a significant impact on the health of the population. Examples: minimum wage legislation, no-smoking bylaws, and helmet and seatbelt legislation.

2. *Create supportive environments for health.* Supportive environments include the physical, social, economic, cultural, and spiritual environments in which people live, work, and play. In addition to direct action to create supportive environments, all of the other action strategies described here can help create environments that support health. Examples: clean air and water, healthy workplaces, and safer playgrounds.

3. *Strengthen community action.* This strategy ensures that people in communities have the necessary skills and are actively involved in setting priorities and making decisions on issues that affect their health. Examples: community-driven crime prevention programs, school communities, involving students, parents, teachers, and community groups.

4. *Develop personal skills that enable people to meet the challenges of daily life and to participate as active members of society.* These include life skills, such as decision making, problem solving, critical thinking, and coping skills, that help people take greater responsibility for their own health. Examples: basic literacy skills, ability to advocate for health needs, pre-employment training for women.

5. *Reorient health services to focus on the needs of the whole person and on service delivery.* Reorienting health services might mean redistributing resources across the continuum of care, from treatment and rehabilitation to prevention, protection, and promotion. It could also mean moving services into communities and providing services that are relevant to a community's needs. Examples: primary health care, inner city health centre, and older adult friendly environments within health care settings.

Evaluating Outcomes

The ultimate goal of a population health approach is to improve the health of the population. As this improvement is typically a result of changes throughout a complex web of influences on health, evaluation of outcomes is challenging. It also can be very difficult to show how the various changes and strategies that have been implemented are having an impact in the short term. In spite of these challenges, evaluation is critically important to ensure that resources are being used in the most effective ways to produce the greatest improvement in the health of the population.

Ongoing evaluation and tracking of outcomes should provide the necessary information to assess whether or not the strategies are having the desired effect. For example, how effective (if at all) are the actions being taken to reduce premature institutionalization of frail older adults? Are health professionals more actively involved in encouraging health promoting behaviours? Are changes being made in community environments and public policy to make it easier to choose healthy behaviours and reduce the incidence of heart disease and stroke? Is a coordinated approach to reducing motor vehicle accident morbidity and mortality in place, and is it resulting in a reduction in the rate and severity of injuries? Are the changes effective?

These are just some examples of the kinds of questions that should be addressed through the continuous long-term evaluation of population health strategies. With answers to these questions, strategies can be revised, adjusted, expanded, or eliminated based on sound evidence of their effectiveness in improving health.

Leadership Implications

Canada has led the world in the development and application of the population health approach. Although the concepts and principles of this approach were originally associated exclusively with the field of public health, they are now recognized as essential to setting goals and measuring outcomes in all sectors of the health system. When there is competition for resources, it is important to be able to assess whether expenditures are resulting in demonstrable improvements to the health of individuals and groups. Health economists have demonstrated the effectiveness of population-level interventions to improve sanitation and public health, control or eradicate communicable diseases, and proactively prevent or manage chronic illness. In recent decades, there has been a growing recognition of the need to apply population health principles in the planning and evaluation of services provided in hospitals and all other care settings in order to assure long-range financial sustainability of the health system. However, population-level interventions are usually long-term investments with outcomes that are not readily apparent within the annual budgeting cycle or the four-year election cycle during which funding priorities are most frequently decided.

In the past, structural and financial incentives enabled, and often encouraged, the governing boards and senior leaders of individual health agencies or sectors of the health system to compete with one another for available funds. These traditional arrangements and the restriction of public insurance coverage to hospital and medical services are disincentives to intersectoral cooperation in addressing the needs of vulnerable and disadvantaged populations. In a climate of scarce resources and political realities, the expansion of traditional hospital and medical services or the adoption of new treatments and technologies with popular appeal has often been favoured over longer-range, population-level health investments. Strong professional advocacy and organizational leadership are needed to lobby for the adoption of population-level initiatives oriented to the improvement of health status outcomes. The implementation of regional governance structures has reduced intersectoral competition within individual health regions, but resource allocation is still heavily weighted toward hospitals and the infrastructure and technology costs associated with specialized medical practice. The developing field of health technology assessment is of particular importance in providing health policy and decision makers with evidence about the efficacy and effectiveness of specific technologies and interventions so that they can make informed resource allocation decisions.

All nurses are oriented to a broad view of human needs and the determinants of health in their basic education and therefore possess the values and knowledge to help advance the health of populations. Resource allocation decisions at the level of the health system, or even a health region, may seem far removed from the day-to-day realities of practicing nurses and first-line or middle managers. At the level of specific programs, care units, or agencies, an analysis of the common characteristics of the client population, the reasons for their admission to the program, and the reasons for non-compliance with treatment leads to the development of interventions such as patient teaching programs and materials, programs for pre-hospital or follow-up care, employee wellness programs, or well-baby programs offered in languages and locations that make them accessible and understandable to new Canadians or vulnerable populations.

Leaders, managers, and population health specialists all focus on the needs of groups, whether these are the clients and employees of an organization, a particular patient population, a neighborhood, or a geographic area. Therefore, the principles and practices of the population health perspective can be applied to many leadership situations and are now part of the essential knowledge and skill base for all health service managers.

Summary

- A population health approach is not new to Canada. In fact, Canada is known as a leader in understanding and emphasizing the importance of addressing a broad range of factors that determine health.

- In recent years, implementation of a population health framework has frequently taken a back seat to more pressing concerns about introducing new technologies and treatments or reducing waiting times for surgeries and diagnostic tests.

- Looking ahead to the future of Canada's health care system, there is a growing recognition that the overall health of Canadians and the future sustainability of the health care system cannot be adequately addressed by focusing on the health care system alone. By taking a broader population approach, we have an opportunity to identify the most pressing priorities and take comprehensive concerted action to prevent health problems, decrease inequities in health among different groups in our society, and improve the health of Canadians for generations to come.

Applying the Knowledge in this Chapter

Exercise

1. Select and briefly describe a population or subpopulation of interest to you in your current area of practice.

2. Obtain information about health determinants and risks that apply particularly to the population you have selected.

3. Develop a short proposal for a program or intervention to improve the health of the group you have selected, using the population health approach.

4. Consider how the program you have proposed should be evaluated. What health indicators and outcomes are relevant?

Resources

evolve Internet Resources

Canadian Community Health Survey (CCHS):
  www.statcan.ca/english/concepts/health/
Canadian Health Network:
  www.canadian-health-network.ca/
Canadian Institute for Health Information:
  www.cihi.ca
Canadian Policy Research Network (CPRN)—Ekos Changing Employment Relationships Survey:
  www.jobquality.ca
Health Canada–Population and Public Health Branch:
  www.hc-sc.gc.ca/pphb-dgspsp/new_e.html
Institute of Population and Public Health (IPPH)–Canadian Institutes of Health Research (CIHR):
  www.cihr-irsc.gc.ca/institutes/ipph/index_e.shtml
Statistics Canada:
  www.statcan.ca

Further Reading

Canadian Institute for Health Information and Statistics Canada:
  Health Indicators, Volume 2002, No. 2: October 2002.
  Health Indicators, Volume 2002, No. 1: May 2002.
  Health Indicators, Volume 2001, No. 3: December 2001.
  Health Indicators, Volume 2001, No. 2: June 2001.
  Health Indicators, Volume 2000, No. 1: December 2000.

Canadian Institute of Child Health. (1994). *The health of Canada's children: CICH profile* (2nd ed.). Ottawa, ON: Author.
Hanselmann, C. (2001). *Urban aboriginal people in Western Canada: Realities and policies*. Calgary, AB: Canada West Foundation.
Hawaleshka, D. (2002, June 17). Measuring health care. *Maclean's*, 23–31.
Health Canada. (1999, November). *A second diagnostic on the health of First Nations and Inuit people in Canada*. p. 21. Available from http://www.hc-sc.gc.ca/fnihb-dgspni/fnihb/cp/adi/publications/second_diagnostic_fni.htm
Health Canada. (2000, March 10). *Diabetes among aboriginal people in Canada: The evidence*. Available from http://www.hc-sc.gc.ca/fnihb-dgspni/fnihb/cp/adi/publications/the_evidence.htm#Executive%20Summary
Health Canada. (2002). *Economic burden of illness in Canada, 1998*. Minister of Public Works and Government Services Canada. (Catalogue No. H21-136/1998E). Available from http://www.hc-sc.gc.ca/pphb-dgspsp/publicat/ebic-femc98/index.html
Health Canada. (2003). *A statistical profile on the health of First Nations in Canada*. (Catalogue No. H35-4/30-2002). Ottawa, ON: Health Canada. Available from http://www.hc-sc.gc.ca/fnihb-dgspni/fnihb/sppa/hia/publications/statistical_profile.htm
Health Care Renewal Accord. (2003). *Agreement of Canada's first ministers*. Available from http://www.hc-sc.gc.ca/english/hca2003/index.html

Lavis, J., & Stoddart, G. (1994). Can we have too much health care? *Daedalus, 123*(4), 43–60.

Shields, M., & Tremblay, S. (2002). The health of Canada's communities. *Health Reports, 13*(Suppl), 1–24.

References

Black, D. J., Smith, C., & Townsend, P. (1982). *Inequalities in health: The Black report.* New York: Penguin Books.

Canadian Census Geograhpy, Highlights and Analysis. (2003). Retrieved April 15, 2003, from http://geodepot.statcan.ca/Diss/Highlights/Page2/Page2_e.cfm

Canadian Institute for Health Information (CIHI). (2003). CIHI profile. Retrieved April 15, 2003, from http://secure.cihi.ca/cihiweb/dispPage.jsp?cw_page=profile_e

Commission d'etude sur les services santé et les services sociaux. (2000). *Les solutions émergentes: rapport et recommandations.* Commission Clair. Quebec (Province): Gouvernement de Quebec.

Commission on Medicare. (2001). *Caring for medicare: Sustaining a quality system.* Commissioner: K. Fyke. Regina, SK: Government of Saskatchewan.

Commission on the Future of Health Care in Canada. (2002, November). *Building on values: The future of healthcare in Canada – Final report.* Commissioner: R. Romanow. Ottawa, ON: Parliament of Canada.

Epp, J. (1986). *Achieving health for all: A framework for health promotion.* (Catalogue No. H39-102/1986E). Ottawa, ON: Health and Welfare Canada.

Evans, R.G., Barer, M.L., & Marmor, T.R. (1994). *Why are some people healthy and other people not? The determinants of health of populations.* New York: Aldine de Gruyter.

Evans, R.G., & Stoddart, G.L. (2003). Consuming research, producing policy? *American Journal of Public Health, 93*(3), 371–379.

Federal, Provincial and Territorial Advisory Committee on Population Health. (1994). *Strategies for population health: Investing in the health of Canadians.* (Catalogue No. H39-316/1994E). Ottawa, ON: Health Canada.

Federal, Provincial and Territorial Advisory Committee on Population Health. (1999). *Toward a healthy future: Second report on the health of Canadians.* (Catalogue No. H39-468/1999E). Ottawa, ON: Health Canada. Retrieved April 10, 2003, from http://www.hc-sc.gc.ca

Frank, J., & Mustard, F. (1994). The determinants of health from a historical perspective. *Daedalus, 123*(4), 1–19.

Frankish, J., Kwan, B., & Flores, J. (2002). *Assessing the health of communities: Indicator projects and their impacts.* University of British Columbia, BC: Institute of Health Promotion Research. Retrieved April 10, 2003, from http://www.ihpr.ubc.ca

Hamilton, N., & Bhatti, T. (1996). *Population health promotion: An integrated model of population health and health promotion.* Ottawa, ON: Health Canada.

Health Canada. (2002). *Healthy Canadians: A federal report on comparable health indicators.* (Catalogue No. H21-206/2002). Ottawa, ON: Health Canada. Retrieved April 15, 2003, from http://www.hc-sc.gc.ca/iacb-dgiac/arad-draa/english/accountability/indicators.html

Kindig, D., & Stoddart, G. (2003). What is population health? *American Journal of Public Health, 93*(3), 380–383.

Lalonde, M. (1974). *A new perspective on the health of Canadians.* (Catalogue No. H31-1374). Ottawa, ON: Minster of Supply and Services Canada.

Lowe, G.S. (2002). High-quality healthcare workplaces: A vision and action plan. *Hospital Quarterly, 5*(4), 49–56.

Lowe, G.S., & Schellenberg, G. (2001). *What's a good job? The importance of employment relationships.* Ottawa, ON: Renouf Publishing.

Macdonald, P., & Fraser, N. (1989). *Dimensions of health in Edmonton.* Edmonton, AB: Edmonton Board of Health.

Marmot, M.G., Kogevinas, M., & Elston, M.A. (1987). Social/economic status and disease. *Annual Review of Public Health, 8*, 111–135.

McKeown, T. (1979). *The role of medicine: Dream, mirage or nemesis?* Oxford, UK: Basil Blackwell.

National Forum on Health. (1997). *Canada health action: Building on the legacy, Volumes I & II.* Ottawa, ON: Minister of Public Works and Government Services. Retrieved April 10, 2003, from http://www.hc-sc.gc.ca/english/care/health_forum/forum_e.htm

Ottawa Charter for Health Promotion. (1986). *Canadian Journal of Public Health, 77*(6), 425–430.

Premier's Advisory Council on Health. (2001). *A framework for reform. Report of the Premier's Advisory Council on Health.* Chair: D. Mazankowski. Edmonton, AB: Government of Alberta.

Raphael, D. (2003, March). Addressing the social determinants of health in Canada: Bridging the gap between research findings and public policy. *Policy Options,* 35–40. Retrieved February 28, 2004, from http://www.irpp.org/po/archive/mar03/raphael.pdf

Roberge, R., Berthelot, J.-M., & Wolfson, M. (1995). Health and social-economic inequalities. *Canadian Social Trends, 37,* 15–17.

Ross, N.A., Wolfson, M.C., & Dunn, J.R. (2000). Relation between income inequality and mortality in Canada and in the United States: Cross sectional assessment using census data and vital statistics. *British Medical Journal, 320,* 898–902.

Saskatchewan Health. (1999). *A population framework for Saskatchewan health districts.* Regina, SK: Author.

Standing Senate Committee on Social Affairs, Science and Technology. (2002). *The health of Canadians – The federal role. Final report on the state of the health care system in Canada. Volume 6, Recommendations for reform.* Chair: The Honorable M.J.L. Kirby. Ottawa, ON: Parliament of Canada. Retrieved April 5, 2003, from http://www.parl.gc.ca/common/Committee_SenRep.asp?Language=E&Parl=37&Ses=2&comm_id=47

Statistics Canada. (2002). *Population projections for Canada, provinces and territories 2000-2026.* (Catalogue No. 91-520). Retrieved April 15, 2003, from http://labour.hrdc-drhc.gc.ca/worklife/aw-overview-diagnostic-01-en.cfm and http://www.statcan.ca/english/Pgdb/demo23a.htm

Statistics Canada. (2003a). *Animated population pyramid.* Retrieved November 11, 2004, from http://www12.statcan.ca/english/census01/products/analytic/companion/age/pyramid.cfm

Statistics Canada. (2003b). *A profile of the Canadian population: Where we live.* Retrieved April 15, 2003, from http://geodepot.statcan.ca/Diss/Highlights/Page2/Page2_e.cfm

University of Alberta. (1994). *Strategic directions for local environmental health programs in Alberta.* Edmonton, AB: University of Alberta Department of Health Sciences Administration and Community Medicine.

US Department of Health and Human Services. (2000, November). *Healthy people 2010.* (2nd ed.). Washington, DC: US Government Printing Office. Retrieved February 27, 2004, from www.health.gov/healthypeople

Wilkinson, R.G. (1992). Income distribution and life expectancy. *British Medical Journal, 304,* 165–168.

Working Group on Community Health Information Systems and Chevalier, S., Choiniere, R., Freland, M., Pageau, M., & Sauvageau, Y. (1995). (Directions de la sante publique Quebec). *Community health indicators. Definitions and interpretations.* Ottawa, ON: Canadian Institute for Health Information.

CHAPTER 4

IMPLEMENTING PRIMARY HEALTH CARE THROUGH COMMUNITY HEALTH CENTRES

John Church and Sheila Gallagher

Learning Objectives

In this chapter, you will learn:

- That community health centres are an organizational form designed to implement the principles of primary health care
- Historical and political contexts within which community health centres operate
- What constitutes a community health centre model
- Current community health centre developments in Canada
- The impact of regional health structures on community health centres
- The benefits of community health centres
- Unique characteristics of a community health centre model, including the role of nurse practitioners within this model
- Opportunities for nurse managers offered by the community health centre model

Traditionally, delivery of health care services in Canada has been organized around the needs of health providers within a biomedical view of the world. Introduction of universal health insurance in Canada during the late 1960s entrenched this bias in the delivery, organization, and financing of primary health care services. Health services continue to be delivered with a distinct biomedical focus in hospitals, individual physician practices, and sometimes in group practice. Individuals and communities have had relatively little input into health policy and the design of health care services.

Despite this reality, Canada is home to significant innovation in the organization and delivery of primary health care services through an organizational model generically referred to as the community health centre (CHC). For the purposes of this chapter, a CHC is defined as a community-based health organization that provides an integrated range of primary health and social services, including, but not limited to, "clinical diagnostic, therapeutic, and preventive services to regular, special care and transient patients as well as participatory health promotion to a defined geographic or demographic community" (Birch, Lomas, Rachlis, & Abelson, 1990, p. 1). These services are provided by a broad multidisciplinary team of health and social service professionals and allied workers through various payment mechanisms. Professionals and allied workers include, but are not limited to, nurses, physicians, chiropodists, nutritionists, and social workers (Birch et al., 1990; Hastings, 1972; Ontario Ministry of Health, 1993). The definition of CHC chosen for this chapter, then, excludes other forms of primary health services delivery such as "nurse-centred" or "physician-centred" models because these models are, by definition, focused on a particular provider (Abelson & Hutchinson, 1994).[1]

The CHC model has long been found in the organizational landscape of international health, and CHCs can be found throughout Europe, North America, and Australia. In the North American context, the CHC model has been most closely associated with the efforts of community activists, public health workers, and medical activists to ensure that the poor and other disadvantaged populations receive adequate primary health and social services. CHCs also have been associated with the preventive paradigm of health care because they emphasize a broader range of services than conventional medical practice. In recent years, they have become an increasingly attractive option for health care policy makers because, unlike other possible models, they address the five principles of primary health care espoused by the World Health Organization (WHO): accessibility, public participation, health promotion and illness prevention, appropriate technology, and intersectoral and interdisciplinary collaboration (WHO, 1978). In addition, CHCs allow for the provision of services in lower-cost community settings.

The purpose of this chapter is to examine the CHC as an organizational model that offers health care managers and provides significant opportunities for innovation in the management of programs and delivery of services. This discussion will include a description of the model, an overview of CHCs in Canada, a CHC profile to highlight the uniqueness of the model, research on outcomes associated with CHCs, and the implications for managers. Although reference will be made to research findings and experiences in other Western democracies, the focus is on the experience in Canada.

---

[1]In the second edition of this book, we adopted a more traditional (narrow) definition of CHC: "a non-profit health corporation or association, controlled by an elected community board of directors" (Church & Lawrence, 1998, p. 220). Health reforms in Canada over the past decade have caused us to rethink this position.

The Community Health Centre Model

The CHC model offers a means for integrating and coordinating health and social services at the community level. Development of CHCs often is initiated by representatives of community groups, defined either by geography or population. Early community involvement is designed to encourage ownership. Objectives of CHCs include the following:

- Improving access to appropriate primary care services
- Empowering individuals and communities in health and health services delivery
- Developing coordinated primary health and social services that make the most appropriate and efficient use of service providers and resources
- Promoting health and preventing illness
- Promoting an interdisciplinary or team approach to meeting health and social needs
- Providing primary health services such as treatment, health promotion, health education, mental health care, disease prevention, dental care, and dietary, placement, and coordination services
- Providing social services such as information, referrals, crisis and emergency services, counselling services, legal services, and community services (e.g., food banks, daycare centres, recreational services)

Funding for CHCs is provided through a variety of mechanisms, including global budgeting, program budgeting, and capitation. Within these organizational funding arrangements, health care providers are usually paid through some combination of capitation, salary, fee-for-service, or sessional arrangements.

Adoption of CHCs by Canadian Provinces

With very few exceptions, most provinces and territories have experimented with CHCs over the past 50 years. In 1995, the Canadian Alliance of Community Health Centre Associations (CACHCA) was created to improve health services for individuals and their families and to promote the CHC as a successful and cost-effective delivery model. As CHCs have grown in number within provinces, provincial associations have increased in number as well. At the time of this writing, Newfoundland and Labrador had not yet established any CHCs. The distribution of CHCs by province is presented in Table 4.1.

Traditionally the health policy innovator, Saskatchewan introduced CHCs during the height of a doctors' strike in 1961 (Tollefson, 1963). In this context, community activists organized health cooperatives staffed by imported physicians in order to maintain access to basic services during the strike (Badgley & Wolfe, 1967). By the mid-1990s, there were three varieties of CHCs in operation: community clinics, community health and social centres, and wellness centres. Saskatchewan currently has five independent CHCs, 10 community health and social centres, and 36 community health centres (hospital conversions). Each of these variations reflects chang-

Table 4.1 Community Health Centres in Canadian Provinces

Province	Number of Centres
Nova Scotia	7
New Brunswick	4
Prince Edward Island	4
Quebec	147
Ontario	55
Saskatchewan	5
Manitoba	13
Alberta	5
British Columbia	25

ing government preferences over time. Quebec, Ontario, and British Columbia followed suit in the early 1970s.

Quebec introduced community health and social centres, that is, centres locales de service communautaire (CLSCs), during the 1970s to provide "basic health and social services with a community orientation" (Bozzini, 1988, p. 349). Again, the arrival of the model coincided with a doctors' strike. CLSCs provide a range of integrated health and social services, including primary health and mental health care, home care, health care in the workplace, community programs for special needs populations, and diagnostic and prevention services. Although the government has been attempting to standardize the range of services provided through CLSCs, these centres also provide emergency health services in some rural areas where hospital services are not available (Bozzini, 1988). What differentiates Quebec from other provinces is that its 147 CLSCs serve the entire geographic area of the province and make services available to 100% of the population. In addition, CLSCs are formally and informally linked to other organizations in a fashion unequalled in other provinces.

British Columbia also began developing CHCs during the 1970s. Although commitment from successive provincial governments with ideological differences has vacillated, 13 independent centres were operating by 1997. Provincial efforts in the mid-1990s to reform the health care system have placed a renewed emphasis on the development of CHCs as a single point of access for a range of health services that will "encourage community participation and provide integrated, client-centred services at the local level" (British Columbia Ministry of Health, 1993, pp. 1–3). More recently, regional health authorities have begun to develop CHCs as a means of integrating the delivery of primary health care services. In 2004, there were 25 CHCs operating in the province.

Beginning in the early 1970s as pilot projects, CHCs in Ontario have evolved to program status. Currently, Ontario has 55 CHCs and 10 Aboriginal Health Access Centres (AHACs) with over 100 communities hoping to establish new centres in the future. In 2001, CHCs served approximately 330,000 residents (3.5% of Ontario's population) and employed about 140 of the province's 6,500 licensed physicians (2.2%). At that time, CHCs and AHACs also utilized 128 nurse practitioners, more than any other employer in Ontario. CHCs and AHACs serve populations facing barriers to access as a result of many socioeconomic, health, and equity factors. They provide services in primary care, health promotion, disease prevention, community development, chiropody, dental care, social services, and legal aid. The mix of services varies according to the needs of the client populations.

In Alberta, three community-based CHCs have developed since the 1970s. These centres emphasize provision of primary health and related social and community services to underserved and disadvantaged urban populations. The centres provide a range of primary care medical services, referral services, mental health and public health care, health promotion and disease prevention services, community nursing outreach services, well-baby clinics, counselling, and social services. Although funding had been provided directly by the provincial ministry of health through a variety of arrangements, the three CHCs now negotiate their budgets with regional health authorities (Alberta Ministry of Health, 1993). As is the case in British Columbia, regional health authorities have launched their own CHC initiatives to develop a number of additional centres.

Manitoba lays claim to the oldest CHC in Canada. Launched in 1926, the Mount Carmel Clinic has continued to serve the evolving needs of its surrounding neighbourhood (Rizzo, n.d.). Rural CHCs have been integrated into regional access models, which may include existing buildings or networks of community health services. CHCs in Winnipeg tend to serve marginalized populations from either a geographic or special needs perspective (e.g., Aboriginals, people with HIV, low-income populations). By 2004, the province had developed 13 CHCs.

Nova Scotia has seven CHCs, which provide varying levels of primary health care, social services, and health promotion and disease prevention programs. Of these CHCs, six included nurse practitioners in 2004. Although CHCs are funded through contracts with district health authorities, they continue to maintain their independent governance structures. An additional four health centres in the province provide physician services.

In 2002, the New Brunswick government adopted the CHC model and introduced nurse practitioners to enhance the delivery of primary health care, and by 2004, three urban and one rural CHC were under development. Nurse practitioners also are involved in 20 other "health centres," mainly in rural areas of the province.

Prince Edward Island had developed four CHCs, called "family health centres," by 2004. At these CHCs, physicians, primary care nurses, public health nurses, and other providers offer a range of disease prevention, health promotion, mental health, home care, and addiction and legal services.

The operation, staffing, and programming of a CHC are illustrated in more detail in the case example presented in Box 4.1.

Box 4.1

Case Example

The North East Community Health Centre

The North East Community Health Centre (NECHC) in Edmonton is a unique agency located in a demographically diverse neighbourhood. This centre is modelled on the WHO's philosophy of primary health care (PHC). The presence of the NECHC is a testament to the long-standing community activism to acquire health care services in this quadrant of the city. The community's commitment to increase local access to health services influenced the NECHC's original planning team to incorporate the WHO's PHC philosophy in the centre's conceptual model.

All NECHC services are ambulatory. They include a pediatric asthma clinic; services for women, families, older adults, children, and adolescents; mental health services; community health (also known as public health) services; and emergency services. NECHC outreach programs include home visits, shared care consultations with community-based family physicians and other service providers, and outreach clinic activities to high needs neighbourhoods. Multicultural health brokers and interpreters work extensively with NECHC care providers to support clients with cultural or linguistic barriers to health services. As part of the Capital Health Authority's regional network, the NECHC is linked to a range of comprehensive services to which referrals are made.

Professional Roles in the NECHC

At the NECHC, the conceptual model drives the function and evolution of professional roles. The three foci in the centre's conceptual model are:

- the five PHC principles;
- formative and summative program evaluation; and
- integrated, client-focused service delivery.

The PHC principles provide philosophical guidance, the evaluation program supports NECHC's commitment to a learning organization, and the client-centred approach moves staff members outside their respective services in ever-changing combinations. NECHC professionals take on independent roles when providing services to clients and assume collegial supporting roles for interdisciplinary team efforts.

A key to NECHC's approach to working with medically and socially complex families is using health care providers from various services to form an integrated interdisciplinary team tailored to meet the needs of the individual or family. For example, depending on the person's needs, a client in Women's Health Service may receive services from the obstetrician/gynecologist and a registered nurse from that team, and she also may receive support from an addictions counsellor who is part of the mental health team. The preschooler accompanying this woman to her appointments may be directed to the Community Health Service for immunization updates or to the nurse practitioner in Child and Adolescent Service for a developmental assessment.

Nursing Roles

Registered nurses (RNs), registered psychiatric nurses (RPNs), nurse practitioners (NPs), and licensed practical nurses (LPNs) are included on the teams. All RNs, RPNs, and NPs are encouraged to develop their full scope of practice in individual and team-based roles. Some LPNs work in a specialized role as orthopedic technicians on the Emergency Service's multidisciplinary team. Community members are able to directly access the services of RNs and NPs without a physician referral.

Currently, two NPs practice in the NECHC—one in Family Health and one in Child and Adolescent Health Service. Both of them (like the centre's RNs) carry individual client loads and work collaboratively with other team members in supporting roles to provide client care. These NPs provide primary care and consultant pediatric services. Plans are now underway to introduce the NP role into the centre's Emergency Service.

Physician Roles

Family physicians and physician specialists are integral members of NECHC services and multidisciplinary teams. Physicians are paid by an alternate payment plan rather than the fee-for-service model. Because they are paid by session rather than by client volume, physicians are able to spend more time with each client. The payment structure also supports necessary non-clinical activities in which physicians can participate fully with other team members, including case conferences (both on and off site) and shared care work in which the physician or psychiatrist supports the practice of other professionals to the maximum degree of their scope of practice. Through shared care, the patient has increased points of access to more advanced levels of care in a primary health care setting.

The Research Context of Community Health Centres

Since the mid-1960s, governments in Canada have been interested in CHCs for a variety of reasons, including their ability to increase access to services for underserved populations, their emphasis on health promotion and disease prevention, and their potential to provide cost-effective services. Governments are becoming increasingly interested in the potential cost savings of the CHC model.

When examining the political context within which CHCs operate, studies in Canada, the United States, and the United Kingdom suggest a similar pattern in the development of health centres, with competing coalitions of stakeholders: organized medicine and its supporters; local, provincial/state, or federal administrators and their supporters; and members of the community and their supporters. The absence of medical opposition and/or the alignment of the interests of administrators and community advocates appear to be key to the development of CHCs. Dependency on public resources has made CHCs vulnerable to wavering political support and financial cuts (Allen, 1984; Church, 1994; Hall, Land, Parker, & Webb, 1975; Sardell, 1988).

Since the mid-1980s, a variety of literature reviews have been published on community-based health services models. These reviews encompass studies examining the cost, quality, and outcomes of the CHC model in the international and Canadian context. The term HSO was originally used to refer to a government-funded program in Ontario that encompassed health service organizations similar to CHCs in the fact that physicians are paid through capitation payment. A critical appraisal of the research on the performance of these organizations identified that, when compared to fee-for-service practice, HSOs are generally assumed to have:

- lower hospital utilization rates;
- comparable use of ambulatory care;
- greater patient loads for physicians;
- more ancillary health personnel;
- higher quality care;
- structures that facilitate more preventive services;
- physicians who believe that the method of payment favours the delivery of more preventive services; and
- less patient satisfaction.

In examining the evidence for these assumptions in the literature, the authors concluded that, with the exception of hospital utilization and personnel substitution, the level of supportive evidence was not high. This conclusion is attributed to a lack of methodologically rigorous or consistent studies on the performance or outcomes of the CHC model (Birch et al., 1990).

A more recent appraisal of primary care models contradicted findings of the earlier reviews. These authors suggested that the evidence to support lower hospital utilization or lower overall costs when compared to the cost of fee-for-service models is weak. Despite the apparent lack of rigorous and consistent evidence for the cost-effectiveness of CHCs, a closer look at some of the international and Canadian literature indicates the potential of CHCs to fulfill the requirements of current government thinking on health policy (Abelson & Hutchison, 1994).

A review of the evaluative literature on neighbourhood health centres in the US concluded that, in general, health centres have succeeded in "delivering good comprehensive care, including preventive services and health supervision through a team approach...at a reasonable cost" (Seacat, 1977, p. 168). Two US surveys on neighbourhood health centres indicated that access to ambulatory care for low-income and minority populations is enhanced, utilization of hospital ambulatory care is reduced, and patients have measurably lower hospital utilization rates when compared to hospital outpatient populations (Freeman, Kiecolt, & Allen, 1982). An impact assessment of the federally funded CHC program in the US showed that CHCs have had a significant impact on the infant mortality rate among certain target populations (Goldman & Grossman, 1988).

In the European setting, studies of CHCs in Finland, the Netherlands, and Sweden indicated that CHCs provide a quality of care that is comparable to fee-for-service methods. Health centres in which services are delivered by "small teams consisting of a GP, two nurses, and an assigned social worker" are most successful in terms of responsiveness to population needs, collaboration among health care providers, service integration and coordination, methods of reimbursement, and financial management and accountability practices (Abelson & Hutchison, 1994, p. 26).

Studies of CHCs in Canada are perhaps the most intriguing. A study of two CHCs matched to two fee-for-service practices in Saskatchewan (Prince Albert and Saskatoon) indicated that hospital costs were 23% lower for the Prince Albert CHC and 30% lower for the Saskatoon CHC. Furthermore, overall costs were 13% and 17% lower for the Prince Albert and Saskatoon CHCs, respectively, than for the comparative fee-for-service practices. This significant cost difference is attributed to lower admission rates to hospitals and fewer prescriptions (Birch et al., 1990).

Research on CLSCs in Quebec indicates that patients are likely to receive a higher quality of care for the treatment of certain ailments and more appropriate prevention services than in other practice settings (Battista & Spitzer, 1983; Renaud, Beauchemin, Lalonde, Poirier, & Berthiaune, 1980). Additional research suggested that physicians practicing in CLSCs might do so because of already internalized values and preferences that favour preventive activities and quality time with patients. The chosen medical pathway (e.g., family medicine) may influence these attitudes. Age and gender also affect practice patterns, with young female physicians on salary being more likely to engage in cancer detection and prevention activities and encourage patient involvement in treatment. The CHC context may reinforce this predisposition (Pineault, Maheux, Lambert, Beland, & Levesque, 1991).

In summary, the literature on CHCs identifies some methodological shortcomings of the research conducted on this model, but it generally concludes that CHCs have shown promise in their potential to make the principles of primary health care a reality and to address the cost concerns of government. Factors in the political context within which CHCs operate, especially in North America, have limited the wholesale adoption of the model.

Leadership Implications

CHCs offer unique opportunities for innovation in management and service delivery. They are smaller in scale, have a flatter administrative structure, embrace a determinants of health framework, and are more organic in nature than traditional health care organizations such as hospitals. Philosophically, they are committed to redressing the traditional power imbalance between service providers and lay individuals and to facilitating individual and community empowerment. These attributes are reflected in the accountability of all health providers to the board of directors, the accountability of the board to the community, and the variety of opportunities for community participation in the development and delivery of programs. However, as the organizations grow, the emphasis on organic participation by clients and staff may be displaced by an institutional culture. In the case of CHCs established by regional health authorities, the board structure resides at the regional rather than the neighbourhood level, and board members may be elected, appointed, or both. Thus, some advocates would say that the link to the community is weaker.

Nevertheless, regional health authorities have created new opportunities for collaboration through integration of the administration and the delivery of a broad spectrum of health services at the local level. In effect, regions have enhanced the capacity to coordinate the delivery of primary health care services through the infusion of new physical, financial, and political resources. For example, regional health authorities have entered into arrangements with CHCs to provide infrastructure upgrades (e.g., office equipment, Internet access) in exchange for the delivery of complementary regional programs and services through health centres. Through interagency collaboration, regions and CHCs have begun to identify and address the needs of the common populations they serve.

The multidisciplinary team approach to the delivery of services requires all health providers to function as equal partners. With health reform, this has become increasingly common since the 1990s. This approach is fundamental to the CHC setting. In at least one case, this has resulted in an experimental partnership between a physician and nurse practitioner "that is based on mutual respect for the other's experience, knowledge and skills" (Birenbaum, 1994, p. 77). Increasingly, the manager must facilitate these emerging, nontraditional interdisciplinary arrangements.

The commitment of CHCs to a framework that emphasizes the determinants of health and the principles of primary health care results in partnerships with existing agencies and new or fledgling community groups. These partnerships increase the potential to address a wide range of health issues that go beyond health care and engage community development.

Leaders and managers operating in this environment need to be creative, flexible, adaptable, responsive, and visionary. It is particularly essential that they be skilled in creating and sustaining the culture of collaboration and teamwork that is fundamental to the principles and effective outcomes of CHCs. They also must be skilled in collaborating with a wide range of external stakeholders, including federal and provincial funding agencies, providers from diverse professional backgrounds, community board members, clients, and local agency partners. Increasingly, nurses are finding new opportunities as program and facility managers within regional structures.

CHCs have been a part of the health care landscape for a long time. In more recent years, governments in Canada have become increasingly interested in the CHC model because it offers an innovative means of delivering integrated and coordinated primary health care through interdisciplinary teams. While research to date has not provided conclusive evidence of the benefits of the model, there is growing evidence that CHCs provide greater access to appropriate primary care for the populations they serve. There also is evidence to suggest that CHCs provide services in a more cost-effective manner when compared to other methods of service delivery. In addition, CHCs have, in some cases, achieved better clinical and population health outcomes for the prevention or treatment of certain ailments.

In most jurisdictions, either the provincial government or regional health authorities have established CHCs to facilitate primary health care reform. This trend suggests that CHCs will offer both opportunities and challenges for new managers in the future. If they are to survive and thrive, community-based CHCs will have to adapt to the changing environment in health care. The introduction of regional governance and administrative structures for health care in most jurisdictions of Canada is proving to be a double-edged sword for some CHCs. On the one hand, regional structures and a broadened policy mandate are bringing the rest of the health care system more in line with the broad philosophical approach of the CHC movement. On the other hand, individual CHCs, which have operated largely as highly autonomous community-based organizations accountable to local communities, are now faced with the prospect of surrendering some or all of their autonomy through integration into regional systems. Past experience has suggested that, where CHCs are integrated with hospitals, the hospital culture dominates the new organizational form (Begin, 1977).

If CHCs are to play a significant role in the future health care system, governments must invest in research into the potential of CHCs to provide cost-effective services that contribute to improvements in population health. This will involve establishing pilot projects across Canada and conducting rigorous and comparative evaluations of the benefits of the CHC model in different population settings. Governments also will have to commit to adequate and stable funding to ensure that existing and future CHCs can fulfill their mandate.

Summary.

- Community health centres are a service delivery model based on the five principles of primary health care defined by the WHO: accessibility, public participation, health promotion and illness prevention, appropriate technology, and intersectoral and interdisciplinary collaboration.
- CHCs are non-profit agencies that deliver a range of primary health and social services through multidisciplinary teams.
- Currently, most provincial governments and/or regional health authorities in Canada are developing CHCs as a mechanism for reforming and delivering primary health care.
- Although the research on CHCs is incomplete and has had some methodological shortcomings, it has demonstrated that CHCs have the capacity to achieve cost savings while allowing communities to achieve improvements in health outcomes.
- CHCs are an employment setting in which nurse practitioners can apply the full range of their knowledge and skills in collaboration with other professionals, and increasing numbers of nursing practitioners are being employed in these centres.
- Both the philosophical underpinnings and organizational design of CHCs offer unique opportunities for nurse managers to develop innovative strategies for service delivery and human resource and program management.

Applying the Knowledge in this Chapter

Case Study

Members of the Valdez family, who recently immigrated to Edmonton, Alberta, from South America, came to the Abbotsfield Outreach Clinic for primary health care services. Some of the family's issues were addressed in the outreach clinic, but the family also was directed to the North East Community Health Centre (NECHC) for other services. The family was struggling with a variety of issues, including financial, cultural, and general adjustment issues; primary health care needs; and pediatric neurological and behavioural needs.

Once at the NECHC, the family members were referred to a variety of the centre's care providers. Coordination of the family's challenges was discussed at Complex Client Rounds, a monthly meeting of health care providers from all services (including Emergency Services) who are involved with a given family. Multicultural health brokers worked with the family and the NECHC to facilitate access to other community-based agencies and services.

Recently, a follow-up check provided some good news: Mr. Valdez is now employed, and Mrs. Valdez is enrolled in an English language program. With her increasing ability to speak English, Mrs. Valdez is communicating with other mothers in her community, thereby decreasing her isolation. These other mothers also are sharing information on neighbourhood resources that the Valdez family now accesses. The oldest of the Valdez children is enrolled in a Head Start program, which provides comprehensive preschool and family support services for low-income families five days a week. In addition to the program's educational focus, strengthening children's self-esteem and enhancing developmental capacities are essential goals. The younger child, who is followed by pediatric neurologists, is mildly delayed but steadily achieving developmental milestones.

Questions for discussion:

1. If the NECHC had not been available, where would the Valdez family have obtained the services they needed?

2. How many different settings or locations would they have had to visit?

3. How would information have been shared among the care providers in these various settings?

4. What would have been the costs of these services if not provided in a CHC?

5. How are the CHC objectives illustrated in this case example?

Resources

evolve Internet Resources

Association of Ontario Health Centres:

   www.aohc.org

Citizen Participation Partnership Project:

   www.cippp.ualberta.ca

Further Reading

ARA Consulting Group. (1992). *Evaluability assessment of Ontario's Community Health Centre Program. Final report*. Toronto, ON: Ministry of Health.

   This is an assessment of the potential to evaluate the CHC Program in Ontario, conducted by the ARA consulting group for the Ontario Ministry of Health.

Ginzberg, E., & Ostow, M. (1985). The community health center: Current status and future directions. *Journal of Health Politics, Policy and Law, 10*(2), 245–267.

   This is a descriptive assessment of the Robert Wood Johnson Foundation's Municipal Health Services Program.

Pong, R., Saunders, LD., Church, W.J.B., Wanke, M.I., & Cappon, P. (1995). *Health human resources in community-based health care: A review of the literature. Building a stronger foundation: A framework for planning and evaluating community-based health services in Canada, Component 1*. Ottawa, ON: Health Promotion and Programs Branch, Health Canada.

   This is a systematic review of the literature on health human resources in community-based settings, including policy recommendations, conducted for the Federal/Provincial Advisory Committee on Health Human Resources.

Wanke, M.I., Saunders, L.D., Pong, R., & Church, W.J.B. (1995). *Building a stronger foundation: A framework for planning and evaluating community-based health services in Canada*. Ottawa, ON: Health Promotion and Programs Branch, Health Canada.

   This is a discussion paper of issues relating to community-based health delivery and presents a framework for evaluating community-based models. It was prepared for the Federal/Provincial Advisory Committee on Health Human Resources.

Weiner, J. (1988). Primary care delivery in the United States and four northwest European countries: Comparing the "corporatized" with the "socialized." *The Milbank Quarterly, 65*(3), 426–461.

   This article provides a descriptive comparison of primary care delivery models in the United States, Sweden, Finland, Denmark, and the United Kingdom.

References

Abelson, J., & Hutchison, B. (1994, September). *Primary health care delivery models: A review of the international literature*. McMaster University Centre for Health Economics and Policy Analysis Working Paper 94–15. Hamilton, ON: McMaster University.

Alberta Ministry of Health. (1993). *Sessional payment manual*. Edmonton, AB: Alberta Ministry of Health.

Allen, D. (1984). Health services in England. In M. W. Raffel (Ed.), *Comparative health systems: Descriptive analyses of fourteen systems* (pp. 197–257). University Park, PA: Pennsylvania State.

Badgley, R., & Wolfe, S. (1967). *Doctors' strike: Medical care and conflict in Saskatchewan*. Toronto, ON: Macmillan.

Battista, R., & Spitzer, W. (1983). Adult cancer prevention in primary care: Contrast among primary care practice settings in Quebec. *American Journal of Public Health, 73*(8), 1040–1041.

Begin, C. (1977). Can the HCs and CLSCs co-exist? *Mental Health in Canada, 5*(4), 11–15.

Birch, S., Lomas, J., Rachlis, M., & Abelson, J. (1990, January). *HSO performance: A critical appraisal of current research*. Centre for Health Economics and Policy Analysis Working Paper 90-1. Hamilton, ON: McMaster University.

Birenbaum, R. (1994). Nurse practitioners and physicians: Competition or collaboration? *Canadian Medical Association Journal, 151*(1), 76–78.

Bozzini, L. (1988). Local community services centres (CLSCs) in Quebec: Description, evaluation, perspectives. *Journal of Public Health Policy, 9*(3), 346–375.

British Columbia Ministry of Health. (1993). *Community health centres*. Victoria, BC: Author.

Church, W.J.B. (1994). *Health politics and structural interests: The development of community health centres in Ontario*. Unpublished doctoral dissertation, University of Western Ontario, London, Ontario, Canada.

Church, W.J.B., & Lawrence, S. (1998). Community health centres: Innovation in health management and delivery. In J.M. Hibberd & D.L. Smith (Eds.), *Nursing management in Canada* (2nd ed., pp.219–235). Toronto, ON: W.B. Saunders Canada.

Freeman, H.E., Kiecolt, K. J., & Allen, H.M., II. (1982). Community health centers: An initiative of enduring utility. *Milbank Memorial Quarterly, 60*(2), 245–267.

Goldman, F., & Grossman, M. (1988). The impact of public health policy: The case of community health centers. *Eastern Economic Journal, 14*(1), 63–72.

Hall, P., Land, L., Parker, R., & Webb, A. (1975). Change, choice and conflict. In P. Hall, L. Land, R. Parker, & A. Webb (Eds.), *Social policy* (pp. 277–310). London: Heinemann.

Hastings, J.E.F. (1972). *The community health centre in Canada: Report of the community health centre project to the conference of health ministers*. Ottawa, ON: Queen's Printer.

Ontario Ministry of Health. (1993). *Community health centres: A picture of health*. Toronto, ON: Author.

Pineault, R., Maheux, B., Lambert, J., Beland, F., & Levesque, A. (1991). Characteristics of physicians practising in alternative primary care settings: A Quebec study of local community service centre physicians. *International Journal of Health Services, 21*(1), 49–58.

Renaud, M., Beauchemin, J., Lalonde, C., Poirier, H., & Berthiaume, S. (1980). Practice settings and prescribing profiles: The simulation of tension headaches to general practitioners working in different practice settings in the Montreal area. *American Journal of Public Health, 70*(10), 1068–1073.

Rizzo, D.D. (n.d.). *Mount Carmel Clinic: A history (1926-1986)*. Winnipeg, MB: Mount Carmel Clinic.

Sardell, A. (1988). *The U.S. experiment in social medicine: The community health center program, 1965-1986*. Pittsburgh, PA: University of Pittsburgh.

Seacat, M.S. (1977). Neighborhood health centers: A decade of experience. *Journal of Community Health, 3*(2), 156–170.

Tollefson, E.A. (1963). *Bitter medicine*. Saskatoon: Modern Press.

World Health Organization. (1978). *Primary health care: Report of the International Conference on Primary Health Care*. Alma-Alta, USSR: WHO.

Acknowledgments

The authors wish to thank Jeanette Edwards, Terry Kaufman, Gary O'Connor, Heather McCleave, Monica Chaperlin, Donna MacAusland, and Juanita Barrett for providing input on various aspects of this chapter.

CHAPTER 5

CONTINUITY OF CARE, SERVICE INTEGRATION, AND CASE MANAGEMENT

Donna Lynn Smith, Jane E. Smith, Cora Newhook, and Bernadette Hobson

Learning Objectives

In this chapter, you will learn:

- Why continuity of care is important to citizens and to the health system

- Why clients with complex, long-term needs are particularly susceptible to problems arising from fragmented delivery systems

- The extent to which Canada's health system is integrated, and about case management as an intervention for integrating health and human services

- Definitions, core components, and various models of case management

- Factors that influence the way case management services are designed and implemented

- Elements of a case manager's role, and similarities and differences between the roles of case managers and other health services managers

- About case management in the context of the Canadian health system

- About research and resources for improving case management models and practice

Continuity of care is important to people only when they need it and it is absent. Without it, people who require a variety of health and human services over a period of time may experience gaps or duplications in service, inconvenience, added expense, and the personal and financial consequences of health care mistakes. Taxpayers and the health care system are subject to inefficiency, liability, loss of public confidence, and increased costs because of policies and management practices that contribute to discontinuity of care.

People who need health and human services encounter a bewildering array of service providers and arrangements. They must often find the services they need through a process of trial and error in a system where such services are delivered in different geographic and program settings, provided by an array of health professionals, and funded or paid for in a variety of ways. As a person's health or social problems become more complex, it often becomes difficult to locate or obtain access to services or to make transitions between service providers and locations. Vulnerable client groups are particularly susceptible to the problems arising from fragmented service delivery systems and multiple payers. One goal of health reform efforts in the early 1990s was to achieve better integration of services and assure that people were directed to the right care provider or service at the right time and in the service setting most appropriate to their needs. Therefore, the broad purpose for improving the integration of health and human services is to improve continuity of care. The concepts of integration and continuity of care, and the relationship between them, are now discussed, providing a context for the more detailed discussion of case management that is the focus of the latter part of this chapter.

Integrated Health Services: Concepts and Characteristics

The importance of improving the integration of health services in Canada is illustrated by the fact that in the spring of 2000, the entire issue of the journal *Healthcare Papers* was devoted to a discussion of this issue in the Canadian health system. This collection of articles by distinguished scholars and leaders was distributed to all 3500 members of the Canadian College of Health Service Executives, an organization of senior health care leaders in Canada. In the introductory paper of this issue, Leatt and colleagues (Leatt, Pink, & Guerriere, 2000) unequivocally stated that Canada does not have integrated health care:

> Canada has a series of disconnected parts, a hodge-podge patchwork healthcare industry comprising hospitals, doctors' offices, group practices, community agencies, private sector organizations, public health departments and so on. Each Canadian province is experimenting with different types of organizational structures and processes with the intent of improving the coordination of services, facilitating better collaboration among providers and providing healthcare to the population. However regional health authorities and their variants in Canada do not possess most of the basic characteristics of integrated health care (p. 13).

Based on a review of literature and experiences in other countries, these authors (Leatt, Pink, & Guerriere, 2000) recommended that, in order to achieve more integrated health care, Canada needs to

- focus on the individual,
- start with primary health care,
- share information and exploit technology,
- create virtual coordination networks at local levels,
- develop practical, needs-based funding methods, and
- implement mechanisms to monitor and evaluate.

In their discussion, the authors posed the important question: How will patients know when integrated health care exists? They also presented a set of person-centred indicators that can be used to evaluate the level of integration and the progress being made toward improving it. These indicators are listed in Box 5.1.

Box 5.1

Person-Centred Indicators of Integrated Health Services

- People do not have to repeat their health history for each provider encounter.
- People do not have to undergo the same test multiple times for different providers.
- People are not the medium for informing their physician that they have been hospitalized, have undergone diagnostic or treatment procedures, have been prescribed drugs by another physician, have not filled a previous prescription, or have been referred to a health agency for follow-up care.
- People do not have to wait at one level of care because of incapacity at another level of care.
- People have 24-hour access to a primary care provider.
- People have easy-to-understand information about quality of care and clinical outcomes in order to make informed choices about providers and treatment options.
- People can make an appointment for a visit to a clinician, a diagnostic test, or a treatment with one phone call.
- People have a wide variety of primary care providers who are able to give them the time they need.
- People with chronic disease are routinely contacted to have tests that identify problems before they occur, are provided with education about their disease process, and are provided with in-home assistance and training in self-care to maximize their autonomy.

Source: Adapted from Towards a Canadian Model of Integrated Healthcare, by P. Leatt, G.H. Pink, and M. Guerriere, 2000, *Healthcare Papers*, 1(2), p. 16.

Functional and clinical integration are related concepts (Shortell, 1993, 1996 as cited in Leatt, Pink, & Guerriere, 2000) that are helpful in understanding the conditions necessary for continuity of care and the role that integration strategies such as case management can play in achieving it. Functional integration is "the extent to which key support functions, such as financial management, human resources strategy planning, information management, marketing and quality improvement are coordinated across operating units so as to add the greatest value to the system. Integration involves shared or common policies and practices for each of these functions, but does not mean the centralization or standardization of these activities" (Leatt, Pink, & Guerriere, 2000, p. 15). Clinical integration is an umbrella concept "including the notion of continuity of care, disease management, good communication among caregivers, smooth transfer of information and records, elimination of duplicate testing and procedures and, in general making sure things don't fall between the cracks" (Leatt, Pink, & Guerriere, 2000, p. 15). A lack of functional integration can create barriers to clinical integration. The need to integrate medical care and physicians' activities with other health services has also been extensively discussed by experts in this field of study. Many of the initiatives to develop and improve primary health care and population health are designed to address this issue.

Continuity of Care

In 2001, the Canadian Health Services Research Foundation, the Canadian Institute for Health Information, and the Conference of Deputy Ministers of Health's Federal/Provincial/ Territorial Advisory Committee on Health Services recognized that, although policy reports worldwide identify the need to improve continuity of care as a priority, efforts to achieve improvements are hampered because continuity has been defined and measured in many different ways (Reid, Haggerty, & McKendry, 2002). To better understand this problem, Reid and colleagues (2002) conducted a search of selected literature to see how the phrase "continuity of care" was used. The results of this search were presented to 59 researchers and decision makers from across Canada in a two-day workshop in June 2001. A report of these activities entitled *Defusing the Confusion: Concepts and Measures of Continuity of Healthcare* was published in March 2002 and is available from the Canadian Health Services Research Foundation (Reid, Haggerty & McKendry, 2002, or see Internet Resources at the end of the chapter). One of the key conclusions was that studies of continuity of care are weakened by a lack of conceptual clarity. Most measures have been developed with a single aspect of continuity in mind, and few examine continuity of care across settings. Reid and colleagues (2002) suggest that there are two core elements and three types of continuity that bridge the domains of health care. The first core element is the experience of care by a single patient with his or her provider(s). The second is that the care continues over time, which is sometimes referred to as longitudinal or chronological continuity. These authors concluded that, although both of these elements must be present for continuity to exist, their presence alone does not constitute continuity. They also discuss the following three types of continuity:

- *Informational continuity* is the use of information on prior events and circumstances to make current care appropriate for the individual and his or her condition;

- *Relational continuity* refers to an ongoing therapeutic relationship between a patient and one or more providers, which bridges past and current care and provides a link to future care;
- *Management continuity* refers to the provision of timely and complementary services within a shared management plan. These authors note that "disease specific literature emphasizes the content of care plans to ensure consistency, but nursing and mental health literature goes further, emphasizing the importance of consistent implementation, especially when patients cross organizational boundaries" (Reid et al., 2002, p. iii).

The authors concluded that no single measure captures the whole concept of continuity and that new measures are needed for continuity of care across organizational and disciplinary boundaries.

Some years before this work was completed, nursing scholars had reached similar conclusions. As this book goes to press, the extensive review of literature focusing on the definition and measurement of continuity of care by Sparbel & Anderson (2000a, 2000b) is the most comprehensive work of its kind with a focus on nursing research literature. No consensus on the conceptual definition of continuity of care was found in the studies reviewed by these scholars. Continuity was defined as a "multifactorial concept affected by environmental influences, communication, patient, professional and system factors" (Sparbel & Anderson, 2000a, p. 17). In examining the various ways that continuity had been studied, Sparbel and Anderson noted that conceptual models were not widely used as a basis for research, and when models were used, they were from case management, discharge planning, or organizational theory literature. Because well-developed frameworks and defined standard terminology are essential for conceptual understanding, strong research design, and communication of findings, these authors recommended that priority be given to the development of conceptual definitions and frameworks associated with continuity of care. Although Reid and colleagues (2002) did not refer to the findings of Sparbel and Anderson in their work, they reached a similar conclusion about the need for stronger conceptualizations to guide research in this area.

In the context of these more recent reviews, an earlier concept analysis of continuity of care conducted by Glenn (1996) must now be recognized as a significant contribution to continuity of care research. In this study, the formal methodologies of concept analysis were applied to an extensive review of literature from nursing and other disciplines from the 1960s onward. Data regarding the attributes of the concept of continuity were collected. Surrogate terms and concepts, such as discharge planning, were identified and their relationships to continuity explored. For example, discharge planning is seen as "a mechanism which may contribute to continuity of care, rather than an embodiment of continuity of care" (Glenn, 1996, p. 78). The analysis of data included interdisciplinary and temporal comparisons, and a model case of the concept of continuity was identified. Antecedents, attributes, and consequences of continuity were also described. The first antecedent is *recognition of need and first contact*; the second is *availability and accessibility of service*. Five attributes of continuity were identified in this study: (a) availability and accessibility, (b) responsibility shifts, (c) singularity, (d) the presence of care and caring, and (e) planning and unidirectionality. The consequence of continuity is the ability to achieve a state of self-care, which may include care by family members and others if illness or disability remains. Glenn (1996) concluded that a lack of conceptual clarity has been a fundamental barrier to progress in this area.

In 2004, Newhook conducted an analysis of seven literature reviews of continuity of care. Her research included an examination of the work of Glenn (1996); Sparbel and Anderson (2000a, 2000b); Reid, Haggerty, and McKendry (2002); Freeman, Sheppard, Robinson, Ehrich, and Richards (2000); Branson, Badger, and Dobbs (2003); and two Canadian reviews (Hollander & Prince, 2002; Beaupre et al., 2003). From her analysis of this body of work, Newhook (2004) concluded that research in this field is broadly based but has two major shortcomings. First, there continues to be a need for improved conceptual clarity, definition of variables, and valid measurement. Second, all scholars who have evaluated continuity of care research agree that most work in this field to date has been developed from the perspective of the health system and health care providers with under-representation of the patient perspective. This bias must be corrected in future research in order to answer the critical question posed by Leatt and colleagues (2000): How will patients know when an integrated health care system exists?

The LINCS (Listen, Innovate, Navigate, Connect, and Share) Research Program, based in the Faculty of Nursing at the University of Alberta, was initiated in 2001 to study how person-centred continuity of care can be improved by policy and management decisions in the health system. This program was funded by the Canadian Health Services Research Foundation, the Alberta Heritage Foundation for Medical Research, and organizational partners in Alberta and Saskatchewan. Within this research program, continuity of care is conceptualized as an outcome of health services (Smith & Birdi, 2002). Therefore, continuity of care is not an end in itself, but rather a means for achieving the larger and more important goal of improved health status that enables people to go about their lives without the undue burdens associated with trying to locate and access services or navigate complex transitions between them.

In the LINCS Research Program, the characteristics of a number of different strategies and interventions to integrate services are being described. Explicit descriptions of these interventions are needed because service integration strategies differ from one another in their scope, complexity, and maturity. It is necessary to understand the characteristics and contexts of the integration strategies if they are to be accurately and successfully implemented in other settings to achieve similar results. For example, provincial and regional policies may create either incentives or barriers for the implementation of particular integration strategies, and the LINCS Research Program is designed to document contextual factors of this kind. Following an analysis of the strengths and limitations of existing continuity of care research, a model to structure this research was developed. In this model, continuity of care is conceptualized as a *health service outcome* within a population health framework that acknowledges the importance of contextual factors including those identified by Starfield (1998) in her work on primary care. In the LINCS Research Model, continuity of care is considered to be a consequence of antecedent factors, including the determinants of health, the characteristics and operation of interventions for integrating services, and organizational variables such as administrative practices and the way professional roles are structured. These are among the many factors that affect the ability to achieve the *health status outcomes* that are the end goal of continuity of care. Doctoral work being conducted by Leona Zboril-Benson, MN, will contribute to conceptual and theoretical foundations of continuity of care research by empirically testing the relationships between some of the variables illustrated in the LINCS Research Model depicted in Figure 5.1.

Figure 5.1 Continuity of Care in a Population Health Perspective

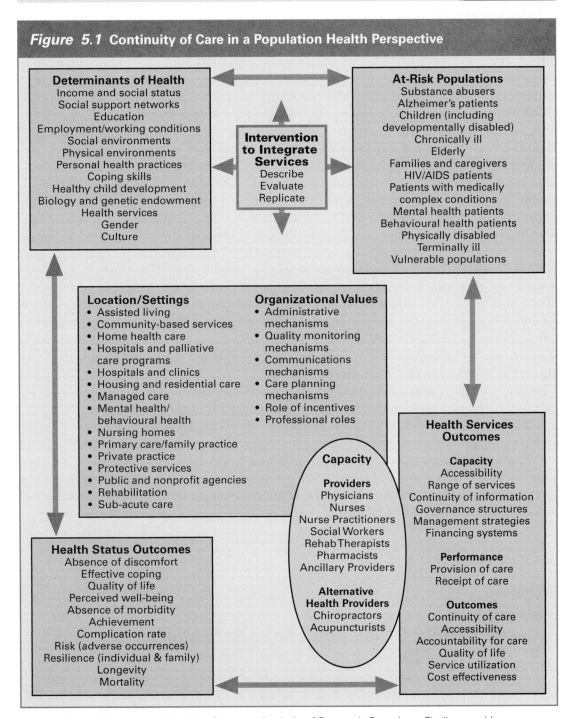

Determinants of Health
Income and social status
Social support networks
Education
Employment/working conditions
Social environments
Physical environments
Personal health practices
Coping skills
Healthy child development
Biology and genetic endowment
Health services
Gender
Culture

**Intervention
to Integrate
Services**
Describe
Evaluate
Replicate

At-Risk Populations
Substance abusers
Alzheimer's patients
Children (including
developmentally disabled)
Chronically ill
Elderly
Families and caregivers
HIV/AIDS patients
Patients with medically
complex conditions
Mental health patients
Behavioural health patients
Physically disabled
Terminally ill
Vulnerable populations

Location/Settings
• Assisted living
• Community-based services
• Home health care
• Hospitals and palliative
  care programs
• Hospitals and clinics
• Housing and residential care
• Managed care
• Mental health/
  behavioural health
• Nursing homes
• Primary care/family practice
• Private practice
• Protective services
• Public and nonprofit agencies
• Rehabilitation
• Sub-acute care

Organizational Values
• Administrative
  mechanisms
• Quality monitoring
  mechanisms
• Communications
  mechanisms
• Care planning
  mechanisms
• Role of incentives
• Professional roles

Capacity

Providers
Physicians
Nurses
Nurse Practitioners
Social Workers
Rehab Therapists
Pharmacists
Ancillary Providers

**Alternative
Health Providers**
Chiropractors
Acupuncturists

**Health Services
Outcomes**

Capacity
Accessibility
Range of services
Continuity of information
Governance structures
Management strategies
Financing systems

Performance
Provision of care
Receipt of care

Outcomes
Continuity of care
Accessibility
Accountability for care
Quality of life
Service utilization
Cost effectiveness

Health Status Outcomes
Absence of discomfort
Effective coping
Quality of life
Perceived well-being
Absence of morbidity
Achievement
Complication rate
Risk (adverse occurrences)
Resilience (individual & family)
Longevity
Mortality

Source: From *A Conceptual Model to Structure Analysis of Research Questions, Findings and Issues Pertaining to Continuity of Care in a Population Health Context* (p. 2), by D.L. Smith and T.K. Birdi, 2002, Edmonton, AB: LINCS Research Program. Reprinted with permission.

Various clinical and management interventions have been designed as strategies to achieve functional and clinical integration. Four case examples of evidence-based integration strategies are presented in Boxes 5.2 to 5.5. Care maps are one such strategy, illustrated by the published Canadian case described in Box 5.2. Strategies to integrate access to services through what is often called a "single point of entry" have been found to improve continuity of care. In Box 5.3, the example of a coordinated access service based in Saskatoon is described. Boundary-spanning care management is another intervention that has been shown to improve continuity of care, and a case example of this in an organ transplant program is presented in Box 5.4. The example in Box 5.5 describes the evidence-based CHOICE™ program, in which there is a high level of functional and clinical integration and in which physician services are also integrated. In this trademarked program designed to serve a specific population at risk for discontinuity of care, the elements of the intervention are clearly specified and include case management. This precise description enables an accurate replication of the program elements, and also its results, if contextual and organizational variables are similarly supportive. Such highly integrated and well-documented programs are rare in the Canadian health system, which has not adopted the systematic approach to the development of demonstration, evaluation, and replication projects that is a feature of programmatic innovation in the American health system. Repeated "one-of-a-kind " program innovations and evaluations occur in Canada because of the complex federal-provincial funding arrangements, and many experts have identified the need to overcome this problem in order to achieve consequential and lasting improvements in the delivery and outcomes of health services in Canada.

In summary, interventions designed to achieve service integration are intended to achieve a person-centred outcome—continuity of care—that is critically important to the people who use and pay for health services. Integration and continuity of care are particular needs of people with chronic illnesses, who make up an increasing percentage of the population and whose service requirements account for about 70% of all health care costs. Case management is one of many possible interventions that can be used to improve continuity of care, and because it has been widely implemented in most Western countries, the remainder of this chapter is devoted to a detailed discussion of this subject.

Box 5.2

Case Example: Development of a Care Map for Transurethral Resection of the Prostate

This article describes the development of a care map that was designed to deliver a continuum of care between hospital and community services in Edmonton, Alberta. The development and implementation of this care map required extensive collaboration, planning, and evaluation by members of many professions from a variety of different program and service settings (Raiwet, Halliwell, Andruski, & Wilson, 1997).

Box 5.3

Case Example: Case Management by Client/Patient Access Services in Saskatoon, Saskatchewan

Saskatoon Health Region is the regional governing authority for all health services in the city of Saskatoon. The corporate structure has been designed to support increased integration of services for groups of clients who have similar needs. All services are provided through 12 care groups, eight of which receive case management services provided by the Client/Patient Access Services (CPAS).

The case management services provided by CPAS are offered independently of various programs such as acute care, continuing care, or home care. Case managers in CPAS are responsible for arranging services for clients in the various care groups as they move from one program, service provider, or site to another, and back again. In some cases (e.g., many clients within the surgery care group), involvement by the case manager is time-limited by the client's needs. For other care groups, such as continuing care, geriatrics, palliative care, or rehabilitation whose clients include people with brain injuries, the case manager's involvement will be ongoing and may include providing continued attention over a period of months or years as the needs of the client and family change. Case managers in CPAS share responsibility for resource allocation and utilization with the managers of the programs that provide services.

CPAS calls upon a variety of services, including home care (both professional services and personal or homemaking services), community day programs, social work, physiotherapy, occupational therapy, and various housing, community support, and private services. Waiting lists for special care homes and continuing care facilities are managed by CPAS.

Further information about the program can be obtained from the Saskatoon Health Region Web site: www.saskatoonhealthregion.ca/your_health/ps_cpas.htm

Source: Personal communication from Sue Melrose, registered social worker and manager of CPAS, Saskatoon, Saskatchewan.

Box 5.4

Case Example: Boundary-Spanning Care Management with Organ Transplant Recipients

The specialized course of organ transplantation has expanded in volume and importance over the last decade. For example, organs now transplanted at the University of Alberta Hospital site of Capital Health in Edmonton, Alberta include heart, lungs, liver, kidney, pancreas, islet cells, intestine, and on occasion, a combination of two of these organs. In 2002, 289 transplants were done. Most transplant candidates live at home until hours before their transplant. Some transplant recipients, for example those receiving islet cells, return to their homes within 24 hours following the transplant procedure. Others return to their homes or community care settings within six days to three weeks. Before transplantation, the life span of many transplant candidates is uncertain or limited. While uncertainties remain following transplant procedures, approximately 75% of recipients survive the first five years, and many live for 10 to 20 years following their procedure.

Over 20 registered nurses, in a combination of full- and part-time positions, work with transplant candidates and their families to integrate care before, during, and following transplantation. Although their role title is not "case manager," the recipient transplant coordinators and nephrology nurse clinicians who work with transplant recipients are fulfilling a boundary-spanning or beyond-the-walls case management role. The transplant process can be overwhelming to people and their families, and the transplant coordinator sees them safely through the process as part of the dedicated health care team. The multidisciplinary team consists of transplant physicians, the nursing staff on the inpatient transplant unit, social workers, physiotherapists, occupational therapists, and a dietician. The RN coordinator maintains a relationship with the patient and family and all members of the care team over time, acting autonomously to make adjustments to the care plan within written policies and protocols. These adjustments may be highly specific, for example, deciding to refer the patient for alteration of a medication dose. The coordinator also communicates with a number of outside agencies to facilitate care. These include home care support (nursing, housekeeping, or nutrition support), government assistance programs, and other physician groups for the management of diabetes, renal failure, or other long-term medical complications of transplantation. In these beyond–the-walls communications, the RN coordinator is a resource to the community-based agency and its staff, as well as to the transplant recipient and family. The multiple health problems of the transplant recipient and the many side effects of the immunosuppressive drugs used can be overwhelming to care providers outside the transplant program.

The goal of the transplant program is to achieve successful outcomes for all transplant recipients so that they are able to manage their own health care and participate fully in their communities. The RN coordinator is often the pivotal health care provider as this process occurs over a period of years. Through this process, transplant recipients and their families often become independent, proactive, health care consumers.

Source: This case example was prepared by Bernadette Hobson, RN, BScN.

Box 5.5

Case Example: CHOICE™ — The Comprehensive Home Option of Integrated Care for the Elderly

CHOICE™ offers a systematic and integrated approach to meeting the health and social needs of older people who are at risk for admission to a continuing care facility in

Edmonton, Alberta. Established in 1995, CHOICE™ is modelled on the Program for All-Inclusive Care (known as PACE) that was developed through a series of demonstration and evaluation projects in the United States. The goal is to maintain frail older persons in their own homes for as long as possible, within the bounds of medical, social, and economic feasibility. Participants are usually functionally or medically frail, have chronic mental illness, or are in various stages of dementia. Care is provided by a multidisciplinary team using a case management approach.

The core program elements include a day health centre, health clinic, home support services, transportation, overnight treatment, and respite beds. Medical services are provided by a salaried physician who becomes responsible for the clients' medical needs when they are admitted to the program. A consulting psychiatrist provides enhanced support to the mental health clients. Because CHOICE™ services are provided from a day health centre, transportation is a key element of the program. Participants are picked up from their homes each morning and returned at the end of the day.

There are five program sites—three are owned and operated by the Capital Care Group (a publicly owned multi-site provider of continuing care services), and the other two by the Good Samaritan Society (a voluntary continuing care provider). Within the five sites there are two smaller specialty programs: The Good Samaritan Society operates a program for elders with advanced dementia, and the Capital Care Group has established an innovative program, based in a shopping mall, to provide service to elders with chronic mental illness.

Admission to the CHOICE™ program is through the Regional Single Point of Entry for Community Care Services. Participants are accepted for trial admission following an interdisciplinary team conference. During the trial admission, assessments are conducted in the core service areas of nursing, social work, medicine, physical therapy, occupational therapy, nutrition, home support, recreational therapy, and pharmacy. The interdisciplinary team then meets to discuss the assessment results and make the admission decision.

A registered nurse is the coordinator of the CHOICE™ Clinic. Once a participant is admitted, an interdisciplinary care plan is developed. All team members are responsible for implementing the plan and contributing to the achievement of the established goals. If a participant requires services beyond those offered directly through the program, staff of the CHOICE™ program would organize access to these services; for example, the program is closely coordinated with a respite unit. In this innovative program, the core elements of case management are vital to the achievement of objectives for individual clients and for the program.

Further information about the program can be obtained from the Capital Health Web site: www.capitalhealth.ca/default.htm

Source: From Community Care Services, Capital Health Group, Edmonton, Alberta.

What Is Case Management?

Definitions of Case Management

Case management is an integration strategy that is both a process and a professional service intended to achieve the goal of more integrated and cost-effective care. The role, skills, and organizational base of the case manager are best determined by the needs and characteristics of particular client groups whose needs are sufficiently complex to warrant the need for case management services. In this chapter, case management is introduced from a historical perspective and is also examined in current contexts so that leaders and managers in the health system can assess its appropriateness and potential benefit for the client groups they serve.

The term "case management" arose in an earlier era, and today, the term itself presents some problems. One client admonished health professionals by stating, "We're not cases and you're not managers" (Everett & Nelson, 1992, p. 60). In response to this concern, many health professionals and organizations now describe case management in a more client-centred way, preferring terms such as "care coordination," "service coordination," and "care management." The term *case management* is used in this chapter because it continues to provide a convenient entry point to the professional literature on the subject; however, *care management* and other terms appear in more recent literature.

Case management is a generic term with multiple definitions. It has been said that "case management...derives its definition in large part from the nature and needs of a system whose component parts it will be coordinating and integrating. It must be a creature of its environment, tuned to the specific characteristics and needs of its host system" (Beatrice, 1981, p. 124). For example, Austin (1993) defines case management as "an intervention whereby a human-service professional arranges and monitors an optimum package of long-term care services" (p. 452). In a slightly different vein, the American Public Welfare Association describes it as the "brokering and co-ordination of the multiple social health, education, and employment services necessary to promote self-sufficiency and strengthen family life" (as cited in Pearlmutter & Johnson, 1996, p. 179). The Case Management Society of America (1994) describes case management as "a collaborative process which assesses, plans, implements, co-ordinates, monitors and evaluates options and services to meet an individual's health needs through communications and available resources to promote quality cost-effective outcomes" (p. 60). Case management has also been defined as "a process or method for ensuring that consumers are provided with whatever services they need in a coordinated, effective and efficient manner" (Intagliata, 1982, p. 657), and as "a service that links and co-ordinates assistance from both paid providers and unpaid help from family and friends to enable consumers with chronic functional and/or cognitive limitations to obtain the highest level of independence consistent with their capacity and their preference for care" (Geron & Chassler, 1994, p. v). While these definitions have commonalities, they also illustrate some differences in perspective.

In this chapter, case management is defined as an intervention undertaken to facilitate access to, and integration of, services, including assessment, planning, coordination, delivery, and monitoring of the services that are provided to individuals and families. By assuring that these services are appropriate and accountable, case managers contribute to positive health outcomes and cost-effectiveness in the service delivery system. The degree of integration in any health and human services system can be improved if increased continuity of attention is provided to clients and families as they make their way across the boundaries that separate programs, service settings, care providers, and geographic locations where services are provided. Ideally, a single case manager assists a client or family throughout an entire episode of illness and the many transitions that must be managed by people who require support over long periods of time because of chronic illness or disability.

Origins of Case Management

Many disciplines have contributed to the evolution of case management practice. At the turn of the century, nurses implemented public health programs and visiting nurse services, and Lillian Wald established the Henry Street Settlement for individuals requiring home care. Family physicians also arranged and coordinated services for patients requiring care, and in the 1940s, the American worker's compensation board inaugurated a more formal approach to medical case management (Henderson & Collard, 1988). Community-based social work can be traced back to groups of ministers in the 1830s, charity boards in the late 19th century, and settlement houses in the early 20th century (Austin & McClelland, 1996).

In the mid-1970s, the term "case management" began to be used in North America to refer to a formal process through which professionals responded to the needs of the mentally ill, the aged, and other groups for whom services were fragmented or unavailable. Deinstitutionalization of the mentally ill in the 1950s resulted in the discharge of these clients into communities that were unprepared to meet their needs. Problems escalated as these clients attempted to access a network of services that was highly complex, fragmented, duplicative, and uncoordinated (Intagliata, 1982). At the same time, long-term care for the elderly in nursing homes was becoming too expensive for the aged population, whose numbers were rapidly growing, and community-based models were developed to address this issue (Austin, 1996). In the late 1970s, the role of case manager was usually filled by social workers who were working with the mentally ill and the aged in the community.

By the mid-1980s, case management had become prominent in hospital-based systems in the United States as one approach to containing the escalating costs of high-tech health care. A nursing case management model at the New England Medical Center Hospitals (NEMCH) in the early 1980s is generally credited with inaugurating the practice of case management by nurses in acute care settings. This model incorporated critical paths (Zander, 1988) and became a prototype for many subsequent hospital-based case management initiatives, including one at the Toronto Hospital (Lamb, Deber, Naylor, & Hastings, 1991).

Case management continues to be used as an intervention to integrate services for people with mental health needs and the elderly living in the community, as well as for an increasing number of other client populations with complex health and rehabilitation needs, as illustrated earlier in the LINCS Research Model (see Figure 5.1). Case management practice has expanded into home care and other human service settings, such as worker's compensation, child welfare programs, and the justice system. More recently, persons with AIDS or substance abuse problems; victims of spinal cord, brain, and other traumatic injuries; and children with developmental disabilities have also received case management services.

There are powerful financial incentives to control costs, for example, by restricting access to high-cost services, by promoting early discharge of patients from acute care hospitals through improved hospital utilization management, and by ensuring that discharged patients (especially those with chronic illnesses) are able to manage their care at home. For these reasons, the benefits of case management, and particularly of boundary-spanning case management roles, have received increasing recognition from insurance companies, health care agencies, and health policy makers in most Western countries, some of which have legislated requirements for this service.

Core Components of Case Management

Although definitions sometimes emphasize different aspects of case management, there is widespread agreement about the core activities in the case management process:

1. *Targeting:* Case management services begin by identifying, or targeting, individuals who need case management services. Clients are usually people with complex, long-term needs, requiring a variety of services over an extended period of time. Not all clients require case management services, and case management can be expensive; therefore, targeting case management services to those clients most likely to benefit from them is particularly important.

2. *Assessment:* Assessment requirements vary among organizations and can include measurement of the physical, cognitive, psychosocial, functional, and financial status, as well as the caregiver support system. An in-depth assessment provides the information necessary to determine needs and service priorities. When an interdisciplinary team is involved, assessments can become repetitive and sometimes exhausting for clients. The goal should be to develop an integrated interdisciplinary assessment in which information needed by all participating disciplines is gathered only once to create a cumulative database that is specific to each client.

3. *Care planning:* Information gathered in the assessment phase is formulated into a multidisciplinary care plan that indicates how each of the identified needs will be met. A working knowledge of services and resources is required at this stage.

4. *Implementation:* At this stage, formal and informal providers are contacted to arrange needed services. The case manager authorizes services, allocates resources, and coordinates service delivery.

5. *Monitoring:* Monitoring ensures that services are achieving the agreed-upon goals and are available as required by the client. This is particularly important in case management as clients are usually dependent on services over long periods of time. Ongoing contact with the client enables the case manager to respond quickly as needs and priorities change.

6. *Reassessment:* A client's need for case management services changes over time. During the reassessment process, the case manager determines what services are still needed and makes any necessary changes to the care plan in consultation with those receiving and providing services.

The case management intervention is shaped by (a) each client's needs and circumstances, (b) the availability of resources in the community, (c) the worker to client ratio, (d) the system of case management, (e) the education and background of case managers, (f) the budgets of service agencies, and (g) the organizational structure. Ideally, the case manager will work proactively with each client and/or family to develop a realistic and attainable service plan. The core activities of case management can be adapted in response to differences among client groups, organizational changes, environmental influences, and fiscal requirements.

Models of Case Management

Rapid growth in the popularity of case management has resulted in a profusion of models and frameworks for implementing this intervention. One group of models is defined by the different ways in which the role of the case manager is designed and the way services are funded and administered. A second group of models is defined by the setting or provider of case management services, and a third group is defined in terms of the range and scope of case management services. These three types of models are now discussed in more detail.

Models Defined by the Role of the Case Manager

Brokerage, Service Management, and Managed Care Models

In their classic discussion, Applebaum and Austin (1990) described the characteristics of three models that are differentiated from one another by the way the roles of case managers are structured and the way services are funded:

1. *Brokerage Model:* In brokerage models, case managers serve as links between consumers and the system, making referrals and allocating existing services, but not providing or monitoring care. In a brokerage model, case managers generally do not have funds to purchase services for their clients. These models are widely used by insurance companies and private practices, and increasingly in public programs such as home care, in which an approved array of services is provided to eligible clients by various contracted agencies.

2. *Service Management Model:* In the service management model, case managers have the authority to order services for their clients within set limits and develop care plans with predetermined cost caps or allocation limits. Managers are fiscally responsible for the care plans they develop, although they may not provide services directly to the client.

3. *Managed Care Model:* In managed care models, fiscal responsibility has been shifted from the funder to a care provider agency. Providers are pre-paid a specific amount and are liable for any excess costs. Case managers in this model are accountable for their care plans and for keeping the costs of these plans below a capitated payment.

Generalist Model

In 1993, a generalist model, in which one case manager performs a majority of case management activities, was described by Roberts-DeGennaro (1993). This model focuses more on the role of the case manager than on the organizational and administrative arrangements for care management services.

Advanced Models

Four models that extended the work of Applebaum and Austin were described by Raiff and Shore in 1993. They refer to these models as "new" or "advanced" because they are applicable to a wider series of populations, such as children with special needs and persons with mental health conditions. They make the case that case management is more than just the coordination of care and authorization of services, arguing that it is an essential service in the care continuum. Their concept of advanced case management is particularly applicable to difficult-to-serve clients or those with multiple and/or very complex conditions or life circumstances. These authors emphasize the distinction between client-focused and system-focused case management. The advanced case management models are as follows:

- *Expanded Broker Model:* This model is similar to the brokerage model, but the case manager's responsibilities extend beyond making referrals to ensuring the availability and delivery of services.
- *Personal Strengths Model:* This is a client-centred model in which case managers act as advocates, guides, and facilitators to assist clients to improve their quality of life.
- *Rehabilitation Model:* This model is part of a broader discharge planning framework that focuses on identifying the client's strengths, goals, and deficits in order to teach the client the skills needed for successful community living.
- *Full Support Model:* This model combines service planning and coordination, advocacy, supportive care such as psychotherapy, clinical case management, and proactive direct provision of treatment and rehabilitation services.

As Dill (2001) observed, case management is becoming a much more broadly based phenomenon, and there is increasing diversity in the professions that are involved with case management.

Models Defined by Setting and Provider

Other case management models have been described in terms of the settings or programs from which they have developed, and there are numerous examples in the literature to illustrate how the core components of case management have been applied in a variety of settings. Seven examples have been described by DeSimone (1988):

- *Social Case Management* is a multidisciplinary approach geared to a relatively healthy population, and it is used to delay hospitalization by emphasizing long-term community care services.
- *Primary Care Case Management* is a model in which the physician has traditionally assumed the role of gatekeeper to services.
- *Medical/Social Model* focuses on the long-term client, coordinating health and social resources, both formal and informal, in the community.
- *Health Maintenance Organization (HMO) Model* coordinates a limited number of services to treat an episode of illness.
- *Independent (Private) Case Management* services have evolved to meet the needs of clients outside the publicly funded systems of care.

- *Insurance Case Management* is usually a pre-paid service, including an incentive to manage costs of service.
- *In-House Case Management models* are developed by internal or intrafacility settings within an institution or organization.

Models Defined by Range and Scope of Services

Distinctions can also be made between case management models that involve working within specific program settings and those that are intended to bridge many settings.

Vertical Models

This term refers to case management that occurs within one specific program, service, or care setting. This type of case management was described as "internal case management" by More and Mandell (1997) and as "within the walls" by Cohen and Cesta (1997). In such models, the case manager is employed and based in a single health care organization or program, such as an acute care hospital, a rehabilitation program, or a home care program. Narrower vertical case management roles are usually seen in specific units or interventions that are part of larger programs.

Horizontal Models

This term describes case management services designed to manage a client's transition from one program, service, or setting to another. Discharge planning is an element of the horizontal case management model. "External case management" takes place outside the health care network, and external case managers may work for insurance companies, workers' compensation programs, or private companies. Cohen and Cesta (1997) referred to case management outside of hospitals in primary care, community, and home care settings as being "beyond the walls".

Boundary-Spanning Models

This term describes case management services that follow clients as they move between various service settings and care providers over an extended period of time. Boundary-spanning case management models are advocated by experts as a key element for achieving appropriate and cost-effective care for people with chronic illness. Dill (2001) explains the need for boundary-spanning care management roles by saying: "Making case management everyone's responsibility ensures that it becomes no one's. Clients end up with multiple case managers, but with none of them able to span the system of care" (p. 181).

Nursing Models

In the past decade, the nursing profession has become actively involved in the development of models for case management. Pelletier and Blouin (1990) define nursing case management as "a system of patient care which strategically positions nursing and recognizes the key role nursing plays in the allocation of resources, consumer perceptions and the overall profitability of health-care organizations" (p. 55). Lamb (1992) identifies three categories of nursing case management models: hospital-based, hospital-to-community, and community-based.

The nursing literature provides a number of examples of programs with a nursing case management focus (see Bower, 1992; Brett & Tonges, 1990; Ethridge & Lamb, 1989; Gibson, Martin, Johnson, Blue, & Miller, 1994; Olivas, Del Togno-Armanasco, Erickson, & Harter, 1989). These examples illustrate the growing recognition of the role case management can play in the integration of nursing care with other services across more than one setting.

As can be seen from the above discussion, there are substantive differences among the various models of case management. Some programs contain elements of more than one model; thus, it is important to understand how the roles of case managers are designed, how funding for services is allocated and administered, what settings or care providers are involved in a case management service, and how the range and scope of services have been defined. An American health care administrator has made a strong case for a comprehensive case management system. The following quotation from her (Satinskty, 1995) work is included here because it succinctly summarizes the trends that can be expected to influence the evolution of case management in Canada:

> Most so-called case management programs deal with separate components of care, not the continuum of patient care. For example, hospital-initiated case management programs usually deal with the inpatient component, leaving the events that give rise to the hospitalization and the issues surrounding post-discharge to somebody else, or worse yet, to nobody else.
>
> By design, some case management programs deal with a partial component of care. Obstetrical case managers, for example, generally deal with new mothers, but not with medical problems unrelated to childbirth. Thus, if the new mother develops a cardiac problem the obstetrical case manager may not be involved in the case. Also, by design, some case managers focus on a particular pay class—for example, Medicaid clients—and if the patient is no longer eligible for Medicaid, the case manager's responsibility may terminate. Finally, case managers may deal with a subset of "high-risk" patients—regardless of how the term is defined—only for as long as specific criteria are met.
>
> How far can and should case management extend? The most progressive case management programs focus on the patient *wherever* he or she receives care; they also deal with the patient and family *prior to and after* initiation of the episode of care that warranted the involvement of the case manager. Progressive case management is ongoing— that is, in periods of health as well as sickness—although the levels of care intensity differ depending upon need. Some HMOs and some employers, particularly those that are self-insured, have taken this approach.
>
> Two current health care trends, the shift of financial risk from payers to providers and the integration of payers and providers into single systems, will change the rules. Case management in the future is more likely to be comprehensive than limited in scope (Satinskty, 1995, pp. 1–2).

The Role of the Case Manager

Role descriptions for case managers vary considerably and encompass diverse responsibilities. Some of these are summarized in Box 5.6. The role of a case manager is determined, and may be limited by, the type of case management model in use. Despite these differences in models and practice, there is a high level of consensus in the professional literature as to what a case manager's role entails. The goal of case management in an integrated system is to provide the client with continuity, consistency, and coordination of care across service settings and boundaries, to assist the client with daily coping skills, and to advocate for resources that are unavailable in the community.

At present, hospital-based case management and community-based case management are the two main areas of practice, and although they have some common features, there are also some differences in the approaches used. These two care settings have the following features in common:

Box 5.6

Roles and Responsibilities of a Case Manager

1. **Clinical Expert** provides in-depth assessment, care planning, and consultation regarding the client's needs and issues.

2. **Facilitator** eases the client's interaction with the system.

3. **Liaison** brings services/resources to the client/family level.

4. **Supporter** promotes the client's confidence in becoming the "insider expert" (Lamb & Stempel, 1994) of her or his own care.

5. **Educator** provides information so that the client/family can make informed decisions.

6. **Researcher** identifies areas of concern and initiates research to aid in the development of evidence-based practice.

7. **Negotiator** intercedes and/or brings problems to the attention of others so that change can be initiated.

8. **Monitor** ensures that the client and services are doing what they have agreed to do, and identifies problems, gaps, and/or necessary changes at an early stage.

9. **Advocate** provides support and/or assists the client to identify goals and objectives that ensure a client-driven plan of care.

10. **Manager** develops care plans that are creative and innovative.

- Promoting interdisciplinary practice among health professionals
- Ensuring that all participating care providers coordinate and collaborate in their efforts to meet the goals of the care plan as efficiently as possible
- Promoting quality care for the client
- Ensuring the appropriate and efficient use of resources and services

Hospital- and community-based case management often differ in the following respects:

- *Duration of care:* Hospital-based case management has usually been limited to coordination of services during the episode of care or immediately afterward. Care plans developed for clients with complex needs in the community must often provide for case management and certain other services to continue for a longer period and, sometimes, indefinitely.
- *Standardization of care:* The overall plan of care in hospital-based case management (which is sometimes called a care map or a clinical pathway) is standardized from pre-admission to discharge, although it may sometimes be individualized to reflect preferences of individual physicians or the programmatic interests of some service providers. Case management plans for community care are usually developed individually after in-depth assessments, and the goals, objectives, and service plan are more likely to be developed with the involvement of the client and family.

The degree of integration within hospital- or community-based case management systems may vary considerably. From the client's perspective, a high degree of integration in either of these two sectors is desirable, and the integration of hospital and community services with each other is even more important.

Case managers' actual activities "are shaped ultimately by the constraints of the environment within which they work, not by their formal job descriptions" (Intagliata, 1982, p. 670). Today, case managers come from a variety of professional backgrounds, including nursing, social work, rehabilitation therapies, and medicine. In many instances, and particularly in Canada, family members or informal caregivers often have no choice but to act as case managers without the support of a formal or insured case management service.

Qualifications and Education for the Role of Case Manager

Comprehensive case management practice requires professionals with the knowledge and skills to work with clients who have complex needs, within existing bureaucratic and organizational service systems. Kanter (1989), for example, recognized the need for case managers to have generic interdisciplinary training augmented by years of continuing education and clinical supervision. All members of an interdisciplinary team contribute their expertise to enhance the appropriateness, quality, and coordination of services provided.

As the importance of the case manager role becomes more widely recognized, educational requirements are changing. Many case managers have acquired the specialized knowledge and skills they need through a combination of on-the-job experience and in-service education provided by their organizations. More recently, structured continuing education and certificate programs in case management have been established.

It is becoming increasingly obvious that the specialized knowledge and skills required by case managers should be built upon a foundation of professional education in a health or human service discipline. Many organizations and health agencies now require a minimum standard of a baccalaureate degree and relevant clinical experience with the client group to be served as prerequisites for the case management role. Cronin and Maklebust (1989) described a project at the Detroit Medical Center in which BScN-prepared nurses piloted the role of case manager. It was found that, although the nurses reported an increase in the quality of care provided and in job satisfaction, they felt ill prepared to collaborate and delegate with their level of educational preparation. The next project in this setting was successfully initiated with master's-prepared nurses.

More recent literature suggests a trend toward employing nurses with advanced preparation as case managers, for example, nurse practitioners and clinical nurse specialists. Some educational institutions offer specific preparation for case management at the graduate level; for example, the University of San Francisco implemented a master's program that focuses on the case management needs of older people (Haw, 1995). In Canada, continuing education to prepare case managers has been offered at the University of Western Ontario and McMaster University, and the Ontario Case Managers Association has, for some years, provided other professional development and networking opportunities.

Case Management and Traditional Management Roles

Case management involves responsibility for individual clients and groups of clients, but it may also include responsibilities at the level of programs, organizations, or service delivery systems. A case management role that focuses on gatekeeping, care planning, or clinical activities may require superior organizational skills, but it may not be designated as a management position if it does not entail responsibility for supervising staff or managing a budget. However, it has already been noted that the effectiveness with which gatekeeping and utilization management functions are carried out will have a direct effect on expenditures. Some case management roles incorporate responsibility for obtaining, training, supervising, and evaluating the workers who will deliver direct services, whereas others may involve only authorization and payment for direct services provided by collaborating agencies.

When case managers function in situations where there is a high level of ambiguity and uncertainty, the decision-making dilemmas they face in locating and mobilizing services for clients with complex needs may be as complex as those faced by managers in more conventional roles. The noted organizational theorist, Charles Perrow (1970), has used the term "unanalysable search" (p. 83) to describe the requirement for high-level discretionary decision making in some professional roles. There is clearly a high requirement for personal initiative, high-level communications skills (including the ability to influence others), and discretionary decision making in case management roles in which many boundaries must be crossed in the process of locating, coordinating, and monitoring the services provided by many different disciplines and workers from a variety of programs, organizations, and geographic locations. Clinical nurse specialists, nurse practitioners, and advanced practice nurses have broadly based and specialized knowledge and skills that equip them to practice effectively in boundary-spanning case management roles that require high levels of discretionary decision making.

Usually, management positions are defined as such because the people who hold them have responsibilities for supervising and assessing the performance of other workers and because they have discretionary decision-making responsibilities with regard to the allocation of funds. Such positions are often referred to as "out of scope," meaning that they are not among the positions and classifications covered by collective agreements. When positions with case management responsibilities can be shown to have such managerial dimensions, these positions may be defined as out of scope and subject to the conditions and remuneration of management work. Grisham, White, and Miller (1983) distinguished among case management models by placing them on a continuum depending on the level of authority and responsibility of the case manager. They suggested that case management services are not present when each health professional controls some of the resources and is independently responsible for the services he or she provides. The intensity of case management service changes as authority and responsibility for total client care and financial resources increase. Because case management roles vary in complexity and other dimensions, the extent to which a case manager's role has elements in common with more traditional managerial roles depends upon the authority, financial accountability, and discretionary decision making expected of a case manager within a particular organizational context. Managers at various levels of the health and human services system may find it helpful to understand the role of a case manager by comparing it with other specialist roles that cut across functional or departmental boundaries to accomplish defined tasks.

Case Management in the Canadian Health System

Since the introduction of the *Hospital and Diagnostic Services Act* in 1957 and the *National Medicare Insurance Act* in 1966, Canada has had a "single payer" for hospital and physician services through its universal health insurance system. As discussed earlier in Chapters 1, 2, and 4, the availability of universal public insurance coverage for hospital and medical services has created incentives for overuse of acute care services. Not surprisingly, Canada lagged behind Scandinavian countries and Britain in developing and funding such services as home care, community mental health, and community-based home and family support services. In general, although vertical case management has traditionally been a feature of mental health and home care programs, boundary-spanning case management interventions for integrating services are less established in Canada than in most other Western countries.

In the last few decades, chronic mental and physical illnesses have been more widely recognized and effectively treated. As the Canadian population ages, the prevalence of chronic illness in the population is also increasing, and it is estimated that about 70% of health care costs result from chronic conditions. These developments have created a need for services not provided by doctors or in hospitals. In response, a variety of services have been developed under the auspices of religious and voluntary groups, community organizations, and other not-for-profit organizations, as well as by businesses that market health and personal care services. Some agencies provide their services free of charge, others charge fees based on clients' ability to pay, while others require full payment, either directly or via private insurance plans. The more vulnerable people are, or the more complex their health or social problems, the more likely they are to need these community-based services. The problems created by a scarcity of these community services and the economic benefit of using such services (where appropriate) in place of higher cost, medically-oriented care have been well documented (Angus, Auer, Cloutier, & Albett, 1995; Hollander & Prince, 2002).

Case management services in Canada were first widely used in the area of mental health. Goering and colleagues conducted a number of studies of mentally ill clients in a community outreach program in Toronto, Ontario. They found that, although the rate of hospitalization did not change, clients in the program had higher occupational functioning (Goering, Wasylenki, Farkas, Lancee, & Ballantyne, 1988), improved role performance (Goering, Farkas, Wasylenki, Lancee, & Ballantyne, 1988), and decreased gender differences in social skills, supportive networks, and housing conditions (Goering, Wasylenki, St. Onge, Paduchak, & Lancee, 1992).

In an intensive case management program in the Waterloo region of Ontario, differences were found in the hospitalization rates of clients who had received case management services (i.e., lower rates for case-managed clients). The study associated the differences in rates with the ratio of clients to case managers, program philosophy, and the availability of hospital beds (Nelson, Sadler, & Cragg, 1995).

Mercier and Racine (1995) surveyed 25 homeless women with substance abuse problems in Montreal to determine the frequency, type, nature, and location of the contacts that case managers had with these women. They found that developing and maintaining a significant relationship with the clients constituted a major part of the case manager's work. A high staff-to-client ratio was necessary to respond adequately to the multiple needs of homeless people. This conclusion is supported by Pyke, Clark, and Walters (1991) who suggest three themes in providing case management services to clients with long-term mental illness: (a) the relationship between the case manager and the client is essential, (b) the case manager must respect the client's values and choices, and (c) the case manager must keep in mind that she or he has a number of clients, including not only the client, but also the client's informal and formal networks. When 17 nurses practicing case management in publicly supported community-based agencies across Canada were interviewed, they placed high value on nurse-client relationships (Rheaume, Frisch, Smith, & Kennedy, 1994).

In recent decades, case management services have expanded into other areas of health and human services as the shift to community-based care continues. Most health regions in Canada will be forced to provide services at lower cost in community settings that were once provided within institutions. Given the diverse demographics in Canada, case managers will require advanced educational programs to prepare them with the knowledge, skills, and cultural competency necessary for this complex role. When clients with complex needs receive continuity of attention, unnecessary costs can often be avoided. To achieve service integration, or what is often wistfully referred to as a "seamless system," a single case manager (or a case management team) should work on behalf of clients and their families to assess their needs on an ongoing basis and assist them to obtain, plan, coordinate, and monitor services for as long as they are needed, irrespective of the client's location within the system. When this is not possible, incentives and procedural mechanisms to improve the accountability of one service provider or program for what happens in the next program or care setting can help make incremental improvements in the continuity of care and integration of services.

All provinces have taken measures to restrict health spending, and these have had the effect of reducing access to hospital services by creating financial incentives for hospitals to screen and restrict admissions, shorten lengths of stay, and discharge clients to their homes or community services even when they still have extensive health care needs. Clients now pay out of pocket for many services, supplies, and drugs that were formerly provided to them without charge in or by hospitals. One outcome of these trends has been an increase in the number and variety of uninsured services available, particularly those provided by the for-profit sector. As they directly assume more health care costs, clients in the Canadian health system have become intolerant of the personal inconveniences and the costs of fragmented care and mistakes in the health system. These contextual developments help to explain why the need for case management services in Canada is now greater than ever before.

Research on Case Management

Case management is one of many interventions that can be used to improve the integration of health and human services and to achieve improved continuity of care. Research on case management and its outcomes has been compromised by imprecise descriptions of the characteristics of case management models in their organizational and policy contexts. Most research has been undertaken to address questions of interest at the level of health systems and providers. As with other health services research, problems of design and measurement have resulted in inconclusive findings, and the characteristics of case management as an intervention, or independent variable, may be unclear or not precisely documented in research proposals and reports. Nevertheless, there is broadly based evidence to support the use of case management as an intervention for improving cost-effectiveness by reducing duplication of service, avoiding mistakes, and improving access and timeliness of care and treatment. As with continuity of care research, there is widespread agreement that research on case management needs to be undertaken from the client and family perspective. Some client-focused evaluation criteria for case management programs have been proposed by Dill (2001), who believes that client's self-determination and attention to the whole of their lives should be considered the hallmarks of service quality for case management services, and that trusting relationships between human service workers and clients should be the norm. As discussed at the beginning of this chapter, this view is reinforced by the conclusions of researchers and scholars who argue that measurement of continuity of care should be person-centred and that continuity of relationships, information, and support are all important from the client's perspective.

Although research on case management has mainly been focused on cost savings, early indications also indicate other positive outcome measures. Health care becomes more cost-effective as duplication and mistakes in services are reduced. Proactive care leads to early intervention and prevention of costly complications. As clients become more confident in a responsive and proactive community-based care system, hospital utilization decreases (Hollander, 2001; Hollander Analytical Services, 2001). Increased client confidence can lead to a reduction in family burnout and to stronger, longer lasting, informal networks. This can result in decreased usage of the health care system by family members as they experience decreased physical and emotional symptoms of burnout (Smith & Smith, 1997).

Leadership Implications

The purpose of this chapter has been to illustrate how particular strategies for integrating health and human services contribute to the broader health service outcome of continuity of care. Continuity of care is not an end in itself or simply a means for achieving administrative efficiencies in the health system. Rather, it is required to achieve the broader social goal of improved health status for the population, particularly for people with chronic illness or other conditions that require the services of different providers in multiple settings over a protracted period of time.

In the past, the leaders of health programs and organizations operated within distinct sectors of the health system such as acute care, home care, community health, mental health, and long-term care. Traditionally, these sectors were in competition with one another for funds. The prestige, visibility, and influence in the acute care and medical sectors dominated health policy discourse and funding practices at the expense of the other sectors in which people with chronic illness receive non-medical or preventive services. Unfortunately, this has continued to be the case. Health reform efforts in the 1990s were intended to improve the integration of care between the various health sectors and to address disparities among them so that the health of the population could be improved and the costs of the health system managed. However, as Leatt and colleagues (2000) point out, structural changes in the system, including the creation of health regions, have not dramatically improved integration in the Canadian health system. Some policies and practices have changed and improved, but many have not. Traditional sources of power and influence in the health system continue to create inertia that prevents the introduction of evidence-based strategies that could improve integration and continuity. The slow progress in introducing boundary-spanning case management roles in the Canadian health system is one such example of delayed knowledge utilization. Another current example is the slow progress being made toward introducing roles for advanced practice nurses within various health sectors and settings. It is doubtful whether any other occupational group has been subjected to such rigorous evaluation of capability and outcomes. Despite a body of evidence that has been accumulating since the 1980s in Canada and other countries, the institutionalization of these roles, so necessary for the achievement of integrated and boundary-spanning care in all sectors, continues at a snail's pace in Canada. Evidence-based policy and decision making is required to correct these and other barriers in order to improve the integration of health and human services in Canada.

A growing and persuasive body of knowledge now exists to guide policy and decision making for the improvement of service integration and continuity of care for people with chronic illness. Best practices for achieving clinical and functional integration of services are particularly well documented, and leaders can learn more about these by consulting the references in this chapter (see Dill, 2001; Health Canada, 2002; Hollander, 2001; Hollander Analytical Services, 2001, 2002; Leatt et al., 2000; National Chronic Care Consortium, 2001; Pakarinen & Saranummi, 1999; Satinsky, 1995). Health system leaders must initiate the changes needed to implement and sustain evidence-based integration strategies.

Leaders and managers have particular responsibility for the factors required to achieve functional and clinical integration. Human resources policies and practices, and the design of roles and responsibilities of professionals, are exclusively management prerogatives. Nursing education programs have prepared nurses to plan, implement, and evaluate strategies to achieve clinical continuity since the 1970s, but few clinical nursing positions are designed to enable nurses to apply this knowledge. The creation of task-oriented roles and the arbitrary movement of professionals from one work setting to another have become common practices that have the inevitable effect of interrupting relational and informational continuity. Management continuity (i.e., to achieve shared interprofessional and inter-agency care plans) only can be achieved in organizational settings and cultures where teamwork is valued and the knowledge and contributions of all team members are respected and applied. The creation of client-centred cultures that value all professional contributions and create the conditions for effective teamwork is a leadership responsibility. Leaders must find ways to respect and use the expert knowledge of all clinical professionals, which is so necessary to the achievement of health system goals and cost-effectiveness. When human resources management practices, program planning, and quality monitoring systems operate at a distance from clinicians and without respect for their expert knowledge, health outcomes for individuals and the health system are compromised. Leaders and managers are the only people who can create the policies, infrastructure, and culture required to integrate services and improve continuity of care.

Summary

- The need to improve continuity of care has been identified as a health policy and leadership priority in all Western countries including Canada.
- Experts have concluded that despite the structural changes of the 1990s, often referred to as "health reform," Canada's health system is not integrated when assessed in terms of specific indicators of importance to patients or consumers.
- Research on continuity of care, service integration, and case management is proliferating but continues to have certain shortcomings. The patient or consumer perspective has been

under-represented in this research. There has also been a lack of conceptual clarity, imprecise definitions of variables, and problems of measurement. Improvements in these areas are needed so that studies and interventions can be replicated and generalized with confidence. Nursing scholars in Canada are contributing to the development of knowledge in this area.

- Case management (now often called care, or service, management) is a widely used, patient-centred intervention for integrating services and improving continuity of care.

- The core components of case management include targeting, assessment, care planning, implementation, monitoring, and reassessment.

- There are many models for the organization and delivery of case management services. These can be described and compared in terms of the way the case manager's role is defined, the settings and providers of case management services, or the range and scope of services provided. Specific descriptions of these dimensions of case management models and the testing and comparison of various models with different populations and in different settings are necessary to advance knowledge and improve case management outcomes.

- There is widespread agreement on the role requirements of case managers. Advanced knowledge of both the population to be served and the service delivery system, and high levels of discretionary decision-making skills are needed for effective performance in case management roles, particularly those that span boundaries between settings and sectors in the health and human service systems.

- Experts agree on the need to introduce formal, boundary-spanning case management roles within the formal delivery systems for health and human services in order to improve the integration of services for persons with complex needs and chronic illness. This service is necessary to manage costs, to assure appropriate access to and provision of service, and to support family caregivers who now deal with increasing burdens in the restructured health system. The introduction of such roles has been delayed in Canada for various reasons, but this can be expected to change in the years ahead. As this occurs, new career opportunities will be available for registered nurses in roles that enable the full application of nursing knowledge and skill across the continuum of care.

Applying the Knowledge in this Chapter

Exercise

1. Use your professional or personal experience to describe a case situation involving discontinuity of care.

2. Select one of the analytic perspectives presented in this chapter, for example, the definitions and typology identified by Reid, Haggerty, and McKendry (2002) or the LINCS Research Model (Smith & Birdi, 2002).

3. Apply the analytic perspective you selected to the case situation you described in order to explain and interpret the events in the case.

4. Make recommendations for how continuity of care could have been improved in the case situation. Consider changes that might be necessary at the clinical level and at the level of the organization and health system.

5. What actions and decisions would be necessary to implement the recommendations you have made for change? Who would have to make these decisions? Who would have to implement the decisions?

Resources

evolve Internet Resources

Alberta Heritage Foundation for Medical Research. State of the Science Review: Continuum of Care and Integration of Services for Treatment of Elderly Patients with Hip Fracture: www.ahfmr.ab.ca/grants/docs/state_of_science_reviews/Saunders_Review.pdf

Canadian Health Services Research Foundation. Defusing the Confusion: Concepts and Measures of Continuity of Healthcare: www.chsrf.ca/funding_opportunities/commissioned_research/projects/pdf/defusing_e.pdf

Hollander Analytical Services Ltd. The National Evaluation of the Cost-Effectiveness of Home Care:
www.homecarestudy.com/reports/

National Chronic Care Consortium:
www.nccconline.org/

Ontario Case Managers Association:
www.ocma.on.ca

Further Reading

Aubry, T., Farrell, S., O'Connor, B.V., Kerr, P., Weston, J., & Elliott, D. (2000). Family-focused case management: A case study of an innovative demonstration program. *Canadian Journal of Community Mental Health, 19*(1), 63–78.

This community-based mental health service at the Royal Ottawa Hospital evaluated a new family-focused case management program nearly one year after its inception. This model is unique in that it not only provides intensive case management of individuals with mental health care needs, but also includes meeting the needs of the primary support persons in the family unit, whether or not they are residing together.

Berube, D., & Carefoote, R. (2002). Canadian forces seek out civilian nurses for case managers. *Canadian Journal of Nursing Leadership, 15*(4), 26–32.

The Canadian Forces Health Services in Ottawa has established the role of a civilian nurse case manager. A large number of military personal are disabled and require complex care and/or release from the military every year. In the past, these people have experienced discontinuity in their care and have reported feelings of abandonment by the military. The Canadian Forces saw the case management model as a way to address these issues. Civilian nurses were chosen as case managers because they are not deployed like military health personnel, but can be a constant fixture on a military base.

Callwood, J. (1986). *Twelve weeks in spring*. Toronto, ON: Key Porter.

When case management services are not provided through the formal system, family members and friends often become case managers. This book describes a situation in which a group of individuals in Toronto, many of them strangers to each other, came together to help a dying friend remain in her home during the last three months of her life.

Dobbelsteyn, J., & Dupuis, M.E. (2000). Investigating the viability of case management in LTC. *Canadian Nursing Home, 11*(3), 13–17.

This article reports on the perceptions of staff and family on case management two years after its implementation at a 30-bed nursing home in New Brunswick. The investigators found some differences between the perceptions of staff and families. They concluded that staff and families need to be aware of the organizational structure and be given clear direction about appropriate lines of communication. The paper includes an extensive literature review of case management, outlining the potential benefits to staff and patients.

Lawlor, D., Vandewater, D., & Ur, E. (2002). Diabetes case management: a newly emerging health care strategy at the Queen Elizabeth II Health Sciences Centre in Halifax ensures improved delivery of care. *Canadian Nurse, 98*(1), 27–30.

The Queen Elizabeth II Hospital in Halifax implemented a diabetes case management program in February 1999. A Clinical Initiatives Group designed the diabetes case management strategy to provide better service to patients while controlling health care costs. The program has been so successful that the QEII added a second diabetes case manager and implemented similar programs for orthopedics and respiratory care in 2000.

McClaran, J., Lam, Z., Franco, E., & Snell, L. (1999). Can case management be taught in a multidisciplinary forum? *Journal of Continuing Education in the Health Professions, 19*(3), 181–191.

This report comes from the Centre for Continuing Medical Education at McGill University in Montreal. Their interest is in educational interventions that enhance perceptions of the importance of case management to the multidisciplinary team. This group developed a workshop explaining the benefits of case management, including patient needs, family education, community liaison, and cost monitoring. The purpose was to determine if there was any change in the participants' perceptions of the value of the case management model for patient care.

McWilliam, C., Stewart, M., Desai, K., Wade, T., & Galajda, J. (2000). Case management approaches for in-home care. *Healthcare Management Forum, 13*(3), 37–44.

An exploratory descriptive study of community-based case managers in Southwestern Ontario is presented in this report. The purpose of the study was to determine the characteristics of clients who were assigned to one of three models of case management: the brokerage model, the integrated team model, or the consumer-managed model. This report describes a useful methodology for examining decision making by case managers and provides an interesting insight into the factors that influenced decision making in this group of case managers.

More, P.K., & Mandell, S. (1997). *Nursing case management: An evolving practice*. New York: McGraw-Hill.

This introductory text describes the role of the nurse case manager in the institutional setting, the community, and the insurance field. The authors describe key components of case management and the skills required by case managers.

Pyke, J. (1996). Case management and mental health services. *The Canadian Nurse, 92*(7), 31–35.
The author of this article, a case management consultant in Toronto, provides a review of case management services for mental health clients in Canada and suggests criteria that can be used to assess whether case management is appropriate within a particular organizational context.

References

Angus, D.E., Auer, L., Cloutier, J.E., & Albett, T. (1995). *Sustainable health care for Canada: Synthesis report*. University of Ottawa Economics Project. Ottawa, ON: Renouf.

Applebaum, R.A., & Austin, C.D. (1990). *Long-term care case management: Design and evaluation*. New York: Springer.

Austin, C.D. (1993). Case management: A systems perspective. *Families in Society: The Journal of Contemporary Human Services, 74*(3), 451–459.

Austin, C.D. (1996). Aging and long-term care. In C.D. Austin & R.W. McClelland (Eds.), *Perspectives on case management practice* (pp. 73–98). Milwaukee, WI: Families International Inc.

Austin, C.D., & McClelland, R.W. (1996). Introduction: Case management—everybody's doing it. In C.D. Austin & R.W. McClelland (Eds.), *Perspectives on case management practice* (pp. 1–16). Milwaukee, WI: Families International Inc.

Beatrice, D.F. (1981). Case management: A policy option for long-term care. In J.J. Callahan & S.S. Wallack (Eds.), *Reforming the long-term-care system* (pp. 121–161). Toronto, ON: Lexington.

Beaupre, L.A., Johnston, D.W.C., Jones, C.A., Majumdar, S.R., Buckingham, J., & Saunders, L.D. (2003). *State of the science review: Continuum of care and integration of services for treatment of elderly patients with hip fractures*. Edmonton, AB: Alberta Heritage Foundation for Medical Research.

Bower, K.A. (1992). *Case management by nurses*. Washington, DC: American Nurses Publishing.

Branson, C., Badger, B., & Dobbs, F. (2003). Patient satisfaction with skill mix in primary care: A review of the literature. *Primary Health Care Research and Development, 4,* 329–339.

Brett, J.L., & Tonges, M.C. (1990). Restructured patient care delivery: Evaluation of the ProACT model. *Nursing Economics, 8*(1), 36–44.

Case Management Society of America. (1994). CMSA proposes standards of practice. *The Case Manager, 5*(1), 59–71.

Cohen, E.L., & Cesta, T.G. (1997). *Nursing case management: From concept to evaluation* (2nd ed.). St. Louis, MO: Mosby.

Cronin, C.J., & Maklebust, J. (1989). Case-managed care: Capitalizing on the CNS. *Nursing Management, 20*(3), 38–47.

DeSimone, B.S. (1988). The case for case management. *Continuing Care, 7*(6), 22–23.

Dill, A.E.P. (2001). *Managing to care: The care management and service system reform*. Hawthorne, NY: Aldine De Gruyther.

Ethridge, P., & Lamb, G.S. (1989). Professional nursing case management improves quality, access and costs. *Nursing Management, 20*(3), 30–35.

Everett, B., & Nelson, A. (1992). We're not cases and you're not managers: An account of a client-professional partnership developed in response to the "borderline" diagnosis. *Psychosocial Rehabilitation Journal, 15*(4), 49–60.

Freeman, G., Sheppard, S., Robinson, I., Ehrich, K., & Richards, S. (2000). *Continuity of care: Report of a scoping exercise for the SDO programme of NHS R & D*. London, UK: NHS Service Delivery and Organization (SDO), Research and Development Programme.

Geron, S.M., & Chassler, D. (1994). The quest for uniform guidelines for long-term care case management practice. *Journal of Case Management, 3*(3), 91–97.

Gibson, S.J., Martin, S.M., Johnson, M.B., Blue, R., & Miller, D.S. (1994). CNS-directed case management: cost and quality in harmony. *Journal of Nursing Administration, 24*(6), 45–51.

Glenn, M.R.E. (1996). *Continuity of care: A concept analysis*. Unpublished master's thesis, Faculty of Nursing, University of Alberta, Edmonton, Alberta, Canada.

Goering, P.N., Farkas, M., Wasylenki, D.A., Lancee, W.J., & Ballantyne, R. (1988). Improved functioning for case management clients. *Psychosocial Rehabilitation Journal, 12*(1), 2–17.

Goering, P.N., Wasylenki, D.A., Farkas, M., Lancee, W.J., & Ballantyne, R. (1988). What difference does case management make? *Hospital and Community Psychiatry, 39*(3), 272–276.

Goering, P., Wasylenki, D., St. Onge, M., Paduchak, D., & Lancee, W. (1992). Gender differences of a case management program for the homeless. *Hospital and Community Psychiatry, 43*(2), 160–165.

Grisham, M., White, M., & Miller, L.S. (1983). Case management as a problem solving strategy. *Pride Journal of Long Term Home Health Care, 2*(4), 21–28.

Haw, M.A. (1995). State-of-the-art education for case management in long-term care. *Journal of Case Management, 4*(3), 85–94.

Health Canada. (2002). *Determinants of health. What makes Canadians healthy or unhealthy?* Retrieved May 14, 2003, from http://www.hc-sc.gc.ca/hppb/phdd/determinants/index.html#determinants

Henderson, M.G., & Collard, A. (1988). Measuring quality in medical case management programs. *Quality Review Bulletin, 14,* 33–39.

Hollander, M.J. (2001). *Substudy 1: Final report of the study on the comparative cost analysis of home care and residential care services*. Victoria, BC: National Evaluation of the Cost-Effectiveness of Home Care.

Hollander, M.J., & Prince, M.J. (2002). *Analysis of interfaces along the continuum of care: Final report: "The third way": A framework for organizing health related services for individuals with ongoing care needs and their families*. Victoria, BC: Hollander Analytical Services.

Hollander Analytical Services Ltd. (2001). *Analysis of interfaces along the continuum of care: Technical Report 1: Literature review*. Victoria, BC: Author.

Hollander Analytical Services Ltd. (2002). *Final report of the analysis of interfaces along the continuum of care project. "The third way": A framework for organizing health related services for individuals with ongoing care needs and their families*. Victoria, BC: Author.

Intagliata, J. (1982). Improving the quality of community care for the chronically mentally disabled: The role of case management. *Schizophrenia Bulletin, 8*(4), 655–674.

Kanter, J. (1989). Clinical case management: Definition, principles, components. *Hospital and Community Psychiatry, 40*(4), 361–368.

Lamb, G.S. (1992). Conceptual and methodological issues in nurse case management research. *Advances in Nursing Sciences, 15*(2), 16–24.

Lamb, G.S., & Stempel, J.E. (1994). Nurse case management from the client's view. Growing an insider-expert. *Nursing Outlook, 42*(1), 7–14.

Lamb, M., Deber, R., Naylor, C.D., & Hastings, J.E. (1991). *Managed care in Canada: The Toronto Hospital's proposed comprehensive health organization*. Ottawa, ON: Canadian Hospital Association Press.

Leatt, P., Pink. G.H., & Guerriere, M. (2000, Spring). Towards a Canadian model of integrated healthcare. *Healthcare Papers, 1*(2), 13–35.

Mercier, C., & Racine, G. (1995). Case management with homeless women: A descriptive study. *Community Mental Health Journal, 31*(1), 25–37.

More, P.K., & Mandell, S. (1997). *Nursing case management*. New York: McGraw-Hill.

National Chronic Care Consortium. (2001). *SASI (Systems Assessment for Services Integration): Section 3: Global measures*. Bloomington, MN: Author.

Nelson, G., Sadler, C., & Cragg, S.M. (1995). Changes in rates of hospitalization and cost savings for psychiatric consumers participating in a case management program. *Psychosocial Rehabilitation Journal, 18*(3), 25–37.

Newhook, C. (2004). *Analytical perspectives in research on continuity of care*. Unpublished master's project, University of Alberta, Edmonton, Alberta, Canada.

Olivas, G.S., Del Togno-Armanasco, V., Erickson, J.R., & Harter, S. (1989). Case management—A bottom-line care delivery model. Part I: The concept. *Journal of Nursing Administration, 19*(11), 16–20.

Pakarinen, V., & Saranummi, N. (1999). *System integration in health care.* Retrieved April 5, 2004, from http://www.vtt.fi/virtual/hl7/ si-opas/si-main.html

Pearlmutter, S., & Johnson, R. (1996). Case management in the public welfare system. In C.D. Austin & R.W. McClelland (Eds.), *Perspectives on case management practice* (pp. 175–202). Milwaukee, WI: Families International Inc.

Pelletier, M.G., & Blouin, A.S. (1990). Case study: Case management success in a community hospital. *Definition, 5*(3), 55–56.

Perrow, C. (1970). *Organizational analysis: A sociological view.* Belmont, CA: Wadsworth.

Pyke, J., Clark, S., & Walters, J. (1991). Case management. *The Canadian Nurse, 87*(1), 22–25.

Raiff, N.R., & Shore, B.K. (1993). *Advanced case management: New strategies for the nineties.* Newbury Park, CA: Sage Publications.

Raiwet, C., Halliwell, G., Andruski, L., & Wilson, D. (1997). Care maps across the continuum. *The Canadian Nurse, 93*(1), 26–30.

Reid, R., Haggerty, J., & McKendry, R. (2002). *Defusing the confusion: Concepts and measures of continuity of healthcare.* Ottawa, ON: Canadian Health Services Research Foundation.

Rheaume, A., Frisch, S., Smith, A., & Kennedy, C. (1994). Case management and nursing practice. *Journal of Nursing Administration, 24*(3), 30–36.

Roberts-DeGennaro, M. (1993). Generalist model of case management practice. *Journal of Case Management, 2*(3), 106–111.

Satinsky, M.A. (1995). *An executive guide to case management strategies.* Chicago, IL: American Hospital Publishing Inc.

Smith, D.L., & Birdi, T.K. (2002). *A conceptual model to structure analysis of research questions, findings and issues pertaining to continuity of care in a population health context.* Unpublished Review (pp. 1-4). [Mimeograph]. (Available from D.L. Smith, LINCS Research Program, University of Alberta.)

Smith, J.E., & Smith, D.L. (1997, February). Achieving evidence-based case management nursing practice. Paper presented at the Canadian Association of University Schools of Nursing Conference, Edmonton, Alberta, Canada.

Smith, J.E., & Smith, D.L. (1999). Service and case management. In J. Hibberd & D. Smith (Eds.), *Nursing Management in Canada.* Toronto, ON: W.B. Saunders.

Sparbel, K.J.H., & Anderson, M.A. (2000a). Integrated literature review of continuity of care: Part 1: Conceptual issues. *Journal of Nursing Scholarship, 32*(1), 17–24.

Sparbel, K.J.H., & Anderson, M.A. (2000b). A continuity of care integrated literature review: Part 2: Methodological issues. *Journal of Nursing Scholarship, 32*(2), 131–135.

Starfield, B. (1998). A framework for measuring primary care. In B. Starfield (Ed.), *Primary care: Balancing health needs, services and technology* (pp. 19–34). New York: Oxford University Press.

Zander, K. (1988). Managing care within acute care settings: Design and implementation via nursing case management. *Health Care Supervisor, 6*(2), 27–43.

THE NURSING WORKFORCE IN CANADA

Jennifer Dziuba-Ellis, Jennifer Blythe, and Andrea Baumann

Learning Objectives

In this chapter, you will learn:

- The past and present context that shapes the profession and how nurses work

- The composition of the Canadian nursing workforce in terms of care providers, age, gender, and education

- The impact and prevalence of nursing employment arrangements in Canada

- The work environment needs of Canadian nurses

- Nursing administration, management, and leadership strategies for improving the work lives of Canadian nurses

Traditionally, most Canadian nurses have worked in hospital environments. Today, they work in diverse settings, ranging from hospitals to communities and even through telecommunication networks. Wherever they work, political, economic, and social factors influence their status, roles, and activities. It is essential for nurse leaders to understand how national, provincial, and local governments and organizational policies of the past and present influence the nursing workforce and the nursing profession.

The Changing Health Care Environment

The last two decades have demonstrated how economic forces and the work environment are interconnected. In the 1980s and early 1990s, the health care system was well funded. Health care budgets increased in many countries, including Canada, and health care workforces grew. With the downturn of the world economy in the mid-1990s, funding decreased, and the creation of a more efficient and effective Canadian health care system became the goal of policy makers.

Around 1985, Canada experienced one of its periodic nurse shortages. There had previously been an over supply, but low pay for registered nurses (RNs) relative to other professions led to fewer people joining the profession (Friss, 1994). Cutbacks in community colleges in Canada in the mid-1970s also contributed to the shortage of nurses. Employers said that they could not fill full-time jobs and that nurses preferred to work part-time. In response, organizations focused on improving working conditions, supporting nursing leadership, and providing continuing education in efforts to retain experienced staff and recruit new nurses (Meltz, 1988). Due to the shortage, nurses' salaries eventually rose again (Friss, 1994).

The hospital sector in Canada engaged in voluntary restructuring from the late 1980s, but by the 1990s, provincial governments throughout Canada had become more serious about reducing expenditures. In the mid- to late 1990s, cutbacks in government funding occurred, leading to radical health care system restructuring and reform. An interesting case occurred in the province of Ontario where a restructuring commission was created. As in other Canadian jurisdictions, downsizing was the major restructuring strategy. By 1999, more than 200 hospitals in Ontario had been reconfigured into 171 corporations. The merged hospitals were reorganized to consolidate services and eliminate duplication. Overall, hospitals increased their rates of day surgery and decreased the average length of stay, transferring much of the patient care burden to the community (Baumann & Blythe, 2003a). Other provinces, such as Alberta, created regional health authorities in attempts to coordinate health services.

The Impact of Restructuring on Canadian Nurses

In the 1990s, nurses were laid off, relocated, or redeployed as a result of restructuring. Between 1991 and 1998, Canada experienced the largest nursing employment displacement in its history (Grinspun, 2002). Human costs included loss of employment opportunities, job dissatisfaction, a less satisfying work environment, and reduced professional growth and development. Vahtera and colleagues (1997) found that workers undergoing radical change suffered psychological strain and personal insecurity, which disrupted group performance, reduced productivity, and increased turnover. A study exploring nurses' experiences of restructuring in three hospitals in Ontario showed how restructuring compromised nurses' individual, team member, and hospital employee roles and affected their ability to provide patient care (Blythe, Baumann, & Giovannetti, 2001).

Survivors of restructuring faced many challenges. In unionized organizations, collective agreements included a layoff and recall article. Senior nurses were permitted to take a more junior nurse's position in situations with "similarity of function, skills or operations" (Brown & Beatty, 2003, p. 6-32). Baumann and colleagues coined the term redeployment to describe this phenomenon. Redeployment describes the reallocation of workers to other clinical units due to factors such as seniority, retirement substitution, and unit closures (Baumann & Silverman, 1998; Baumann et al., 1996). Nurses were uncomfortable about taking someone else's position, which resulted in anxiety and a strained work relationship. Studies documented how "bumping" weakened collaboration and disrupted tacit agreements in stable work teams (Brawn, 1992; Lyall, 1991). Restructuring limited professional growth and development, and nurses were faced with unfamiliar patient populations. Expertise was marginalized. Nurses worried about competence and identified the need for increased knowledge of hospital policies and procedures, patient protocols, nursing interventions, and technical procedures in their new positions (Butt et al., 2002).

There was a transition from a workforce with a relatively high rate of full-time employment to one characterized by part-time and casual work. Working full- or part-time in the past had been a personal choice, but now nurses had little control over their careers because the jobs available did not match their goals or work preferences. The casualization of the nursing workforce weakened the nursing team. A study of 12 Ontario hospitals reported on the disruptive effects of massive rounds of downsizing on the skill level and age mix of nursing teams (Richard Ivey School of Business, 1997). Blythe and colleagues reported that downsizing affected the age mix of the nursing teams. The average age of nurses rose when junior nurses were laid off. The older nursing team became exhausted and used more sick time. Many nurses found that increased pressures at work made it difficult to balance work and home life. There was decreased socialization among team members, and "the nursing team became less integrated and members became more individualistic" (Blythe et al., 2001, p. 70).

Organizational Commitment and Productivity

Numerous studies demonstrate a relationship between job satisfaction and organizational commitment (Acorn, Ratner, & Crawford, 1997; Bishop & Scott, 1997; Brooks & Swailes, 2002). Armstrong-Stassen, Cameron, and Horsburgh (1996) found that nurses expected job security from the organization in return for performing their work well. The lay-offs, redeployment, and casualization of the nursing workforce that resulted from restructuring broke what is commonly referred to as the "psychological contract." Solomon (as cited in Blythe et al., 2001) found that employees considered job cuts a betrayal of trust and began to place their own interests ahead of those of the organization. As well, there was lower organizational commitment among redeployed nurses compared to those who retained their positions (Baumann, Giovannetti, et al., 2001).

During the mid-1990s, program management became the common model for restructured hospitals. Middle managers in specific health care professions were dismissed and replaced by managers of multidisciplinary teams who might be nurses from any specialty or members of any health care discipline. Blythe and colleagues (2001) suggested that the elimination of middle managers occurred at a time when leaders were most needed. Communication between managers and front-line nurses became more distant, and performance appraisals lapsed. Decisions were made with less input from front-line nurses, making them feel devalued as employees and as professionals. The damage done to nursing leadership during this restructuring era has not yet been repaired. The number of registered nurses in management positions has declined in the last five years; the Canadian Institute for Health Information (CIHI) reports that the percentage of RNs employed as managers fell from a national rate of 8.5% in 1998 to 7.2% in 2002 (CIHI, 2003a). Nurses have taken on many administrative roles, but few are managers.

The Nursing Shortage

The emergence of another nursing shortage in the new millennium resulted from the interaction of many variables, such as demography, restructuring, employment practices, and increased demand. Zimmerman (2000) predicts that the current shortage will be more extreme than past shortages due to emerging demographic and social trends. Factors include an aging workforce, declining nursing school enrolments, older nursing graduates, and the preference of "greying" nurses to work part-time. The aging of the RN workforce has been attributed to the decline in the number of young people entering the nursing profession during the last 20 years. "Unless this trend is reversed, the RN workforce will continue to age, and eventually shrink, and will not meet projected long-term workforce requirements" (Buerhaus, Staiger, & Auerbach, 2000, p. 2948). Many authors, including the Canadian Nursing Advisory Committee (CNAC), have noted a growing demand for nursing services due to increasing patient acuity and the care needs expected for the aging baby boomers (Zimmerman, 2000; CNAC, 2002; Baumann, O'Brien-Pallas, et al., 2001).

How many nurses do we need? While there is no consensus about the extent of the future shortage, Ryten (1997) identified an RN shortage ranging between 59,000 and 113,000 by the year 2011. A problem with most projections is that they assume previous or current patient care ratios are both optimum and applicable to future circumstances. In a review of health human resource planning in five different countries, Bloor and Maynard (2003) found that workforce planning policies tend to assume that existing health care delivery systems are efficient. They argue that, in reality, workforce planning is driven by health care expenditures, with resources dictating the volume of provision. The Canadian Nursing Advisory Committee advises similar caution when assessing projections: "We do not know if the number of nurses per capita in 1990 was the right one, and since then, the system has undergone dramatic changes in its structure and operations. However, rising rates of absenteeism, excessive overtime and decaying morale suggest strongly that the number of nurses is too low to deliver the care required" (CNAC, 2002, p. 9).

A variety of frameworks should be used to explore the issues of nursing supply and demand. In their review of forecasting models, O'Brien-Pallas and colleagues (2001), found that different modelling approaches and assumptions provide varying estimates on future nursing resource needs. They warn that health human resource planning is iterative and requires continuous updating. It is clear that human resource planning should be proactive rather than reactive and that it should be ongoing at government, organization, and unit levels, using a variety of planning models and frameworks.

Composition of the Nursing Workforce

Effective human resource management and leadership require an understanding of the nursing workforce. Workforce demographics and nursing roles change constantly in response to their political, economic, and social context.

Nursing Care Providers

Nurses are the largest health care workforce in Canada (CIHI, 2001). They include three regulated occupational groups: licensed practical nurses (LPNs), registered psychiatric nurses (RPNs), and registered nurses (RNs). This chapter focuses on the work life and demographics of RNs, the largest nursing profession; however, LPNs and RPNs are an integral part of the health care team in many work environments. In 1999, RNs made up 76% of the workforce, LPNs 22%, and RPNs 2% (CIHI, 2001). In addition, nursing care delivery is supported by a number of unregulated workers such as health care aides and personal support workers.

Licensed practical nurses were established during the second World War and are the second largest regulated health care provider group in Canada. They are registered health care providers, professionally regulated, who work within established standards of practice and codes of ethics (CIHI, 2003b). They are "a distinct and separate nursing profession in all provinces and territories, except Ontario where they fall under the same regulatory body" (CIHI, 2003b, p. 36) as RNs. In Ontario, LPNs are known as registered practical nurses.

Registered psychiatric nurses are regulated as a distinct profession in Saskatchewan, Alberta, Manitoba, and British Columbia. RPNs have provided professional mental health services in Canada for 80 years, and they work in a variety of settings. In 2002, there were approximately 5285 RPNs working in Western Canada (CIHI, 2003c).

In Canada, provincial and territorial professional nursing associations regulate registered nurses' practice in keeping with the regulation principles endorsed by the International Council of Nurses (ICN) in 1985. In Ontario, however, "self-regulation" is the responsibility of the College of Nurses of Ontario, which is independent of the professional association, (i.e., the Registered Nurses Association of Ontario). The registered nurse category includes advanced practice nurses, for example, nurse practitioners (NPs). The ICN (2002) defines a nurse practitioner as "a registered nurse who has acquired the expert knowledge base, complex decision-making skills and clinical competencies for expanded practice, the characteristics of which are shaped by the context and/or country in which s/he is credentialed to practice," (p. 1) and it recommends a master's degree for entry to practice. However, there is no prescribed education level for NP practice in Canada. The Canadian Nurses Association (CNA) describes the nurse practitioner as an advanced practice nursing role, regulated under provincial and territorial nursing regulatory bodies. Nurse practitioners practice in a variety of autonomous and collaborative roles

(CNA, 2003). The demand for NPs is increasing, and most Canadian provinces are currently passing relevant legislation. The Canadian Institute for Health Information estimates that there are 912 NPs employed in Canada, including 681 in Ontario (CIHI, 2003a).

Nursing Supply

The Canadian nursing workforce increased by 1.4% between 1998 and 2002, from 227,814 to 230,957 RNs. This increase occurred unevenly across the country, with Alberta reporting a substantial increase and the Yukon reporting a decrease in RNs. Although the nursing workforce is growing, it has not kept pace with population growth. There are currently 74.4 RNs per 10,000 Canadians, a decrease from 74.9 in 1998. Among individual provinces, Ontario reports the lowest RN to patient ratio with 65 RNs per 10,000 Canadians (CIHI, 2003a). Figure 6.1 illustrates the distribution of RNs across Canada. On a more positive note, the percentage of RNs actually working in nursing has increased from that of earlier years (Table 6.1).

Approximately 4863 RNs currently work outside Canada but maintain a Canadian licence. Of these nurses, 81.2% are in the United States, and 12.9% are in Saudi Arabia, Hong Kong, and the United Kingdom (CIHI, 2003a). Nurses who do not maintain a Canadian licence are not tracked; therefore, the total number of Canadian nurses working abroad is unknown.

Nursing Demographics in Canada

Although more men are entering the profession, most nurses are women. In 2002, 5.1% of the Canadian nursing workforce was male compared to 4.4% in 1998. The distribution of male nurses varies across the country with almost half of all male RNs working in Quebec. The Northwest Territories and Nunavut have the highest percentage of male nurses, and Prince Edward Island, the lowest (CIHI, 2003a).

The nursing profession is experiencing a radical shift in age distribution. In 1990, the average age of a nurse was 39 years (CNAC, 2002); in 2002, it was 44.2 years (CIHI, 2003a). A major concern is that fewer nurses are entering and remaining in the profession; furthermore, nurses are graduating at an older age, thus reducing their potential years in the workforce. The shift in the average age of Canadian nurses between 1998 and 2002 is demonstrated in Figure 6.2. The age distribution of nurses varies across Canada, with British Columbia having the oldest workforce, and Newfoundland and Labrador, the youngest nursing workforce.

Table 6.1 Percentage of RNs Employed in Nursing				
1998	**1999**	**2000**	**2001**	**2002**
89.4%	89.1%	91.3%	91.5%	90.7%

Source: © (2003a) Canadian Institute for Health Information (CIHI). Adapted from Table 5 on page 45 of *Workforce Trends of Registered Nurses in Canada, 2002* as published by CIHI. Used with permission.

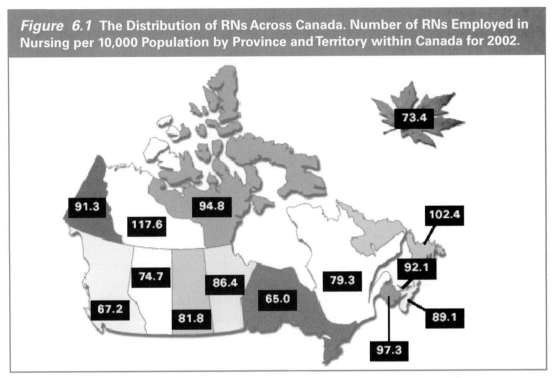

Figure 6.1 **The Distribution of RNs Across Canada. Number of RNs Employed in Nursing per 10,000 Population by Province and Territory within Canada for 2002.**

Source: © (2003a) Canadian Institute for Health Information (CIHI). Reproduction of Figure 3 on page 48 of *Workforce Trends of Registered Nurses in Canada, 2002* as published by CIHI. Used with permission.

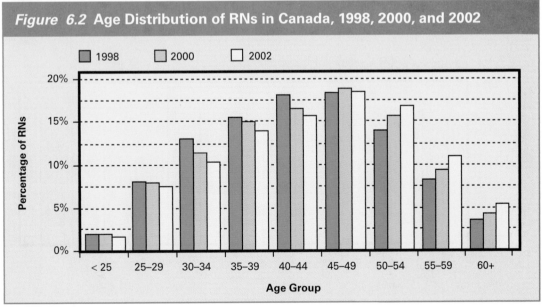

Figure 6.2 **Age Distribution of RNs in Canada, 1998, 2000, and 2002**

Source: © (2003a) Canadian Institute for Health Information (CIHI). Reproduction of Figure 6 on page 53 of *Workforce Trends of Registered Nurses in Canada, 2002* as published by CIHI. Used with permission.

The retirement of RNs will pose a major challenge to the health care system in the near future. In 2002, 16.2% of the Canadian nursing workforce was 55 years or older. While no data is available on the average age of retirement for Canadian nurses, Baumann and O'Brien-Pallas (2001) estimated it to be between 55 and 58 years of age. Early retirement is common in health care (O'Brien-Pallas, Alksnis, & Wang, 2003); for example, 48.9% of health care professionals retired before age 65 between 1997 and 2000. The percentages of Canadian nurses who were eligible for retirement in 2002 are presented in Figure 6.3. Based on the number of nurses working in 2001, O'Brien-Pallas and colleagues (2003) estimated that if RNs retired at 55 years of age, Canada could lose up to 28% of its current workforce by 2006. Efforts to retain nurses who are eligible for retirement could prevent a sudden and significant reduction in the nursing workforce and therefore need to be explored.

The Evolution of Nursing Education

In the 1960s and 1970s, hospital-based programs offered diplomas in nursing. By the 1990s, three-year college diploma programs and four-year university degree programs were the standard education for nurses. University degree programs, first introduced in British Columbia in 1919, are gaining favour. In 2002, 13.2% of the nursing workforce entered with a degree, compared to 10.6% in 1998 (CIHI, 2003a). As Canadian provinces begin to require a bachelor's degree, diploma programs are closing or merging with university programs (CIHI, 2002). The Canadian Nurses Association stresses that the competencies for practice for new registered nurses "are most effectively and economically achieved through baccalaureate education" (CNA, 1999, p. 1).

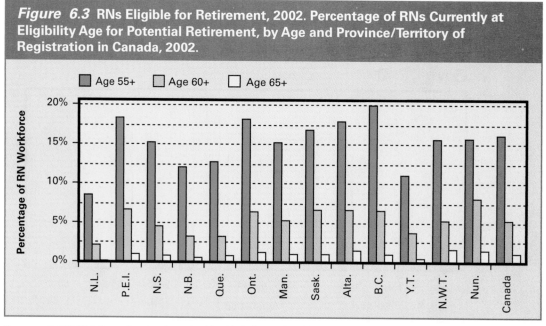

Figure 6.3 RNs Eligible for Retirement, 2002. Percentage of RNs Currently at Eligibility Age for Potential Retirement, by Age and Province/Territory of Registration in Canada, 2002.

Source: © (2003a) Canadian Institute for Health Information (CIHI). Reproduction of Figure 9 on page 57 of *Workforce Trends of Registered Nurses in Canada, 2002* as published by CIHI. Used with permission.

Following this trend, the College of Nurses of Ontario will require nurses to have a degree in nursing for entry to practice in the year 2005 (Schofield, 2001). RNs with diplomas will not be required to upgrade but may pursue nursing degrees in programs tailored to their needs. In 2002, 72.7% of nurses had a diploma, 27.3% had a bachelor's degree, and only 1.9% of nurses had a master's degree or a doctorate as their highest educational qualification (CIHI, 2003a).

Advances in nursing education include distance education and Internet-based education. These strategies provide greater accessibility and flexibility for nursing students. In the rural RN workforce, baccalaureate-educated nurses have increased from 12.5% in 1994 to 18.0% in 2000 (CIHI, 2002).

As nurses are entering the profession later, they are working fewer years (CIHI, 2002). As previously mentioned, it now takes longer to graduate as a nurse, and the average age of graduation for RNs has increased since the 1970s. The average age of university nursing graduates rose from 22.0 years in 1970 to 26.7 years in 1990; the average age of diploma graduates rose from 22.0 years to 27.2 years in the same period. At graduation, 24.4% were aged 30 years or older, compared to 2.9% in 1970. Overall, the number of nurses entering nursing programs is decreasing. In 1990, there were 12,170 admissions to basic entry RN programs; by 2001, there were 8790 admissions (CNA, 2002).

Nurse educators also are aging—the average age of a nurse educator is nearly 49 years. An Ontario environmental scan in 2001 suggested cumulative retirement rates to the year 2010 of 49.6% for university professors and 37.7% for college instructors (CNAC, 2002). The need to foster the development of young nursing faculty and recruit educators is apparent.

Nurses' Employment Status

To estimate the employment status of Canadian nurses, the CIHI created a measure known as the derived employment status. This measure presents the employment status (full-time, part-time, or casual) of nurses together, as shown in Table 6.2 (CIHI, 2003a).

Table 6.2 Percentage Distribution of Canadian RNs Employed in Nursing by Derived Employment Status

	1998	1999	2000	2001	2002
Full-time	49.1%	49.2%	51.7%	52.1%	54.1%
Part-time	32.2%	32.5%	33.2%	33.9%	33.8%
Casual	18.6%	18.2%	14.8%	12.7%	11.8%
Unknown	0.1%	0.2%	0.3%	0.3%	0.3%

Source: © (2003a) Canadian Institute for Health Information (CIHI). Adapted from Table 12 on page 64 of *Workforce Trends of Registered Nurses in Canada, 2002* as published by CIHI. Used with permission.

Part-time employment in nursing increased from 29.3% in 1970 to 42.7% in 1995, a growth much higher than that of the female proportion of the profession as a whole (Baumgart, 1997). More recently, part-time employment has remained relatively stable compared to casual and full-time arrangements. Registered nurses working in full-time positions increased from 49.1% in 1998 to 54.1% in 2002. Casual employment decreased during those years, except in the Yukon where there was an increase. Currently, casual employment varies throughout the country, ranging from 6.5% in Manitoba to 24.9% in Nunavut (CIHI, 2003a).

Voluntary casual employment is offered as a reason for the shift towards casual employment by senior nursing staff (CIHI, 2002); however, nurses who graduated in the past six years have a much higher casual employment rate (23.6%) than those who graduated 20 to 30 years ago (7.1%). This is likely the result of an established policy of recruiting nursing graduates to part-time jobs. Nurses constrained to part-time work are considered to have involuntary employment, a hidden form of underemployment. Underemployment is more prevalent in junior workers (Barret & Dorion, 2001), and it is hypothesized that most new nursing graduates who work casually do so involuntarily. Presently, the rates of casual employment are highest among recent nursing graduates. In fact, it is the high casual employment rates for new graduates that are considered to have led to the decline in enrolment in nursing education programs in the late 1990s. In 1997, more than half of newly graduated nurses were employed casually, with less than 20% employed on a full-time basis (CIHI, 2002). Currently, newly graduated nurses have less difficulty securing full-time employment than in 1997.

Branine (as cited in Zeytinoglu, 2002) argues that the main rationale for employers offering part-time work is cost reduction and flexible working practices. Grinspun (2002) reflects upon the management concept of the late 1980s—the so-called just-in-time employee—which benefits employers by allowing labour to be paid on an as-needed basis. However, for the nurse, part-time work has disadvantages. McBride and others argue that nurses may be confined to the lowest qualified clinical grades and disadvantaged in terms of career development (McBride; Branine & Glover as cited in Zeytinoglu, 2002). Conversely, some nurses may find part-time work beneficial in terms of work schedule flexibility and the pursuit of opportunities for professional growth.

The Registered Nurses Association of Ontario (RNAO, 2003) reported that deterrents to working full-time included family responsibilities, workload, scheduling, and insufficient professional development. However, there still was involuntary part-time employment. If all respondents had their preferred employment status, the RNAO study suggested that there would be a shift of about 11% to full-time employment from non-full-time employment. The study found 54% of part-time and casual nurses continued to decline full-time employment; however, many of these nurses said they would accept full-time work under different circumstances. This confirms that "nurses need responsive, flexible and innovative schedules that allow a female-dominated workforce to balance home and working lives and to meet unpredictable family care needs" (CNAC, 2002, p. 12).

Where Nurses Work

Approximately 85.9% of employed RNs provide direct patient care (CIHI, 2003a). Just over 60% of nurses are employed in hospitals. Hospitals remain the biggest employer of nurses, although small increases in the community health agency and nursing home sectors have been noted

(CIHI, 2002). Nurses working in hospitals are younger, having an average age of 42.8 years compared to 45.0 years for nurses in community health. Employment status in each sector is somewhat comparable in terms of full-time employment rates, but it varies more in part-time employment rates, as shown in Table 6.3.

Table 6.3 **Percentage Distribution of Canadian RNs by Employment Status and Place of Employment, 1997–2001**			
	Hospitals	**Community Health**	**Nursing Homes**
Full-time	53.1%	56.9%	46.5%
Part-time	34.8%	28.0%	40.7%
Casual	12.1%	15.1%	12.8%

Source: © (2002) Canadian Institute for Health Information (CIHI). Adapted from page 141 of *The Supply and Distribution of Registered Nurses in Canada, 2001* as published by CIHI. Used with permission.

The New Workforce

The major issues in the contemporary nursing workforce are supply, recruitment, and retention. The question is whether or not it will be possible to meet the demands for nursing services in the future, particularly since the Canadian population is aging. Because nurses have become a scarce commodity, they are now receiving attention. Discussions of the nursing shortage are prominent in the media, the pronouncements of national and provincial governments, and the publications of professional nursing associations. Federal and provincial governments have made funds available for research to support the nursing profession, have appointed chief nursing officers, and have provided supportive infrastructure to enable nurses to be more fully engaged in decision making (Health Canada, 2000).

Recruitment and retention of nurses has become a priority for governments and organizations. Discussions of these problems resemble those that occurred during the shortage in the 1980s, and many of the strategies to deal with these problems also resemble those of that period. Health care organizations are employing recruitment and retention specialists and are undertaking recruitment campaigns. Nursing associations have attempted to persuade nurses working outside the country to return to work in Canada. Organizations are attempting to retain staff by improving the quality of nursing work life; for example, urban hospitals are offering inducements such as parking subsides, overnight hostels, childcare facilities, and security measures. Organizations with sufficient resources are offering educational support and may pay up to 100% of tuition costs, and initiatives such as staged retirement are being contemplated to keep nurses working. Flexible scheduling is being explored to allow nurses to work longer hours while still fulfilling their personal and family obligations (Baumann, O'Brien-Pallas, et al., 2001).

It is easier to fill full-time rather than part-time jobs, and evidence suggests that generous staffing policies are more cost-effective than excessively lean ones (Flood & Diers, 1988; Robertson, Dowd, & Hassan, 1997). Managers in some health care organizations are creating more full-time jobs and seeking greater commitment from employees. Unfortunately, in other health care organizations, managers still conform to staffing guidelines internalized during the restructuring era and are reluctant to adopt policies that emphasize high proportions of full-time employment (Baumann, O'Brien-Pallas, et al., 2001).

Many nurses are unable to find full-time employment, and during recent years, they have adopted more entrepreneurial strategies in order to survive. Many part-time nurses work full-time hours, either because they work beyond agreed hours or because they have an additional job or jobs. For the employer, the consequence is that casual and part-time nurses rarely are available for extra shifts. Recently, some hospitals have set up float pools of full-time nurses in order to decrease their reliance on casual staff; however, the extent of staffing shortfalls is such that it is often necessary to make use of expensive agency staff.

New Nursing Roles

The nursing workforce is characterized by polarities of older and younger nurses, by more male nurses, and by greater ethnic diversity. Nurses' roles are becoming increasingly diverse. More of the burden of care is moving from acute care hospitals to communities, and nurses must follow their clients. There are new ways of providing care, such as through telephone services and jobs in private industry. Nurses must be familiar with new technologies and the use of evidence to support practice. Their clients and patients are better informed about health care due to the widespread use of the Internet.

Promoting Quality Workplaces

A health care environment characterized by rapid change poses challenges for nursing management and opportunities for leadership. To exploit change, leaders must use their formal knowledge and intuitive understanding of the workforce to plan for future directions. They require a clear vision so that they can anticipate change and create strategies and action plans responsive to the needs of nurses. Both professional practice and operational issues challenge the ability of managers and leaders to maintain a healthy workforce. The final report of the Canadian Nursing Advisory Committee (2002), *Our Health, Our Future: Creating Quality Workplaces for Canadian Nurses,* identifies specific operational, managerial, and professional practice issues affecting the nursing workforce (Table 6.4).

Researchers report that nurses suffer the highest stress levels of all health professionals (Sullivan, Kerr, & Ibrahim, 1999 as cited in CNAC, 2002), and they have identified issues related to nurses' work and work environments as key factors, including heavy workloads, long hours, injuries, and poor relations with other professions. As well, "long periods of job strain affect professional

Table 6.4 Operational, Managerial, and Professional Practice Issues Facing the Canadian Nursing Workforce

Operational and Managerial Issues	Professional Practice Issues
Workload Overtime Absenteeism Employment status Scope of practice and non-nursing tasks	Secondary to the effects of downsizing: Leadership Education Violence and abuse The search for respect

Source: Adapted from *Our Health, Our Future: Creating Quality Workplaces for Canadian Nurses: Final Report of the Canadian Nursing Advisory Committee* (p. 12), by the Advisory Committee on Health Human Resources, 2002, Ottawa, ON: Advisory Committee on Health Human Resources.

and personal relationships and increase sick time, turnover and inefficiency" (Baumann, O'Brien-Pallas, et al., 2001, p. iv). The policy synthesis *Commitment and Care: The Benefits of a Healthy Workplace for Nurses, Their Patients and the System* provided a wide variety of recommendations to increase the health and productivity of the Canadian nursing workforce (Baumann, O'Brien-Pallas, et al., 2001). Box 6.1 presents seven categories of recommendations for employers that some organizations have used as a template for change.

Address Staffing Issues

Nurse managers must address staffing challenges and put forth strategies to ensure an appropriate supply of care providers. This involves hiring an appropriate number of nurses for

Box 6.1

Areas of Recommendation for Employers

Address Staffing Issues

Reward Effort and Achievement

Strengthen Organizational Structures

Support Nursing Leadership and Professional Development

Promote Workplace Health and Safety

Ensure a Learning Environment

Promote Recruitment and Retention

Source: Adapted from *Commitment and Care: The Benefits of a Healthy Workplace for Nurses, Their Patients and the System* (pp. 16–17), by A. Baumann, L. O'Brien-Pallas, M. Armstrong-Stassen, J. Blythe, R. Bourbonnais, S. Cameron et al., 2001, Ottawa, ON: Canadian Health Services Research Foundation.

current and anticipated workload and ensuring that the staffing complement includes a high proportion of full-time nurses. The RNAO (2003) suggests that at least 70% of RNs should have full-time employment and that the government of Ontario should fund 15,000 more positions to return the RN to population ratio to its 1986 levels. The development and routine use of work-load measurement tools that are current, accurate, and appropriate are essential for nurse staffing. Developing efficient staffing strategies is paramount. Steps to improving efficiency might include assessing whether the costs incurred by agency use and overtime hours could be used more effectively for permanent full-time and part-time positions. Float pools might be considered as a means of providing casual workers for permanent employment opportunities. Hiring additional support staff would conserve nursing resources by enabling professional nurses to spend more time at the bedside and less time on administrative tasks. The implementation of more flexible scheduling and innovative staffing strategies, developed in collaboration with nursing unions, would enable more nurses to take full-time jobs (RNAO, 2003).

Reward Effort and Achievement

The relationship between effort and reward was outlined by the Siegrest effort and reward model. Recent work by Siegrist and colleagues in a study of German nurses found that burnout was associated with high work demands and low levels of reward (Bakker, Kilmer, Siegrist, & Schaufeli, 2000). Employers can recognize and reward nursing excellence and experience by offering competitive pay, rewarding seniority with increments and benefits, and recognizing seniority gained elsewhere. Career ladders, which are programs that recognize achievement, reward nurses for their professional contributions, and promote professional growth, can also be implemented (Day, 1995). Most clinical ladder programs have defined criteria or competencies that must be met in order for advancement. Nurses who act as preceptors or mentors to junior nurses should also be recognized. Non-monetary forms of recognition include provision of childcare, staff lounges, access to hot food for all shifts, health programs, and awareness of quality of work life issues.

Strengthen Organizational Structures

The early work by McClure, Poulin, Souvie, and Wandelt (1983) explored the impact of organizational culture and management on nursing staff and patient outcomes in one of the most influential studies of the 1980s. The study identified hospitals in the United States that had reputations for being good places for nurses to work. These "magnet hospitals" were measured using indices of retention and turnover, skill mix, and nurse/patient ratios. Despite the nursing shortages of the time, these hospitals had no recruitment problems. They also had lower rates of nurse burnout than comparable non-magnet hospitals (Aiken, Sloane, & Klocinski, 1997). Subsequent studies confirmed that investments in nursing yielded returns in terms of both retention and nurse and patient care outcomes (Aiken, Clarke, & Sloane, 2002; Aiken, Smith, & Lake, 1994). In the late 1990s, the magnet hospital concept was revived in the US and became the basis of credentialing by the American Nursing Association (Aiken, Havens, & Sloane, 2000). Aiken and colleagues have demonstrated that adequate organizational and managerial support and adequate staffing can improve nurse retention and quality of care (Aiken et al., 2002; Clarke & Aiken, 2003). Kramer and Schmalenberg (2003) continued the work on magnet hospitals and found that reorganization and mergers can negatively affect nurses' control over their practice. The need for nursing leadership at the organizational level is obvious. It is essential for nursing leadership to promote supportive work environments for nurses in order to benefit patients.

Multidisciplinary teams, nurse decision making, and effective communication strategies are required for managers and staff to clarify roles of regulated and unregulated workers and to explore the impact of board policies on staff and patients. Nurse executives and decision makers must foster a culture that encourages strong nursing leadership.

Support Nursing Leadership and Professional Development

The importance of nursing leadership cannot be underestimated. Nurse leaders provide the disciplinary perspective to senior management and professional role modelling to the staff. Both these roles are critical in order to preserve the integrity of the provision of nursing care. Leaders have to be responsive to changes in staffing, care delivery, and diffusion of new technology and treatment modalities. The recent emergence of new diseases challenges nurses and the health care system. Nursing leadership can become more prominent through the integration of nurses into management and administrative positions in the organizational hierarchy. Decision making at both the individual clinician and professional practice levels would also be beneficial. For example, in magnet hospitals, strong nursing leadership and decision making were facilitated by flat organizational structures with unit-based decision-making processes. These hospitals had influential nurse executives and invested heavily in nurse education (Kramer & Schmalenberg, 1993). Baumann and Blythe (2003b) challenge governments and employers to invest in human capital and abandon the costs approach to human capital. An investment in the knowledge, skills, competencies, and attributes of nurses is past due.

Ensure Workplace Health and Safety

Nurse safety is a prerequisite for effective care. The presence of nurses on occupational health and safety committees would allow their needs to be addressed. A participatory action approach would facilitate the identification of precursors to injury or harm and the support of management in promoting and ensuring a safe work environment. Access to adequate supplies, properly working equipment, and appropriate support personnel should be evaluated and monitored. Safety programs, such as walking partners to after-hours parking lots, as well as other work-safe initiatives should be available. The violence and abuse that continues to be reported by nurses in their workplaces is a serious concern. Nurses in leadership and management positions must insist on the implementation and enforcement of institutional policies of zero tolerance for all forms of abuse in the work setting (CNAC, 2002).

Make the Work Environment a Learning Environment

A dynamic work environment with rich educational and staff development opportunities fosters professional satisfaction. The provision of educational and professional development opportunities in isolation is not enough. Nurses must have the flexibility and support from management to pursue and participate in career building education and skill acquisition. A culture supportive of education must be instilled in the organization through preceptor and mentorship programs and through support for performance evaluations. Recognition of the value placed on staff development is needed. Tuition assistance programs, career ladders, education leaves, and remuneration for on-site education may be effective.

Evidence-based practice is changing the provision of care. The work environment must become a learning environment in which nurses are able to access evidence of all kinds and critically appraise what they find. Managers must nurture a flexible environment where staff are able to participate in educational activities, updating their skills to provide the most current care. Employers must look at innovative ways to support education and offer opportunities for professional development. Employers, educators, and government ministries should inform nurses and nursing students about educational opportunities and encourage them to apply for financial support. Examples of current initiatives include the following:

- The Nursing Education Initiative, a tuition reimbursement program funded by the Ontario Ministry of Health and Long-Term Care, provides grants to support continuing education of nurses for advancement of knowledge and professional skills (RNAO, 2003);
- Tuition assistance programs have been sponsored by some provincial organizations, universities, and employers (Ontario Ministry, 2003; St. Michael's, n.d.; RNAO, n.d.; University of Saskatchewan, 2002);
- The Prince Edward Island Nursing Recruitment and Retention Strategy campaign offers a student sponsorship program to assist students with employment and tuition costs and provide further assistance to the health regions to secure more new nursing graduates (Prince Edward Island, Health and Social Services, n.d.);
- In 2003, the Ontario Ministry of Health and Long-Term Care created the Free Tuition Program for Nurses, which will reimburse tuition costs in exchange for working a corresponding number of years in an eligible underserviced community (Ontario Ministry, 2003).

Education opportunities are particularly important because new graduates are being recruited to specialty units. Mentoring programs can assist nurses to develop additional skills and socialize them into the work team. Oermann and Garbin (2002) stress that new graduates need mentors, especially in organizations without preceptor programs. In today's chaotic work environment, employees rarely have the opportunity to meet with managers to discuss their performance. Bloor and Maynard (2003) note that lack of performance appraisal results in difficulties in measuring efficiency. They suggest that poor access to information, weak management, and lack of systematic continuing education and reaccreditation aggravate poor performance monitoring. Nurse leaders and managers must allocate time for performance appraisal and career planning for nurses.

Emphasize Recruitment and Retention

The potential severity of the nursing shortage makes recruitment and retention of nurses a priority. Employers are actively seeking ways to recruit new nurses, but emphasis on retention is even more vital given the recent estimated number of nurses who will soon leave the profession. O'Brien-Pallas and colleagues (2003) suggest that retention incentives could lead to a 52.8% reduction in retirement of Canadian RNs. Unfortunately, we have yet to identify truly successful incentives for retention. It is imperative that governments, employers, and nurse leaders make every effort to devise and implement innovative recruitment and retention strategies.

Leadership Implications

New work patterns have emerged. Many nurses work in more than one institution, have full-time hours but not full-time jobs, and have little job security. Nurse burnout and fatigue due to ramifications of health care re-engineering also are limiting the number of hours nurses are able to work.

Organizations must continually review their plans and progress. One strategy is the use of tools to assist planning. Performance indicators and hospital report cards can provide front-line managers with evidence on how to support their workers and create work environments conducive to client and employee health (Pink et al., 2001). Managers and leaders also must be responsive to workforce need so that nurses, in turn, can respond effectively to patient care needs.

The challenges of the evolving health care system require new styles of leadership and management. McDaniel (1997) suggests that the current health care system was designed to face past problems. Today, there are new challenges, and the system must adapt to address them. Nurse leaders must facilitate this movement. Traditional models of management are created for an orderly and predictable world; however, this is no longer the case, and strategic leaders should help organizations focus on the concept of "learning" rather that "knowing." This will help leaders cope with "the turbulent unfolding of the health care world" (McDaniel, p. 27).

Summary

- The nursing workforce is comprised of three regulated occupational groups: registered nurses (76%), registered psychiatric nurses (2%), and licensed/registered practical nurses (22%). There are also advanced practice nurses (e.g., nurse practitioners, clinical nurse specialists) and, depending on the setting, various categories of unregulated support workers.
- Widespread restructuring in the health care system during the 1990s resulted in many disruptions in the working lives of nurses, including layoffs, redeployment, involuntary changes in full-time and part-time employment status, loss of work preferences, interruption of careers, and loss of nursing management positions.
- Following restructure and redeployment, nurses reported feeling devalued, dissatisfied with their jobs, less commitment to their places of work, and declining morale.

- There is currently a shortage of RNs in the health care system brought about by an aging workforce, decreased enrolment in schools of nursing, and increased demand for RN services. The average age that nurses graduate and enter the workforce is rising.

- In 2002, there were 74.4 RNs per 10,000 Canadians; the average age of RNs was 44.2 years; 5.1% of RNs were male; 54.1% worked full time, 33.8% part time, and 11.8% casually.

- In 2002, approximately 72.7% of nurses held diplomas in nursing, 27.3% held bachelor's degrees, and 1.9% held master's degrees or higher.

- Most employed RNs (85.9%) provide direct nursing care, and over 60% are employed in hospitals.

- Ensuring the supply of nurses to meet the future health care needs of the population will require multifaceted recruitment and retention strategies, with increased attention to providing work environments that are professionally rewarding, healthy, and safe.

Applying the Knowledge in this Chapter

Exercise

Systems Level

1. What government initiatives and policies do you think may impact the nursing profession?

2. As a nurse leader, how would you advise a politician interested in improving nursing work conditions?

3. How might future restructuring of health care impact nursing care delivery?

4. What challenges may face the nursing profession in a shift toward primary health care?

5. How has the change toward baccalaureate education affected nursing recruitment and supply?

6. Where should efforts in recruitment and retention of nurses from a national level be directed?

Organizational Level

1. How is nursing leadership visible in your organization? What would make it more visible?

2. Where are there opportunities for flexibility in nursing resource utilization?

3. Are the work arrangements (e.g., employment contracts, scheduling, staffing) in your organization flexible or conducive to balancing home and work life?

Individual Level

1. What leadership characteristics make a successful nurse manager?

2. What personal and professional characteristics make a successful nurse leader?

3. What areas of growth do you see facing the profession?

4. What educational opportunities are available to present and future leaders?

5. What challenges do you foresee facing the profession?

Resources

evolve Internet Resources

Canadian Institute for Health Information (CIHI):
  http://secure.cihi.ca/cihiweb/splash.html
Canadian Nursing Advisory Committee (CNAC):
  www.hc-sc.gc.ca/english/for_you/nursing/cnac.htm
  The 2002 CNAC final report entitled *Our Health, Our Future: Creating Quality Workplaces for Canadian Nurses* can be found on this site.
International Council of Nurses (ICN):
  www.icn.ch/

References

Acorn, S., Ratner, P.A., & Crawford, M. (1997). Decentralization as a determinant of autonomy, job satisfaction, and organizational commitment among nurse managers. *Nursing Research, 46*(1), 52–58.

Aiken, L.H., Clarke, S.P., & Sloane, D.M. (2002). Hospital staffing, organization, and quality of care: cross-national findings. *Nursing Outlook, 50,* 187–194.

Aiken, L.H., Havens, D.S., & Sloane, D.M. (2000). The Magnet Nursing Services Recognition Program: A comparison of two groups of magnet hospitals. *American Journal of Nursing, 100*(3), 26–36.

Aiken, L.H., Sloane, D.M., & Klocinski, J.L. (1997). Hospital nurses' occupational exposure to blood: Prospective, retrospective, and institutional reports. *American Journal of Public Health, 87,* 103–107.

Aiken, L.H., Smith, H.L., & Lake, E.T. (1994). Lower medical mortality among a set of hospitals known for good nursing care. *Medical Care, 32,* 771–787.

Armstrong-Stassen, M., Cameron, S., & Horsburgh, M.E. (1996). The impact of organizational downsizing on the job satisfaction of nurses. *Canadian Journal of Nursing Administration, 9,* 8–32.

Bakker, A., Killmer, C., Siegrist, J., & Schaufeli, W. (2000). Effort-reward imbalance and burnout among nurses. *Journal of Advanced Nursing, 31,* 884–891.

Barret, G.F., & Doiron, D.J. (2001). Working part time: By choice or by constraint? *Canadian Journal of Economics, 34,* 1042–1065.

Baumann, A., & Blythe, J. (2003a). Restructuring, reconsidering, reconstructing: Implications for health human resources. *International Journal of Health Administration, 26,* 1563–1581.

Baumann, A., & Blythe, J. (2003b). Nursing human resources: Human costs versus human capital in the restructured health care system. *Health Perspectives Quarterly, 3,* 27–34.

Baumann, A., Giovannetti, P., O'Brien-Pallas, L., Mallette, C., Deber, R., Blythe, J., et al. (2001). Healthcare restructuring: The impact of job change. *Canadian Journal of Nursing Leadership, 14,* 1420.

Baumann, A., O'Brien-Pallas, L., Armstrong-Stassen, M., Blythe, J., Bourbonnais, R., Cameron, S., et al. (2001). *Commitment and care: The benefits of a healthy workplace for nurses, their patients and the system.* Ottawa, ON: Canadian Health Services Research Foundation.

Baumann, A., & O'Brien-Pallas, L. (2001). *The status of the nursing workforce in Ontario: The numbers and the worklife issues in November 2001* (Rep. No. Report submitted to the Ontario Nurses' Association, December 2001). Ottawa, Ontario: Ontario Nurses Association.

Baumann, A., & Silverman, B. (1998). De-professionalization in health care: Flattening the hierarchy. In L. Groake (Ed.), *The ethics of the new economy: Restructuring and beyond* (pp. 203–209). Waterloo, ON: Wilfred Laurier University Press.

Baumann, A., O'Brien-Pallas, L., Deber, R., Donner, G., Semogas, D., & Silverman, B. (1996). Downsizing in the hospital system: A restructuring process. *Health Care Management Forum, 9*(4), 5–13.

Baumgart, A.J. (1997). Hospital reform and nursing labor market trends in Canada. *Medical Care, 35,* OS124–OS131.

Bishop, J.W., & Scott, K.D. (1997). How commitment affects team performance. *HR Magazine, 42,* 107–111.

Bloor, K., & Maynard, A. (2003). *Planning human resources in health care: Towards an economic approach. An international comparative review.* Ottawa, ON: Canadian Health Services Research Foundation.

Blythe, J., Baumann, A., & Giovannetti, P. (2001). Nurses' experiences of restructuring in three Ontario hospitals. *Journal of Nursing Scholarship, 33*(1), 61–68.

Brawn, S. (1992). Surviving in tough times: Adventures in downsizing. *The Nursing Report, 47,* 1–8.

Brooks, I., & Swailes, S. (2002). Analysis of the relationship between nurse influences over flexible working and commitment to nursing. *Journal of Advanced Nursing, 38,* 117–126.

Brown, D.J.M., & Beatty, D.M. (2003, November). *Canadian labour arbitration.* (3rd ed.). Release No. 41. Agincourt, ON: Canada Law Book.

Buerhaus, P.I., Staiger, D.O., & Auerbach, D.I. (2000). Implications of an aging registered nurse workforce. *Journal of the American Medical Association, 283,* 2948–2954.

Butt, M., Baumann, A., O'Brien-Pallas, L., Deber, R., Blythe, J., & DiCenso, A. (2002). The learning needs of nurses experiencing job change. *Journal of Continuing Education in Nursing, 33,* 67–73.

Canadian Institute for Health Information. (2003a). *Workforce trends of registered nurses in Canada, 2002.* Ottawa, ON: Canadian Institute for Health Information.

Canadian Institute for Health Information. (2003b). *Workforce trends of licensed practical nurses in Canada, 2001.* Ottawa, ON: Canadian Institute for Health Information.

Canadian Institute for Health Information. (2003c). *Workforce trends of registered psychiatric nurses in Canada, 2002.* Ottawa, ON: Canadian Institute for Health Information.

Canadian Institute for Health Information. (2002). *The supply and distribution of registered nurses in Canada, 2001.* Ottawa, ON: Canadian Institute for Health Information.

Canadian Institute for Health Information. (2001). *Health care in Canada 2001: A second annual report.* Ottawa, ON: Canadian Institute for Health Information.

Canadian Nurses Association. (2003). *Position statement: The nurse practitioner.* Ottawa, ON: Author.

Canadian Nurses Association. (2002). *Highlights of 2002 nursing statistics.* Retrieved November 21, 2004, from http://www.cna-nurses.ca

Canadian Nurses Association. (1999, June). *Post-basic RN baccalaureate programs in nursing.* Retrieved November 11, 2003, from http://www.cna-nurses.ca/pages/education/educationframe.htm

Canadian Nursing Advisory Committee. (2002). *Our health, our future: Creating quality workplaces for Canadian nurses.* Final report. Ottawa, ON: Advisory Committee on Health Human Resources.

Clarke, S.P., & Aiken, L.H. (2003). Failure to rescue: Needless deaths are prime examples of the need for more nurses at the bedside. *American Journal of Nursing, 103,* 42–47.

Day, D. (1995). A career ladder program designed by perioperative staff nurses. *AORN, 62,* 805–809.

Flood, S.D., & Diers, D. (1988). Nurse staffing, patient outcomes and cost. *Nursing Management, 19,* 34-35, 38-39-42.3.

Friss, L. (1994). Nursing policies laid end to end form a circle. *Journal of Health Politics, Policy and Law, 19,* 597–631.

Grinspun, D. (2002). A flexible nursing workforce: Realities and fallouts. *Hospital Quarterly, 6*(1), 79–84.

Health Canada. (2000). *Office of nursing policy strategic priorities.* Ottawa, ON: Health Canada.

International Council of Nurses. (2002). ICN announces position on advanced nursing roles. Retrieved November 11, 2003, from http://www.icn.ch/pr19_02.htm

Kramer, M., & Schmalenberg, C. (2003). Securing "good" nurse physician relationships. *Nursing Management, 34,* 34–38.

Kramer, M., & Schemalenberg, C. (1993). Learning from success: Autonomy and empowerment. *Nursing Management, 24,* 58–64.

Lyall, J. (1991). Shut out. *Nursing Times, 87,* 9.

McClure, M.L., Poulin, M.A., Sovie, M.D., & Wandelt, M.A. (1983). *Magnet hospitals: Attraction and retention of professional nurses.* Washington, DC: American Academy of Nursing.

McDaniel, R.R., Jr. (1997). Strategic leadership: A view from quantum and chaos theories. *Health Care Management Review, 22*(1), 21–37.

Meltz, N. (1988). *Sorry no care available due to nursing shortage.* Toronto, ON: Registered Nurses Association of Ontario.

O'Brien-Pallas, L., Alksnis, C., & Wang, S. (2003). *Bringing the future into focus: Projecting RN retirement in Canada.* Ottawa, ON: Canadian Institute for Health Information.

O'Brien-Pallas, L.L., Baumann, A., Donner, G.J., Murphy, G.T., Lochhaas-Gerlach, J., & Luba, M. (2001). Forecasting models for human resources in health care. *Journal of Advanced Nursing, 33,* 120–129.

Oermann, M.H., & Garbin M.F. (2002). Stresses and challenges for new graduates in hospitals. *Nursing Education Today, 22,* 225–230.

Ontario Ministry of Health and Long-Term Care. (2003, November). *Ontario's investment in nursing.* Retrieved October 16, 2003, from http://www.health.gov.on.ca/english/public/updates/archives/hu_03/docnurse/nursing_fs.html

Pink, G.H., McKillop, I., Schraa, E.G., Preyra, C., Montgomery, C., & Baker, G.R. (2001). Creating a balanced scorecard for a hospital system. *Journal of Health Care Finance, 27*(3), 1–20.

Prince Edward Island, Health and Social Services. (n.d.). *Nursing recruitment and retention strategy.* Retrieved October 16, 2003, from http://www.gov.pe.ca/hss/recruitment/nursing.php3

Registered Nurses Association of Ontario. (2003). *Survey of casual and part-time registered nurses in Ontario.* Ottawa, ON: Registered Nurses Association of Ontario.

Registered Nurses Association of Ontario. (n.d.). *Nurse education initiative.* Retrieved October 16, 2003, from http://www.rnao.org/projects/nei.asp

Richard Ivey School of Business. (1997). *Leading the management of change: A study of 12 Ontario hospitals.* London, ON: University of Western Ontario.

Robertson, R.H., Dowd, S., & Hassan, M. (1997). Skill-specific staffing intensity and the cost of hospital care. *Health Care Management Review, 22*(4), 61–71.

Ryten, E. (1997). *A statistical picture of the past, present and future of nursing in Canada.* Ottawa, ON: Canadian Nurses Association.

Schofield, J. (2001). Raising the requirements. *Maclean's, 114,* 48.

St. Michael's Hospital. (n.d.). *Tuition assistance program.* Retrieved October 16, 2003, from http://www.stmichaelshospital.com/content/careers/tuition_assistance.asp

Vahtera, J., Kivimaki, M., & Pentti, J. (1997). Effect of organizational downsizing on the health of employees. *Lancet, 350,* 1124–1128.

University of Saskatchewan. (2002, May). *U of S board announces 2002-03 operating budget.* Retrieved 16, 2003, from http://www.usask.ca/events/news/articles/20020510-1.html

Zeytinoglu, I. (2002). *Flexible work arrangements: Conceptualizations and international experiences.* London, UK: Kluwer Law International.

Zimmerman, P.G. (2000). The nursing shortage: What can we do? *Journal of Emergency Nursing, 26,* 579–582.

SECTION II

STRUCTURE AND ORGANIZATION

The structure of an organization dictates how work is divided and coordinated. The formal structure of an organization illustrates how power, authority, and the responsibility for managing resources are allocated, and it prescribes the channels of communication that are expected of, and available to, employees of the organization. Section II provides an understanding of the ways in which systems, organizations, and work are structured, which is important for nurses in clinical practice and leadership roles within these complex work environments.

As explained in Section 1, health agencies exist within a complex external environment in which shifting political, social, and economic factors directly and indirectly affect their ability to carry out their mission. In Chapter 7, *Health Agency Boards and Regional Governance*, the roles of the board and chief executive officer (CEO) are described, and the development and challenges of regional governance of health services are discussed. A key role of the governing boards of health agencies is to monitor the external environment, approve policies, and manage external relationships to enable the agency they represent to obtain the resources and other support necessary to achieve its mission. The governing board directly employs and supervises the CEO, who is responsible for leading and managing the organization in implementing the policies and strategies adopted by the board, thereby achieving the mission and goals of the agency. The author of this chapter, Professor Susan Wagner, is uniquely qualified to present this material, having been appointed by the Saskatchewan Minister of Health to serve on the first regional health board established in Canada in February 1992. In 1995, she was a successful candidate in health board elections and served as chair of the Saskatoon Health Board. Her leadership on community boards and as board chair for the Saskatoon Health Region is evidence of the ability and opportunity nurses have to provide visionary policy leadership for health agencies at the highest levels.

Structure in Health Agencies is discussed in Chapter 8. At the level of individual health regions or agencies, the CEO is responsible for recruitment of an executive team and for adopting a structure for the overall organization. However, in hospitals, some aspects of organizational structure are prescribed through provincial legislation that confers unique responsibilities upon physicians through the medical staff organization and which enables them, like the CEO, to report directly to the governing board. This unusual arrangement is one reason why hospitals have been called the most complex of modern organizations. The discussion of structure in this chapter is intended to help readers understand some of these complexities and, particularly, why members of the medical staff may behave autonomously and occasionally with disregard for the policies and procedures that govern the behaviour of other employees. There is an intentional emphasis on hospitals in this chapter because of their complexity and because the traditional relationships and communication patterns embedded in the organizational structure of hospitals have often influenced the design of agencies in other sectors of the health system.

Various approaches to the *Structure and Organization of Nurses' Work* are described in Chapter 9 and will be of direct interest to nurses in clinical positions. Position descriptions and day-to-day organizational arrangements are sometimes taken for granted, but, in fact, they are a way of operationalizing values, setting priorities, and allocating resources. These decisions also affect the ability to optimize and document nursing contributions to health outcomes. Historically, the organizational structures of hospitals and most other health services reflected the centrality of nursing services to the mission of the organization. There was traditionally a functional division, or department, of nursing directed by an individual whose superior professional qualifications and leadership ability commanded the respect of nursing colleagues within and outside the organization. This traditional form of organization enabled the senior nursing leader to articulate and implement a vision for the contribution of nurses and the standards of practice within the agency. It also allowed coordination of the efforts of a team of middle and first-line nursing managers to distribute human resources in a manner appropriate to the nursing care requirements of the populations being served. Various models or systems of nursing care delivery were devised in response to the availability of registered nurses, the resources available, and the care requirements of various patient populations.

In Chapter 10, *Organization Design and Strategic Management: A Critical Analysis*, theoretical perspectives from the areas of scholarship known as organization design and strategic management theory are used to explain and predict the consequences of changes in the structure of health agencies that have occurred since the mid-1980s. This critical analysis of organization design and strategic management may be challenging to undergraduate students or novice managers, but the design of nursing roles at all levels of a health agency has a direct bearing on nursing and health outcomes. Although nurses still constitute the largest group of employees in the health system, the visibility, power, and influence of the nursing profession have been diminished in most health agencies since the mid-1980s. The number of nursing leaders in health agencies in Canada steadily and significantly decreased in the 1990s. The responsibility for the design of nursing roles, the organization of nurses' work, or the allocation of nursing human resources no longer rests exclusively with a nurse who has advanced educational preparation and professional experience, and in some organizations, managers who are not nurses have this authority. The analytical approach exemplified in this chapter illustrates how theoretical perspectives can be used to explain and predict the consequences of structural changes in health organizations. This critical analysis will stimulate reflection on the values and assumptions inherent in the structuring of nursing services in the past, present, and future. This issue of particular interest in the context of concern about safety and quality of health care that has marked the beginning of the 21st century.

HEALTH AGENCY BOARDS AND REGIONAL GOVERNANCE

P. Susan Wagner

Learning Objectives

In this chapter, you will learn:

- Differences between governance and management of an organization and the role of a governing board

- Roles of site- or service-specific boards compared with roles of a regional health board

- Successes and challenges of regional governance

- Ways provincial policies affect functioning of regional health boards

- The relationships of health service providers and stakeholders to health boards

- Relationships between regional health boards and first-level or middle managers in relation to the board's strategic directions, monitoring, and linkage with stakeholders

In this chapter, differences between the governance and management functions of health agencies are described. The roles of governing boards will be explored. The role of traditional site- or service-specific boards is contrasted with the role of regional health boards in relation to scope of governance, membership, and the relationship between the boards and the agencies. The influence of provincial policies on regional health boards and the advantages and disadvantages of regional governance will be described. Nurse managers are affected by regional health boards, but they also have opportunities to influence them. A goal for the reorganized system is the two-way exchange of information to achieve the common goal of effective planning of health care services for the future.

A revolution has taken place in Canadian health care, and the impetus came from governments, health organizations, professionals, and consumers. With health reform as the goal, there has been widespread restructuring and reorientation of health care delivery systems. Pressure for increased effectiveness and efficiency of health care services stimulated exploration and implementation of new structures and options in care delivery, and most provinces have implemented regionalization of health care governance in response to fiscal pressures. The approach in each province is different because health is within provincial jurisdiction in Canada. Continuing regional and hospital merger developments across the country require vigilant monitoring as each change has an impact on health, human resources, and the efficiency and effectiveness of the services delivered.

Governance and Management

There is widespread confusion about the difference in meaning between "governing" and "managing," which is further complicated by the fact that dictionaries use the words "control" and "direct" in both definitions. The secondary meanings provide more assistance. To "govern" means to "exercise a directing or restraining influence over" (de Wolf, Gregg, Harris, & Scargill, 1997, p. 666). To "manage" means to "succeed in accomplishing" (p. 912). A board of directors governs an organization and sets policies that direct what the agency should and should not do. The role of management is to implement the policies set by the governing board.

Many organizations in business, health care, non-profit volunteer work, and advocacy have boards of directors at the helm. Boards are common in both public and non-profit organizations. Generally, the public view is that organizations with boards tend to be less self-interested than organizations with only one person responsible. A board of directors distributes responsibility for the policy decisions of an organization among a group of different individuals. If there were no boards of directors, decisions would be made by single individuals as is done in privately owned companies. A single individual may not possess all of the information or perspectives that are necessary to make informed decisions, and judgment may be influenced by subjectivity. If, for example, the actions of an individual decision maker are driven by the prospect of monetary gain, the impact on clients, staff, or the mission of the organization may not be adequately considered. Groups of people can make better decisions than individuals, because the discussion is balanced and informed by various opinions. A group may also tend to take more risks than a single person, so innovation is more likely to be encouraged.

Almost without exception, boards of health care organizations are established under provincial or national legislation, such as the Non-Profit Corporations Act or the Cooperatives Act. These boards are required to have bylaws or constitutions that articulate rules for the governance of the organization. Such rules include the purpose of the organization, roles of the board and its officers, qualifications required for membership on the board, terms of office, methods of attaining a board seat, and expectations of board members. In some organizations, representatives of the users of the services are board members. Sometimes, people perceived to have a conflict of interest are prohibited from being board members (e.g., an employee of the organization, an owner of a company that does contract work for the organization). Legislation may also include conflict of interest guidelines, expectations for financial reporting to the supervisory body, and processes for dissolution or amalgamation of the agency should this become necessary. Accountability is clearer if a group has an approved set of rules of conduct and attempts to make its decision-making processes open to its members and the public.

Because most organizations are created under provincial or federal legislation, their boards of directors are legally responsible. Members of the governing board are accountable not only for all board decisions and actions, but also for decisions and actions of all staff and volunteers within the organization. Board members as individuals, and the board as a whole, can be held liable by parties who feel wronged; therefore, most boards hold liability insurance to protect individual members from financial loss. The member is protected if he or she acted with the best interests of the board in mind. Then, if a lawsuit is successful, the assets of the board or organization will be affected rather than those of the individual.

Role of the Board

The board of directors establishes what services will be offered, to whom, and at what cost. According to the classic work by Carver (1990), a board of directors for any organization has several roles:

- To make decisions on the strategic direction of the organization
- To monitor activities of both management and the board itself
- To establish and maintain linkages with stakeholders
- To develop and review policies to guide itself and the organization.

The board's primary responsibility is to articulate a purpose and vision for the future of the organization. It sets the strategic direction for the organization, establishing goals and budget allocations. To fulfill these goals, most organizations hire a chief executive officer (CEO) to lead and manage. The second important function of a board is to monitor the performance of the CEO to ensure that the organization is fulfilling its vision and goals and that the policies of the board are followed. The board also must monitor its own ability to function and follow board policies. The third function of a board is to establish linkages with other organizations offering similar or complementary services and linkages with the owners. The owners could be public taxpayers who may be users of the service in the future. The final function of a board is to develop policies and to review and revise them as necessary. Relationships between boards and managers in the organization arise from these functions of boards and will be discussed later in the chapter.

A major conference on Canadian health care mergers concluded that "a board should be the liaison between the hospital and the community, the public face that wins support from government, patients, the business community and the public in general" (Canadian Health Services Research Foundation [CHSRF], 2000, p. 8). Leadership by the board and the CEO is critical, particularly in times of stress and change.

Role of Management

The primary responsibility of the CEO and all management personnel is to implement the goals and vision of the board. In doing so, the CEO is expected to follow the policy and strategic direction set by the board and to accomplish the work of the organization within the framework of relevant provincial and federal legislation and regulations. It is important that the board and the CEO have a similar understanding of their respective roles and responsibilities. For example, they should agree that it is the board's responsibility to establish goals, but it is the CEO's responsibility to decide how to attain them. Board members should not be involved in the operational activities or decisions required to implement board decisions, such as hiring particular people, deciding which computer to buy, or choosing colours of carpet. In the same way, CEOs should not control the agenda for board meetings, determine the direction of the organization, or maintain relationships with boards of other organizations.

Because the boundaries of their roles merge and are often ambiguous, CEOs and boards must continually explore role expectations with one another. Effective governance relies upon similar understandings of each other's roles. The board informs the organization of its strategic directions, managers within the organization report activities to the board so it can monitor success, and there is two-way communication about linkages with other community providers. Organizations that have problems are often those with poor communication between the board and the CEO.

Traditional Health Care Boards

Historically, most governing boards in health care were responsible for a single organization that delivered only one type of service or a variety of services from only one site. Boards of such organizations have little difficulty in defining the services they deliver, to whom, and how, because the role of the organization or facility determines the board's purpose.

Scope of Governance

Most hospitals in Canada are owned by provincial governments or by private non-profit groups. Both public and private non-profit types of ownership use boards to govern the affairs of the agency. Indeed, most provincial health legislation requires that there be boards of directors and specifies certain responsibilities for ensuring quality care and stewardship of the human and financial resources within the organization. No private for-profit hospitals existed in Canada until 1997, when the first one was established in Calgary, Alberta.

Long-term care facilities in Canada are a mix of publicly owned, private non-profit, and private for-profit organizations. Provincial or municipal governments are usually the owners of the public facilities. In recent years, the federal government has divested itself of direct ownership of most of its health care facilities; hospitals and long-term care homes built for veterans have been transferred to provincial or local control. Religious groups or community-based groups frequently own private non-profit facilities, as in the case of long-term care facilities owned by such groups as the Lutherans, Seventh Day Adventists, Jews, and various orders of the Catholic faith.

Both publicly owned and private non-profit facilities are managed by boards of directors who are accountable for the nature and scope of services and for the stewardship of the resources within the organization. For-profit facilities, particularly if they are small operations, will likely be governed and managed by a single owner. In the for-profit facilities, one person or family may own a group of similar organizations (usually small) and govern them directly without a board, although managers may be hired. For-profit, long-term care facilities are more likely to have a board of directors if they are owned by a large corporation that is involved with several branches or facets of the business. Extendicare, for example, is a large corporation that owns both long-term care facilities and community-service agencies across Canada, and it is governed by a board of directors that acts on behalf of the owners.

The major advantages of governing boards for site- or service-specific organizations include the expertise of board members in a particular site, service, or client population served; a clear organizational identity that is a source of pride for both staff and clients; and an ability to attract both volunteers and donor dollars. A variety of providers in a community or region add depth and breadth to the network of social and health supports available and can strengthen the civic pride of local citizens in the community. Smaller organizations may also be able to respond more quickly to client or community needs, provide more personalized care, and be more creative.

A main disadvantage of having governing boards for site-specific or service-specific agencies is that a multiplicity of boards will cost taxpayers or clients more because there are multiple administrations. As well, there are often duplications in client programs (e.g., several maternity services within one local area) or in support services (e.g., several laundry or purchasing departments). Furthermore, governing boards of extremely small site- or service-specific organizations often face challenges in attracting and maintaining competent managers and staff because their small organizations may have fewer opportunities for career advancement. Another disadvantage is the human tendency to guard territory and expand both influence and control (e.g., empire building). This tendency means that the commitment of both board members and staff may be directed to enhancing the status, the number of clients served, or the budget of the organization. It follows that the vision of such an organization is often restricted to the site, the service, or the specific client group involved, and broader goals concerning the collective good for the community or the region may not be considered. The resulting competition is accentuated if each governing board has access to the provincial Minister of Health for funding. This tendency for organizations to be self-serving discourages cooperation, increases fragmentation of care for clients, and does not address gaps within the larger health service system.

Because of these disadvantages, most provinces are moving away from the traditional site- or service-specific model for health care agencies. By 2003, this model existed in only one province, Ontario.

Board Membership

Membership on many health care boards is open to anyone who expresses an interest. Boards often look for balanced representation, ensuring that membership includes both men and women and people from a variety of ages, professions, and work experience. Board members with an admirable community reputation may be desirable if fundraising is a major activity of the board. Boards that anticipate vacancies among their membership will often canvass friends and acquaintances looking for those who may be interested in contributing to the good work of the organization by volunteering to be a board member. When a list of interested people is obtained, the selection will be made according to the bylaws or constitution either by board vote or by a vote of the general membership of a non-profit corporation or cooperative. Sometimes, the board of a provincial health care organization is appointed by the Minister of Health through an order-in-council of the provincial cabinet. There are so many boards involved in the governance of health, social service, charitable, and sports organizations in Canadian communities that many boards consider themselves lucky to have the required number of members, regardless of particular ability and experience.

The vast majority of these traditional boards are established as volunteer boards, without any financial compensation to directors for the work or time given to the organization. Some of the organizations are so small and short of funds that board members actually perform the work of the organization for no pay. As an organization grows, it begins to assign responsibilities to employed staff, although the board role usually continues to be a volunteer position. Health care boards that have honoraria available for their members tend to be larger organizations with a high profile in the community, such as university teaching hospitals.

Relationship Between Boards and Management

Many traditional health care boards govern small organizations, some with annual budgets of less than $100,000 and only one or two staff members. In these organizations, it is almost impossible for the board not to become involved in the operational details of day-to-day management. In fact, board members may be required to do the work. The board may hire a CEO as the only employee, and then the board members will follow the CEO's instructions and do the work of the organization themselves. In this situation, roles between board and management personnel blur, become confused, and create many emotional and organizational problems. As the organization becomes larger, there are more staff members and more activities. It becomes more difficult for board members to know all of the details of daily operations. It is then easier for the board to focus on vision and goals and easier to give the CEO the independence required to get the daily work done without interference. Differences in size do not, however, determine the quality of the relationship between boards and management. Small organizations are just as likely to have good or poor governance as larger ones.

Regional Health Care Boards

In the last decade, all provinces but Ontario established geographic health regions governed by lay health boards. It was recognized that the delivery of health care services was too complex to be controlled from provincial capitals. Health care was no longer just illness treatment of the individual, and local communities wanted more control over services (Lewis, 1997). The governing boards of regional health authorities are responsible for the delivery of previously separate services offered in the region, such as acute care, long-term care, community health, home care services, and perhaps, mental health and substance abuse programs. The new boards were intended to increase efficiency and reduce health care costs by avoiding duplication in care and by reducing bed usage in both acute and long-term care. Another mandate of these new regional boards was promotion of local community services and increased illness-prevention initiatives, both of which improve the health of the population, thereby increasing the effectiveness of all local health programs. The purpose of a regional board approach was to achieve more integration and be more responsive to community and client needs through increased public participation in health care decision making (Wagner, 1996).

Although there are differences in the number of health authorities per province, as well as differences in their size, scope of governance, and structure, the Canadian Centre for the Analysis of Regionalization and Health (CCARH, 2003) identifies several features held in common by regional health authority boards:

- Autonomy and responsibility for the majority of health services in a region
- Appointed, or combined appointed and elected boards
- Responsibility for funding and delivery of community health services
- Responsibility for funding and delivery of institutional health services
- An increased focus on prevention
- An aim to integrate services
- An aim to reduce duplication and overlap.

Scope of Governance

Regional health boards across Canada have varying scopes of governance responsibilities. Provincial governments have the major responsibility for funding health care services, including physician services and drugs. Some services, such as cancer care and ambulance services, are delivered outside the regional health authority structure in some provinces. The major difference among the models of regional health care governance is the number of organizations that receive funding and power directly from the provincial government. In the territories, the transition from federal government control to territorial control of the delivery of health care services is ongoing. The Northwest Territories has had regional health and social service authorities since 1988. The Yukon is not regionalized. In Nunavut, the regional health and education boards have been replaced by centralized territorial control (CCARH, 2003).

The type of regional health board closest to the traditional site- or service-specific structure is the sector-based regional board. Within health care, *sectors* are clearly defined settings for service delivery. Major health sectors are acute care institutions, long-term care institutions, community-based services, and mental health services. A regional health board that is sector specific governs more than one site, but includes all regional services provided in that sector of health care. For example, New Brunswick established sector-based regional hospital corporations in

1992 to govern acute care services. At that time, home care services, long-term care facilities, mental health agencies, and services in other sectors were still governed separately, usually by site-specific or service-specific boards.

A variation on this sector model is a parallel structure of regional boards (by sector or type of service) in which there is an acute care board and a community services/long-term care board for the same geographic region. This approach reflects an attempt to give each regional health care sector independence in working out the difficulties of amalgamating its own site-specific boards. The sector-specific regional boards then negotiate linkages and common goals for the client populations who require services from both sectors. Newfoundland's first regional boards were sector-specific boards for institutional and community services. Sometimes this model was used developmentally to ease the transition from site-specific boards to regional health authority structures. In Winnipeg, Manitoba, for example, two parallel regional sector boards preceded the creation of a regional board with responsibilities for both acute care and long-term and community services.

In a nesting model, one regional board with governance responsibility for a wide range of health care services allocates money to another regional board that governs one sector of health services in that region. In 1991, legislation passed in Quebec created regional boards with control over both the hospital regional boards and the community health and social service centre boards (Pineault, Lamarche, Champagne, Contandriopoulos, & Denis, 1993). Thus, Quebec had a nesting model because two levels of governance existed.

The single regional health authority is the type usually associated with the regional governance model. In this model, the regional health board has governance responsibility for a wide range of health care services for its geographic population, including acute care and long-term care facilities, community-based home care, and health promotion services, as well as, in some instances, ambulance, mental health, and addiction services (Figure 7.1). The provinces of Saskatchewan and Alberta have had single regional health authorities since 1992 and 1993, respectively, although the services controlled in each province differ. A variation in the single regional authority model is a board with governance over other human services, such as housing or social services, in addition to health care. Prince Edward Island has been the only provincial example of this model.

Most provinces with regional health care governance actually have combined models in which there is a mixture of types of authorities. There may be site- or service-specific boards existing as affiliates that receive their funding from a regional health authority board. There may be site- or service-specific boards, such as large specialized teaching hospitals or merged acute care facilities, which continue to receive funds from the provincial government alongside the regional health boards in the same province. Boards of these organizations communicate extensively with the co-existing regional boards, and staff work closely with regional staff to plan and deliver client care. Another combined model includes two types of regional authorities with differing scopes of governance, such as large regional health authority boards with smaller more local boards, both receiving their funds directly from the province. These small boards have governance control over local services such as community health and long-term care. Some additional responsibilities may include conducting needs assessments, doing public consultation and education, and providing local advice to the regional health boards on

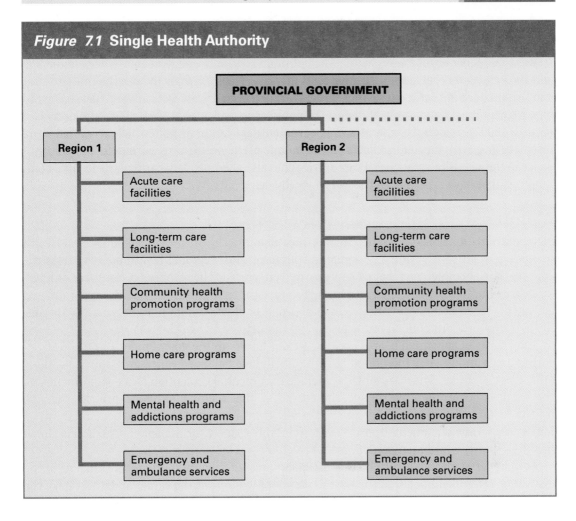

Figure 7.1 **Single Health Authority**

health service planning and evaluation. One iteration of health reform in British Columbia used this model. Some regional boards have created community health committees to provide advice on local needs, but without responsibility for governance; this model would be classified as a single regional health authority structure with advisory committees.

This pluralistic approach is supported as "the only sensible approach" by policy experts who have reviewed the literature (Forest, Gagnon, Abelson, Turgeon, & Lamarche, 1999, p. 3). They maintain it is too early to tell which model is the most effective and has the most public support.

How Big Is Too Big?

In all provinces and territories, there have been legislative changes since the onset of regionalization in health care governance. Arguments over the optimum size of a health authority continue. Most provinces have reduced the number of regional health authorities, creating imbalances in the budgets and power of authorities within the same province. Rural regions can include 10,000 to 20,000 people, while an urban region in the same province may include 300,000 to over 1 million people. The little research that has been completed on hospital merger demonstrates that bigger is not always better. The optimum size for hospitals seems to be between 200 and 400 beds. After that, administrative costs increase. Mega-mergers in both the United States and Britain have not achieved savings targets (or have even driven costs up) and have had trouble with decreased staff morale; therefore, responsiveness and quality of care have also decreased (CHSRF, 2002). Successive changes in government legislation or policy have triggered more restructuring, with inevitable effects on the morale of the health care workforce. Public confidence in the accessibility of health care services has also been affected, particularly in rural communities that have experienced the loss of locally delivered services.

Membership: Appointed or Elected?

Members of regional health boards can be either appointed by the provincial Minister of Health or elected by citizens within a geographic boundary. Most regional health boards across the country have appointed members. Many boards were preceded by planning committees or interim boards that were established as a foundation for the first governing boards. Appointments are usually made after consultation with local people or after a call for nominations and are confirmed by an order-in-council of the provincial cabinet.

Advantages of appointed boards include greater loyalty to the government's health restructuring goals and greater likelihood that there will be a balanced representation of genders, ethnicities, and ages. The disadvantages include the potential perception that appointments are the result of government patronage, the possibility that regional and local priorities will be less important than provincial goals, and public concerns regarding board accountability. A national resource document reports "overwhelming" support for the appointment of regional health authority board members (Forest et al., 1999, p. 14).

Advantages of elected health boards include increased accountability to the citizens of the district, greater likelihood that the board's decisions will reflect the values and interests of the residents, more community involvement in the selection process, and more opportunity for anyone interested in the position to run for the office (Orlikoff & Totten, 1996). Disadvantages include the potential for special interest groups to field and financially support single-issue candidates. Because elected members would represent geographic areas or specific communities, chances increase that a board might be dominated by people interested in only one issue (Lomas, 1997). In addition, a balance of genders, ethnic minorities, and ages cannot be guaranteed with a wholly elected board, and political issues may be more important than the mission of the organization in improving health. Whereas the government has the authority to remove any board member it appoints, the behaviour of elected members has no restrictions because the power to remove them rests with the electorate.

Regional governance in all provinces began with appointed health board members. Some provinces have tried or are moving to public elections for board members. A couple of provinces that tried elections have gone back to appointing members. In October 1995, Saskatchewan became the first province with elected members of regional health boards— two-thirds (12 out of 14) of the total members were elected, the remainder appointed by the health minister. Only 14% of the electorate voted in the 1995 health board elections, and only 10% in the 1999 elections. In 1999, 84 of the 127 positions were filled by acclamation ("Health Boards," 1999). In 2003, the government made further revisions to regional health authority boundaries and also suspended health board elections, returning to provincially appointed members. Other provinces have stated their intention to have elected boards in the future or have been silent on the issue.

Board Member Eligibility

The qualifications of people considered eligible to be regional health authority board members is another issue where provinces have differed. Sometimes, the only people restricted from board membership were the CEO, any person reporting to that position, and members of a provincial legislature or parliament. Health care providers and employees of health regions were permitted to be on the boards as long as they declared any conflicts of interest. This created some challenges for board processes and relationships when the health care providers and staff on one Saskatchewan board outnumbered the other members. In some provinces, health care providers and staff were specifically prohibited from board membership. There was a fear that, if health providers or employees were members of the board, they would have undue influence on decisions. As an alternative means of involving these people, volunteer technical advisory committees of health professionals were established to advise these regional boards.

On this item, as well, provincial governments have changed policy, depending on feedback from the public, board members, and government officials. Forest and colleagues (1999) maintain that trust and a good working relationship between managers and health professionals is more important in achieving board goals than giving these internal stakeholders membership on the board. Involvement of health care providers is recognized as essential for issues related to the quality of care.

Are Board Members Representative of their Communities?

In spite of the intent that regional health authority boards be representative of their communities, the reality is different. A study was conducted of the sitting members of regional health boards in five provinces during 1995 (Lomas, Veenstra, & Woods, 1997). The response rate was 65%, with 514 people completing the survey. The responding board members, who were all appointed members, "spent 35 hours per month, on average, on work for their board. Members were largely middle-aged, well educated, and well off. Only 36 percent were employed full time. Nine out of ten had previous experience on boards, more often in health care than in social services" (p. 513). Although the members considered themselves to be representative of their regions and citizens, their personal characteristics did not match those of the citizens of most communities.

Relationship Between Boards and Management

When a new board is established, the relationship with senior administration takes time to develop. Board members also need time to orient themselves to their roles and responsibilities and to the purpose of the board. A regional board must focus on major policy issues because it is impossible to be familiar with all of the detail related to service delivery. Management of organizational activities should be left to the CEO, and the board's role should be to monitor the CEO's effectiveness. The CEO is responsible for ensuring that the board's goals are met and its decisions are carried out.

The most difficult task for a regional health board is deciding priorities among its goals, sites or services, and special population groups and then ensuring that the budget allocations follow those priority decisions. Those decisions on priorities require knowledge about the health of the population and community preferences, information that is sometimes not available. The study of regional health boards carried out by Lomas and colleagues (Lomas et al., 1997) reported the following:

> The information for decision-making most available to them [regional health boards] was information on service costs (68%), and utilization (64%); the least available information was that on key informants' opinions (47%), service benefits (37%) and citizens' preferences (28%). Board activity was dominated by setting priorities and assessing needs, secondarily occupied with ensuring the effectiveness and efficiency of services and allocating funds, and least concerned with delivering services and raising revenue (p. 513).

Influence of Provincial Policies

Provincial governments have jurisdictional responsibility for health services in Canada. They create the context in which health boards operate through policies and legislation. Boards must stay within those expectations as the provincial governments are the major funders of health services in Canada. In turn, the provinces must ensure that federal legislation and policies are followed if they wish to retain the federal cash transfers and federal tax points received for health services. Each province has moved at a different pace in legislating health service restructuring, and each has tackled the aspects in different order.

The basic elements of provincial policy that influence regional health boards are described briefly in this section, with one or two provincial examples.

Vision

A vision is the perception of a future not currently visible. During the 1990s, visions for the future of health services were developed in most provinces. Provincial commissions or task forces studied their respective health services and articulated plans for the future. Provincial governments then adopted that vision, modified it, or created health councils to define health and establish provincial health goals. In most provinces, these health councils were disbanded as soon as their work was completed, despite recommendations that they continue as watchdogs during restructuring of the health care system. Saskatchewan, however, created a Provincial Quality Council in 2002 to monitor the effectiveness of health services on improving the health of the population. Health Canada has followed the Romanow Commission's suggestion that a Canadian Health Council be established to monitor and publicly report on the quality of health services and foster collaboration across government jurisdictions (Commission, 2002).

The provinces vary in how closely these visions and the restructuring reality are linked. In 1992, the government of Saskatchewan published the first of a series of documents for the new regional health boards that clearly stated why the restructuring was necessary, what the future system would be like, and how it would be better than the old health care system (Saskatchewan Health, 1992). Alberta followed its commission's recommendations to establish regional health boards but imposed massive budget cuts at the same time without articulating a vision or goals for future care.

If the provincial government does not articulate a vision for the future, regional health boards in that province vary enormously in their goals and priorities and provide inconsistent levels and types of health care services. When a vision exists, the regional health boards have clearer guidelines for both long- and short-term decisions. Consistency of service delivery across the province is much more likely where there is an overall provincial vision because goals and philosophies of those boards will be more similar.

Many provinces explicitly stated that these new regional boards would address the determinants of health. The challenge with that expectation is that the health authority, even with an expanded scope to include housing and social services, still has little control over societal factors like general poverty and unemployment. An additional challenge is that when funds are diverted from treatment services to "upstream" activities such as health promotion or community development, health care providers lobby strongly against the reductions in their budgets. Regional health boards, to keep their providers happy, often make decisions which support the status quo rather than working towards the provincial or regional vision.

An additional hope for the regional health boards was that communities would be empowered through increased involvement in decision making related to their health services. The reality is that many small, local health care boards have disappeared, reducing community influence and control. Some small communities are still in competition with one another rather than working together to address common issues. Rural-urban tensions still exist; however, there are opportunities and examples across Canada where communities, social and health agencies, and members of the public are working together to improve the quality of life and health in their area (Kouri & Hanson, 2000). Some boards are putting systems in place to enhance "citizen access to the board, board receptivity to communities and constituents, the capacity to communicate, board members' openness in addressing issues, willingness to take a public stand on those issues, and board flexibility in working with a variety of groups" (Kouri & Hanson, 2000, p. 29).

Jurisdictional Boundaries: Governments and Health Authority Boards

The autonomy of regional health authorities continues to be a "major bone of contention" across the country (Fooks & Lewis, 2002). Some government officials and politicians believe that the boards do not make good decisions and need to be under greater control. One way of achieving this is through specially targeted funding that must be accounted for separately from the global budget. Boards and senior managers, on the other hand, feel that the government is "micromanaging," telling the health authorities what to do with specific issues rather than establishing policy direction. Some health authorities feel like line departments of government and attribute this to their inability to tax citizens directly for a portion of board revenues, like school boards or municipal councils. A survey of Saskatchewan health board members found "more than three-quarters feel their boards are legally responsible for things over which they have no control, with almost two-thirds feeling too restricted by provincial government rules" (Kouri, Dutchak, & Lewis, 1997, p. ii). A prime example is the improvement of the health status of the population; it has been repeatedly shown that the determinants of health such as poverty, housing, and income have far more influence than board-controlled health services on that outcome. Forest and colleagues (1999) identify some principles of accountability for integrated health system boards, including relevance, public control, and self-administration. The self-administration principle is the one violated when governments begin to interfere with board autonomy.

Information Systems

Provincial policies and priorities related to information systems are extremely important for health services because almost all of the infrastructure costs for new systems are borne by the province. The commitment of provincial governments to the evaluation of health system changes is shown by decisions made to invest or not invest in a provincial health information system. The ability of regional health boards to fulfill their legislated mandate of assessing health needs and monitoring the effectiveness of programs will be determined by the availability of client-specific and aggregate population health data. The provincial priority given to health information system design and funding will determine how comprehensive that database is.

Technology has begun to change the way information is gathered and used in all fields. In health care, the most radical technological transformations also include how care is provided. The transmission of X-rays images and other diagnostic data over telephone lines is now more common. Telehealth technology makes expert services such as psychiatry, dermatology, and cardiology more accessible to clients and family physicians in rural areas. Most provinces are continually assessing their health information needs, the linkages required, and the type of infrastructure needed to support an integrated provincial health care information and delivery system.

Baseline data on the health of provincial populations do not exist in most provinces, so the impact of health care system changes on the health status of people cannot easily be determined. Health departments and ministries must decide which information is important if an integrated health care information system is to be centralized to improve access to client health information. Some provinces have even passed legislation to protect the privacy of personal health care information to prepare for the creation of large central stores of data. Every organization collected its own health information in the past. Clearly, policies on confidentiality of health records must be developed. Provincial databases on drug use, service utilization, and physician services have all developed separately, but they need to be linked for evaluation of system efficiency. Some health promotion activities take more than a decade to show results, so health system effectiveness may be proven only if data from the education, social services, and justice sectors can be meaningfully linked to the health data at some point in the future.

Most provinces have established research centres that evaluate health policy and study health care utilization patterns. Examples include the Centre for Health Economics and Policy Analysis in Ontario and the Manitoba Centre for Health Policy and Evaluation. These units play an increasingly important role in obtaining the information to support decision making by both regional and provincial bodies.

Funding

Methods of funding health care organizations determine how services are provided. Most provincial governments used to fund both acute care and long-term care facilities based on their numbers of occupied beds. That funding policy encouraged indiscriminate use of those beds. Clients were admitted to acute care on Friday, given a weekend pass, and told to go home until Monday. The bed was "occupied," and the hospital made money because no meal, housekeeping, or care costs were incurred on the weekend.

Provincial health departments used to approve budgets for health organizations in detail, line by line. More recently, hospitals have been funded on global budgets, although the previous year's utilization statistics may still be used as a basis for the allocation. This system allowed hospitals some freedom to move money between departments and support innovation. Unfortunately, many of these funding policies still compensated hospitals only for the provision of acute care, severely limiting ventures in outpatient, day program, or community outreach services.

Many people were admitted permanently to long-term care facilities before community support services in their homes had first been considered or attempted. These facilities may have been funded according to the classification of the "bed," as light or heavy care, regardless of the needs of the person who filled the bed. This practice created an incentive to admit people requiring very light care, whenever possible, to keep staff workloads at a reasonable level. If the province funded facilities on a line-by-line basis, flexibility across departments was discouraged; if budgets were global, more freedom occurred in programming during the year. However, funding policies tied to the total number of beds still severely limited the ability of a long-term facility to offer day programs or community outreach services for seniors and the disabled.

Most provinces now fund both hospitals and long-term care facilities according to the resource intensity weighting of client needs in addition to utilization data. The specificity and accuracy of this measure is not good, but it provides some recognition of the higher costs and resource levels needed for high-need clients.

Some provinces are funding regional health authorities using a "needs-based" funding formula. This formula bases funding on the population of a region but is adjusted according to several variables specific to health care sectors. In acute care, for example, a higher number of elderly people and women of childbearing age in the community will mean an increase in the funding allocation because these groups require more care. In the long-term care envelope, more money is provided when there are greater numbers of young disabled people and single women over the age of 65 years because these groups have higher rates of admissions. In the home care sector, the formula is richer for regions that must serve sparse populations over greater distances in order to compensate for the increased costs of providing service. Even though the model is more population-based than needs-based, this funding policy has given health authority boards freedom to allocate resources to areas of greatest need within each sector. The disadvantage of this approach is that it appears to reward health authorities for higher utilization of services and poorer health status (Lewis, 1997). To support the intent of moving services to the community, Saskatchewan Health established a "one-way-valve" policy that permitted movement of money from institutional sectors to community programs, but prevented transfers from the community side to prop up the retention of institutional beds in acute or long-term care. Successive provincial budgets and policies have supported the provincial goals of reducing institutional services and enhancing community services.

A complicating factor is that all mergers and reorganizations create immediate and direct costs, both in actual terms as services are consolidated and in terms of staff time and costs for retraining (CHSRF, 2000). Unfortunately, most provinces announced regional governance structures as a means of saving money and promptly reduced budget allocations for health services. This meant that health authority boards claimed to be following a vision for an improved system at the same time as they were forced to reduce services and downsize the health workforce. The cynicism created back then continues to exist years later.

Physicians

The influence of physicians is powerful because they are essential to the delivery of effective health services, but most practice outside the system, often in independent businesses. Because physicians are the primary gatekeepers to the health care system, they generate many of the costs. They directly control admissions to hospital, use of drugs, and use of surgical, laboratory, and some therapy services. Most provinces have a human resource plan in place in an attempt to control the supply and distribution of physicians, particularly specialists, who generate high costs to the health care system and tend to locate only in large urban centres.

All provinces have retained the direct responsibility for physician payment, even where regional health authority boards have been established for as long as 10 years. The most common method is fee-for-service payment for individual services. Physician earnings under the government health insurance plans comprise about 16% to 18% of the overall provincial health budget. Provincial medical associations bargain with provincial governments for changes to fee schedules.

Provinces vary in their use of alternative methods for paying physicians. In some, nearly all doctors are paid on a fee-for-service basis. In Saskatchewan, nearly 20% of doctors receive some alternative method of payment instead of, or in addition to, fee-for-service payment, including a combination of individual or group practice contract payments, salary, and per-capita reimbursement. (See Chapter 2 for further discussion of this subject.)

Regional boards are often preoccupied with physician-related issues because so many of the health services offered in the region are dependent on the availability and cooperation of physicians. Coordination of efforts and development of policies on physician recruitment, retention, and compensation must occur at the provincial level to be fair to all parts of the province. Physician payment policies have often reflected attempts to keep physicians content or to retain medical services in remote areas. Quebec influenced physician distribution by paying less than the negotiated fee schedule to urban physicians, and more than the fee schedule to rural physicians when both do the same procedure. Saskatchewan provided a one-time $25,000 incentive to physicians who established practices in rural communities.

Regional board policies also have an enormous influence on physician practice because health facilities and operating rooms are required as a base for many doctors to provide care. Surgeons, oncologists, and pathologists, for example, all practice primarily in larger regional facilities. Regional boards and management make many decisions that affect physician opportunities to practice and earn a living. Some of these decisions include acute care bed closures, summer bed reductions or "slowdowns," the renovation of facilities, new equipment purchases, and even the quantity of artificial hips or cataract lenses available per year. If physicians are not included in these decisions, their antagonism toward changes to their practice patterns may be communicated directly to both patients and the media. Provincial and regional health board policies regarding physician payment and practices have a tremendous influence on the delivery of health services. For health care restructuring to work effectively, there must be collaboration with, and cooperation of, physicians. Some analysts maintain that regional boards will not be able to control resources effectively or truly integrate services until they control the budgets for physicians and drugs (Fooks & Lewis, 2002; Lomas, 1997) or the fee-for-service system is abandoned (Lewis, 1997). Lomas (1997) makes the additional point that the wide diversity, numbers, and funding structures of community-based agencies make it almost impossible for a regional health board to effect any significant difference in that sphere. The coordination or integration of services within that sector is also complicated by the lack of consistent information about services or client populations. Most analysts, and all of the recent reports on health care in Canada, have agreed that additional money is required to achieve many of the goals of the health care system, including the integration of community and institutional services. Both the Kirby and Romanow Commissions insisted that the new money had to buy changes in how health care is delivered, not just more of the status quo (Standing Senate Committee, 2002; Commission, 2002).

Unions

Health care worker unions are another major factor that must be considered in the restructuring of health services. These unions are powerful, particularly if they are organized provincially or federally. Their mandate is to protect jobs and benefits for their members, so changes to the health care system are often mistrusted. Provincial policies and legislation affect the negotiations, jurisdiction, and involvement of unions in health care system change. Because approximately 80% of health system operating costs is salaries, a provincial decision not to fund a provincially negotiated contract increase has an enormous and immediate effect on regional health authority boards. The money for contract increases must then be found in existing budgets and by reducing other expenses.

Regional board decisions frequently have implications for employees or unions. Any decisions to consolidate services mean that staff positions may move to other sites and people may have new job descriptions. Any decision to reduce acute care or long-term care beds means that jobs disappear, in both direct care positions and in support services such as housekeeping and laundry. A regional health board decision to offer a new service or program creates new staff positions, but the board has to decide whether to offer the new program directly through its own employees, usually unionized, or to contract it out.

Because each site or health service agency used to have its own board of directors, there were hundreds of employers in the health care system. Since the advent of regional health boards and amalgamations, the number of employing organizations has been dramatically reduced. Historically, unions have organized themselves in local units that correspond to the settings or programs created by the employer in order to provide for the opportunity of face-to-face contact between employees and managers and thus facilitate the resolution of issues. Sometimes, the same category of workers was represented by more than one union within the same region.

To complicate matters, locals of the same union were so separate that sometimes a member from one site would not have access to jobs at a different site. If two different unions (or a union and a non-union site) were involved, the seniority of a staff member transferred to a different site to do the same work would seldom be recognized. These jurisdictional problems created have difficulties for regional boards that want to move programs, consolidate services, and have staff with the same skills relieve one another on different sites. Some boards and union locals have been able to negotiate letters of understanding, which enable some of these system changes to benefit both management and workers. Long-term flexibility for both management and worker, however, rests entirely with provincial government policy.

In Saskatchewan, the Dorsey Commission developed solutions to the jurisdictional issues in health care, and the major unions supported the process even though it was likely that some would lose membership. The recommendations of this commission established only three categories of workers in health care: nurses, other licensed health workers, and health workers who do not need professional licences to work (e.g., maintenance workers and office clerks). The first two categories bargain provincially as separate unions. The non-professional category negotiates as locals with each health region; the union affiliation will be the same within a region but may be different across regions. For each health region, there are only three union categories of workers, and all workers doing the same job in the same region will be in the same union.

Union jurisdiction will continue to be a problem in all provinces where a provincial solution to the multiplicity of health care unions and union locals is not adopted in collaboration with these important stakeholders.

Health Boards and First-Level Managers

The role of first-level managers is to focus on the delivery of services from a particular unit, program, or health centre. They have responsibilities for direction and supervision of staff, quality of services delivered to patients and clients, hiring and firing of staff, budgeting, and professional development activities. Their relationship to the health board is usually indirect. Only in a small health agency would a first-level manager's report go directly to a board; in larger institutions, it would be channeled through one or more administrators. Unit-level issues would only be of importance to the board when those issues are common across several parts of an agency.

In a policy governance model, the board role includes establishing the mission and goals of the organization, monitoring their achievement, maintaining linkages with stakeholders, and developing and reviewing policy (Carver, 1990). Establishing strategic directions for the organization includes framing the mission and goals and articulating values and vision. Monitoring the application of those values and the achievement of those goals is an important part of the board's accountability to the public and to the Minister of Health. The process of maintaining linkages with both internal and external stakeholders brings the board full circle, using the broadly based information obtained through those linkages to re-evaluate strategic directions. Figure 7.2 shows that the direction of flow and type of information are different for each of the three responsibilities: strategic directions, monitoring, and maintaining linkages.

Figure 7.2 Communication Flow Between Boards and Nurse Managers

Strategic directions	Board	>>>	Nurse Manager
Monitoring	Board	<<<	Nurse Manager
Linkages to community	Board	←→	Nurse Manager

With respect to strategic directions, the communications flow is from board to managers. Managers are expected to review all activities of their units or programs in light of the values, vision, goals, and mission statements articulated by the board, as well as to interpret them to the staff.

In the case of monitoring, the flow of communication is from management to the board once the board has indicated the type of information it needs. The best example is the budget because the board will want to know how money has been spent and whether it was spent in accordance with the values and goals of the board. Boards are also keenly interested in outcome data. The effect of the care provided on client health is the most important aspect to monitor but also the most difficult to demonstrate due to the multiple factors contributing to health status.

And finally, in relation to linkages with external and internal stakeholders, communication between board and managers flows both ways. External stakeholders include the general public, physicians, professional associations, the provincial government, and other provider organizations. Communication with internal stakeholders usually occurs through the CEO. Mechanisms must be in place to ensure that dialogue and feedback are maintained between the board and all stakeholders in relation to values, vision, goals, the budget, and organizational activities.

Conclusion

A major purpose of regionalization was to reorient the health care system away from costly institutional care to an increased emphasis on population and community-oriented services. In most provinces, little change has been evident in budgets for long-term care and community sectors, particularly in health promotion and mental health services. Demands for institutional services, particularly surgery, have continued to climb. Regional health authority boards continue to work towards budget allocations that are no longer based on historical funding patterns. Priorities for budgets and service delivery are increasingly driven by the population health goals of the board and the needs of the community. Regional health boards have the potential to increase community capacity and thus contribute to the community's overall health status (Kouri & Hanson, 2000). The delicate balance of power between government and stakeholders, including health care providers and citizens, is the challenging context for regional health boards in Canada today (Lomas, 1997).

Leadership Implications

To govern effectively, boards need to have good information and evidence upon which to base their decisions. Whether or not they have direct contact with the board, all managers in an organization or region are likely to be involved in the preparation of material that will be distributed to or discussed by the board. By understanding the policy-making role of the board, managers can anticipate the types of information that may be relevant to board members and which senior executives may request it.

As representatives of the community, board members have a legitimate interest in how the policies and operation of health services are serving citizens and how services could be improved. In their contacts with the community, board members may learn of the individual experiences and stories of recipients of health care and may occasionally make inquiries to management about matters raised by these stories. Managers may be asked to respond to such inquiries and, in doing so, have an opportunity and responsibility to place the individual's experience in a context of other relevant information. To be of value to board members, written information needs to be concise, factual, free of "insider" jargon, and oriented to the strategic plan and goals of the organization.

Although the relationship of middle and first-line managers to the board is usually indirect, resource people from the organization are sometimes asked to participate in board committees or committees attended by one or more board members, such as a quality council. In these instances, managers have the opportunity to directly provide information relevant to the mandate of the committee.

Summary

- The board of directors governs an organization and establishes what services will be offered to whom and at what cost. Management exists to accomplish those activities.
- A board of directors distributes the responsibility for decisions related to the organization across a variety of different individuals.
- The role of the board is to make decisions on the strategic direction of the organization, to monitor activities of both management and the board itself, to establish and maintain linkages with stakeholders, and to develop and review policies to guide itself and the organization.
- The traditional structure of governance in health care consisted of many boards for site- or service-specific organizations.
- Most provinces have now established regional health boards that are responsible for the delivery of a combination of health services offered in the region, such as acute care, long-term care, ambulance, home care, mental health, substance abuse, and community health services. The major difference between the various models of regional health care governance is the number of organizations that receive funding and power directly from the provincial government.

- Provincial governments have jurisdictional responsibility for health services and create the context in which health boards operate through policies and legislation.
- Regional health authority boards have shown some benefits by reducing expenses and duplication through integration of services, but there are still challenges related to structure, jurisdiction, funding, relationships with health care providers, and long-term impact on population health status.
- The relationship between health boards and first-level or middle management is generally indirect. The board informs the organization of its strategic directions, people within the organization report activities so the board can monitor success, and there is two-way communication about linkages with other community providers.

Applying the Knowledge in this Chapter

Exercise

You have been invited to attend the quarterly meeting of the Quality Council of a regional health authority (RHA). You are a nurse and the manager responsible for all nursing personnel in the continuing care division of the RHA. The Director of Long-Term Care and Community Services to whom you report has selected you to represent her division. The local press has been running a series of articles on patient and staff abuse in Canadian health facilities, and one of the board members wants to know if this is an issue in this region. You have had to deal with several incidents of resident abuse during your career, and you are considered to be the best person to brief the council on this topic.

Using the material on writing briefs in Chapter 30, draft a suitable paper for distribution at the Quality Council meeting. Identify relevant information you will need to consider for inclusion in this brief. Outline the steps you will take prior to your attendance at the meeting to ensure your brief contains the information the board members need.

Resources

evolve Internet Resources

Canadian Policy Research Networks:
  www.cprn.org
The Canadian Centre for the Analysis of Regionalization and Health:
  www.regionalization.org/Centre.html
The Romanow Report (2002):
  www.healthcarecommission.ca

Further Reading

Health and Welfare Canada. (1993). *Planning for health: Toward informed decision-making*. Ottawa, ON: Health and Welfare Canada.

Lomas, J., Veenstra, G., & Woods, J. (1997). Devolving authority for health care in Canada's provinces: 3. Motivations, attitudes and approaches of board members. *Canadian Medical Association Journal, 156,* 669–676.

Lomas, J., Woods, J., & Veenstra, G. (1997). Devolving authority for health care in Canada's provinces: 1. An introduction to the issues. *Canadian Medical Association Journal, 156,* 371–377.

Rachlis, M., & Kushner, C. (1994). *Strong medicine: How to save Canada's health care system*. Toronto, ON: Harper Collins.

Zander, A. (1993). *Making boards effective: The dynamics of non-profit governing boards*. San Francisco: Jossey-Bass.

References

Carver, J. (1990). *Boards that make a difference*. San Francisco: Jossey-Bass.

Canadian Centre for the Analysis of Regionalization and Health (CCARH). (2003). Retrieved October 16, 2003, from http://www.regionalization.org/Centre.html

Canadian Health Services Research Foundation. (2000). *The merger decade: What have we learned from Canadian health-care mergers in the 1990s?* Ottawa, ON: Author.

Canadian Health Services Research Foundation. (2002). *Myth: Bigger is always better when it comes to hospital mergers*. (Mythbusters series). Ottawa, ON: Author.

Commission on the Future of Health Care in Canada. (2002, November). *Building on values: The future of healthcare in Canada – Final report*. Commissioner: R. Romanow. Ottawa, ON: Parliament of Canada.

de Wolf, G.D., Gregg, R.J., Harris, B.P., & Scargill, M.H. (Eds.). (1997). *Gage Canadian dictionary*. Vancouver, BC: Gage Educational Publishing.

Fooks, C. & Lewis, S. (2002). *Romanow and beyond: A primer on health reform issues in Canada*. (Discussion Paper No. H/05). Ottawa, ON: Health Network, Canadian Policy Research Network.

Forest, P-G., Gagnon, D., Abelson, J., Turgeon, J., & Lamarche, P. (1999). *Issues in the governance of integrated health systems*. (Library Series Documents. Project PS-002-05). Ottawa, ON: Canadian Health Services Research Foundation.

Health boards need to be fixed. [Editorial]. (1999, October 16). *The Saskatoon StarPhoenix*.

Kouri, D., Dutchak, J., & Lewis, S. (1997). *Regionalization at age five: Views of Saskatchewan health care decision-makers*. Saskatoon, SK: HEALNet Regional Health Planning.

Kouri, D. & Hanson, L. (2000). *Exploring health care regionalization and community capacity*. (Regionalization Research Centre Occasional Paper No. 5). Saskatoon, SK: Regionalization Research Centre.

Lewis, S. (1997). *Regionalization and devolution: Transforming health, reshaping politics?* (HEALNet Regional Health Planning Occasional Paper No.2). Saskatoon, SK: HEALNet Regional Health Planning.

Lomas, J. (1997). Devolving authority for health care in Canada's provinces: 4. Emerging issues and trends. *Canadian Medical Association Journal, 156,* 817–823.

Lomas, J., Veenstra, G., & Woods, J. (1997). Devolving authority for health care in Canada's provinces: 2. Backgrounds, resources and activities of board members. *Canadian Medical Association Journal, 156,* 513–520.

Orlikoff, J.E., & Totten, M.K. (1996). *The future of health care governance: Redesigning boards for a new era*. Chicago: American Hospital Publishing.

Pineault, R., Lamarche, P.A., Champagne, F., Contandriopoulos, A-P., & Denis, J-L. (1993). The reform of the Quebec health care system: Potential for innovation? *Journal of Public Health Policy, 14,* 198–219.

Saskatchewan Health. (1992). *A Saskatchewan vision for health: A framework for change*. Regina, SK: Saskatchewan Health.

Standing Senate Committee on Social Affairs, Science and Technology. (2002). *The health of Canadians – The federal role. Final report on the state of the health care system in Canada. Volume 6, Recommendations for reform*. Chair: The Honorable M.J.L. Kirby. Ottawa, ON: Parliament of Canada.

Wagner, P.S. (1996). Quality management challenges in Canadian health care. In J. Schmele (Ed.), *Quality management in nursing and health care* (pp. 245–277). New York: Delmar Publications.

8

STRUCTURE IN HEALTH AGENCIES

Donna Lynn Smith, Hester E. Klopper, Anita Paras, and Anita Au

Learning Objectives

In this chapter, you will learn:

- The fields of study that have contributed to health services and nursing administration

- Highlights in the evolution of management and organizational theories

- Definitions and terminology associated with organizational structure

- Sources of complexity in organizations

- About the organizational variables of environment, raw materials, technology, leadership, and culture

- About traditional, matrix, and program management structures in health service organizations

- About structural sources of conflict in health service organizations

- Reasons why health service organizations are unstable

- About accountability within, and for, the structure of health service organizations

- How theories and evidence can be used to assess the appropriateness and effectiveness of organizational structure

Management and organizational theories originated in the early part of the 20th century as Victorian views of human nature, and their corresponding values, were combined with ideas from the rapidly expanding fields of engineering and manufacturing. By the 1940s, concepts and methods from the disciplines of sociology, political science, psychology, and social psychology were being applied to the study of complex organizations. As this continued, new domains of scholarship took shape. The foundational disciplines of sociology and political science contributed to the domain now known as organizational theory, and the disciplines of psychology and social psychology were the foundation for what is now called administrative behaviour. In the period following the depression and World War II, governments in Western countries began to design and implement large-scale social programs. The need for public accountability in determining the goals and values that would shape these programs, and a related need to assure that programs were meeting their political and practical objectives, led to the development and professionalization of policy science (Dunn, 2004). Studies of leadership began to be oriented toward testing and comparing leadership theories, leadership styles, and organizational outcomes.

Knowledge from these relatively new domains became the basis for the professionalization of leadership and management. The field of health services administration emerged as a more specialized branch of administrative studies in the 1960s and 1970s. In North America, the prestigious Robert Wood Johnson Foundation dedicated funding to advance the development of this specialized field, and graduate programs to prepare health administrators were established in major universities in the United States and Canada. Similar programs were established in other Western countries.

This chapter begins with an introduction to early management theories. The assumptions and precepts of these theories have had an influence on the way health organizations and the nursing work within them have been structured. As more recent theories and organizational variables such as environment, raw materials, technology, and leadership are discussed, it will become obvious that the structure in some dimensions of health care organizations has changed frequently and rapidly, while, in others, it has remained relatively constant. Unique features of hospital organizations are considered, including structural sources of conflict in hospitals.

Structure in organizations affects how work is done, how opportunities and influence are distributed, and even how organizational outcomes are measured and reported. It is important for leaders at all levels of an organization to have an understanding of what structure is, how it develops, how it can be changed, and how it interacts with other organizational variables and outcomes. A basic understanding of management theories, and organizational variables such as the environment, technology, leadership, structure, and culture, enables nurses to understand and influence organizational decision making and other processes. Since a central purpose of this chapter is to help readers understand the nature and effects of structure, a basic definition is presented here. "The structure of an organization can be defined simply as the sum total of the ways in which it divides its labour into distinct tasks and then achieves coordination among them" (Mintzberg, 1979b, p. 3). Traditional and contemporary theories of management and organization have incorporated definitions, principles, and concepts of structure, and some of these theoretical ideas are now highlighted.

The Evolution of Management and Organizational Theories

Writings on management and organization, in some form or another, can be traced back thousands of years (George, 1972). However, the year 1886 marked several important turning points in business and management history. In his paper *The Engineer As an Economist*, Henry R. Towne (1844–1924) proposed that the American Society of Mechanical Engineers create an economic section to act as a clearinghouse and a forum for "shop management" and "shop accounting." Shop management would deal with the subjects of organization, responsibility, reports, and the executive management of industrial works and factories. Shop accounting would deal with time and wage systems, cost determination and allocation, bookkeeping methods, and manufacturing accounting. The society would develop a body of literature, record members' experiences, and provide a forum for exchanging managers' ideas (Hellriegel & Slocum, 1996). During the past century, theorists have attempted to understand the most effective ways to structure and manage organizations. It is valuable to understand how management theory developed because current ideas about management often incorporate earlier ideas and conclusions (Mullins, 1999).

There are different ways of categorizing the theoretical perspectives about management and organizational theories. The approaches discussed here include traditional (classical) theories, behavioural (human relations) theories, systems theory, and contingency theory.

Traditional, or Classical, Theories

Traditional, or classical, theories are the oldest of the four principal viewpoints of management (Hellriegel & Slocum, 1996). The classical theorists thought of the organization in terms of its purpose and formal structures and assumed that people in the organization would behave rationally and predictably. They emphasized the planning of work, the technical requirements of the organization, principles of management, and the assumption of rational and logical behaviour (Mullins, 1999). Bureaucratic, or administrative, management and scientific management are two branches of classical management theory that reflect what has been described as a mechanistic view of organizations (Morgan, 1997).

Bureaucratic Management

As he observed the exercise of power and authority in Germany's governmental bureaucracy, Max Weber developed a theory of bureaucracy based on a rational-legal authority system. He recognized that the definition of tasks and responsibilities and the standardization of work procedures created administrative continuity that was uninterrupted as individuals entered and left positions in organizations (Mullins, 1999). The seven characteristics of bureaucratic management can be summarized as follows (Hellriegel & Slocum, 1996):

1. *Rules*: Rules are formal guidelines for the behaviour of employees while they are on the job. Weber (1964) argued that it is very important for managers to develop a well-defined

system of rules, standard operating procedures, and norms so that they can effectively control behaviour. *Rules* are formal written instructions that specify actions to be taken under different circumstances. *Standard operating procedures* (SOPs) are specific sets of written instructions on how to perform tasks or processes. *Norms* are informal codes of conduct that govern the behaviour of employees within the existing organizational culture. Rules, SOPs, and norms are the basis for discipline in the organization, and adherence ensures correctness and uniformity of procedures and operations. This contributes to the stability of an organization.

2. *Impersonality*: Employees are treated impersonally if the organization leans towards a reliance on rules. Since all employees are evaluated according to rules and objective data (predetermined indicators), the characteristic of impersonality guarantees fairness to all employees.

3. *Division of labour*: Organizational activities and duties are divided into simpler, more specialized tasks, and this is assumed to enable organizations to use their personnel resources efficiently.

4. *Hierarchical structure*: Most organizations have a pyramid-shaped hierarchical structure in which authority increases at each level of the hierarchy. Weber (1964) believed that a well-defined hierarchy helps to control employee behaviour by making clear exactly what is expected of each staff member.

5. *Authority structure*: The rules, impersonal supervision, division of labour, and hierarchy create structure for communication and coordination in the organization.

6. *Lifelong career commitment*: In a bureaucratic management system, employment is viewed as a lifelong career commitment. There is reciprocity in this relationship as employees are committed to the organization and vice versa. The organization uses job security, step-by-step salary increases, tenure, and pensions to ensure that employees satisfactorily perform assigned duties. Promotion is granted when an employee demonstrates the competence required to handle the demands of the next higher position.

7. *Rationality*: Rational managers are those who use the most efficient means possible to achieve the organization's goals. It is assumed that when activities are goal-directed, financial and human resources are used efficiently.

In the bureaucratic management model, individual employees are viewed impersonally and are expected to respond to the rules. Morgan (1997) has pointed out that Weber was concerned about the effects bureaucracy would have on the "human side" of society, and that, considered in their entirety, Weber's writings are "pervaded by a great skepticism" (p. 17).

Scientific Management Theory

In the early 20th century, Taylor (Morgan, 1997) defined the techniques of scientific management as the study of relationships between people and tasks for the purpose of redesigning work processes to increase efficiency. This approach involved careful specification, standardization, and measurement of all organizational tasks and appeared to work well for organizations with assembly lines and other mechanistic and routine activities. In the writings of contemporary organizational theorists, the term *machine bureaucracy* is used to describe structures that incorporate the scientific management view (Morgan, 1997).

Taylor advocated the following four principles to increase efficiency in the workplace:

- *Principle 1: Develop a science for each individual's work.* This implied detailed study of the way workers perform their tasks, gathering of information about the informal job knowledge possessed by workers, and experimentation with ways of improving the way tasks are performed to increase efficiency. New and improved methods of performing tasks were codified into written work rules and standard operating procedures.

- *Principle 2: Improve production efficiency through work studies, tools, and economic incentives.* This was achieved through the establishment of a fair and acceptable level of performance for particular tasks, followed by the development of a pay system that provided a higher reward for performance above the acceptable minimum level.

- *Principle 3: Ensure scientific selection, training, and development of the workers.* This process was intended to make sure that workers possessed the skills and abilities necessary to meet the demands of their tasks and that they were trained to perform the tasks according to the rules and procedures.

- *Principle 4: Divide work and responsibilities between management and the workers.*

Fayol's Classical Management Theory

Henry Fayol (1841–1925) was a French engineer who extrapolated from his experiences in French mining organizations to theorize about what worked well in organizations. He aspired to develop an "administrative science" with a consistent set of principles that all organizations could apply in order to run properly (Morgan, 1997). Fayol specified five functions that are still relevant to management practices today:

1. *Forecast and plan:* Examine the future and draw up plans of action.
2. *Organize:* Build the structure, material, and human resources of the undertaking.
3. *Command:* Maintain activity among personnel.
4. *Coordinate:* Bind together, unify, and harmonize activities and efforts.
5. *Control:* Ensure that everything occurs in conformity with policy and practice.

The principles of classical management theory are summarized in Box 8.1.

Many of the precepts from the scientific management and classical approaches remain obvious in the structural and supervisory arrangements for support departments and nursing in modern health care organizations. When the structural arrangements for nursing are contrasted with those of other health professions, it is readily apparent that much of nursing work is divided into discrete tasks through arrangements devised by administrative officials, as though the provision of professional nursing services were a production process in a machine bureaucracy.

Behavioural, or Human Relations, Theories

The mass production in American industry during the 1930s sparked radical social and cultural changes that resulted in a second industrial revolution. Workers did not always exhibit what the early management theorists had thought was rational economic behaviour, and they did not always

Box 8.1

Principles of Classical Management Theory

Unity of command: an employee should receive orders from only one superior.

Scalar chain: the line of authority from superior to subordinate, which runs from top to bottom of the organization. This chain, which results from the unity-of-command principle, should be used as a channel for communication and decision making.

Span of control: the number of people reporting to one superior must not be so large that it creates problems of communication and coordination.

Staff and line: staff personnel can provide valuable advisory services but must be careful not to violate line authority.

Initiative: to be encouraged at all levels of the organization.

Division of work: management should aim to achieve a degree of specialization designed to achieve the goal of the organization in an efficient manner.

Authority and responsibility: attention should be paid to the right to give orders and to exact obedience; an appropriate balance between authority and responsibility should be achieved. It is meaningless to make employees responsible for work if they are not given appropriate authority to execute that responsibility.

Centralization (of authority): always present in some degree, this must vary to optimize the use of faculties of personnel.

Discipline: obedience, application, energy, behaviour, and outward marks of respect in accordance with agreed rules and customs.

Subordination of individual interest to general interest: through firmness, example, fair agreements, and constant supervision.

Equity: based on kindness and justice, to encourage personnel in their duties, and fair remuneration, which encourages morale yet does not lead to overpayment.

Stability of tenure of personnel: to facilitate the development of abilities.

Esprit de corps: to facilitate harmony as a basis of strength.

These principles, many of which were first used by Frederick the Great and other military experts to develop armies into "military machines," provided the foundation of management theory in the first half of the 20th century. Their use is very widespread today.

Source: From *Images of Organization* (2nd ed., p. 19), by G. Morgan, 1997, Thousand Oaks, CA: Sage.

perform to their physiological capabilities as Taylor predicted rational people would do. Not all effective managers consistently followed Fayol's principles (Hellriegel & Slocum, 1996), and it was inconsistencies such as these that created the conditions for the development of behavioural theories. The turning point in the development of the behavioural approach, also called the human relations movement, was when Elton Mayo discovered through the Hawthorne studies that the informal organization, social norms, acceptance, and sentiments of the group were determinants of individual work behaviour (Mayo, 1933). These famous experiments at the Western Electric Company's Hawthorne plant in Chicago (1924–1932) accelerated the development and acceptance of the principles of human relations theory (Roethlisberger & Jackson, 1939; Landsberger, 1958).

The Hawthorne Experiments

In these early experiments, employees were divided into two groups: a test group, subjected to deliberate changes in lighting, and a control group, for which lighting remained constant throughout the experiment (Hellriegel & Slocum, 1996). When lighting conditions for the test group were improved, the group's productivity increased, as expected. However, the engineers were surprised by a similar jump in productivity when the lighting for the test group was reduced to the point of twilight. The output of the control group also kept rising, even though its lighting conditions were not changed. Faced with these surprising results, Western Electric consulted Harvard professor and psychologist Elton Mayo. In a new experiment, Mayo, Roethlisberger, and Dickson placed two groups of six women in separate rooms. They changed various conditions for the test group, such as shortening coffee breaks and allowing the test group to choose its own rest periods, but left the conditions unchanged for the control group. Once again, productivity increased in both the test group and control group. There were no changes to the payment schedule for either group, so financial incentives could be ruled out as an explanation. The researchers concluded that the increases in productivity were not caused by any physical events, but rather by complex emotional factors. As employees in both groups had been singled out for special attention, they had developed a group pride that motivated them to improve their performance (Hellriegel & Slocum, 1996). This led to the important discovery that when employees are given special attention, productivity is likely to change regardless of whether working conditions change. This phenomenon became known as the Hawthorne effect.

These and related experiments gave rise to the human relations movement which emphasizes that when managers behave toward workers in ways that elicit their cooperation, productivity may increase. Maslow's widely accepted theory of a hierarchy of human needs provided a foundation for the development of human relations theories of management (Morgan, 1997).

The Motivation-Hygiene Theory

The motivation-hygiene theory described by Frederick Herzberg in 1959 classifies *motivational factors*, such as achievement, recognition, the work itself, responsibility, and advancement, as *job satisfiers* because they are more likely to motivate individuals to excel in performance and produce positive attitudes. The factors required to prevent job dissatisfaction were termed *hygiene factors*. They include organizational policy, administration, supervision, salary, interpersonal relations with co-workers, and working conditions. This theory has had far-reaching effects because many motivational factors are within the direct control of first-line and middle managers. Many continuing education programs for managers are designed to teach them to use interpersonal skills and adapt their own behaviour to constructively influence the attitudes and performance of those they supervise and work with.

McGregor's Theory X and Y

Another well-known human relations theory influenced by organizational psychologists Maslow, Herzberg, and others was McGregor's "Theory X and Y" (McGregor, 1957). *Theory X* is the term used to describe a set of negative assumptions about human nature and managerial responsibilities. The *Theory X* perspective incorporates a negative view of human nature, assuming that most people are inherently lazy and unambitious and that managers must assure workforce productivity by either the promise of reward or the threat of punishment. McGregor proposed alternative managerial assumptions and practices that emphasized releasing potential, encouraging growth, removing obstacles, creating opportunities, and providing guidance. These propositions, described as *Theory Y*, provided for a more humanistic approach and popularized a participatory style of management. Other major contributions to the human relations approach led to research into different systems of management, organizational learning, and effective leadership styles.

Managerial Roles

Additional insights into the nature and importance of various managerial roles and functions arose from the research of Dr. Henry Mintzberg based at McGill University. Roles have been defined as organized sets of behaviours (Hellriegel & Slocum, 1996). Mintzberg concluded that 10 common managerial roles could be classified into three categories: interpersonal, informational, and decisional, as summarized in Table 8.1.

These managerial roles are interdependent and may be enacted simultaneously (Hellriegel & Slocum, 1996). For example, a nursing manager may disseminate information to staff in her program or to more senior managers, allocate human resources through staffing and scheduling, or liaise with staff, patients, families, and colleagues from other disciplines. She thus fulfills the figurehead role, representing the organization to the public and to the staff. Mintzberg's theoretical ideas have been used to structure many studies about the roles of nursing managers.

Much of the contemporary continuing education for leadership and management continues to focus on the application of human relations theories, emphasizing the application of interpersonal and management skills in order to convey respect for employees, encourage involvement and participation, practice effective coaching and mentoring, and meaningfully involve them in change management and quality improvement processes. Human relations theories

Table 8.1 Managerial Roles		
Interpersonal Roles	**Informational Roles**	**Decisional Roles**
■ Figurehead	■ Monitor	■ Entrepreneur
■ Leader	■ Disseminator	■ Disturbance handler
■ Liaison	■ Spokesperson	■ Resource allocator
		■ Negotiator

help to explain and validate many issues and concerns of nursing mangers today, such as retention, job satisfaction, effective communication, empowerment, and leadership.

Systems Theory

Systems theory was proposed in the 1940s by the biologist Ludwig von Bertalanffy who applied metaphors and ideas from the biological sciences to the analysis of organizations. This approach can be contrasted with the classical theories that emphasized the requirements of the organization, and with the human relations theories that focused on the psychological and social aspects of the employee in the organization. Within the systems perspective, organizations are perceived as sets of "interacting subsystems" (Morgan, 1997, p. 43).

A helpful introduction to the core concepts of systems theory is provided by Hellriegel and Slocum. They explain that an organization is an association of interrelated and interdependent teams, departments, and levels that are linked to achieve the organization's goals. The systems viewpoint is an approach to solving problems by diagnosing them within a framework of inputs, transformation processes, outputs, and feedback (Hellriegel & Slocum, 1996). The system involved can be an individual, a work group, a department, or an entire organization. *Inputs* are defined as the physical, human, material, financial, and information resources that enter the transformation process. At the input stage, an organization acquires resources from the environment. *Transformation processes* (also referred to as the conversion stage) comprise the technologies used in the organization (Hellriegel & Slocum, 1996). At the *output* stage, the organization releases its goods or services to the environment. *Feedback*, or information about the performance of the organization, provides guidance for ongoing actions and decisions.

There is potential for constant exchange between organizations and their environments. As Charns and Schaefer (1983) observe, "What happens outside affects a health care organization. In turn, what a health care organization does or fails to do exerts an influence on its external environment: its community, region, or possibly the entire nation" (pp. 8–9). A *closed system* limits its interactions with the environment and is self-limiting. In contrast, an *open system* interacts with the environment to survive. The extent to which an organization depends on and interacts with its environment determines the degree of its openness. Systems that do not interact with their environment can be expected to *entropy* or reach limits. There are very few, if any, totally closed social organizations. It has been hypothesized that systems tend to seek balance with their environments and that there is an optimum size for a system. This recognition has contributed to the development of the strategic management approach that is discussed in more detail in Chapter 10.

One of the tools of systems analysis is systems thinking. Systems thinking requires that organizations be viewed from a broad perspective that acknowledges the interactions of structures, patterns, and events rather than individual events. Individual departments such as human resources and finance, or processes such as marketing, production, and quality assurance, can be thought of as organizational *subsystems*. Because the overall behaviour of a system is more than the sum of its parts, managers need to see the broader scheme of things. This is sometimes described as "seeing the big picture," strategic thinking, or "thinking outside the box." The application of systems theory to modern health care organizations is visible through planning and evaluation activities such as environmental scanning, consultation with community stakeholders, needs assessments, and customer satisfaction surveys.

Contingency Theory

Contingency theory (also called the situational approach) was developed in the mid-1960s to apply concepts from earlier theories to solve managerial problems. In this approach, the particular characteristics, or contingencies, of each management situation or groups of situations are recognized. The central premise of contingency theory is that there is no one best structure and management viewpoints can be used independently or in combination to respond to the contingencies in different situations (Hellriegel & Slocum, 1996). This means the following:

* Managers must allow organizations or departments to organize and control their activities in ways that best allow them to obtain the resources they need.
* The characteristics of the organizational environment will influence the way managers design the hierarchy, choose a control system, or decide how to lead.
* Conceptual skills are needed to apply contingency theory in order to diagnose and understand a situation thoroughly and to determine the approach most appropriate to the motivational level and abilities of workers in specific situations (Hellriegel & Slocum, 1996).

An understanding of the contingencies (or variables) can help the manager make choices about which leadership approach is most appropriate (Smit & Cronje, 1997). These variables include

* the organization's external environment (its rate of change and degree of complexity),
* the organization's own capabilities (its strengths and weaknesses, including the knowledge and attitudes of staff),
* the managers and workers (their values, goals, skills, and attitudes), and
* the technology used by the organization.

Laurence and Lorch conducted important studies demonstrating that styles of organization may need to vary between organizational subunits because of the detailed characteristics of the sub-environments. They also demonstrated that organizational structure and management approaches should vary accordingly (Morgan, 1997).

Contingency theory has many theoretical and practical applications. For example, Kanter (1993) developed the Theory of Structural Power, which explains that work behaviours and attitudes are not individual or personal characteristics. Rather, they are shaped by organizational contingencies, including power and access to what she termed the "opportunity structure," that is, the ability to obtain power by mobilizing support, information, and resources within an organization. Kanter also studied the processes of adaptation and innovation in organizations. Her theoretical concepts have been operationalized in management practice and research, such as that conducted by Dr. Heather Spence Laschinger and colleagues in the School of Nursing at the University of Western Ontario. Practical applications of contingency theory are also discussed in other chapters in this book (Chapters 14 and 21). Contingency theory provides a framework for thinking about issues such as staff mix, role design, care delivery models, and the allocation of care providers to patients or clients through the work schedule or daily work assignment process. These issues are discussed in greater depth in Chapter 9.

Bridging Classical and Contemporary Theories

Classical, human relations, systems, and contingency theories were all concerned with organizational structure and leadership behaviour, and by the latter part of the 20th century, research and theory on organizations and management had become grounded in an awareness of the complexities of modern organizations. Contemporary views of organizations are informed by theoretical perspectives from sociology and anthropology, which acknowledge the existence of organizational cultures and subcultures. Morgan (1997) points out that the word culture is derived metaphorically from the idea of cultivation and the process of tilling and developing land. Therefore, the concept of *organizational culture* refers to the "pattern of development reflected in a society's system of knowledge, values, laws, and day to day ritual" (Morgan, 1997, p. 120). The realization that organizational leaders have a role and responsibility to develop organizational culture in the form of "appropriate systems of shared meaning (Morgan, 1997, p. 147)" arose in the 1980s and has had a far-reaching impact on organizational practice. The awareness of organizational culture and its importance highlighted the fact that the behaviour of executives and the way they are seen and experienced by others in the organization have the powerful effect of shaping organizational reality. As Morgan (1997) puts it, the strength of the culture metaphor is that it "makes people own their impact on the way things are and shows that it is their responsibility to change when appropriate. They can no longer hide behind formal structures and roles or excuse themselves for having unfortunate personality traits. From a cultural standpoint, shared meaning is all important" (p. 148).

Organizations and organizational subsystems differ from one another in variables such as their environment, raw materials, technology, leadership, structure, culture, and outcomes. When these variables are considered, it becomes obvious why health care organizations, particularly hospitals and academic health centres, have been identified as the most complex of modern organizations. The remainder of this chapter is devoted to a discussion of terminology, concepts, and issues that have a bearing on structure in health service organizations and the structure of professional work within them. Since hospitals and their history have influenced structure and management practice in all other sectors of the health system, the structural features of hospitals are emphasized.

Organizational Structure

It is challenging to explain and understand why organizations are structured as they are. Mintzberg (1979b) observed that descriptions of structure in the professional literature do not always seem related to the functioning of organizations, that is, "what really goes on inside the structure, and how work, information, and decision processes actually flow through it" (p. 12). All organizations have *core processes* or basic functions that must be accomplished to achieve the organizational mission and objectives. Core processes encompass the entire work to be accomplished, from beginning to end, rather than individualized job tasks (Robbins, De Cenzo,

& Stuart-Kotze, 1999). One purpose of organizational structure is to support core processes and optimize their outcomes.

The most familiar forms of organizational structure are the functional and divisional forms. A *functional structure* is one in which similar or occupational specialties are grouped together. This produces economies of scale, minimizes duplication of personnel and equipment, and makes employees comfortable and satisfied because they can "talk the same language." Since coordination occurs at the level of top management, the leaders of functional departments do not always have the opportunity to understand the organization as a whole or to develop higher-level managerial skills (Robbins et al., 1999). *Divisional structures* originated in industrial organizations in the 1920s to provide for the development of specialization and to standardize work process and standard operating procedures within functional units. Centralized support departments, such as finance and human resources, provide *horizontal* standardization of common processes across the organization as a whole. Robbins and colleagues (1999) state the advantages of divisional structures are that they focus on results and assure accountability because division leaders have full responsibility for a product or service. Divisional structures are also an excellent vehicle for developing senior executives, since the managers of subunits can initially be coaches for more senior roles within their divisions, and divisional leaders gain a broad range of operational experience in running their autonomous units.

Coordination in organizations is achieved by means of direct supervision, standardization of work processes, and mutual adjustment processes (Mintzberg, 1979b). As organizations become larger or more complex and their external environments become more turbulent, higher levels of internal coordination and responsiveness are needed. Other mechanisms for horizontal coordination, such as matrix structures, networks, taskforces, committees, and horizontal processes such as total quality management, have been developed to address this need. Table 8.2 summarizes various organizational design options, their advantages, and the conditions under which they are likely to be most effective.

Five prototypical organizational configurations have been described by Mintzberg and colleagues at McGill University. The *professional bureaucracy* is a prototype of particular interest in the health field. This organizational form is designed to enable professionals to work relatively independently of their colleagues, but closely with the clients they serve. Coordination is achieved with the development of knowledge, skills, standards, and professional socialization through the education and credentialing programs of the higher education system. Mintzberg (1979b)explains that in simpler or more traditional organizational forms, work and production standards are designed by the organization and enforced by its managers; whereas, in contrast, "the standards of the Professional Bureaucracy originate largely outside its own structure in the self-governing associations its operators join with their colleagues from other Professional Bureaucracies" (p. 351). The professional bureaucracy is designed to give professional specialists control over their own work.

Mintzberg also described a highly flexible form he termed the *adhocracy*, predicting that this form would become more common. Morgan (1997) notes that simple structure and *adhocracy* configurations are found, and tend to work best, in unstable environmental conditions where speedy decision making is required, provided that tasks are not too complex. These highly centralized structures lend themselves to the management of projects and innovations.

Table 8.2 Organizational Design Options

Structure	Advantages	Best Used
Simple	Speed, flexibility, economy	In small organizations during formative years of development; in simple and dynamic environments
Functional	Economies through specialization	In single-product or single-service organizations
Divisional	High accountability for results	In large organizations; in multiple-product or multiple-market organizations
Matrix	Economies through specialization and accountability for product results	In organizations with multiple products or programs that rely on functional expertise
Network	Speed, flexibility, economy	In industrial firms during formative years of development; when many reliable suppliers are available; when low-cost foreign labour is available
Task Force	Flexibility	In organizations with important tasks that are unique and unfamiliar and require expertise that crosses functional lines
Committee	Flexibility	In organizations with tasks requiring expertise that crosses functional lines
Horizontal	Speed, flexibility, customer focus	In large organizations facing complex and dynamic environments; when tasks require expertise that crosses functional lines; when ability to deal with rapid change is paramount

Source: From *Fundamentals of Management: Essential Concepts and Applications* (p. 185), by S.P. Robbins, D.A. De Cenzo, and R. Stuart-Kotze, 1999, Scarborough, ON: Prentice-Hall Canada. Reprinted with permission by Pearson Education Canada Inc.

The functional and divisional forms, the professional bureaucracy and adhocracy, and combinations of these can be identified in hospitals. Traditionally, nursing and medicine were recognized as core processes, and this was reflected in the organizational structure. There was a senior leader for each of these functions, reporting at the highest level of the organization. As these original core processes became more specialized, divisional structures were adopted. Although registered nurses (RNs) are central to the provision of hospital and other health services and have broadly based educational preparation, the structures governing nursing work do not typically provide for professional autonomy. The work of physicians and some other professionals is organized in the form of the professional bureaucracy. Models to structure nursing work as a professional bureaucracy within hospitals have yet to be adopted. Extensive research literature confirms the lack of professional autonomy and empowerment as a fundamental cause of job dissatisfaction and turnover in the RN workforce.

There is a need for coordination in all the organizational structures. The coordination processes of direct supervision, standardization of work processes, and mutual adjustment are now discussed in detail below.

Direct Supervision

The most familiar coordinating mechanism is that of *direct supervision*, in which one individual (the supervisor) takes responsibility for the work of others. The concept of the *scalar chain* describes the "direct line of command from CEO through successive superiors and subordinates to worker," and the term *span of control* refers to the number of subordinates reporting to a single superior (Mintzberg, 1979b, p. 9). The position of chief executive officer (CEO) is at the top of the scalar chain. The CEO is the direct supervisor of members of the senior or executive management team. Each member of this group, in turn, supervises other individuals. The concepts of *line* and *staff* refer to the type of supervisory authority held by managers. Managers directly above and below one another in the line of authority in the hierarchy, and who have the formal authority to make decisions and control resources, are referred to as *line*, or *operational*, *managers*. The positions of managers who provide specialized advice, and who exercise power through specialized knowledge and influence rather than operational decision making, are traditionally termed *staff*. Departments such as human resources and positions such as patient representative illustrate the concept of staff departments and positions.

Generally speaking, three levels of line management have been described. *Senior, or executive, managers* include the CEO and the small number of positions at the "strategic apex" or upper level of an organization. In traditional hospital organizations, the position of director or vice-president of nursing was part of the strategic apex. Managers or supervisors who direct and control workers in the operating core of the organization are usually called *first-line or frontline managers*. In traditional health care organizations, position titles such as "head nurse" or "charge nurse" described the first-line nursing manager. More recently, position titles such as "unit manager" or "patient care manager" have become popular, and it can no longer be taken for granted that such positions will be held by RNs. *Middle managers* supervise and coordinate the work of first-line managers and report to the senior level of management. In complex organizations, there may be several levels of middle management, including staff positions such as the internal auditor or clinical nurse specialist.

Standardization of Work Procedures

A second familiar way of coordinating work in organizations is the standardization of work procedures. This approach is reflected in the principles of the classical theories discussed earlier in this chapter. Work processes can be standardized by machines and also by specifying and programming the work done by people. If it were not possible to categorize, classify, and stereotype many tasks and operations in organizations, volume production or volume services would be impossible (Perrow, 1970). Therefore, bureaucratic organization is appropriate for some kinds of activities. For example, in materials management departments, the sterilization, packaging, and delivery of supplies for the surgical suite is structured and coordinated through a combination of machinery, standardized processes, and work routines. Workers are usually trained on the job and are supervised directly by more knowledgeable and experienced staff. When more complex work must be done, organizations have the option of proliferating rules and procedures to maintain control, or of using professional personnel whose education prepares them to do complex work and whose professional socialization makes them likely to be trustworthy in acting in the best interests of the organization (Perrow, 1970). Rules and professionalization are often used in combination. An example of this can be seen in the way that surgeries are performed. The work of anesthetists, surgeons, operating room nurses, and other assistants is coordinated around a series of repetitive steps for specific surgical procedures. Expert knowledge and discretionary decision making are required by each professional in their own realm of responsibility.

Coordination through Mutual Adjustment

The third process for coordinating work in organizations is *mutual adjustment*, which is achieved by informal communication. Mintzberg (1979b) explains that this mechanism is used in the most simple organizations, for example, as two people paddle a canoe, but it is also "the only one that works in difficult circumstances" in which "knowledge develops as work unfolds" (p. 3). He further notes that many studies have demonstrated that formal and informal structures in organizations are intertwined and indistinguishable. This can be seen in the earlier example of the surgical suite. If an unexpected complication arises, discretionary decision making by the anesthetist may determine that the procedure must be shortened or interrupted. In this situation, mutual adjustment will be the only process that can coordinate the newly emerging work presented by the complication and the need to respond to it. Obviously, processes of mutual adjustment will work best when individuals respect the expertise of others with whom they work and when there are established processes for collegial problem solving. It is now widely recognized that the absence of interprofessional respect, organizational norms, and standardized processes to support interdisciplinary teamwork is a factor that contributes to the occurrence of adverse events in hospitals.

Factors Affecting the Choice of Coordinating Mechanisms

A number of organizational variables affect the outcomes of organizations. *Environmental variables* are factors such as the geographic location, the external environment, ownership type, and funding. Another variable is the characteristics of the client population and the health care workforce, who can be thought of as the *raw materials* that are the *inputs* of health service organizations. The specialized knowledge and skill required to carry out the mission of the organization and its subsystems constitute the organization's *technology or technical system*. The variables of environment, raw materials, and technology have particular relevance in health service organizations and account for the complexity of such organizations. These variables, or contingencies, are therefore important considerations in the design of organizations.

Enviromental Variables

Health service organizations and the individual units or programs within them exist within multi-layered environments or contexts. Characteristics and issues in the external contexts of Canadian health agencies are discussed in Section 1 of this book. The features of these contexts have a bearing on the way organizations, work units, programs, positions, and tasks are structured. Environmental factors such as stability, predictability, and turbulence all affect structural requirements. Since the 1990s, the environments of health service organizations have become increasingly more susceptible to direct political influence. It therefore requires intense effort by the governing board and senior executives to manage the external relationships and the image of the organization. This changes the role expectations for other leaders and managers within the organization. The environmental variables of mission, size, and revenue sources are discussed in greater detail below.

Mission and Size

The mission of a health care organization is determined by its owners and funders, as represented by the governing board. Size and complexity of an organization are closely associated with its purpose or mission. A certain size and base of resources are necessary to achieve viability and stability over time, and without a critical mass of resources, organizational survival is in jeopardy. It is commonly thought that economies of scale, or efficiencies, can be gained when organizations are larger, and this may be true up to a point. However, research on hospital mergers suggests that bigger is not necessarily better (Canadian Health Services Research Foundation, 2002).

Complexity in organizations usually increases with their size. When organizations are very large, centralized decision-making processes are often used to achieve standardization and control. This limits the options in day-to-day decision making for unit and program level managers and also limits opportunities for participatory decision making. In regional health organizations, there are usually multiple sites, which would have previously been independent organizational units with unique features of identity and culture. In larger and more central-ized organizations, it is more challenging to sustain the loyalty and personal commitment of individual workers, managers, volunteers, and donors.

Organizational Type and Revenue Sources

There are three primary types of ownership of health services organizations in Canada.

1. *Public not-for-profit organizations* are publicly owned and accountable and have tradition-ally received most of their revenues from government sources. At the time of this writing, most hospitals in Canada continue to be public and not for profit.

2. *Voluntary organizations* are owned by religious or charitable groups and often have distin-guishing features that arise from the traditions and beliefs of the owners. Such organiza-tions originally developed in response to social needs and were often particularly concerned with vulnerable or underserved populations. In the past, such organizations have often been leaders in health system innovation, raising and investing their own funds to champion community needs. More recently, voluntary organizations have become reliant on government funding to achieve their objectives, and many are now indistin-guishable from public or private organizations except for their religious insignia and state-ments of philosophy. Many nursing homes and some hospitals in Canada are voluntary organizations. The Victorian Order of Nurses is an example of a non-sectarian voluntary health care organization.

3. *Private for-profit organizations* exist to make profit for owners and shareholders. Many are directly subsidized by government funds or receive predictable revenues through long-term government contracts. For example, they may be contracted to perform diagnostic services such as MRI examinations for government agencies such as Workers Compensation Boards, or they may receive subsidized operating grants or long-term con-tracts that guarantee government revenue for each occupied bed, as in the case of privately owned nursing homes. Some private for-profit health organizations are small businesses owned by a family or corporation, such as individual or group physician practices, owner-operated pharmacies, some physiotherapy practices, and nursing or home care agencies. Other private for-profit organizations are large internationally owned companies that are traded on the stock exchange, whose mission is to make profit for shareholders. Many nursing homes and seniors housing organizations in Canada are owned by for-profit organizations. Diagnostic facilities, such as private MRI clinics; surgical facilities for cataract surgery and other eye care; laboratory services; and some community or home care services are other Canadian examples of for-profit organizations. Some hospitals are also privately owned, and this matter remains controversial.

Raw Materials and Technology

The human inputs of patients, clients, staff, and other stakeholders are a source of complexity in organizations and are referred to as *raw materials* in some theories. The term *technology*, as it is used in organization design theory, refers to the nature of the work to be done and the knowledge and skills required to do the work. Mintzberg (1979b) points out that the concept of technology is very broad and prefers the term *technical system*, which can be described in terms of several dimensions, including the rate of change and how easily the work can be divided into smaller technical systems. The dimension of *regulation* describes the influence of the technical system on the work of people and, particularly, the extent to which work is controlled or regulated by instruments, or vice versa. The dimension of *sophistication* describes the complexity or intricateness of the technical system, that is, how easy or difficult it is to understand.

When the human inputs or raw materials are known, similar and predictable task-oriented roles, work assignments, and assembly line production processes may be appropriate and effective. When work is non-routine and there is more uncertainty, workers' roles need to be more flexible and autonomous so that they can readily apply their specialized knowledge, problem solving, and interpersonal skill (Perrow, 1973). It is advisable to hire knowledge workers (i.e., professionals and specialists) to do complex and non-routine work because their education prepares them to engage in an "unanalyzable search" for a succession of new and complex problems (Perrow, 1970).

The people who constitute the raw materials of health service organizations are unique and have varying degrees of similarity and predictability over time. Therefore, organizational structure must accommodate complex and readily adaptable work technologies required to deliver clinical care and make non-routine clinical decisions in a timely fashion. As illustrated in Table 8.3, the level of discretionary decision making in health agencies is a dimension of work technology that is determined by the characteristics of patients and the nature of their health problems.

The nature of work and the knowledge and problem-solving skills required to perform it are contingencies to be considered as policy decisions about organizational structure are being made. Decisions about organizational structure have financial consequences. If role descriptions and the organizational context and culture do not enable and encourage the autonomy and empowerment of knowledge workers such as RNs, the value that can be gained by employing them is lost.

Public criticism of health services has often centred on issues of depersonalization, the experience of being in an assembly line, fragmentation or discontinuity of care processes, and errors

Table 8.3 Determinants of Discretionary Decision Making in Health Agencies		
	Few Exceptions (uniform and stable)	**Many Exceptions (non-uniform and stable)**
Unanalyzable Search (not well understood)		Elite psychiatric agency
Analyzable Search (well understood)	Custodial institutions, vocational training	

Source: Adapted from *Organizational Analysis: A Sociological View* (pp. 78–79), by C. Perrow, 1970, Belmont, CA: Wadsworth.

arising from inadequate communication among individuals, professions, departments, and agencies. Patients and employers expect nurses to individualize care and to respond appropriately to unexpected clinical and organizational occurrences. Paradoxically, the work of RNs is often structured by administrative officials through specific task assignments and rigid work schedules designed to substitute one nurse for another. This issue is discussed in more detail in Chapter 9. The growing research literature that links magnet hospital characteristics and RN availability to hospital outcomes provides evidence to support the view that designing more appropriate roles and structural arrangements for RNs would reduce mortality and adverse occurrences in hospitals. This would also be more closely aligned with public expectations of the health system. Rachlis (2004)directly addressed this issue in his book about innovations that can improve the Canadian health system. In a chapter entitled "Reengineering for Excellence," one section is subtitled "Extra! Extra! Researchers Discover the Obvious! Nurses Are Good for Your Health!" (p. 343).

Leadership

The leadership of organizations is another variable that affects structure and organizational outcomes. The interdependent roles of the CEO and other administrators are summarized in Table 8.1 (Kovner, 1984a; Mintzberg, 1982). Studies of managers have shown that their work tends to be "at an unrelenting pace; activities are characterized by brevity, variety, and discontinuity; managers are strongly oriented to action and dislike reflective activities" (Mintzberg, 1982, p. 32). Managers prefer verbal communication and tend not to write information down, and decision making and information processing occur within the manager's head (Mintzberg, 1982). Usually, the manager is working with "informal and soft data" (Morlock & Nathanson, 1983, p. 45). Employees expect that administrators will make quick and wise decisions and be aware of employees' needs (Snook, 1981b).

As health care delivery became more complex, the expert and positional power of the CEO increased, particularly during the 1970s. The CEO became part of the hospital board (Morlock & Nathanson, 1983), and control over resources shifted to management (Schulz & Johnson, 1990c). In modern health service organizations, the CEO manages many complex relationships. She or he is the individual most directly responsible for creating and influencing the norms, culture, and structure of the organization. The CEO is expected to be responsive to the community in which the hospital functions (Harvey, 1982), and by ignoring problems and needs of the organization, becomes "less and less able to creatively respond to the needs of constituents" (Veninga, 1982a, p. 51). In particular, the CEO is supposed "to help move the organization to meet the health needs of the community; that is, to improve access to health services, improve quality of service, [and] contain costs" (Schulz & Johnson, 1990a, p. 109).

The CEO has been described as the conscience of the organization, who must support managers and provide "an overriding and consistent personal values–driven leadership" (Schulz & Johnson, 1990d, p. 319). The values and behaviour of the CEO exemplify and informally communicate the norms and culture of the organization (Morgan, 1997). These can be thought of as an invisible infrastructure of values that set the tone for the way mutual accommodation processes will occur in the complex organizational environment.

Leadership Competence

Textbooks on health services administration describe the skills needed to become a competent executive manager. These include the ability to control structure and process, develop well-functioning teams, link executives to constituents, articulate values, direct communication, and increase physicians' and nurses' participation in decision making (Scott & Shortell, 1983). Competent administrators "think in terms of the interests and needs of consumers" (Veninga, 1982c, p. 12) and create healthy work environments characterized by a sense of "belonging, respect, and achievement" (p. 13). The Canadian College of Health Service Executives has specified expected competencies for health service managers. The designation Certified Health Executive (CHE) indicates that an individual has passed a national examination designed to test these competencies.

Administrators need to coordinate both physicians and employed staff and include these people in decisions that affect job satisfaction (Schulz & Johnson, 1990c). It is also important that administrators be able to solve conflicts within departments that might include many staff because conflicts affect the delivery of patient care (Veninga, 1982b).

Coordination and cooperation may be enhanced when committees are used to make decisions. Certain hospital committees are required by legislation and regulations. In other cases, executive managers or their designates establish committees. In these instances, they are accountable for structuring the terms of reference and scope of authority for the committee, as well as its membership. Committee work requires the investment of organizational resources and can be time-consuming. Resources are wasted when committee decisions are made out of politeness or because one faction dominates another (Haimann, 1991a).

Communication is a vital skill for administrators and may be compromised by stereotyping, suspicion, a lack of understanding of professional values and processes, the use of professional jargon, contradictory nonverbal cues, and status differences (Veninga, 1982b). Communication moves in four directions: downward, usually directive; upward, to a higher level; horizontal, across departments; and diagonal, from one level of one department to another level in another department (Haimann, 1991b). Although much of administrative communication is verbal, appropriate written communication is expected of executive managers. Written words have a formality that is often lacking in oral communication, provide a permanent record, and are usually more accurate and effective when communication with many people is necessary (Haimann, 1991b). Administrators have been advised to keep written files to protect themselves when dealing with physician complaints (Kovner, 1984b).

Executive Managers and Medical Staff

Managing relationships with medical staff is a specialized area of professional competence for health service executives. CEOs and their designates work with medical staff and the board in order to maintain "required standards of medical performance" (Harvey, 1982, p. 251). It has been suggested that a good relationship between medical staff and the hospital administrator is characterized by mutual respect, understanding and trust, and a willingness to learn from each other (Snook, 1981b). Physicians are accustomed to working autonomously with review by their peers and not by administrators. There is little guidance available to assist administrators in understanding the way the process of medical peer review works or what administrators should do if it does not work. However, administrators are accountable to the board for monitoring the outcomes of medical care (Schulz & Johnson, 1990a), and when there is a "violation of law, of medical ethics or morals, or of the hospital rules and regulations" (Snook, 1981b, p. 33), the administrator must intervene and inform the board. Administrators are expected to change physician behaviour in order to improve practice and to motivate physicians to support hospital organizational goals (Schulz & Johnson, 1990f). However, they are also advised to defer to physicians when conflicts occur and physicians will not yield (Kovner, 1984b). This idea is at variance with research demonstrating that when there was a perception of high physician influence, the death rate was higher (Morlock & Nathanson, 1983; Shortell, 1982).

Structure in Health Service Organizations

Policy choices about organizational structure are among the many discretionary decisions made by executive managers. Ideally, such decisions are governed by objectivity, rationality, application of theoretical principles, evidence, expert advice, and stakeholder consultation. However, they can also be unproven fashions or fads (Abrahamson, 1996) driven by vested interests, and political and ideological considerations. Executive level managers, and ultimately the governing board, are accountable for the outcomes of decisions about how health organizations are structured.

The documented official relationships of an organization are referred to as its *formal structure*. Organizational structure is usually depicted in a graphic format or *organizational chart* that illustrates the major vertical and horizontal relationships and channels of communication. Within an organization, individuals are placed in groupings for reporting purposes. These groupings may be based on common functions, professional affiliations, or on other factors such as common tasks or customers. However, as Mintzberg (1979a) has pointed out, there is no single basis for groupings that can account for all interdependencies in an organization, and each approach to structure has its strengths and shortcomings.

Matrix Structures

As explained earlier, mutual accommodation is an important coordinating mechanism in organizations, and the need for this process increases with the complexity of work to be done. Matrix organizations are intended to improve coordination or liaison between the separate functional or divisional units of organizations and to achieve "a balance of power between managers responsible for technical standards and those responsible for maintaining an adequate work flow" (Morlock & Nathanson, 1983, p. 255). There are two kinds of matrix structures: "a permanent form, where the interdependencies remain more-or-less stable and so, as a result, do the units and people in them; and a shifting form, geared to project work, where the interdependencies, the market units and the people in them shift frequently" (Mintzberg, 1979a, p. 171).

The principle of unity of command is violated in matrix structures because they disperse accountability. In some hospitals, "functional managers are in charge of their professional function, with an overlay of project managers who are responsible for the end product" (Haimann, 1991c, p. 133) in which there might be a traditional chain-of-command structure, but employees might answer to more than one supervisor. Matrix organizations are characterized by "delicate balances of power" (Mintzberg, 1979a, p. 170) and require that conflicts be resolved by "negotiation among equals rather than recourse to formal authority" (Mintzberg, 1979a, p. 170). Therefore, working in a matrix structure requires "highly developed interpersonal skills and considerable tolerance for ambiguity" (Mintzberg, 1979a, p. 174). More time and effort are required for processes of planning, coordination, and communication in matrix organizations, with a corresponding increase in administrative support (Kimberly, Leatt, & Shortell, 1983). Some matrices are permanently embedded in the structure of hospitals and others are added through the decisions of executive managers concerning changes to the formal structure of the organization.

The organizational arrangements for physicians in hospitals have been described as an "informal matrix" that results in multiple responsibilities (Kimberly, Leatt, & Shortell, 1983). Individual physicians are not part of the official hospital organizational structure. Nurses, in contrast, are employees who are accountable to their supervisor within the traditional organizational chain of command. However, it is taken for granted that nurses will also take direct orders from physicians regarding the medical aspects of patient care and answer to physicians for the care provided (Morlock & Nathanson, 1983). The literature on health services administration describes an "administrative triad" in which the organized medical staff is authorized to report directly to the hospital board, enabling them to bypass the CEO and other bureaucratic structures of the organization. The effects of this triad are far reaching and will be discussed in greater depth in the following section.

Organizational Structure in Hospitals

The origins of hospital organizational structure are found in religious and military organizations. Bureaucratic control of employed hospital staff has been presumed necessary because of the need to adhere to certain standards and to manage particular kinds of uncertainty. However, the arrangements for medical practice in hospitals have always been beyond the control of the organization for structural reasons that are explained by the hospital administration triad.

The Hospital Administration Triad

It is clear from historical and current literature about hospital and health service administration that a triad of groups holds the power in hospital organizations. The three groups are the hospital board, the CEO, and the medical staff. The existence of this triad explains why physicians, who are not typically employees of the hospital, have "substantial influence, arising from their exclusive control over diagnosis and treatment processes" (Munson & Zuckerman, 1983, p. 61). As explained in Chapter 7, the governing board is ultimately responsible for the functioning of the hospital and for hiring and evaluating the performance of the chief administrator (Schulz & Johnson, 1990b). Boards have the "ultimate legal responsibility for quality of care to patients" (Haimann & Morgenstern, 1991, p. 143; see also Morlock & Nathanson, 1983; Schulz & Johnson, 1990b; Snook, 1981a). A board must "establish, maintain, and support, through the hospital's administration and medical staff, an ongoing quality assurance program that includes effective mechanisms for reviewing and evaluating patient care, as well as an appropriate response to findings" (Joint Commission on Accreditation of Hospitals, 1982, p. 229). The hospital board is usually made up of individuals from the community. In the past, board membership excluded the CEO and physicians; however, during the 1970s, CEOs and physicians frequently became board members (Morlock & Nathanson, 1983). The hospital board is responsible for ensuring that the medical staff is providing quality patient care, including medical care, and has "an obligation to purge the hospital of inadequate physicians" (Snook, 1981a, p. 28).

Although the CEO is the most senior employee of the hospital and reports directly to the board, the medical staff, through the medical staff organization, have traditionally had a legislated reporting channel that enables them to bypass the CEO and interact directly with the governing board.

Medical Staff Organization

Hospital medical staff consists of physicians who are not employees, but who provide patient care within the hospital. It has been acknowledged that neither the board nor the CEO typically has much influence over physicians because physicians are outside of the hospital administrative structure (Georgopoulos & Mann, 1982). Although a hospital board is ultimately responsible for the activities of all employees and physicians and for clinical outcomes, the relationships of physicians with other health care professionals and hospital administrators within hospitals is an example of a deeply embedded matrix structure superimposed on all other structures of the hospital, and one in which accountability is dispersed. The board delegates responsibility for clinical care and quality to the medical staff, who meet these obligations through their committee structure (Joint Commission on Accreditation of Health Care Organizations, 1989 as cited in Schulz & Johnson, 1990f, p. 164).

During the 1970s, there were changes to hospital administration, and the position of a salaried medical administrator, sometimes called the chief of staff, was added to enforce medical staff bylaws and rules and regulations and to represent medical staff to the board and to the CEO (Morlock & Nathanson, 1983). In larger hospitals or health regions, there is now usually a salaried position of vice-president of medicine. Medical department or division heads may also receive remuneration for their administrative responsibilities. Although these positions carry formal organizational responsibilities, the incumbents usually maintain some form of clinical practice in the organization and therefore also belong to the organized medical staff. This structure carries the potential for conflict of interest, defined as a situation in which someone has two sets of obligations and meeting one makes it difficult to meet the other (Darr, 2002). The potential for a conflict of interest does not mean one will occur, and conflicts of interest can sometimes be avoided by disclosure and recusing oneself from particular decisions being made.

Supervision and Evaluation of Medical Staff

The board is legally responsible for the quality of care provided by medical staff, for selecting which physicians are given practice privileges, and for intervening when a physician does not provide quality care (Haimann & Morgenstern, 1991). Carrying out this duty can be difficult. Medical department chairs or chiefs of service have accountability delegated from the board and medical staff organizations for "all professional activities within the department. [They must] provide continuing surveillance of professional performance [and] assure that the quality and appropriateness of patient care provided within the department are monitored and evaluated" (Schulz & Johnson, 1990f, p. 165). However, if department heads are elected by the medical staff or appointed on a rotating basis, this prevents adequate supervision of subordinates' work and makes it difficult to hold the department head accountable (Kovner, 1984b). Thus, according to Schulz and Johnson (1990e), the quality of medical peer review is highly variable. Medical staff can be disciplined by the organization through the withdrawal of admitting privileges, but this happens rarely. Complaints about the practice of individual physicians are dealt with through peer review by the College of Physicians and Surgeons, using processes that are completely independent of administrative processes in health service organizations.

Medical Staff Relationships with Hospital Employees

The relationships between physicians and hospital employees have a direct effect on patient outcomes. When there is less tension between physicians and nurses, when physicians and nurses understand each other's roles, and when there is better coordination of care, patient outcomes are better (Scott & Shortell, 1983). Nurses and other professional staff expect to be viewed as colleagues rather than as subordinates (Schulz & Johnson, 1990c). Inadequacies in the medical peer-review process create tensions or problems of liability for other professionals and ultimately for the board.

Program Management

In the 1990s, the costs of health services became a highly political issue. Because physicians "drive" more than 70% of all costs generated in hospitals, they began to emerge as new factors in management structure (Lemieux-Charles & Wylie, 1992), and attempts began to involve them more closely in the management of critical resources, such as budget and staff allocations. In this process, program management structures replaced previous divisional and discipline-based structures. *Program management* is defined as a type of management structure in which services are grouped into programs by medical specialty, specific diagnosis, or population groups. It is therefore a type of matrix structure, but, unlike the permanent matrix dictated by traditional legal relationships between the board and medical staff, program management has been introduced into health service organizations through the discretionary decisions of senior executives.

In general, the RN workforce has been most affected by the introduction of the program management model. As one advocate of this approach explained, most organizations that adopt program management structures typically continue to separate and centralize corporate services such as financial management, strategic planning, human resources, and information systems (VanDeVelde-Coke, 1999). Most also have maintained the position of vice-president of medicine. However, in programmatic structures, the nursing discipline has been displaced from a traditional position of formal power and influence (Lemieux-Charles & Wylie, 1992). Statistics from the Canadian Institute of Health Information (CIHI) confirm that, between 1992 and 2002, the total number of nursing management positions at all levels in the Canadian health system declined from 25,458 to 16,681. This reduction does not arise from a shortage of qualified nursing leaders. During this decade, the number of nurses with graduate level preparation steadily increased, providing a larger pool of qualified applicants available to fill senior nursing leadership positions than ever before. Executive level and first-line nursing management positions were most affected by changes to organizational structure that eliminated nursing leadership positions. Detailed figures are shown in Table 8.4.

The former role of vice-president of nursing with line authority for management of nursing human resources and the associated budget has usually been eliminated. In some organizations, professional practice leader positions have been introduced in the middle management level of the organization. In this model, the professional practice leader for nursing holds a position parallel to the professional practice leader of other professional groups such as social work, occupational therapy, or respiratory therapy. Some organizations have reintroduced a senior nursing position such as chief nursing officer, whose role is often a staff position with policy influence and limited decision-making authority.

Program management is an intuitively appealing way of dealing with the complexities, including complex communications, inherent in professional coordination in hospitals, and many benefits of it have been promised or claimed. It is not clear whether it has had any significant

Table 8.4 **RNs in Management Positions in Canada, 1992–2002**

Position	1992	1993	1994	1995	1996	1997	1998	1999	2000	2001	2002
CNO/CEO	4,116	3,924	3,822	3,566	3,192	3,306	3,158	3,150	2,233	2,013	1,754
Diploma (%)	65.8	64.1	63.1	60.0	57.6	57.9	56.7	55.7	53.3	50.5	49.7
BScN (%)	27.7	28.8	29.4	32.0	33.5	33.8	34.9	35.6	37.5	39.8	40.1
Master's/PhD (%)	6.5	7.1	7.5	8.0	8.9	8.3	8.4	8.8	9.2	9.7	10.1
Director/Assistant Director	1,193	1,108	1,027	897	976	887	814	799	2,057	2,244	2,452
Diploma (%)	57.8	54.1	50.8	50.2	48.7	49.7	49.9	51.3	56.4	55.1	53.3
BScN (%)	33.6	35.2	38.6	38.9	40.1	39.1	38.6	37.4	33.7	34.9	36.2
Master's/PhD (%)	8.6	10.7	10.6	10.9	11.3	11.2	11.5	11.3	9.9	10.0	10.4
Manager/Assistant Manager	20,149	19,888	18,952	17,445	16,838	16,223	15,426	14,974	13,624	12,540	12,475
Diploma (%)	76.8	74.5	72.7	70.4	68.9	67.0	65.8	64.1	61.0	58.4	56.3
BScN (%)	21.8	24.0	25.4	27.4	28.4	30.5	31.4	32.9	35.4	37.6	39.8
Master's/PhD (%)	1.3	1.5	1.9	2.2	2.7	2.5	2.7	3.0	3.6	4.0	3.9
Total Managerial Positions	25,458	24,920	23,801	21,908	21,006	20,416	19,398	18,923	17,914	16,797	16,681
Diploma (%)	74.1	71.9	70.3	67.9	66.3	64.8	63.7	62.2	59.5	57.0	55.2
BScN (%)	23.3	25.3	26.6	28.7	29.7	31.4	32.3	33.5	35.5	37.5	39.3
Master's/PhD (%)	2.5	2.8	3.1	3.5	4.0	3.8	4.0	4.3	5.0	5.5	5.5

Source: © (2003) Canadian Institute for Health Information (CIHI). The contents of Table 8.4 is adapted from data supplied by CIHI. Used with permission.

impact on physician-driven hospital costs. Other structural arrangements for physicians remain unchanged. Their expert power is very strong, and governing boards and executive level leaders have difficulty controlling or reducing the costs of medical procedures, technology, and drugs that are driven by structural economic incentives, such as the fee-for-service reimbursement system. Because additional administrative and liaison support are needed to effectively operate matrix structures, it is counterintuitive to think that program management structures implemented concurrently with reductions in middle management positions will achieve improved quality or savings in the long term. Justice Sinclair directly attributed negative patient outcomes to the introduction of a program management structure at the Winnipeg Health Sciences Centre after he conducted an extensive inquiry into the causes of unexpected infant deaths there. He explicitly identified structural issues associated with the program management model and a lack of administrative accountability in this model as factors that contributed to the deaths (Sinclair, 2001; Paras, 2004).

Structural Sources of Conflict in Health Care Organizations

It has been suggested that the incidence of intra-organizational strain, defined as tension and conflict among organizational subgroups, is "produced by, if not inherent to the basic structure of hospitals" (Christman & Counte, 1981, p. 28). The main problem with matrix structures is that employees must take orders from more than one source and answer to more than one supervisor, which carries a high risk of conflict (Charns & Schaefer, 1983). It has been generally accepted that policy development in hospitals must maintain the "professional prerogatives of the physician and the integrity of the total organization" (Rakich, Longest, & O'Donovan, 1977, p. 194). Towards the end of the 20th century, it was common for medical staff organizations to have voting members on hospital boards (Snook, 1981c), and medical staff department heads became involved in making policy decisions (Schulz & Johnson, 1990f).

Tensions have traditionally arisen within the administrative triad. The most common tension occurs when administration becomes involved in clinical practice and clinicians become concerned with efficiency and effectiveness (Shortell, 1982). Kovner (1984b) noted that physicians might not always be aware of trespassing out of the medical domain and into the domain of administration. A second cause of conflict may occur if physicians want self-governance and administrators are expected to support that need (Snook, 1981b). Quality performance is best when there are regular interdepartmental meetings, department heads and medical staff are involved in decision making, there is less perceived physician autonomy, and there is medical participation on the board (Scott & Shortell, 1983).

Meilicke (1999) emphasized that health organizations are technologically complex and have high requirements for interdependence, pointing out that there is "a need for high reliability because the cost of error is so high that extraordinary means must be taken to minimize mistakes" (p. 90). One means of assuring this high reliability is the professionalization of work groups, but the autonomy of professional groups does not absolve senior management of the moral and legal responsibility for the actions of physicians and employees who work in health agencies. As independent professionals and as a professional lobby group, physicians enjoy unparalleled autonomy. Their social status also affords them a high degree of access to political decision makers on the boards of health service organizations or in government. Policy makers and decision makers have rarely intervened to directly control the costs of physician-directed care, to curtail unacceptable behaviour of physicians, or to address potential conflicts of interest arising from the direct participation of physicians with clinical responsibilities and entrepreneurial interests in the policy decision-making processes of health organizations.

Instability of Health Care Organizations

At the level of government, health care is rationed by means of price-based reimbursement systems that typically recognize only a portion of operating costs, such as increases in utility rates or salary settlements. At the level of health regions and individual health service organizations, the shrinking value of the dollar is usually dealt with by attempting to achieve greater efficiencies in operating costs associated with nursing and support services. The past two decades have been characterized by unparalleled experimentation in the structure and management of health service organizations. In their search for internal organization-based solutions to financial challenges, health boards and executive managers have eagerly embraced what is sometimes called a business approach to management. Organizational charts are drawn and redrawn, long-standing committees and other mechanisms for coordination and communication are abolished, new taskforces are created, and new departments, administrative arrangements, and terminology appear as the organization is "flattened," "downsized," "right-sized," centralized, decentralized, or restructured (Smith, 1992, p. 126). In 2002, the report of the National Steering Committee on Patient Safety in the Canadian health care system pointed out what seems theoretically obvious: health care is a complex and high-risk enterprise in which broader system issues can significantly impact the number and types of adverse events. This committee identified organizational instability and management experimentation as specific systems issues that are relevant to the study of adverse events, noting that "continual restructuring and non-stop change" compromise an organization's ability "to identify issues and implement timely and appropriate strategies to address deficiencies in a coordinated manner" (National Steering Committee on Patient Safety, 2002, p. 8).

Leadership Implications

The purpose of this chapter has been to introduce readers to key terms, concepts, and ideas from the specialized field of management and organizational theory. Theories are intellectual tools that have value in explaining, predicting, and evaluating the consequences of changes in organizational variables such as the environment, raw materials, technology, leadership, culture, and structure. Theories are derived from and tested through scholarly activity that includes vigorous debate of ideas, peer-reviewed processes of reasoning, and research. When used as predictive tools, theoretical concepts can add objectivity, structure, evidence, and rationality to the processes of policy making and decision making in organizations. As accepted analytical frameworks in the domain of published knowledge, theories also provide structure for reflection and critique of entrenched approaches and fads and fashions in organizational design.

The work conducted in hospitals and other health service organizations is performed on, with, and through human beings who present the organization with "non-standard" raw materials. The work of health professionals, including registered nurses, requires the application of specialized knowledge and skill, and it often demands discretionary decision making to deal with non-routine situations. Clinical processes require high levels of procedural accuracy, and the public expects accountability from health organizations and individual health professionals.

Some structural features reflecting the classical management theories that developed in the manufacturing industry at the beginning of the 20th century are still evident in the organizational structure and design of work in modern health care organizations. Matrix structures have the effect of diffusing accountability and are more expensive than other forms of organization because they intensify requirements for coordination through communication and liaison processes. A permanently embedded matrix creates unique organizational arrangements for the work of physicians and enables them to function within structural arrangements described by theorists as the professional bureaucracy. Historical and legal precedents have created and sustained the hospital administration triad. An understanding of how and why power is concentrated in this triad is critical to the ability of nurses to practice effectively and to influence policies and decisions in health organizations.

Since the early 20th century, when nurses first began to be employees instead of independent professionals, the structures for the organization of nursing services have been determined by administrative officials in response to political and economic contingencies. Traditionally, structural arrangements for nursing have not allowed nurses to act as accountable individual professionals who can autonomously apply their expert knowledge in the service of their clients. More recently, structural changes have interrupted the formal channels for communication and the maintenance of standards and accountability within the nursing discipline.

In the 1990s, changes to the traditional structural arrangements in hospitals were justified on the basis that better teamwork was needed. Program management was introduced as a new type of matrix structure. Although it could be predicted that it would increase the requirements for liaison and horizontal coordination, program management was implemented during a period in which middle management positions were being eliminated to save money. Another justification for the introduction of program management was that it would achieve control or reduction of physician-driven costs in hospitals. As program management was being introduced, the traditional structures and positions for medical administrators, including the role of vice-president of medicine, were maintained as before or expanded. It can be argued that the introduction of the program management model added to physicians' power and increased their potential for conflicts of interest if they continued to practice in a clinical and entrepreneurial capacity while assuming additional administrative authority in hospitals.

Safety and accountability in the health system have emerged as issues of the highest priority in the health policy discourse of the early 21st century. There is strong evidence from these discussions that the improved interdisciplinary "teamwork" that was to have been a result of program management has not materialized and that unequal power relationships and professional disrespect are factors contributing to adverse events for patients.

Until the 1990s, the importance of nursing as a professional function and core process in hospitals was recognized through the positional power of a senior nursing leader who reported at the highest level of the organization and who had line responsibility for financial resources and operational decision making through a functional and divisional structure. In parallel with the introduction of program management, the overall RN workforce and senior and middle level nursing leadership positions have been significantly reduced in hospitals. Some nursing leadership positions were maintained at senior levels with reduced positional and operational power. New staff positions were introduced in some organizations at the middle management level to lead professional practice in various health disciplines.

Nurse leaders in staff positions carry out important figurehead functions on behalf of their employing organization and the nursing profession within it, and they often represent their organizations in external relationships with professional associations, government planning committees, or educational institutions. However, they have limited influence over day-to-day decision making and the allocation of resources. They are in a position to advocate for professional standards, but not to directly make decisions to improve the professional practice environment. They may have the ability to represent the organization in efforts to recruit RNs, but they have limited ability to introduce the measures known to contribute to retention of the professional nursing workforce.

Downsizing of the RN workforce and progressive decreases in the number of nursing leadership positions at all organizational levels are often attributed to the nursing shortage. This view is contradicted by the fact that increased numbers of nurses with advanced qualifications have entered the workforce between 1992 and 2002. Changes in structure to reduce the number and influence of nursing leadership positions are a direct result of discretionary decisions by CEOs and senior management teams. Growing concern about organizational liability for errors may contribute to a reversal of the trend toward program management and the concentration of organizational power with physicians.

Senior nurses within organizations have been participants in and defenders of a succession of structural arrangements for the nursing profession within hospitals. They have often provided strong personal leadership to influence policy and maintain standards of nursing practice despite internal ambiguities and external pressures that affect the supply of RNs and the resources available to provide care. However, at the beginning of the 21st century, the loss of positional power and professional influence of RNs within hospitals is so significant that the ability to provide professional nursing services in hospitals can no longer be taken for granted.

The public clearly regards professional nursing as a core process. Euphemistic communication about teamwork can no longer conceal the reality that without the appropriate structural support for a professional bureaucracy, professional nurses cannot practice appropriately no matter how well educated or professionally committed they may be. Senior health system leaders now face an important choice. They must either acknowledge the growing evidence of the association between professional nursing services and positive health outcomes or assume responsibility for their decisions to deconstruct this service that is widely trusted by the public and valued as essential.

The nursing profession and individual nurses also face important choices about the structure of their work. In the past, they have often been marginalized in the decision-making processes within government and health organizations, even when individual nursing leaders were highly committed and effective. Nurses' unions have wielded significant power and have succeeded in achieving many economic and workplace improvements. Professional nursing associations have provided valuable policy leadership and have had significant policy influence, particularly at the federal level; however, structural problems and political factors have confounded these efforts.

It is daunting to reflect on how nursing services can be more appropriately aligned with the public's confidence in, and expectations of, nurses and with the requirement for appropriate work environments and structure for RN work. These problems must be resolved in order to realize the value of educational investments and assure the safety of patients in hospitals and other health agencies. More radical changes in structure initiated by nurses themselves will need to be considered. These could include the development of nurse-owned and -operated corporations that exist outside of health agencies and are directly accountable to consumers.

Summary

- Knowledge and theories of management, organizational structure, and leadership have developed from foundational disciplines, including engineering, psychology, sociology, political science, and anthropology. A specialized field of health services leadership and administration has developed since the 1960s. Theoretical perspectives from these fields of scholarship and practice can facilitate analysis of the structure and outcomes of organizations including health agencies.

- The structure of organizations is influenced by environmental variables, including mission and revenue sources. Within the Canadian health system, all three types of health service organizations (public not-for-profit, voluntary, and private for-profit) receive most of their revenues from government sources. Other variables of interest to organizational and management theorists include raw materials, technology, leadership, culture, and structure.

- Early management theories emphasized efficiency, standardization of production processes, and the control of employees, giving rise to an organizational form described as the machine bureaucracy.

- The model of the professional bureaucracy recognizes the value of professional and specialized education to the organization, providing structural support to autonomous work and discretionary decision making by professionals in their direct and accountable relationships to clients.

- Other organizational models include the functional and divisional forms, matrix structures, and the adhocracy.

- The coordinating mechanisms of direct supervision, standardization of work procedures, and mutual adjustment are found in all organization types.

- Matrix structures are intended to achieve flexibility and horizontal coordination of organizational processes. They violate the principle of unity of command and diffuse accountability because individuals report to more than one leader or through more than one organizational channel. This characteristic intensifies the requirements for coordination and mutual adjustment.

- Hospitals are among the most complex of modern organizations, and their structure and management have influenced practice in most other types of health agencies.

- The governing board is legally responsible for the actions of all employees and physicians who provide care within a health agency. The most senior employee in a health agency is the CEO, who reports directly to the governing board. The CEO directly selects and leads the individuals who make up the senior management team and who supervise the middle managers in the organization. Middle managers, in turn, supervise the first- or front-line managers.

- Line management positions within the organizational hierarchy have operational authority to make decisions and allocate resources.

- Those in staff positions and departments have an indirect influence on decisions and outcomes of the organization because of their specialized knowledge.

- Legislation governing hospitals has traditionally contained provisions that enable physicians to exercise power because they are entitled to report to, and directly influence, the governing boards of hospitals. This mechanism enables them to bypass the CEO and gives rise to the "hospital administration triad," which creates a source of structural conflict within hospitals.

- Most RNs are employees of health agencies. Their work, particularly in hospitals, has often been structured as though it were a production process and is characterized by fragmentation of tasks, hierarchical supervision, and management decisions to substitute one worker for another. These structural characteristics of the machine bureaucracy interfere with the ability of individual nursing professionals to apply their knowledge and to be directly accountable to patients.

- In hospitals, the organizational arrangements for the work of physicians and some other professionals illustrate the characteristics of a professional bureaucracy, which superimposes a permanent matrix over the other more conventional coordinating mechanisms of the organization and enables physicians to operate more autonomously than other organizational stakeholders, including the CEO.

- In the 1990s, additional matrix structures were created in many hospitals when senior executives made discretionary decisions to introduce program management during a time of fiscal restraint. This discretionary departure from traditional hospital structure was rationalized on the basis that greater involvement of physicians in management would lead to the ability to control the hospital costs driven by physician's activities and behaviour.

- Although the benefits and advantages of program management have been widely touted, these have not been conclusively demonstrated.

- The 1990s were characterized by organizational instability, including downsizing and lay-offs of support personnel and RNs at all levels. During this time, when program management and other structural experiments were introduced in hospitals, the numbers, visibility, and power of nursing leaders and nursing as a profession were substantially reduced. Although sometimes attributed to the "nursing shortage," these reductions took place during a time when the numbers of nurses with advanced preparation had increased. During the 1990s, the safety of patients became a matter of increasing public, professional, and government concern. Organization and management theories can contribute to an understanding of why this might be the case.

Applying the Knowledge in this Chapter

Exercise

Obtain the organizational chart of a health service organization and one subunit within it. Answer the following questions about the organizational structure:

1. What theoretical perspectives are evident in the design of the organization and its subunits?

2. Are the structures and management practices logically related to the technology (i.e., the knowledge and work processes) of professional disciplines?

3. Are accountability relationships clear in the design of the organization?

4. How is nursing work structured within the organization?

5. Is it clear what channel of communication a registered nurse could use to report a safety concern?

6. If a patient or community member wanted to express a concern about care provided by a physician, where in the organization would this be dealt with?

Resources

evolve Internet Resources

Canadian College of Health Service Executives:
  www.cchse.org
Canadian Institute for Health Information (CIHI):
  www.cihi.ca

Readers who want to further their understanding of organizational theory and design are encouraged to examine the influential work and thought of three prominent Canadian scholars in this field.

Dr. Gareth Morgan:
www.schulich.yorku.ca/ssb-extra/ssb.nsf?open

Dr. Morgan is a Distinguished Research Professor at York University in Toronto, Ontario where he teaches at the Schulich School of Business. He is the recipient of many international awards, including election as Life Fellow of the International Academy of Management in recognition of an outstanding contribution to the science of management. A bibliography of his extensive publications and synopses of key ideas are available on this site.

Dr. Heather K. Spence Laschinger:
http://publish.uwo.ca/~hkl/

Dr. Laschinger is Professor and Associate Director, Nursing Research, in the School of Nursing at the University of Western Ontario. She has received many research awards and was awarded Best Paper on the Health Care Management Division at the 2002 Annual Meeting of the Academy of Management. Since 1992, Dr. Laschinger has been principal investigator in a program of research designed to investigate nursing work environments using Kanter's theory of structural power in organizations. Over 40 graduate students have conducted their thesis research within this program. Publications by Dr. Laschinger and her colleagues can be found on the Workplace Empowerment Program page (http://publish.uwo.ca/~hkl/program.html).

Dr. Henry Mintzberg:
www.henrymintzberg.com/

Dr. Mintzberg is Cleghorn Professor of Management Studies at McGill University. His doctoral research, published as The Nature of Managerial Work, was the beginning of a lifelong career of research and teaching on management. The author of a number of widely used texts and reference books on organizational design and management, Mintzberg's extensive publications in the periodical literature include an article in the Journal of Nursing Administration in which he reports his observations of the leadership behaviour of a head nurse in a hospital ward.

References

Abrahamson, E. (1996). Management fashion. *Academy of Management Review, 21*, 254–285.

Canadian Health Services Research Foundation (CHSRF). (2002). *Myth: Bigger is always better when it comes to hospital mergers.* Retrieved May 17, 2004, from http://www.chsrf.ca/mythbusters/pdf/myth7_e.pdf

Canadian Institute for Health Information (CIHI). (2003). Retrieved June 2003, from http://www.cihi.ca

Charns, M.P, & Schaefer, M.J. (1983). Coordination. In M.P. Charns & M.J. Schaefer (Eds.), *Health care organizations: A model for management* (pp. 143–171). Englewood Cliffs, NJ: Prentice-Hall.

Christman, L.P. & Counte, M.A. (1981). *Hospital organization and health care delivery*. Boulder, CO: Westview Press.

Darr, K. (2002). Health services management ethics: A primer. *Hospital Topics, 80,* 30–33.

Dunn, W.N. (2004). *Public policy analysis: An introduction* (3rd ed.). Upper Saddle River, NJ: Prentice-Hall.

George, C.S. (1972). *The history of management thought* (2nd ed.). Englewood Cliffs, NJ: Prentice-Hall.

Georgopoulos, B.S, & Mann, F.C. (1982). The hospital as an organization. In S. Spirn & D. Benfer (Eds.), *Issues in health care management* (pp. 99–106). Rockville, MD: Aspen Systems.

Haimann, C.A, & Morgenstern, L. (1991). Legal aspects of the healthcare setting. In T. Haimann (Ed.), *Supervisory management for healthcare organizations* (pp. 60–69). St. Louis, MO: Catholic Health Association of the United States.

Haimann, T. (1991a). Committees as an organizational tool. In T. Haimann (Ed.), *Supervisory management for healthcare organizations* (pp. 179–194). St. Louis, MO: Catholic Health Association of the United States.

Haimann, T. (1991b). Communication. In T. Haimann (Ed.), *Supervisory management for healthcare organization* (pp. 41–59). St. Louis, MO: Catholic Health Association of the United States.

Haimann, T. (1991c). Division of work and departmentalization. In T. Haimann (Ed.), *Supervisory management for healthcare organizations* (pp. 124–138). St. Louis, MO: Catholic Health Association of the United States.

Harvey, J.D. (1982). Evaluating the performance of the chief executive officer. In S. Spirn & D.W. Benfer (Eds.), *Issues in health care management* (pp. 249–264). Rockville, MD: Aspen Systems.

Hellriegel, D., & Slocum, J.W. (1996). *Management* (7th ed.). Cincinnati, OH: South-Western Publishing.

Joint Commission on Accreditation of Hospitals. (1982). Quality assurance. In S. Spirn & D.W. Benfer (Eds.), *Issues in health care management* (pp. 229–232). Rockville, MD: Aspen Systems.

Kanter, R. (1993). *Men and women of the corporation* (2nd ed.). New York: Basic Books.

Kimberly, J.R., Leatt, P., & Shortell, S.M. (1983). Organization design. In S.M. Shortell & A.D. Kaluzny (Eds.), *Health care management: A text in organization theory and behavior* (pp. 291–332). New York: John Wiley & Sons.

Kovner, A.R. (1984a). Health services managers. In A.R. Kovner (Ed.), *Really trying: A career guide for the health services manager* (pp. 36–56). Ann Arbor, MI: AUPHA Press.

Kovner, A.R. (1984b). Working with physicians. In A.R. Kovner (Ed.), *Really trying: A career guide for the health services manager* (pp. 160–184). Ann Arbor, MI: AUPHA Press.

Landsberger, H.A. (1958). *Hawthorne revisited*. Ithaca, NY: Cornell University Press.

Lemieux-Charles, L., & Wylie, D. (1992). Administrative issues. In A. Baumgart & J. Larsen (Eds.), *Canadian nursing faces the future* (2nd ed., pp. 241–257). Toronto, ON: Mosby.

Mayo, E. (1933). *The human problems of an industrial civilization*. New York: Macmillan.

McGregor, D. (1957). The human side of enterprise. *Management Review, 46*(11), 22–28.

Meilicke, C.A. (1999). Management theory: Critical review and application. In J. Hibberd & D. Smith (Eds.), *Nursing management in Canada* (2nd ed., pp. 81–107). Toronto, ON: W.B. Saunders.

Mintzberg, H. (1979a). Design of lateral linkages: Liaison devices. In H. Mintzberg (Ed.), *The structuring of organization* (pp. 161–180). Englewood Cliffs, NJ: Prentice-Hall.

Mintzberg, H. (1979b). The essence of structure. In H. Mintzberg (Ed.), *The structuring of organization* (pp. 1–16). Englewood Cliffs, NJ: Prentice-Hall.

Mintzberg, H. (1982). The manager's job: Folklore and fact. In S. Sprin & D.W. Benfer (Eds.), *Issues in health care management* (pp. 31–46). Rockville, MD: Aspen Systems.

Morgan, G. (1997). *Images of organization* (2nd ed.). Thousand Oaks, CA: Sage.

Morlock, L., & Nathanson, C.A. (1983). Power and influence. In S. M. Shortell & A. D. Kaluzny (Eds.), *Health care management: A text in organization theory and behavior* (pp. 250–284). New York: John Wiley & Sons.

Mullins, L.J. (1999). *Management organizational behaviour* (5th ed.). London: Financial Times Pitman Publication.

Munson, F.C., & Zuckerman, H.S. (1983). The managerial role. In S.M. Shortell & A.D. Kaluzny (Eds.), *Health care management: A text in organization theory and behavior* (pp. 38–72). New York: John Wiley & Sons.

National Steering Committee on Patient Safety. (2002, September). *Building a safer system: A national integrated strategy for improving patient safety in Canadian health care*. Retrieved May 17, 2004, from http://rcpsc.medical.org/publications/building_a_safer_system_e.pdf

Paras, A. (2004). *Administrative behavior in two cases of unexpected children's deaths*. Unpublished master's thesis, University of Alberta, Edmonton, Alberta, Canada.

Perrow, C. (1970). *Organizational analysis: A sociological view*. Belmont, CA: Wadsworth.

Perrow, C. (1973). The short and glorious history of organizational theory. *Organizational Dynamics, 2*, 2–15.

Rachlis, M. (2004). *Prescription for excellence: How innovation is saving Canada's health care system*. Toronto, ON: Harper Collins.

Rakich, J.S., Longest, B.B., & O'Donovan, T. (1977). The structure of health care organizations. In J.S. Rakich, B.B. Longest, & T. O'Donovan (Eds.), *Managing health care organizations* (pp. 173–202). Philadelphia: W.B. Saunders.

Robbins, S.P., De Cenzo, D.A., & Stuart-Kotze, R. (1999). *Fundamentals of management: Essential concepts and applications*. Scarborough, ON: Prentice-Hall Canada.

Roethlisberger, F.J., & Jackson, W.J. (1939). *Management and the worker*. Cambridge, MA: Harvard University Press.

Schulz, R., & Johnson, A. (1990a). Changing roles of the chief executive officer with special emphasis on the evaluation/control process. In R. Schulz & A. Johnson (Eds.), *Management of hospitals and health services: Strategic issues and performance* (3rd ed., pp. 106–128). St. Louis, MO: C.V. Mosby.

Schulz, R., & Johnson, A. (1990b). Governance of health services organizations. In R. Schulz & A. Johnson (Eds.), *Management of hospitals and health services: Strategic issues and performance* (3rd ed., pp. 142–156). St. Louis, MO: C.V. Mosby.

Schulz, R., & Johnson, A. (1990c). The growing importance of management of institutions, patients, and community health. In R. Schulz & A. Johnson (Eds.), *Management of hospitals and health services: Strategic issues and performance* (3rd ed., pp. 3–16). St. Louis, MO: C.V. Mosby.

Schulz, R., & Johnson, A. (1990d). Managerial performance and ethics for hospitals and health services into the twenty-first century. In R. Schulz & A. Johnson (Eds.), *Management of hospitals and health services: Strategic issues and performance* (3rd ed., pp. 305–321). St. Louis, MO: C.V. Mosby.

Schulz, R., & Johnson, A. (1990e). Organizational arrangements of health services delivery systems. In R. Schulz & A. Johnson (Eds.), *Management of hospitals and health services: Strategic issues and performance* (3rd ed., pp. 129–141). St. Louis, MO: C.V. Mosby.

Schulz, R., & Johnson, A. (1990f). Physicians. In R. Schulz & A. Johnson (Eds.), *Management of hospitals and health services: Strategic issues and performance* (3rd ed., pp. 157–176). St. Louis, MO: C.V. Mosby.

Scott, W.R., & Shortell, S. (1983). Organizational performance: Managing for efficiency and effectiveness. In S. Shortell & A. Kaluzny (Eds.), *Health care management: A text in organization theory and behavior* (pp. 418–456). New York: John Wiley & Sons.

Shortell, S.M. (1982). Hospital medical staff organization: Structure, process, and outcome. In S. Spirn & D. Benfer (Eds.), *Issues in health care management* (pp. 61–72). Rockville, MD: Aspen Systems.

Sinclair, C.M. (2001, May). *Report of the Manitoba pediatric cardiac surgery inquest: An inquiry into twelve deaths at the Winnipeg Health Sciences Centre in 1994*. Winnipeg, MB: Provincial Court of Manitoba.

Smit, P.J., & Cronje, G.J. de J. (1997). *Management principles: A contemporary edition for Africa*. Cape Town, South Arica: Juta.

Smith, D.L. (1992). Nursing practice in acute care hospitals. In A.J. Baumgart & J. Larsen (Eds.), *Canadian nursing faces the future* (2nd ed., pp 111-133). Scarborough, ON: Mosby-Year Book, Inc.

Snook, I.D. (1981a). The governing body. In I.D. Snook (Ed.), *Hospitals: What they are and how they work* (pp. 23–30). Rockville, MD: Aspen Systems.

Snook, I.D. (1981b). The hospital administrator. In I.D. Snook (Ed.), *Hospitals: What they are and how they work* (pp. 31–38). Rockville, MD: Aspen Systems.

Snook, I.D. (1981c). Organization. In I.D. Snook (Ed.), *Hospitals: What they are and how they work* (pp. 17–22). Rockville, MD: Aspen Systems.

VanDeVelde-Coke, S. (1999). Restructuring health agencies: from hierarchies to programs. In J. Hibberd & D. Smith (Eds.), *Nursing management in Canada* (2nd ed., pp. 135–155). Toronto, ON: W.B. Saunders.

Veninga, R.L. (1982a). Understanding the culture of an organization. In R.L. Veninga (Ed.), *The human side of health administration* (pp. 18–54). Englewood Cliffs, NJ: Prentice-Hall.

Veninga, R.L. (1982b). Communicating effectively. In R.L. Veninga (Ed.), *The human side of health administration* (pp. 81–104). Englewood Cliffs, NJ: Prentice-Hall.

Veninga, R.L. (1982c). The pursuit of excellence in health administration. In R.L. Veninga (Ed.), *The human side of health administration* (pp. 1–17). Englewood Cliffs, NJ: Prentice-Hall.

Weber, M. (1964). *The theory of social and economic organization*. London: Collier Macmillan.

STRUCTURE AND ORGANIZATION OF NURSES' WORK

Donna Lynn Smith, Jane E. Smith, Vicki Boechler,
Phyllis Giovannetti, and Bonnie Lendrum

Learning Objectives

In this chapter, you will learn:

- That organizational design, decisions about staff mix, position descriptions, the choice of nursing care delivery model, and documentation practices impose structure on the work of nurses

- That values and assumptions about nursing knowledge and work are reflected in administrative choices about the design of nursing roles and care delivery models

- That patient and nursing outcomes are affected by administrative decisions about staff mix, role design, and the choice of care delivery model

- That care delivery models differ in the extent to which they emphasize or enable the dependent, independent, and interdependent registered nurse (RN) roles

- The historical context and characteristics of various nursing care delivery models, and how the introduction of the nursing process as a key feature of professional nursing practice changed the way nurses view their work

- Criteria and environmental factors to be considered in the design of nursing roles and selection of care delivery models

- About the emergence of patient care delivery models and the rationale for their introduction

- Criteria for evaluating research on nursing and patient care delivery models as management interventions and innovations

- About the problem of invisible work in nursing and the relationship of this problem to the structure of nursing documentation and the measurement of nursing outcomes

- How nursing shortages, the introduction of new categories of health care workers, and legislative changes affecting scopes of practice have all affected the design of RN work, the accountability of RNs, the number of funded positions available to employ RNs, and the way nursing is perceived by the public

The purpose of this chapter is to encourage critical and knowledge-based thinking about aspects of nurses' work and role design that are often taken for granted, but which have direct effects on patient, nurse, and organizational outcomes. Structural arrangements for designing, allocating, and coordinating the work of nurses and others providing direct care are described as *care delivery models*. Until the 1990s, the structural arrangements for nursing work, including the design of nursing roles and position descriptions, the organizational arrangements to coordinate the work of RNs and other levels of nursing personnel, and the division of tasks and allocation of nursing activities, were referred to as *nursing care delivery models* (NCDMs), or systems of nursing care delivery. NCDMs were introduced as *nursing management interventions or innovations*, designed and implemented under the line, or operational, responsibility of a nurse in a senior leadership position who was responsible for the human resources budget for nursing services and for the standards of nursing practice in the agency. In this chapter, NCDMs are distinguished from *patient care delivery models* (PCDMs), which were introduced in the late 1980s and early 1990s. PCDMs, sometimes called patient-focused or patient-centred care models, are defined as *management interventions or innovations* that create structure and organization for the work of RNs, other nursing personnel, and some other health care providers through role and task design and the allocation of work activities and responsibilities.

The roles and utilization of RNs are the main focus of the chapter, and unless otherwise specified, the term *nurses' work* is used to refer to RNs. The chapter begins with a discussion of how social and economic conditions, assumptions, and values have affected the way nursing roles and work are viewed and designed and the way nursing work is documented. The most prominent NCDMs are discussed and compared, and similarities and differences between NCDMs and PCDMs are presented. The published literature contains anecdotal reports and claims of the effectiveness of all of the models discussed. Criteria for designing and implementing management innovations such as care delivery models are presented. These criteria highlight the need for descriptions of the characteristics or elements of the models (the independent variables) and descriptions of the objectives or outcomes (the dependent variables) the models are intended to achieve. Evidence-based decision making is not possible in relation to NCDMs and PCDMs when they are defined only in philosophical terms and descriptions of their characteristics and the indicators for assessment of their outcomes are not specified. Unfortunately, this is the case in much of the published literature in which claims for the effectiveness of one or another NCDM or PCDM are made.

As well, the issues associated with decisions about staff mix, the roles and scope of practice of other levels of nursing personnel, and the substitution of other health care providers for RNs are identified. The chapter concludes with a discussion of invisible work in nursing, emphasizing the importance of documenting nursing assessment, decision making, and outcomes.

Assumptions and Values About the Work of Registered Nurses

A respected Canadian journalist has noted that, when asked, patients identified that nurses cared for them "but when pressed for details, could rarely describe more than superficial tasks" (Picard,

2000, p. 3). Nevertheless, in the annual Public Trust Index, a survey conducted by Pollara to gauge which professionals are the most trusted, "nurses are always on the top, garnering around 97%" (Picard, 2000, p. 4). Assumptions about the nature and value of nursing knowledge and work are reflected in the design of roles for RNs and the way RNs are deployed or assigned to day-to-day work responsibilities. In some organizational cultures, a nurse is thought of as "a pair of hands." Nurses themselves often like this imagery because it seems to reflect the caring dimension that has been a defining feature of professionalized nursing since its earliest beginnings. Other imagery related to nursing, expressed in popular television programs or in get-well cards intended to be humorous, focuses on stereotypic tasks identified with nurses, such as giving "shots," handling bedpans, pushing stretchers, working with technical apparatus, and responding to doctors' commands. Professional nursing associations have attempted to inform the public about the specialized knowledge, intellectual work, and independent roles of RNs through public relations campaigns, but the work of RNs continues to be identified with the performance of observable tasks.

In most acute care hospitals, nursing is organized in ways that emphasize the *dependent nursing role,* in which RNs carry out treatments prescribed by doctors. Extensive published literature, spanning several decades, documents high levels of job dissatisfaction, burnout, and turnover related to RNs' perception of having limited professional autonomy or empowerment to determine *what* nursing care is provided and *how* it will be provided (Laschinger & Wong, 1999; Parsons & Stonestreet, 2003; O'Rourke, 2003).

The cliche "I love nursing but I hate my job" reflects the lack of congruence between the value the public places on RNs and nursing care and the way that employing organizations have designed RN roles and working arrangements. From the 1990s onward, the fragmentation of professional nursing roles that had become common in hospitals has also become more prominent in other settings where nursing care is provided.

Nursing and nursing care are largely invisible in health care records, particularly in hospitals. The limited view that many doctors, employers, and policy makers have of the knowledge base and work of RNs is both a cause and consequence of the this situation. Some tasks performed or observations made by nurses are recorded in checklists, but not all of these are retained in the permanent health care record. *Dependent* nursing activities (i.e., care performed by nurses to support the medical treatment plan) are those most frequently recorded. Discretionary nursing observations have traditionally been recorded in nurses' notes, but these are not coded when health records are abstracted and are usually retained only for the minimum period required by law. The knowledge and expert observation of nurses are reflected in the nursing history or assessment and the resulting care plan, which documents nursing diagnoses, goals, and outcomes of care; however, these are not typically part of the permanent health record. Organizational practices vary, but in general, the *interdependent* activities performed by RNs while collaborating with or coordinating the work of other disciplines are rarely recorded. Other invisible RN activities include coordination of the care provided by other levels of nursing personnel and the activities of interdisciplinary teams. When nursing interventions are not documented, nursing outcomes cannot be measured or differentiated from those of other health care providers.

In reality, limited information about nursing assessments, care plans, or outcomes is documented. In most health care settings, the nursing care plan is a temporary paper record and not part of the patient's chart. In hospitals, the nursing care plan is typically contained in a Kardex, which is written in pencil and can be altered informally, at any time, by nursing or other personnel. The main function of the Kardex is a temporary communications tool that lists the day-to-day medical treatments ordered for the patient by the physician or prescribed by the care map. Most observations and instructions that reflect professional nursing knowledge and judgment are communicated verbally or are written on slips of paper that are inserted into the Kardex to inform the oncoming shift. These informal notes are even more temporary and disposable than the Kardex and are discarded within a few hours. Nurses are assumed to have a dislike of "paperwork," and in many health care settings, charting "by exception" has become the norm (at the direction, or with the approval, of administrative officials). Ironically, legal precedent suggests that if something has not been documented, it is assumed by the court that it has not been done unless there is substantial proof to the contrary (Picard & Robertson, 1996).

More seriously, the view of nurses as "a pair of hands" provides a rationale for substituting other workers for RNs. In some instances, substitution or delegation is a wise use of resources. However, the decision to substitute one level of nursing personnel for another, or another health care provider for a nurse, is often made without direct knowledge of patient characteristics or needs (the "raw materials" or organizational inputs discussed in Chapter 8) and without expert nursing assessment of care requirements. For example, delivering meal trays is a non-nursing activity that is usually delegated to a multi-skilled worker or an aide from the dietary department. However, when a tray is delivered and removed by another worker who has no responsibility to report to the RN, the reasons why the patient did not eat may not be professionally assessed and interventions to assure proper nutrition not initiated. Since inadequate food and fluid intake can delay recovery or lead to complications, this has potentially serious consequences for the patient. "High-tech" examples can also be cited. For instance, it has become common to have technicians, and not RNs, assist physicians during invasive diagnostic procedures such as angiograms or angioplasties. This begs the question of who is available to attend the patient, in a holistic sense, as the procedure is being performed or while the patient is being transported from the cardiac catheterization lab or recovery area to the care unit. If a porter or multi-skilled ancillary worker is transporting the patient and an emergency occurs, it may not be promptly or correctly recognized, and valuable time may be lost before life-saving intervention begins. Substitution of other workers to perform nursing "tasks" also occurs in home care programs and extended care. It remains less common in community health nursing.

If RNs are viewed as easily substitutable when it comes to performing tasks, it is not surprising that they are also seen as easily substitutable from one work setting to another. The disparaging expression "a nurse is a nurse is a nurse" conveys this idea, that nursing work and nurses as individuals are easily replaced. Administrative practices in which the management's right to deploy the workforce is exercised by arbitrarily reassigning RNs (at short notice) from one unit or department to another within a single work setting, or from one setting to another in regional organizations, are now sometimes seen and have emerged as an issue in collective bargaining. Administrative decisions of this nature can be justified in unexpected or emergency situations, but as a routine practice, they reveal a disregard for the importance of continuity of patient care as well as disrespect for nurses as professionals.

The invisibility of the independent and intellectual dimensions of nursing work (i.e., assessment, care planning, coordination, and evaluation of care) and a disproportionate emphasis on the implementation of tasks derived from the dependent nursing role account for the lack, and loss, of *expert power* of RNs and the corresponding trend to substitute other workers for RNs in all health settings (see Chapter 23 for an explanation of these concepts). Values and assumptions about the knowledge and work of RNs are reflected in management decisions about staff mix (i.e., the ratio of RNs to other care providers), role design (i.e., the position descriptions for RNs), organization of nursing work (i.e., the selection of a care delivery model), and the daily resource allocations in which individual care providers are assigned to patients or functional tasks (O'Rourke, 2003). Ideally, these decisions are based on evidence and are made by RN managers who are knowledgeable about patient needs, the characteristics of the available workforce, and management theory. In light of the growing body of evidence concerning the relationship between RN staffing and important health outcomes, including the rate of adverse occurrences (Stanton, 2004; Rachlis, 2004), administrative accountability for decisions about staff mix and substitution of other workers for RNs will be evaluated more critically in the future than in the last two decades. This subject is discussed more extensively in Chapter 12.

Nursing Care Delivery Models as Nursing Management Innovations

In the late 19th and early 20th centuries, nurses were self-employed professionals who operated in directly accountable relationships with patients and doctors who engaged and paid them directly to look after patients at home or in hospitals. Other nurses provided service in the community under the auspices of religious or charitable organizations. It is obvious from the nursing textbooks of that era that a body of independent nursing knowledge had developed and was being systematically transmitted. Professional nursing associations had been formed to coordinate efforts to standardize nursing education, further knowledge development, and promote professional values.

The history of how nurses and nursing as a profession became dependent upon organizational employers is an interesting one, and it offers important insights into some of the structural issues and political dilemmas that face the profession today (McPherson, 1996; Melosh, 1982). In the early 20th century, the work of doctors became more reliant on the availability of hospital infrastructure and workers, and hospital administrators recognized a need for steady affordable nursing labour that was under their direct control. Hospital nursing schools were developed to ensure a continuous supply of this cheap labour, and RNs were hired to supervise the nursing students and manage the care of patients as specified by attending doctors. Models or systems of care delivery were originally developed by nursing leaders to define the roles and to structure the work of nurses. Successive models have reflected the social and economic conditions of their times, including attitudes about women and the value and place of women's work and nursing work.

In early models, work was organized hierarchically as it had been in military and religious organizations, and it was divided into discrete tasks as advocated by the scientific management approach. These characteristics of the machine bureaucracy originated in hospitals but have also affected the design of RN work in long-term care nursing and home care programs. Community health nurses retained greater independence and autonomy in their practice, although, in the past decade, their roles have sometimes become more fragmented and task focused.

By the 1960s, as the number of university-prepared nurses began to expand, nurses were prepared to reflect upon the nature of nursing and the structure of knowledge in their discipline. The scientific method began to be used as a conceptual organizer for curriculum development in schools of nursing and in the care of individuals and groups, resulting in the notion of a "nursing process" that incorporated the activities of assessment, care planning, implementation, and evaluation of nursing care. The nursing process provided a framework and language to describe the intellectual activities of nursing assessment, care planning, and the evaluation of nursing care and distinguished these from the psychomotor skills and other nursing interventions used to *implement* nursing care. At about the same time, knowledge from the social sciences was integrated into the nursing curriculum, and the importance of the therapeutic relationship as a nursing and health care intervention was recognized. These developments provided the impetus for elaboration of an independent nursing role in which nursing knowledge and assessment guided nursing diagnosis, and they led to interventions initiated by RNs that were independent of doctors and other health professionals. Since the mid-1970s, nurses have been prepared to perform this *independent* role through their basic education and professional socialization.

However, most of the intellectual work of nurses remains invisible to others and even to nurses themselves. Therefore, it is not surprising that administrators, consultants, and other health professionals often see a way of saving money by training other workers to do nursing tasks under the supervision of an RN, who takes responsibility for their instruction, supervision, and any mistakes they might make. The substitution of other workers for RNs fragments nursing care, discourages specialization, and deprives patients of the benefits of specialized nursing knowledge.

The introduction of successive NCDMs has been accompanied by prescriptive and anecdotal literature, much of it written by nursing leaders, to explain why each new model makes sense and how it will make things better for patients and nurses. A critical reading of the literature on nursing care delivery models reveals that goals of greater efficiency, decreased labour costs, and control of the workforce were predominant in the development of early models and remain key factors today. Criteria for the selection and evaluation of a care delivery model should be explicit, and the contribution that the model is expected to make to patients, nurses, and the organization should be specified before initial implementation in order to enable assessment of the appropriateness of models that have remained in continuous use. Table 9.1 illustrates the criteria to be considered in the selection and evaluation of an NCDM as advocated by the senior nursing leader of one Canadian hospital in 1992.

The importance of aligning the internal structure and processes of an organization with the characteristics and demands of the external environment is well documented in the organizational literature (Schein, 1993). Factors in the external and internal environments of health care organizations also affect the design of nursing work and the selection of a care delivery

Table 9.1 Criteria for the Selection and Evaluation of a Nursing Care Delivery Model

1. What is good for patients? Does the model
    1.1. have the patient as a central focus?
    1.2. assure that care providers with appropriate knowledge and skills are available to match patient needs and complexity?
    1.3. support continuity of care?
    1.4. highlight patient outcomes?
    1.5. provide for accountability of the nurse to the patient/client?

2. What is good for nursing? Does the model
    2.1. enable nurses to fully apply their knowledge and skills?
    2.2. provide for documentation of nursing assessments, care plans, interventions, and outcomes?
    2.3. maintain control of nursing practice within nursing?
    2.4. minimize non-nursing tasks?
    2.5. promote job satisfaction of nurses?

3. What is good for the organization? Does the model
    3.1. fit with the hospital mission and role?
    3.2. maintain or improve quality of care?
    3.3. promote optimum utilization of human and other resources?
    3.4. promote collaborative practice?
    3.5. provide for safety, continuity, and clinical and administrative accountability?

Source: Adapted from questions developed by S.D. Smith, Vice-President, Nursing Services, Chedoke-McMaster Hospitals, 1992. Used with permission.

model. Senior nursing leaders have taken such factors into account when selecting or designing nursing care delivery models. The environmental factors identified by one Canadian nursing leader as affecting the choice of an NCDM are presented in Table 9.2.

Choices about the design of professional roles and processes for providing and documenting care are important resource allocation decisions and have an impact on patient and nurse outcomes. Organizational and leadership variables, such as the NCDM in use, have been shown to affect the job satisfaction of RNs and other care providers.

Nursing Care Delivery Models

NCDM are management interventions or innovations that create organizational structure for the work of RNs and other nursing and health care personnel through role design and work allocation strategies. NCDMs are designed, chosen, and implemented through decisions by senior nurse executives whose positions in the organizational structure of their agency carry the deci-

Table 9.2 Environmental Factors to Consider when Selecting a Nursing Care Delivery Model

Patients

1. What are the major patient populations supported by the hospital or unit?
   1.1. How would each population be served by each care delivery model?
2. What is the acuity level of this population?

External Environment

Economic

1. What will be the influence of the latest or upcoming contract settlement?
2. How will a new care delivery model be interpreted in light of the current fiscal climate?
3. What other budgetary limitations are imminent?

Health Trends

1. How will the model match consumer expectations of health care services?

Political

1. Which models and their variations have been profiled over the last three years in professional publications?
   1.1. Will there be pressure to adopt one of these models? Which one?
   1.2. Where will the pressure come from and how will it be expressed?

Regulatory

1. How is scope of practice being interpreted by the professional and regulatory bodies?
   1.1. How will that interpretation influence the selection of a care delivery model?

Internal Environment

The Organization

1. How do the values in the organization's mission statement address patients, communication, work, and professionalism?
2. What are the long-term goals of the organization?
3. Which disciplines will need to be included in discussions about a change in patient care delivery?
4. What will promote collaborative practice?
5. What is the floor plan of the unit?

The Nursing Department

1. What are the tenure, skill mix, educational preparation, competency level, and professional orientation of nursing staff and managers?
   1.1. How will each of the above influence the selection of a care delivery model?
2. How do the values in the nursing mission and philosophy address patients, communication, work, and professionalism?
3. What type of model will maintain nursing and, at the same time, promote autonomy and job satisfaction?

Source: Adapted from questions developed by S.D. Smith, Vice-President, Nursing Services, Chedoke-McMaster Hospitals, 1992. Used with permission.

sional and financial authority to make and implement these decisions. NCDMs reflect various values, assumptions, and priorities. They can be appraised and compared in terms of the way they divide and allocate tasks, determine the relationships between RNs and other nursing and health care personnel, make use of the physical environment, or contribute to continuity and accountability for care (Lendrum, 1994; McPhail, 1996). Models differ from one another in the social and economic conditions that fostered their development, the way work is allocated, the types of communication and coordination mechanisms they incorporate, the degree of control nurses have over clinical decision making, the autonomy of RNs, and the role of the first-line manager or head nurse. When viewed in the social, economic, and political contexts in which they originated, and in terms of their strengths and disadvantages, NCDMs can often be seen as responses to shortages of RNs or as efforts to reduce the influence and costs of RNs in the care delivery process. However, in designing or choosing a care delivery model, senior nurse leaders are fully aware of professional nursing standards and are well informed about the knowledge, skills, and work technology of the nursing discipline. These professional leaders are accountable within their organizations for the delivery of nursing services that meet professional standards of care, as well as the standards of the organization, which include expectations of financial management and cost containment. As Lendrum (1999) notes, a lack of clarity in the goals and outcomes of NCDMs can leave nurses "poorly situated" in a time of fiscal restraint.

The characteristics of the NCDMs described most fully in the published nursing literature are summarized and compared in Table 9.3. These models are now described.

The Case Method

In the earliest days of professional nursing, nurses were employed directly by patients or by doctors and received fees for their services. Intricate knowledge of the patient was acquired as the nurse provided individual care in the patient's own home. Care included a variety of nursing and home support activities required by the patient and family, and each nurse transferred the care of the patient directly to another nurse. In this approach, subsequently termed the case method, individual nurses were directly accountable to the patient or the physician who had engaged their services and were paid directly by them. Lemieux-Charles and Wylie (1992) have described how the opening of large numbers of new hospital beds in the 1940s changed the pattern of nursing practice. Whereas, in the 1930s, 60% of RNs were still working as private-duty nurses, in 1960, the number of self-employed or private-duty nurses had decreased to 9%, and there were corresponding increases in the numbers of nurses employed by hospitals. These developments are analyzed in their social, political, and economic context by a Canadian historian (see McPherson, 1996).

Today, nursing students are introduced to clinical care through the case assignment method of learning to assess and care for individual patients holistically. The case method is still seen in some private home nursing. However, very few nurses currently provide direct care services as self-employed professionals, and within hospitals and other care settings, the case method is seen as costly because of its reliance upon one highly skilled RN. Nevertheless, work assignments in some intensive care units continue to reflect features of the case assignment method. Patients and nurses find the direct accountability that is central to this method to be satisfying.

Table 9.3 Characteristics and Comparison of Nursing Care Delivery Models

	Case Method	Functional	Team	Modular	Primary	Case Management	Differentiated Nursing Practice
Date of Origin	1890s	1940s	1950s	1950s–1960s	1960s	1980s	1990s
Work Allocation	All care for the patient.	Specific tasks assigned and supervised by the charge nurse.	RN team leaders assign tasks and responsibilities to other team members.	Modification to team nursing where the unit is divided into modules (geographic location of patient rooms); the same team is assigned consistently to the module.	Care plan developed by RN; direct care responsibilities shared by primary RN and other care providers (associate nurses).	Dependent on the model of case management used; case manager may allocate services and/or provide care.	RN may function as a case manager or nurse practitioner. Work assignment is dependent on educational preparation and competencies (novice, advanced beginner, competent, proficient, and expert); (Benner, 1984) required by the patient population and setting.
Mechanisms of Communication and Coordination	Case notes	Lists Treatment books	Kardex Team conferences	Kardex Team conferences Informal communication	Care plans Nursing progress notes Team meetings Telephone consultation	Service plans Progress notes Team meetings Telephone consultation	Care plans Nursing progress notes

Table 9.3 Continued

	Case Method	Functional	Team	Modular	Primary	Case Management	Differentiated Nursing Practice
Continuity of Care	Per shift by the RN. Day to day when same RN available.	Fragmentation and discontinuity intensified by number of task assignments and workers. Continuity managed through the charge nurse.	Fragmentation reduced when care activities are consistently performed by team members.	Consistent team members perform care in a dedicated module; each module consists of an RN (team/module leader) with other team members.	The primary RN provides informational continuity across the 24-hour period and throughout the episode of care.	By the case manager through the care plan, across settings, and between episodes of care.	By the RN assigned to this responsibility (patient needs are matched with the RN competencies to deliver the full range of nursing services in the key areas of nursing care, management, and communication).
Accountability	Complete for a small group of patients.	Only for the assigned tasks during the one shift.	Shared accountability by the team.	Module leaders are accountable for the assigned tasks performed by the team.	The primary RN is accountable for the plan of care and for assigning and evaluating contributions by associates over the episode of illness.	Case manager is accountable for planning and coordination throughout the episode of care or, in a boundary spanning case management role, for managing care across the continuum for an indefinite period.	RN accountability depends on the client needs, time, and setting where care is delivered.

Table 9.3 Continued

	Case Method	Functional	Team	Modular	Primary	Case Management	Differentiated Nursing Practice
Control of Clinical Decision Making	Per shift by the working RN.	Rests solely with the head nurse who communicates the decisions to the RN on each shift.	Staff participation in team decision making. The team leader coordinates the decisions of other health professionals with the practice of nursing.	Module leader has some decision-making responsibility.	Decentralized to the primary nurse. When the primary nurse is not present, the care is managed by an associate who will contact the primary nurse or designate for any unanticipated clinical decision making required.	Case manager in collaboration with other disciplines involved.	Complexity of decision making increases in relation to client needs and the setting where care is delivered.
Autonomy of RN	Directly accountable to patient, physician, or employing agency.	Limited Top-down management and control.	Some clinical leadership delegated to RN team leaders; still directed by the charge nurse.	Some leadership delegated to the module leaders as directed by the charge nurse.	Discretionary decision making and clinical leadership by the associate to the primary RN for her/his patients.	Primary RN collaborates with other disciplines; coordinates care for her/his patient group.	Accountable to patient and employer; RN is part of an interdisciplinary team.

Table 9.3 Continued

	Case Method	Functional	Team	Modular	Primary	Case Management	Differentiated Nursing Practice
Role of the First-Line Manager (Head Nurse).	Individual RN practices autonomously and is directly accountable to the client.	Schedules and supervises all staff. Assigns tasks, supervises all staff; coordinates care and all communication about the patient.	Schedules and supervises all staff. Assigns and directly supervises team leaders; coordinates communication between team leaders and other health care providers.	Charge nurse expects the module leaders to be accountable; charge nurse may assist in problem solving when necessary; charge nurse may also be a module leader depending on staffing levels; coordinates communication with other health care providers.	Identifies and develops primary RNs; determines the approach for matching primary RNs with patients. Acts as a consultant or coach to primary RNs; provides professional development opportunities; assists in solving complex problems. Defines the roles of associate staff members; schedules and assigns the work of associate staff in consultation with primary RN; provides day-to-day supervision of associate staff.	Determines the approach to assigning a caseload of patients or clients to case managers. May approve service plans that exceed standard funding or time limits for services.	Role change from problem solver to mentor. Develops position descriptions based on educational preparation. Allocates nurses' work based on education, experience, and competence. Fosters collaboration, professional self-development, and accountability. Provides team leadership, team building, and mechanisms to recognize the contributions of all team members so that status differences associated with educational preparation are de-emphasized.

Table 9.3 Continued

	Case Method	Functional	Team	Modular	Primary	Case Management	Differentiated Nursing Practice
Strengths of the Model	Patients receive continuous care by one nurse for an entire shift.	Care can be provided to a large number of people as each person becomes proficient at one task. Required tasks can be easily taught to ancillary workers and supervised, thus increasing efficiency.	The work of team members with different knowledge and skill levels can be delegated, supervised, and coordinated. The team is responsible for a group of patients and can provide continuity of personnel; patients can identify their care providers.	Increased continuity of care; saves nursing time because of physical set up of the module.	Development of a trusting and accountable relationship with patients and families. Designed to achieve continuity of care. Cost-effectiveness is achieved through improved coordination and professional accountability. Enables RNs to fully apply their assessment, care planning, communication, problem-solving, and evaluation skills. Primary RNs directly interact with and observe patients; maintain clinical skills and can identify or prevent adverse occurrences.	Cost-effectiveness is achieved through improved coordination of care, reducing duplications of service and preventing errors. Designed to achieve continuity of care. Enables RNs to fully apply their assessment, care planning, communication, problem-solving, and evaluation skills. Patient/client has a consistent advocate who knows them and is accountable for their care over an extended time period.	Associated with a number of improved client outcomes. Patients have increased access to professional and specialized services. Potential for improved role satisfaction, loyalty, and accountability as team members use full range of their knowledge and skills. Improved efficiency and ability to minimize errors. Decreased lengths of stay and readmission rates. Time savings in work processes.

Table 9.3 Continued

	Case Method	Functional	Team	Modular	Primary	Case Management	Differentiated Nursing Practice
Disadvantages	Requires generalist knowledge and versatility.	Work is task focused, not patient focused, and patient care is fragmented. RNs may lose some of their clinical skills.	Communication is complex. Accountability is only shift by shift.	May require redesign of physical environment; duplication of resources for each module may add costs.	Requires RNs with expert knowledge and high-level communication, care planning skills, and clinical skills. RNs wanting to work part-time, or other levels of nursing personnel, may work in the associate role.	In some models, RNs lose direct care skills. Case manager roles focus on gate keeping and rationing of resources; present challenges to RNs who value patient advocacy.	May accentuate status differences between nurses with different educational levels.

Sources: From Differentiated Nursing Practice: Assessing the State-of-the-Science, by C. Baker, G. Lamm, A. Winter, V. Robbeloth, C. Ransom, F. Conly, et al., 1997, *Nursing Economics, 15*(5), 253–261, 264; Differentiated Interdisciplinary Practice, by G. Hutchens, 1994, *Journal of Advanced Nursing, 24*(6), 52–58; Care Delivery Systems, by J. Komplin, 1995. In P.S. Yoder Wise (Ed.), *Leading and Managing in Nursing* (pp. 422–428). Toronto, ON: Mosby.

Functional Nursing

With the move of patients into hospitals, nursing care became organized to fit the operations of the institution and to support the physicians. The foundations of the functional model were rooted in the classic scientific management of the 1920s (McPhail, 1996), in which the accepted work ethic and culture were centred on efficiency, division of labour, and rigid control (Lendrum, 1994). This care delivery model became popular during World War II when there was a significant shortage of nurses due to recruitment into the military. Nurses were assigned to specific tasks in the roles of "medication nurse" and "treatment nurse." Non-nursing personnel were trained on-site to increase the number of professional staff available for patient care. This model of care delivery has been compared to an industrial assembly line (Lendrum, 1994) in which the charge nurse is the "shift supervisor." Lendrum concluded that the interchangeability of nurses who worked on the "assembly" line was likely the basis for the phrase "a nurse is a nurse is a nurse." Today, this machine bureaucracy approach to the organization of nursing work can be seen in the many examples of functional assignment in hospitals, long-term care, and home care programs. The practice of having a "bath team" make rounds on an extended care unit to bath residents at regularly scheduled times during the week is a common example. Many extended care residents dread and fear bath time, and many critical and adverse incidents occur in association with baths. Statements of philosophy for extended care centres usually contain claims that residents' dignity, privacy, and individuality are respected. Still, the practice of functional bath teams persists despite a high level of rhetoric about how extended care environments are "homelike" and have moved away from a "medical model." Functional nursing has the effect of fragmenting care and focusing workers' attention on tasks rather than patients.

Team and Modular Nursing

Team nursing was developed to ease the pressures of nursing shortages following WWII and to find ways of integrating auxiliary health care personnel trained by the military during the war into the civilian health system. Key features of this model are the role of RN team leader (which decentralized some of the functions previously held by the head nurse) and the assignment of other nursing personnel to teams. Staff schedules were originally organized so that one team routinely worked together. Communication and coordination of care were accomplished through direct supervision by the team leader and through patient conferences in which the care plan was reviewed and updated. Team nursing was an initial step in the development of the "therapeutic relationship" with the patient (Lendrum, 1994), and, although the relationship was short lived within the team nursing model, care could be more patient-centred than in the task-functional model.

Modular nursing is a variation of team nursing in which the geographic location of the patients on the unit determines the work assignment and resources are sometimes decentralized to achieve greater efficiency for workers in each module. If facilitated by scheduling practices and the ratio of full-time, part-time, and temporary (casual) staff, cohesive relationships can be developed between the RN team leader and other nursing staff who work together in a team or module.

Like functional nursing, team nursing incorporates many features of classical management theory, including the division of labour. Because a number of different workers are responsible for different activities for the same patient, there is the potential for fragmentation of care and limited direct accountability. The role of team leader has provided opportunities for clinical leadership development for RNs and is now contained in the language of many collective agreements, perpetuating features of the team nursing model.

Primary Nursing

Primary nursing as a care delivery model should not be confused with the concept of primary health care, which has gained prominence in public policy discourse over the last two decades. In the case of primary nursing, the word primary refers to a directly accountable relationship between one nurse and a group of patients. On the other hand, as explained in Chapter 4, the term primary health care refers to principles and practices governing care at the first, or primary, point of contact that people have with health services and the health care system.

As the number of baccalaureate-prepared nurses increased, and job satisfaction for RNs became a pressing issue during a major nursing shortage, nursing leaders developed the primary nursing model to reduce fragmentation of the professional nursing role, thus responding to the preference of nurses and patients for a more holistic approach to patient care. Manthey's patient-centred care model—primary nursing—was eagerly embraced by North American nurses in the early 1970s. This model brought the RN back to the bedside to provide clinical assessment and direct care and to accept *primary accountability* for planning and managing the care of a small caseload of patients over time. Clinical decision making was thus decentralized, and the role of the first-line nursing manager changed from that of gatekeeper for all information and decision making to that of consultant to primary nurses. In primary nursing, as in the primary medical care provided by doctors, one nurse has 24-hour responsibility for the care provided to the patient. The implementation of nursing care activities (nursing tasks) is assigned to *associate nurses* who are guided in their decision making by the clarity of the nursing care plan developed by the *primary nurse*. When the primary RN has scheduled time off, care is continued by an associate nurse (Manthey, 2003). Delegation arrangements, including telephone consultations, are required to initiate changes to the care plan because it is implicit in this model that the primary decision-making responsibility for the patient lies with one nurse (Lendrum, 1994). These arrangements are similar to those for sharing on-call responsibilities in a general medical practice.

Primary nursing facilitates the development of an accountable therapeutic relationship between the patient and the primary nurse. Thus, as in general medical practice, there is the potential for continuity of care to be achieved through longitudinality, as discussed in Chapter 5. Informational continuity can also be achieved through clarity of the care plan and the direct communication of the primary nurse with associate nurses, the patient, and other care providers, including doctors. The primary nurse can initiate evidence-based nursing interventions in consultation with nursing specialists or experts in other disciplines. Interventions can be systematically assessed for their effectiveness and the care plan formally modified by the accountable RN who then instructs associate nursing staff in the rationale for, and implementation of, the new approach. Written documentation of the care plan, rationale, assessment, goals for nursing, and other interventions enables the evaluation of care outcomes. As Manthey (2003) has concluded, "This revolutionary (both then and now) care delivery system requires a level of competence, personal empowerment, and professionalism that continues to challenge nursing practice within the healthcare hospital environment" (p. 369).

Case Management

In the 1980s in the US, hospital-based RN case management models developed in hospitals where primary nursing had been established. The New England Medical Center model is the best-known prototype. It has been described by Huston (2002) as "an extension of primary nursing methodology called nursing case management and is focused on the acute care hospital episode" (p. 6). In this model, case management is defined as a nursing care delivery model. Huston has explained that, in adopting this NCDM, "principles of concurrent management from engineering and other fields to extend primary nursing into outcomes management in order to balance cost, process and outcomes" (p. 6). In this model, RN expertise in the independent and interdependent domains of the nursing practice is emphasized and exploited to achieve patient and organizational outcomes. The role of RN case managers provided an opportunity for nurses to apply a full range of professional knowledge and skills to coordinate the care of patients throughout an episode of illness, often including transfers from one clinical service to another and preparation of the patient and family for discharge. A compelling argument for the introduction of this model has been cost-effectiveness. A high level of professional coordination of hospital care by RNs minimizes the duplication of services, prevents the omission of critical services, and provides for prompt identification and treatment of complications. Patients feel that an individual professional is taking responsibility for their care, and communication with family members and members of the health team is coordinated and goal-oriented. Care maps or critical pathways provide structure to the interdisciplinary plan of care and can be supplemented and individualized through nursing care plans that incorporate independent nursing activities.

Primary Nursing, Nursing Case Management, and the Nursing Process

Some authors have drawn parallels between case management and the nursing process. Both involve the application of knowledge and skills in a systematic approach to assessing and managing clients' health needs. While the two processes have these and other elements in common, it is important to recognize that the process of planning for, obtaining, coordinating, and monitoring services provided in a succession of settings, by more than one agency, and through more than one funding avenue, is a vastly more complex function than that of developing care plans for one or more individuals within a single unit, program, or agency.

Case management may indeed provide a convenient approach to the organization or assignment of nurses' work, and some of the precepts of primary nursing can certainly be applied to case management. However, in primary nursing, the primary nurse's accountability usually extends only to the point of the client's discharge from one unit or service. Accountability of hospital-based nursing case management usually ends with the episode of care, and the case manager would not typically be expected or empowered to remain involved with the client after discharge.

Those involved in home care programs are often assumed to be more aware of the need for coordination and continuity of care than those employed in hospitals, and many home care professionals take pride in fulfilling a case management role. When examined closely, however, home care and hospital-based case management may prove to be more similar than different. The work of home care nurses is not necessarily structured so they can act as primary nurses or case managers for their clients. In home care programs, the case management function is often limited to planning care and coordinating and monitoring personnel from contracted agencies. Care in the home is delivered by many different workers, disciplines, and agencies and may, therefore, be as task-oriented and fragmented as that provided in hospitals through the functional model.

Fragmentation in the health and human services system is taken for granted to such an extent that if discharge or other service arrangements fail, professionals have not traditionally been held accountable or expected to take responsibility for preventing or rectifying problems outside their own program setting. Ironically, while it is assumed that professionals working within one setting cannot be held responsible for assuring continuity of care when clients move to other settings, it is also assumed that clients and their families can navigate the system on their own without the benefit of "insider" knowledge!

One of the central differences among the roles of primary nurses, hospital nurse case managers, and boundary-spanning case managers is a difference in perspective in which the emphasis shifts from a single episode of illness in one setting to the coordination of services over the entire episode of illness and/or disability (Huber, 2002; Smith & Smith, 1999). Case management can be viewed as an enlargement of the role of primary nurse to include a broader range of assessment, care planning, and other skills. Nursing has a historic tradition of providing and coordinating highly skilled care, 24 hours a day, in many settings. Therefore, nurses are often seen as particularly suited for boundary-spanning case management roles. Huber (2002) describes the community-based nursing service of Carondolet St. Mary's Community Nursing Network (also known as the Arizona Model), explaining that it is "best known for its innovative work in moving beyond the episode of care and truly into the continuum" (p. 215). In this hospital-to-community model, as in other disease management programs, case managers, who are usually RNs with advanced preparation, work with individuals and populations in long-term relationships (Huston, 2002). Professional experience in settings where primary nursing or some other accountability-oriented model of care delivery has been implemented, and in settings where interdisciplinary teamwork has been valued and required, provides nurses with a strong foundation upon which to build the additional skills required to practice in boundary spanning roles within an integrated service delivery system.

Differentiated Nursing Practice

Differentiated nursing practice is described as a personnel deployment model in which the roles of nurses are (re)defined based on education, experience, and competence (Murphy & DeBack, 1990). The concept of differentiated nursing practice "describes the system of sorting roles, functions, and work of RNs according to education, clinical experience, defined competence, and decision making required by the client's needs and the specific setting in which nursing is practiced. This requires matching the skills and core competencies with educational experiences and care" (Felton, Abbe, Gilbert, & Ingle, 1999, p. 275).

This model can be viewed as an application of contingency theory to decisions about the structure and organization of nursing work. It is designed to respond to differences in the needs and complexity of patients and care activities. This means that there is no single nursing care delivery model throughout an organization; rather, the knowledge and skill mix of care providers may be intentionally different from one care setting to another in order to align with the needs of patients. An assumption implicit in this model is the requirement for RNs to supervise care.

Educational programs for RNs and other nursing personnel differ in many respects. These include the length of the course of study, the scientific knowledge base, preparation for critical thinking and ethical judgment in clinical decision making, interpersonal and technological skills, and the use of research and scholarly activities that contribute to the development of a body of knowledge relevant to the profession of nursing. In differentiated practice models, the roles for each level of personnel are defined in terms of proficiency so that structured progress from novice to expert can be managed for each individual staff member (Warzynski, 2001). This model has the potential to add value to patient care processes by bringing the benefits of more advanced nursing preparation to the direct care of patients who can benefit from specialized nursing knowledge. It also provides an avenue for structured progression in clinical careers. For obvious reasons, this model could be expected to work better than others for the transfer of new research evidence into clinical nursing practice.

As noted by Cummings and Estabrooks (2003), the evolution of nursing care delivery models in the 1980s, under the leadership of nurse executives, was motivated by a desire to improve the use of RN time and professionalism. This led to growing recognition that RNs could and should have greater individual accountability for the care management of specific patients from admission to discharge and for the development of professional decision-making structures such as shared governance.

Patient-Centred or Patient-Focused Care

By the late 1980s, maintaining professional practice had become a challenge in cost-contained environments. To obtain improvements in productivity, while containing costs, hospitals began to restructure or redesign systems for providing care (Henderson & Williams, 1991). Nursing roles and care delivery models were affected in this process and PCDMS were introduced. Lendrum (1999) described work redesign as "more than the incremental improvement of tasks," (p. 160) involving an examination of the processes in all disciplines and departments to align them with the needs of patients and the goals of care. Cummings and Estabrooks (2003) explain that the models of this era, termed patient-centred or patient-focused care, were intended to achieve several goals:

1. Realigning hospital resources and processes to bring them closer to the patient
2. Reducing the number of departmental support workers who would interact with each patient on a given day, but introducing a new non-licensed "multi-skilled" worker
3. Eliminating inefficiencies to significantly reduce the length of patient stays, times for diagnostic tests, and redundant processes
4. Improving patient satisfaction, physician-nurse collaboration, nursing autonomy, and job satisfaction

Based on their review of the literature, Cummings and Estabrooks (2003) concluded that "research into the outcomes of implementing patient-focused or patient-centered care models showed that some goals were achieved, but generally results were mixed" (p. 10).

Although there are similarities between these models and team nursing, Schweikhart and Smith-Daniels (1996) contend that patient-centred care is not a return to team nursing because team composition is different, with overlapping job responsibilities to replace traditional nursing roles. Whereas, in traditional team nursing, ancillary workers are under the direction of the team leader, in the patient-centred model, team members are intended to be "mutually accountable" to the patient, who serves as the group's focal point. One example of restructuring that illustrates an attempt to achieve the goals of patient-focused care is that of care production teams (CPTs) (Schweikhart & Smith-Daniels, 1996). In this model, RNs are teamed with one or two non-licensed caregivers to deliver direct patient care services. RNs serve as team leaders and assume responsibility for performing direct patient care services while facilitating the service delivery activities of other team members.

There has been a general tendency for organizations to adopt patient-friendly and euphemistic terminology to describe organizational redesign activities (this is reflected in the terms patient-centred and patient-focused care) that dramatically changed the roles of RNs. A similar tendency is reflected in the paradox of introducing initiatives for total quality management (TQM) or continuous quality improvement (CQI) at the same time as unprecedented downsizing and restructuring were being undertaken in hospitals. Rondeau and Wagar (2004) describe the consequences of some of these initiatives as "disastrous," noting that "whether downsizing has a direct and immediate effect on the quality of medical care or community health outcomes is not yet firmly established, yet its consequences on the emotional health of those who toil in health care organizations remains unassailable" (p. 23). Cummings and Estabrooks (2003) discuss the results of research into this wave of hospital restructuring, which show decreased levels of RN autonomy, increased nursing workloads, increased frequency of adverse patient events and complications, and reductions in quality of care. There is now evidence that "adverse effects on nursing outcomes are directly and explicitly related to increased patient morbidity and mortality" (2003, p. 10). These authors emphasize that reduction in RN positions was a "central feature" of hospital restructuring.

The implementation of patient-focused care models or new quality assurance initiatives has usually stopped short of redesigning organization-wide processes. However, their introduction has had a major impact on the role of RNs and the way nursing work is structured. Typically, in these models, the role of the RN is broadened to coordinate a team of multifunctional, unit-based caregivers. Patients are divided into groups, and RNs are responsible for all the care delivered and for communicating directly with physicians, families, and nursing supervisors, much in the same way the head nurse did in the original functional nursing models. This model is widely used in long-term care facilities and other settings where the number of RN positions has been reduced. The work of RNs in these models often involves supervisory responsibilities without corresponding supervisory authority, and there are sometimes disputes as to whether RNs are eligible for supervisory roles (i.e., case management positions) or should remain within their collective bargaining group. In some settings, administrative decisions have been made to substitute licensed practical nurses (LPNs) for RNs as the leaders of the patient-focused team.

The legal accountability of RNs who work in these models of care is an issue of importance and sometimes of uncertainty. It is problematic for individual RNs if the role description specifies that the RN is responsible for the care provided by other workers but the RN does not have the corresponding authority to assign, direct, and supervise the activities of those workers. As the scope of practice for LPNs has been broadened through legislative and regulatory changes, the traditional assumption that RNs are, or should be, accountable for the practice of LPNs is no longer viable unless the RN has formally delegated administrative responsibility reflected in position descriptions and work assignments.

Research on Effectiveness of Care Delivery Models

Prior to the 1980s, little research was done to demonstrate the effectiveness of nurses' work or to describe and compare service delivery models, such as functional, team, and primary nursing, and their outcomes (Lendrum, 1999). The common outcomes measuring nurses' work during that time period were quality of patient care, job satisfaction, and patient satisfaction (Adams, Bond, & Hale, 1998). For example, Russell, and Beckman (1983) found that patients cared for under a primary nursing model reported greater satisfaction, and their perception of care was more individualized than patients nursed under a more traditional system (i.e., functional nursing). These authors also showed that primary nurses had a greater understanding of the patient, communicated more with the family, showed more concern, and were more proficient in discharge planning.

In this chapter, care delivery models have been described as management innovations, defined by McCloskey and colleagues as "new strategies, structures, or processes for the organization, delivery and financing of quality care" (McCloskey et al., 1996, p. 5). The previous discussion of care delivery models illustrates that each is a complex organizational intervention designed to achieve multiple goals and incorporating many different concepts and characteristics. In Table 9.4, various categories of management innovations, including some care delivery models or features of care delivery models, are described.

The need for systematic evaluation of such management innovation is illustrated by McCloskey and colleagues using the examples of nurse extenders, hospital-based case management, nursing shared governance, and product-line management. They note the following difficulties in evaluating nursing management innovations of this nature:

1. Complex interventions lack clear definition.
2. Innovations are often implemented with other changes, making it difficult to isolate the effect.
3. The group level of measurement makes it difficult to obtain large samples.
4. The intervention variables are not defined, controlled for, or measured.
5. The effects on staff and patients tend to be ignored.

Table 9.4 Categories of Management Innovation

1. Introduction of New Technology
   Bedside computers
   Bedside glucose monitors
   Computerized nursing care plan
   Infusion devices
   Nursing information systems

2. Personnel Development
   Certification
   Cross-training/orientation
   Leadership education for nurse managers
   Preceptor programs

3. Changes in Organization of Work
   Case management
   Critical paths/care maps
   Collaborative practice
   Contracted services
   Differentiated practice
   Flexible scheduling
   Nurse extenders/partners in practice
   Product-line management
   Self-scheduling
   Shared governance

4. Changes in Rewards and Incentives
   Clinical ladders/administrative ladders
   Fee for service
   Incentive pay
   Performance recognition programs

5. Implementation of Quality Improvement Mechanisms
   Competency testing
   Peer review
   Quality assurance program
   Technology/product evaluation
   TQM/CQI

Source: From Nursing Management Innovations: A Need for Systematic Evaluation (p. 6), by J. McCloskey, M. Maas, D. Huber, A. Kasparek, J. Specht, C. Ramler, et al., 1996. In K. Kelly & M. Maas (Eds.), *Outcomes of Effective Management Practice, SONA 8: Series on Nursing Administration* (pp. 3–19), London: Sage Publications.

In a strongly reasoned argument, these same authors recommend indicators for the measurement of five variables: (a) personnel, (b) the organization, (c) patient outcomes, (d) cost, and (e) demographics (McCloskey et al., 1996). Other authors have raised similar concerns, noting that the limitations of previous research on care delivery models include methodological problems such as weak designs, insufficient power, and failure to provide operational details of the work being evaluated (Giovannetti, 1986). A lack of standardization or validity in the psychometric tools used to measure patient outcomes makes it impossible to generalize findings, compare studies (Russell & Beckman, 1983; Thomas & Bond, 1990, 1991), or conduct meta-analyses. Isolated studies that were site specific lacked collaboration, while uncommon variables and different implementation processes further prohibited drawing conclusions about the effectiveness of nursing work (Adams, Bond, & Hale, 1998; Makinen, Kivimaki, Elovainio, Virtanen, & Bond, 2003; Ritter-Teital, 2002). In commenting on this problem, Huber (2002) pointed out that

> There are multiple definitions of case management and a diversity of models for practice. Despite the lack of standardization, the terms *case management* and *case management model* find common usage without a specific description of their meaning. The end result of such a lack of specificity is the inability to accurately compare models, programs, outcomes, and effectiveness. While case management programs generally manage risk and coordinate care as core functions, what is actually done beyond this is highly variable. When the complexity of multiple disciplines interacting to deliver case management is added into the actual practice environment, the potential for communication-related problems increases. Further, confusion and the inability to conduct comparable evaluations diminishes the case managers' effectiveness in clearly demonstrating the value of their individual efforts and their program's outcomes. A method for achieving greater specification is needed (p. 212).

Ingersoll and colleagues go beyond this general problem to comment specifically on methodological limitations of such studies. They build on this point in their comment on studies of professional practice models on the perception of work environments, noting that "a serious limitation of many of these studies is the time frame used to measure effect. Post-intervention testing ranges from 3 to 30 months, with the majority being within 1 year of model implementation. Six months to one year is too short a period of time for determining the true effect of any intervention" (Ingersoll, Schultz, Hoffart, & Ryan, 1996, p. 53).

To rectify problems of this nature, McCloskey and colleagues (1996) have proposed specific guidelines for selecting the variables to measure in order to demonstrate the impact of a management innovation. These guidelines are presented in Table 9.5.

Although there has historically been a lack of well-designed or conclusive studies of nursing care delivery models and the effects of decisions about staff mix and RN role design, this situation is beginning to change. It is beyond the scope of this chapter to discuss and evaluate emerging research in these areas. Readers are encouraged to use the criteria presented in Tables 9.4 and 9.5 to evaluate individual research articles discussing these or other types of nursing or organizational management innovations reported in the periodical literature.

Table 9.5 Guidelines for Selecting Variables in Order to Demonstrate the Impact of a Management Innovation

1. Describe the innovation.

2. What is the desired outcome? What is motivating the innovation?

3. At what level of the organization is the change you wish to measure?

4. Who will be affected by the innovation (e.g., organization, staff, patients, family)? To what extent and in what way will they be affected?

5. What does the research about the innovation demonstrate, that is, what results are known to usually happen?

6. What else is going on in the organization at the same time that might mediate the effects of the innovation?

7. When do the results need to be demonstrated?

8. Are there any natural mechanisms (e.g., regular meetings, evaluation conferences, clinic visits) for collecting data that could be used?

9. What measures are already available? Are these in easily usable form?

Source: From Nursing Management Innovations: A Need for Systematic Evaluation (p. 14), by J. McCloskey, M. Maas, D. Huber, A. Kasparek, J. Specht, C. Ramler, et al., 1996. In K. Kelly & M. Maas (Eds.), *Outcomes of Effective Management Practice, SONA 8: Series on Nursing Administration* (pp. 3–19), London: Sage Publications.

Invisible Nursing Work: Is it a Problem?

The lack of common definitions or classifications for nursing diagnoses and interventions is a barrier to the development of strong research designs to assess the effect of clinical or nursing interventions. The Canadian Nurses Association (CNA) states that these common definitions are needed to measure outcomes and assure generalizability and replicability of individual studies (CNA, 2003). A common classification system would allow nursing data to be collected consistently in order to aggregate and compare data among multiple sites within provincial/territorial, national, and international bodies (CNA, 2003; Maas & Delaney, 2004).

Clearly, the outcomes of nursing management innovations, or nursing services more generally, cannot be measured without data that reflect the demand for nursing care, the response of nurses to that demand, and the contribution of nurses to public health. Such data are generally not available for use in planning, managing, and evaluating the effectiveness of the health system. This may seem surprising since nurses are the largest group of health care professionals, and the need for nursing care is the primary reason for most hospital admissions and home care services. The hospital discharge abstract, which has for so many years been the basis of the permanent record of hospital activities, contains no information about nursing assessment, goals, interventions, or outcomes, and similar deficiencies exist in the data collection systems of community health agencies and other sectors of the health care system. For example, Jeffery (2003) studied the interactions and activities of nurses and patients during the discharge process and pointed out possible consequences of nurses' "hidden work" (as discussed by Wolf, 1990) in this process. These consequences include the patients' perception that no discharge work is being done by nurses (Armitage & Kavanagh, 1998; Cox, 1996; Proctor, Morrow-Howell, Albaz, & Weir, 1992). "Obscure" components of RN work, such as team and system coordination and communication activities that do not include direct contact with patients, were identified by McWilliams and Wong (1994). This work was not accounted for by nurses and therefore remained invisible to patients and other health care providers. This led McWilliams and Wong to conclude that leadership efforts should be directed toward making nurses' hidden work more visible.

Nurses and nursing care are also invisible in large health care and health system databases. This has serious ramifications, as Jacox (1995) points out:

- The nursing care received by patients in most health care settings is not described.
- Much of nursing practice is described as the practice of others, especially physicians.
- The effects of nursing practice on patient outcomes are not described.
- Nursing care within a single setting, or across multiple settings, is not described.
- It is not possible to identify what nurses do so that appropriate reimbursement for nursing services can be calculated.
- It is not possible to tell the difference in patient outcomes and costs when care is delivered by different professional groups (i.e., physicians versus nurses).
- A view of nursing as being indistinct from medicine is perpetuated.

There are two main reasons why the work of nurses has remained invisible. These are (a) the lack of a consensual language that describes the practice of nursing and (b) the fact that data reflecting the practice of nursing are not routinely collected and retained. Clark and Lang (1992) have succinctly stated that "if we cannot name it, we cannot control it, finance it, research it, teach it, or put it into public policy" (p. 109). In view of this, it is of critical importance to identify nursing data elements that should be included in both health agency information systems and in data sets for the health system as a whole. In order to provide the leadership necessary for this process, nursing leaders and all other nurses must become better informed and more concerned about what data are being collected, summarized, reported, and retained in the various practice settings in which they work. They must also become informed about provincial and national initiatives to develop a comprehensive set of data elements for describing nursing diagnoses, interventions, and outcomes and must lend their support to such initiatives.

Professional nursing associations and nursing informatics specialists in the United States began to address this problem with the development of a Nursing Minimum Data Set (NMDS), defined as "a minimum set of items of information with uniform definitions and categories concerning the specific dimensions of professional nursing which meets the information needs of multiple data users in the health care system" (Werley, 1988a, p. 7). Dr. Harriet Werley (1988b), who led this project, defined the benefits of an NMDS as follows:

- Access to comparable minimum nursing care and resources data at local, regional, national, and international levels
- Enhanced documentation of the nursing care provided
- Identification of trends related to patient, or client, problems and the nursing care provided
- Impetus to improved costing of nursing services
- Improved data for quality assurance evaluations
- Impetus to further development and refinement of nursing information systems
- Comparative research on nursing care, including research on nursing diagnosis, nursing interventions, current status of client problems, and referral for further nursing services
- Contributions toward advancing nursing as a research-based discipline

The NMDS consists of nursing care elements, patient demographic elements, and service elements. The nursing care elements identified were nursing diagnosis, nursing intervention, nursing outcome, and nursing intensity. All of these elements arise from the processes employed by nurses as they plan and provide care in any setting. Most of the patient demographic and service elements deemed essential by nurses, with the major exception of a unique nurse-provider identifier, could be accessed through linkages to another data set. In all, 16 essential data elements were identified for the NMDS. Standard classification systems have also been developed for the nursing care data elements to aid the collection of uniform accurate data. These include the North American Nursing Diagnosis Association (NANDA) taxonomy (NANDA, 1996), The Omaha System: Applications for Community Health Nursing (Martin & Scheet, 1992), The Home Health Care Classification (Saba, 1992), the Nursing Interventions Classification (NIC) (Iowa Intervention Project, 1996), and Nursing Outcomes Classification (NOC) (Johnson & Maas, 1995).

Canadian nurses have also been concerned with the task of identifying nursing data elements, referred to as Health Information: Nursing Components (HI:NC) to reflect the intention that nursing data be included with other essential health data. A national conference under the auspices of the Canadian Nurses Association (CNA) brought together an international multi-disciplinary group of experts and RNs from across Canada to deliberate issues related to the development, implementation, and evaluation of a nursing minimum data set for use by Canadian nurses (CNA, 1993). The overall purpose of the working conference was to develop a data set to ensure both the availability and accessibility of standardized nursing data. In the proceedings from this conference, 21 data elements are identified. Subsequently, the Alberta Association of Registered Nurses (AARN) actively pursued the aims of the working conference and developed and endorsed working definitions for the care elements (AARN, 1997). The CNA, along with its provincial counterparts, developed a workbook to assist nurses in reaching a consensus on HI:NC data elements (Sibbald, 1998).

In an effort to recognize the considerable work already completed in developing classification systems for nursing diagnoses, interventions, and outcomes, and the urgent need to develop a uniform international language for nurses, the International Council of Nurses (ICN) began work on an International Classification of Nursing Practice (ICNP). The ICNP would be used to describe nursing practice and compare nursing data across clinical populations around the world and, by doing so, could support the processes of nursing practice and advance the knowledge necessary for cost-effective delivery of quality nursing care. This classification was intended to join the ranks of other well-used classification systems such as the International Classification of Diseases (ICD) and the Diagnostic and Statistical Manual of Mental Disorders (DSM). At its current stage of development, the ICNP provides a detailed integration of the principal international classification systems, including those referred to earlier in this chapter related to nursing diagnoses, interventions, and outcomes. In addition, the ICNP provides cross-mapping to the already developed classification systems. In this way, nursing data can be compared across practice settings regardless of the particular diagnostic, intervention, and outcome classifications in use.

The Canadian Nurses Association has highlighted the need to develop a culture that values nursing informatics and has expressed concern that the failure to implement the common ICNP in Canada has had a profound impact on our ability to measure nurses' work in all arenas in order to improve patient outcomes (CNA, 2003).

In Canada, the Canadian Institute for Health Information (CIHI) has developed a Canadian Classification of Health Interventions (CCI), which was designed to meet the needs of multiple users and care providers. The CCI has several key features that reflect a shift in the development of classification schemes. It is intended to be neutral with respect to service providers and service settings. That is, the same codes are intended to be applicable regardless of whether a physician, nurse, or other provider performs an intervention, or whether the intervention was done in an operating room, emergency department, clinic, or physician's office. It is assumed that information specific to service providers and service settings will be captured as separate data elements in each individual client's record, thus overcoming the problem of "invisibility" of nurses and nursing care. Since the CCI is intended to be "provider neutral," terms such as assessment, counselling, and education can be used by any care provider. Nurses, or any health care provider using the classification, would use the index to search out the term for whatever intervention/service they provided and code it accordingly in their database/abstract.

The CNA was consulted during the development of the CCI, which was first released April 1, 2001. It was updated and re-released in 2003 in English and French and is available on the CIHI Web site. Professional associations, individual health care practitioners, and the general public can make recommendations to the CIHI on enhancements or corrections to the CCI through the public submission process. The cut-off date for inclusion of submissions for version 2006 was February 27, 2004. Submissions received after that date will be considered for version 2008.

The CCI is now the standard for all hospital morbidity data collection and is mandatory throughout Canada with the exception of Quebec, where it is expected to be adopted in 2005. Some provinces are using the CCI in ambulatory care, home care, and other settings. The Insurance Bureau of Canada uses the CCI to capture interventions by all providers for their standard auto insurance claim form. They also use ICD-10-CA to capture the diagnosis and reason for the visit.

Employed RNs in Canada: Issues and Questions

As explained in Chapter 8, the existence of imbedded matrix structures, such as the professional bureaucracy through which physicians' work is organized, intensifies the requirements for horizontal processes of communication and coordination. Management and organizational theory suggest that the introduction of additional matrix structures, such as program management, could logically be expected to further intensify the need for coordination. Historically, RNs have coordinated communication and care activities through their interdependent role. During the decade between 1992 and 2002, as the number of different health care providers involved in the direct care of patients increased, the role and numbers of employed RNs were diminished. Information published by the CIHI shows that there were fluctuations and often decreases in the number of employed RNs in Canada between 1992 and 2002. Decreases in the number of RNs in leadership positions at all levels, and particularly in senior and middle management roles, are illustrated in Table 8.3 in Chapter 8. In this chapter, information about the number of employed clinical nurses and selected other categories of the RN workforce is presented in Table 9.6.

Decreases in the numbers of employed RNs are sometimes explained or rationalized with reference to "the nursing shortage." Therefore, in examining the figures presented in Tables 8.3 and 9.6, it is particularly important to note that the information reflects the number of nurses who reported being *employed* in these positions, and not the pool of nurses available for employment. Authority for determining the number of positions available for RNs is a discretionary prerogative that rests with executive level decision makers in health agencies. The financial priorities of the organization and the value placed on RN work by the senior decision-making group result in decisions about the number of RN positions in the agency. Administrative officials in health agencies are also in control of the factors that create the structure and culture of their agencies, and these, in turn, create the characteristics of the nursing work environment. Conditions in the nursing work environment create either retention or turnover of RNs (Laschinger & Wong, 1999; Parsons & Stonestreet, 2003). Limited professional autonomy, ineffective leadership, the absence of opportunities for professional advancement, and dysfunctional or abusive relationships within the health team have been associated with job dissatisfaction and high levels of burnout and turnover among RNs. Therefore, it is problematic, but important, to separate the causal effects of role design and working arrangements in individual organizations and their subunits from other structural factors contributing to current and projected shortages of RNs and factors affecting RN retention (Upenieks, 2003).

The information in Table 9.6 is now discussed in greater detail. The first row shows that the number of staff nurses (including those in community health positions) who reported being employed fluctuated between 1992 and 2002. Numbers peaked in 1993 and fell to their lowest level in 1996. By 2002, the number of clinical nurses who reported being employed in this category had returned to a few hundred less than in 1992. During this period, there was a steady

Table 9.6 Employed RNs in Canada by Type of Position* and Educational Preparation from 1992–2002

Position	1992	1993	1994	1995	1996	1997	1998	1999	2000	2001	2002
Staff Nurse/ Community Health Nurse	175,909	180,712	183,914	172,450	163,244	170,239	170,383	173,094	178,366	176,681	175,173
Diploma (%)	88.2	87.2	86.4	85.3	84.2	83.4	82.3	81.4	80.6	79.2	78.3
BScN (%)	11.6	12.6	13.3	14.3	15.3	16.2	17.3	18.2	19.0	20.4	21.4
Master's/PhD (%)	0.2	0.2	0.4	0.4	0.5	0.3	0.3	0.4	0.4	0.3	0.4
Other	11,817	12,600	11,817	11,336	9,974	14,339	16,125	16,137	15,552	15,448	15,143
Diploma (%)	77.4	76.9	72.6	70.1	66.4	68.2	67.8	67.4	68.3	66.8	66.7
BScN (%)	21.4	21.5	25.4	27.5	30.9	29.8	29.7	29.9	29.5	30.8	30.9
Master's/PhD (%)	1.3	1.6	1.9	2.5	2.8	2.0	2.4	2.7	2.2	2.4	2.4
Clinical Specialist	1,702	1,535	1,566	1,479	1,876	1,956	2,405	2,391	2,624	2,205	2,064
Diploma (%)	55.2	48.5	46.8	42.7	54.6	54.4	55.1	51.6	51.8	50.7	45.5
BScN (%)	26.6	28.5	29.2	30.6	23.1	23.9	25.1	28.0	28.5	27.5	29.6
Master's/PhD (%)	18.2	23.1	23.9	26.7	22.2	21.7	19.8	20.4	19.7	21.7	24.9
Nurse Practitioner	/	/	/	/	/	/	/	/	/	620	912
Diploma (%)										33.1	38.7
BScN (%)										46.0	41.2
Master's/PhD (%)										21.0	20.1
Instructor/Professor/ Educator	5,915	5,864	5,816	5,532	4,944	4,441	4,506	4,807	5,213	5,658	6,489
Diploma (%)	33.6	30.8	30.2	27.6	27.5	26.9	25.6	25.5	28.3	28.7	28.0
BScN (%)	55.8	56.5	55.9	57.1	55.5	55.0	55.1	55.0	53.3	53.3	54.5
Master's/PhD (%)	10.6	12.7	13.8	15.3	16.9	18.1	19.3	19.5	18.4	18.0	17.5
Researcher	754	877	878	871	1,004	1,016	1,114	1,306	1,394	1,567	1,435
Diploma (%)	68.2	65.7	64.6	61.1	58.5	53.4	54.8	56.7	58.1	57.1	57.6
BScN (%)	27.1	28.3	27.2	31.0	33.8	37.2	37.3	35.1	33.6	35.1	32.4
Master's/PhD (%)	4.8	6.0	8.2	7.9	7.8	9.4	8.0	8.2	8.2	7.8	10.0
Consultant	1,703	1,871	2,017	2,176	2,865	2,871	4,716	5,242	5,949	6,076	6,080
Diploma (%)	56.0	55.2	52.0	51.0	54.3	53.4	51.5	50.5	52.6	49.8	48.8
BScN (%)	35.2	35.7	38.4	39.7	38.2	39.4	43.9	44.5	42.8	45.5	46.5
Master's/PhD (%)	8.8	9.1	9.7	9.3	7.5	7.2	4.6	5.0	4.6	4.7	4.7

*Table contains information about some, but not all, position categories. For complete information, go to www.cihi.ca (Supply and Distribution).
Source: © (2003) Canadian Institute for Health Information (CIHI). The contents of Table 9.6 is adapted from data supplied by CIHI. Used with permission.

increase in the number of nurses in this category with baccalaureate preparation. There were smaller but sustained increases in the number of clinical nurses who held graduate degrees.

The number of nurses who reported being in "other" positions is shown in the second row and follows a similar trend, falling to a low in 1996 and reaching a peak in 1999. The remainder of the table shows the numbers of employed RNs in select other categories: clinical specialist, nurse practitioner (added to the CIHI data dictionary in 2001), instructor/professor/educator, researcher, and consultant.

The figures presented in this table raise more questions than they answer. For example, what are the demographic and educational profiles of the RNs who report being employed in "other" workplaces? How many of these nurses are self-employed? Does this category include nurses who experienced layoffs during the period of hospital downsizing? It is possible that there are RNs in this category who could have been recruited to clinical positions in hospitals, long-term care, or community health agencies if these positions were created and if nursing workplaces were hospitable.

Other information not included in this table is needed to develop a more complete understanding of the effects of managerial decision making on the number of RN positions between 1992 and 2002. It is important to examine the numbers of RNs who held part-time, casual, and temporary positions and to understand whether they had such positions by choice or because full-time positions were not available in health agencies. Other personnel (sometimes euphemistically referred to as members of the "nursing family") are often reported by health agencies as providing nursing services, and for this reason, information about this workforce is also critical to an understanding of trends in the number of employed RNs. Information about the numbers of employed LPNs should be available from their regulatory bodies, health agencies, or provincial ministries of health. However, there is likely to be limited information available about the many unlicensed and unregulated workers who now provide direct patient care. Other questions are raised by the surprising fact that, by 2002, the number of employed RNs (i.e., the number of positions for RNs that are established and funded in health agencies) had gradually returned to 1992 levels, rather than keeping pace proportionally with population growth. The nurse to population ratio during this period is discussed in Chapter 6.

Leadership Implications

Position descriptions for RNs and other health care providers reflect organizational values, policies, and standards. However, once position descriptions are written in one organization, they may influence administrative practice in another. For example, if precedents for the required qualifications of a position are established through the process of grievance arbitration, or if terminology used in position descriptions is incorporated into a collective agreement, organizations other than the one originating the position description may be affected. Because of this, the language and structure of nursing and patient care delivery models that were introduced in response to particular economic or social conditions may be perpetuated and act as barriers to change that might benefit patients and nurses.

Care delivery models can be thought of as management interventions or innovations. Both NCDMs and PCDMs incorporate and operationalize particular priorities and values and have developed in response to, or in parallel with, particular social and economic circumstances. There has been relatively little research to describe, evaluate, or compare care delivery models.

It can be problematic to conduct such research or interpret the results if the objectives to be achieved by the model, the characteristics of the model (the independent variable), and the context in which the model is being implemented are not precisely defined or described (McCloskey et al., 1996).

Decisions about the design of nursing roles and the design and choice of nursing care delivery models were made by senior nursing leaders between the 1920s and the 1980s. Within hospitals, the organizational arrangements derived from the scientific management model became known as functional and team nursing. These arrangements of the machine bureaucracy, and their many variations, still structure the work of RNs in many health care settings today, perpetuating the impression that nursing is nothing more than a series of substitutable tasks.

Auxiliary workers were originally introduced and trained to assist nurses and were called *nurses' aides*. Formal training programs for practical nurses developed in response to nursing labour shortages in the late 1950s and gained increasing prominence in the 1980s and 1990s. Licensed practical nurses are now self-governing and have independent scopes of practice in most jurisdictions. In many settings, unlicensed, multi-skilled workers now provide most of the direct care. Ironically, RNs now have task-oriented roles in which they are called upon to assist LPNs and unlicensed workers by performing specific tasks that the LPN or multi-skilled worker is not legally permitted to carry out.

The assumption that RNs are automatically responsible for the care provided by LPNs and other workers has carried over from the era when the roles of auxiliary workers were designed with the assumption that the workers would take direction and be under the supervision of more knowledgeable RNs while performing delegated tasks. When LPNs have an independent scope of practice, their work assignments and supervision become the administrative responsibility of the organization and should not be assumed to be a professional responsibility of the RN unless the RN role description formally specifies management or supervisory responsibilities. RNs should pay particular attention to the details of position descriptions that deal with their relationships to other categories of nursing personnel, and they should avoid employment situations in which they have responsibility for the work and outcomes of individuals whom they have no authority to select, assign, supervise, or discipline.

Administrative officials (including nursing administrators) are ultimately accountable for the consequences of decisions about staff mix and the design of supervisory and administrative arrangements, including the selection of care delivery models that prescribe how individual care providers are assigned to work with patients. Decisions about work assignments for individual care providers on specific shifts are often treated as a routine matter and made on the basis of habitual practices, such as the assignment of consecutive patient rooms to one worker or team regardless of the acuity or complexity of care requirements of particular patients. First-line nursing managers must recognize that in preparing the daily work assignment and in introducing or maintaining a particular care delivery model, they are making important resource allocation decisions and professional judgments. Although documents such as the daily and shift assignment records are often informal, they can become important evidence in inquests or litigation.

In the absence of conclusive research evidence or regulatory requirements, decisions about staff mix have often been driven by ideology or expediency. Matching the needs of patients and the knowledge and skills of care providers requires professional knowledge and discretionary decision making. Decisions about staff mix are best made by RNs who have expertise to assess the needs and determine the care requirements of the client population being served.

Care delivery models provide organizational arrangements to guide day-to-day decision making about the work assignments of care providers and their collaboration with each other in the care of patients. Since the needs of patients differ from one program or care unit to another, it is illogical to think that the same care delivery model would be appropriate throughout a large program or health care organization. One writer has stated "to believe that only one approach to care delivery is applicable to all patient populations in all care settings is naive as well as potentially dangerous"(Deutschendorf, 2003, p. 58). The principles of contingency theory (situational leadership) provide a useful framework for assessing the appropriateness of a particular care delivery model in specific circumstances.

Summary

- Until the 1990s, the structural arrangements for nursing work were referred to as nursing care delivery models (NCDMs) or systems of nursing care delivery. NCDMs are nursing management interventions or innovations designed and implemented under the line, or operational, responsibility of a nurse in a senior leadership position, who is responsible for the human resource budget for nursing services and for the standards of nursing practice in the agency. Most NCDMs were developed and introduced between the 1920s and the 1990s. The case method was the original and most fully accountable NCDM.

- Patient care delivery models (PCDMs) are sometimes called systems of care delivery or patient-focused or patient-centred care. The stated goals of PCDMs include improved interdisciplinary teamwork and bringing care closer to the patient. PCDMs are defined as management interventions or innovations that create structure and organization for the work of RNs, other levels of nursing personnel, and some other health care providers through role and task design and the allocation of work activities and responsibilities. PCDM were introduced in the late 1980s and early 1990s, often in parallel with organizational restructuring, downsizing, and quality improvement initiatives.

- All NCDMs and PCDMs reflect environmental contingencies such as the availability of resources. They also reflect assumptions and organizational values about nursing work. These assumptions and values affect the way RN work is designed, allocated, and documented. This, in turn, affects that ability to measure nursing outcomes and to understand the contribution of professional nursing services to organizational and health outcomes.

- The principles and practices of scientific management and the machine bureaucracy are evident in the functional and team nursing models which divide nursing work into a series of tasks often performed by different levels of nursing personnel. In these models, coordination of activities and communication and accountability for achieving standards of care rest with a charge nurse and/or RN team leader.

- In the primary nursing model, an RN with expert knowledge of the client population and expert care planning skills has primary responsibility for the development of the nursing care plan and for assessing the outcomes of nursing care. The primary nurse uses the written care plan and other mechanisms of communication and consultation to provide direction to the work of other nursing personnel, referred to as associate nurses, who implement nursing activities throughout the 24-hour period.

- Case management is sometimes used as an approach to allocate nursing work. It builds on the skill set and approaches of primary nursing, but extends the scope for planning and coordinating care to encompass all care activities within an entire episode of care.

- Differentiated nursing practice was designed to make optimum use of the knowledge and skills of RNs with various levels of professional education and experience. Its intent is to assure that patients benefit from advanced nursing knowledge and scientific evidence.

- Evidence-based decision making to select models of care delivery is difficult because in most reports the independent variable (i.e., the model or management intervention) is not described or operationally defined. Therefore, claims for the effectiveness of individual models should be viewed with caution and evaluated in relation to criteria that experts have recommended for appraising reports and research on management interventions and innovations.

- Many issues arise when other health care providers are substituted for RNs in care delivery models and processes. These include how to provide for an accountable relationship between the RN and the patient and accountability for maintaining standards of professional practice and the outcomes of care.

- Nursing is often recognized and defined in terms of its implementation, through the nursing tasks, procedures, and activities that are most visible. Introduction of the nursing process can be viewed as a major paradigm shift within the nursing discipline, providing a conceptual model and language to describe the intellectual activities of nursing assessment, care planning, and evaluation.

- Much of nursing work has traditionally been and continues to be invisible, particularly the conceptual and intellectual activities and activities conducted in the interdependent dimension of the RN role. The structure of health records and organizational approaches to the documentation of nursing care perpetuate the invisibility of nursing services, making it difficult to identify their contribution to organizational and health outcomes.

- Research has shown that factors such as decreased autonomy and increased workloads for nurses are associated with increased patient mortality and morbidity.

- During the period between 1992 and 2002, the numbers of RNs employed in staff nurse positions fluctuated in response to the elimination of positions through organizational restructuring activities, often described as patient-centred, or patient-focused, or for the purposes of quality improvement. The number of employed RNs did not keep pace with population growth during this period. The number of RNs in leadership positions has substantially decreased since 1992.

Applying the Knowledge in this Chapter

Exercise

Observation and Experience: Consider a nursing workplace from your current or past experience.

1. Read the following article with particular attention to the dimensions identified on pages 53 and 54: Deutschendorf, A.L. (2003). From past paradigms to future frontiers: Unique care delivery models to facilitate nursing work and quality outcomes. *Journal of Nursing Administration, 33*(1), 52–59.

2. Now try to describe the care delivery model in use in your area using the dimensions and analytical perspective presented in the article.
   a) Is there a recognizable nursing care delivery model?
   b) What is the role of the RN?
   c) Are the independent assessments and activities of RNs documented in a permanent form?

Appraising Knowledge of Care Delivery Models:

1. Read the following article describing a PCDM: Mitchell, G.J., Closson, T., Coulis, N., Flint, F., & Gray, B. (2000). Patient-focused care and human becoming thought: Connecting the right stuff. *Nursing Science Quarterly, 13*(3), 216–224.

2. Use the categories and guidelines in Tables 9.4 and 9.5 as a framework to evaluate the PCDM described in the article.
   a) What are its strengths and shortcomings?
   b) What is the intervention or innovation?
   c) Are the outcomes described?
   d) Could this model be replicated in other settings based on the information in the article? Should it be replicated? Why or why not?
   e) What is needed to advance knowledge about this or a similar PCDM?

Resources

evolve Internet Resources

Agency for Healthcare Research and Quality (AHRQ):
   www.ahrq.gov/

Canadian Institute for Health Information (CIHI):
www.cihi.ca/
Click on Standards, then Coding/Classification, then CCI.

Further Reading

Deutschendorf, A.L. (2003). From past paradigms to future frontiers: Unique care delivery models to facilitate nursing work and quality outcomes. *Journal of Nursing Administration, 33*(1), 52–59.

O'Rourke, M.W. (2003). Rebuilding a professional practice model: The return of role-based practice accountability. *Nursing Administration Quarterly, 27*(2), 95–105.

References

Adams, A., Bond, S., & Hale, C. (1998). Nursing organizational practice and its relationship with other features of ward organization and job satisfaction. *Journal of Advanced Nursing, 27*, 1212–1222.

Alberta Association of Registered Nurses. (1997). *Client status, nursing intervention and client outcomes classification system: A discussion paper*. Edmonton, AB: AARN.

Armitage, S.K., & Kavanagh, K.M. (1998). Consumer-oriented outcomes in discharge planning: A pilot study. *Journal of Clinical Nursing, 7*(1), 67–74.

Baker, C., Lamm, G., Winter, A., Robbeloth, V., Ransom, C., & Conly, F., et al. (1997). Differentiating nursing practice: Assessing the state-of-the-science. *Nursing Economics, 15*(5), 253–261.

Canadian Institute for Health Information (CIHI). (2003). Retrieved June 2003, from http://www.cihi.ca

Canadian Nurses Association. (1993). *Papers from the Nursing Minimum Data Set Conference*. Ottawa, ON: CNA.

Canadian Nurses Association. (2003). International classification for nursing practice: Documenting nursing care and client outcomes. *Nursing Now: Issues and Trends in Canadian Nursing, 14*(1), 1–4.

Clark, J., & Lang, N. (1992). Nursing's next advance: An international classification for nursing practice. *International Nursing Review, 39*(4), 109–112.

Cox, C.B. (1996). Discharge planning for dementia patients: Factors influencing caregiver decisions and satisfaction. *Health and Social Work, 21*(2), 97–104.

Cummings, G., & Estabrooks, C.A. (2003). The effects of hospital restructuring that included layoffs on individual nurses who remained employed: A systematic review of impact. *International Journal of Sociology and Social Policy, 23*(8/9), 8–53.

Deutschendorf, A.L. (2003). From past paradigms to future frontiers: Unique care delivery models to facilitate nursing work and quality outcomes. *Journal of Nursing Administration, 33*(1), 52–59.

Felton, G., Abbe, S., Gilbert, C., & Ingle, J.R. (1999). How does NLNAC support the concept of differentiated practice? *Nursing & Health Care Perspectives, 20*(5), 275.

Giovannetti, P. (1986). Evaluation of primary nursing. In H. Werley, J. Fitzpatrick, & R. Taunton (Eds.), *Annual review of nursing research* (Vol. 4, pp. 4127–4151). New York: Springer Publishing.

Henderson, J.L., & Williams, J.B. (1991). The people side of patient care redesign. *Healthcare Forum Journal, 34*(4), 44–49.

Huber, D.L. (2002). The diversity of case management models. *Lippincott's Case Management, 7*(6), 212–220.

Huston, C.J. (2002). The role of the case manager in a disease management program. *Lippincott's Case Management, 6*(5), 222–227.

Hutchens, G. (1994). Differentiated interdisciplinary practice. *Journal of Advanced Nursing, 24*(6), 52–58.

Ingersoll, G.L., Schultz, A.W., Hoffart, N., & Ryan, S.A. (1996). The effect of a professional practice model on staff nurse perception of work groups and nurse leaders. *Journal of Nursing Administration, 26*(5), 52–60.

Iowa Intervention Project. (1996). *Nursing interventions classification (NIC)* (2nd ed.). St. Louis, MO: Mosby.

Jacox, A. (1995). Practice and policy implications of clinical and administrative databases. In American Nurses Association (Ed.), *Nursing data systems: The emerging framework* (pp. 161–165). Washington, DC: ANA.

Jeffery, C. (2003). *An exploration of the nursing-patient dyad in acute care discharge.* Unpublished master's thesis, College of Nursing, University of Saskatchewan, Saskatoon, Saskatchewan, Canada.

Johnson, M., & Maas, M. (1995). Classification of nursing-sensitive patient outcomes. In American Nurses Association (Ed.), *Nursing data systems: The emerging framework* (pp. 177–183). Washington, DC: ANA.

Komplin, J. (1995). Care delivery systems. In P.S. Yoder Wise (Ed.), *Leading and managing in nursing* (pp. 422–428). Toronto, ON: Mosby.

Laschinger, H.K.S., & Wong, C. (1999). Staff nurse empowerment and collective accountability: Effect on perceived productivity and self-rated work effectiveness. *Nursing Economics, 17,* 308–316.

Lemieux-Charles, L., & Wylie, D. (1992). Administrative issues. In A. Baumgart & J. Larsen (Eds.), *Canadian nursing faces the future* (2nd ed., pp. 241–257). Toronto, ON: Mosby.

Lendrum, B.L. (1994). Organization of patient care. In J.M. Hibberd & M.E. Kyle (Eds.), *Nursing management in Canada* (pp. 312–330). Toronto, ON: W.B. Saunders.

Lendrum, B.L. (1999). Work process redesign and nurses' work. In J. Hibberd & D. Smith (Eds.), *Nursing management in Canada* (2nd ed., pp. 157–173). Toronto, ON: W.B. Saunders.

Maas, M., & Delaney, C. (2004). Nursing process outcome linkage research: Issues, current status, and health policy implications. *Medical Care, 42*(Suppl 2), II-40–II-48.

Makinen, A., Kivimaki, M., Elovainio, M., Virtanen, M., & Bond, S. (2003). Organization of nursing care as a determinant of job satisfaction among hospital nurses. *Journal of Nursing Management, 11,* 299–306.

Manthey, M. (2003). Aka primary nursing. [Guest editorial]. *Journal of Nursing Administration, 33*(7/8), 369–370.

Martin, K.S., & Scheet, N.J. (1992). *The Omaha system: Applications for community health nursing.* Philadelphia: W.B. Saunders.

McCloskey, J., Maas, M., Huber, D., Kasparek, A., Specht, J., Ramler, C., et al. (1996). Nursing management innovations: A need for systematic evaluation. In K. Kelly & M. Maas (Eds.), *Outcomes of effective management practice, SONA 8: Series on nursing administration* (pp. 3–19). London: Sage Publications.

McPhail, J. (1996). Organization for nursing care: Primary nursing, traditional approaches, or both? In J. Kerr & J. McPhail (Eds.), *Canadian nursing issues and perspectives* (3rd ed., pp. 228–240). St. Louis, MO: Mosby.

McPherson, K. (1996). *Bedside matters: The transformation of Canadian nursing, 1900-1990.* Toronto, ON: Oxford University Press.

McWilliams, C.L., & Wong, C.A. (1994). Keeping it secret: The costs and benefits of nursing's hidden work in discharging patients. *Journal of Advanced Nursing, 19*(1), 152–163.

Melosh, B. (1982). *The physician's hand: Work culture and conflict in American nursing.* Philadelphia: Temple University Press.

Mitchell, G.J., Closson, T., Coulis, N., Flint, F., & Gray, B. (2000). Patient-focused care and human becoming thought: Connecting the right stuff. *Nursing Science Quarterly, 13*(3), 216–224.

Murphy, M., & DeBack, V. (1990). Myths and realities. In American Association of Nurse Executives (Ed.), *Current issues and perspectives on differentiated practice* (pp. 5–16). Chicago: American Hospital Association.

North American Nursing Diagnosis Association. (1996). *NANDA nursing diagnosis: Definitions and classifications.* Philadelphia: NANDA.

O'Rourke, M.W. (2003). Rebuilding a professional practice model: The return of role-based practice accountability. *Nursing Administration Quarterly, 27*(2), 95–105.

Parsons, M., & Stonestreet, J. (2003). Factors that contribute to nurse manager retention. *Nursing Economics, 21*(3), 120–126.

Picard, A. (2000). *Critical care: Canadian nurses speak for change.* Toronto, ON: Harper Collins.

Picard, E.I., & Robertson, G.B. (1996). Medical records. In E.I. Picard & G.B. Robertson (Eds.), *Legal liability of doctors and hospitals in Canada* (3rd ed., pp. 399–419). Toronto, ON: Carswell Thomson Professional.

Proctor, E., Morrow-Howell, N., Albaz, R., & Weir, C. (1992). Patient and family satisfaction with discharge plans. *Medical Care, 30*(3), 262–275.

Rachlis, M. (2004). *Prescription for excellence: How innovation is saving Canada's health care system.* Toronto, ON: Harper Collins.

Ritter-Teital, J. (2002). The impact of restructuring on professional nursing practice. *Journal of Nursing Administration, 32*(1), 31–41.

Rondeau, K.V., & Wagar, T.H. (2004). Implementing CQI while reducing the work force: How does it influence hospital performance? *Healthcare Management Forum, 17*(2), 22–29.

Russell, S., & Beckman, J.C. (1983). Primary nursing: An evaluation of its effects on patient perception of care and staff satisfaction. *International Journal of Nursing Studies, 20*(4), 265–273.

Saba, V.K. (1992). The classification of home health care nursing diagnoses and interventions. *Caring, 11*(3), 50–57.

Schein, E.H. (1993). On dialogue, culture, and organizational learning. *Organizational Dynamics, 22*(2), 40–52.

Schweikhart, S.B., & Smith-Daniels, V. (1996). Reengineering the work of caregivers: Role redefinition, team structures, and organizational redesign. *Hospital & Health Services Administration, 41*(1), 19–35.

Sibbald, B.J. (1998). Nursing informatics. *The Canadian Nurse, 94*(4), 22–30.

Smith, J., & Smith, D.L. (1999). Service integration and case management. In J. Hibberd & D. Smith (Eds.), *Nursing management in Canada* (2nd ed., pp. 175–193). Toronto, ON: W.B. Saunders.

Stanton, M.W. (2004). Hospital nurse staffing and quality of care. *Research in Action, 14,* 1–9.

Thomas, L.H., & Bond, S. (1990). Towards defining the organization of nursing care in hospital wards: An empirical study. *Journal of Advanced Nursing, 15,* 1106–1112.

Thomas, L.H., & Bond, S. (1991). Outcomes and nursing care. *International Journal of Nursing Studies, 28*(4), 291–314.

Upenieks, V. (2003). Nurse leaders' perceptions of what compromises successful leadership in today's acute inpatient environment. *Nursing Administration Quarterly, 27*(2), 140–152.

Warzynski, D. (2001). Is now the time to battle over the issue of differentiated practice??? *Stat: Bulletin of the Wisconsin Nurses Association, 70*(9), 2–3.

Werley, H.H. (1988a). Introduction to the nursing minimum data set and its development. In H.H. Werley & N.M. Lang (Eds.), *Identification of the nursing minimum data set* (pp. 1–15). New York: Springer.

Werley, H.H. (1988b). Research directions. In H.H. Werley & N.M. Lang, (Eds.), *Identification of the nursing minimum data set* (pp. 427–431). New York: Springer.

Wolf, Z.R. (1990). Uncovering the hidden work of nursing. *Nursing & Health Care, 10*(9), 463–467.

ORGANIZATION DESIGN AND STRATEGIC MANAGEMENT: A CRITICAL ANALYSIS

Carl A. Meilicke

Learning Objectives

In this chapter, you will learn:

- The origin and evolution of organization design theory
- Basic theoretical concepts of strategic management theory, including environmental variables and managerial tools
- Perspectives and assumptions about organizations as open and closed systems
- Rational and natural approaches to planning in open and closed systems
- Organizational issues common to all human service organizations
- Six key peripheral concepts to consider in management decision making
- Application of these basic theoretical concepts to events that occurred during the restructuring of typical, large, tertiary health care centres in the l990s

Nursing services are almost always delivered in the context of a formal organization, and this has a profound effect on the quality of these services. Because of this, all nurses should be competent in analyzing the efficiency and effectiveness of formal organizations, and nursing administrators should be highly competent in modifying and managing them.

This chapter provides an overview of organization design theory and indicates how to make use of that knowledge in everyday practice. The material is considered advanced because it is assumed that the reader already has some understanding of organization theory, including the classical, human relations, systems, and contingency theories discussed in Chapter 8. The first and second sections of this chapter will introduce basic theoretical concepts. The third section will provide a conceptual framework for strategic management that will help the reader to apply these theoretical concepts to practical situations. The fourth section will show how to use the conceptual framework to analyze a practical nursing management situation and provide a theory-based critique of what happened in that situation. The chapter begins with an explanation of key concepts that are central to the discussion.

Key Concepts

Organization design theory focuses on the question of how decision makers in enterprises (e.g., governments, health agencies, schools, corporations) create the structures and processes required for achieving their mission and goals effectively and efficiently. Complex organizations such as health care agencies characteristically have multiple goals and offer a range of special-ized services to the public. Decisions must be made about dividing up the work, assigning respon-sibility, and coordinating the efforts of groups and subgroups, in other words, determining the way in which the agency is structured.

Strategic management is a systematic planning process by which decision makers determine the future direction and ongoing administration of an organization. It is based on four steps: (a) assessing the external environment in terms of technical, political, and cultural variables; (b) devising an overall plan based on this assessment that includes goals, structure, and process; (c) establishing a process of day-to-day decision making based on the overall plan; and (d) imple-menting a process whereby the overall plan can be modified in response to environmental changes and internal feedback.

Open and closed system perspectives refer to two ways of understanding the nature of organ-izations and their relationship to the environment. An *open system perspective* assumes that decision making in organizations must involve an assessment of pressures externally imposed by the environment. A *closed system perspective* generally discounts the importance of the envi-ronment in understanding organizations and assumes that management decisions can best be made by analyzing internal structures and processes. (Refer to Chapter 8 for more on systems theory.)

Rational and natural systems approaches refer to schools of thought or ways of thinking about organizations. A *rational* approach to systems is guided by classical bureaucratic princi-ples (e.g., hierarchy, chain of command, rules). Goal setting and achievement of measurable goals and objectives are key features of this approach. A *natural* approach focuses more on the need to respond rapidly and spontaneously to emergent issues to ensure organizational survival, and it de-emphasizes formal goal setting. It is also guided by assumptions about human relations (e.g., worker aspirations, motivations).

Organization Design Theory, Approaches, and Influences

Evolution of contemporary organization theory began at the turn of the 20th century, and the most important developments have occurred since the 1930s. By the late 1970s, the large and varied store of useful ideas that had been developed could be grouped under two general perspectives—open and closed. These were further divided into two distinct approaches, rational and natural, as shown in Table 10.1. Each of these four approaches offered many valuable insights but, as the limitations section of Table 10.1 shows, none offered a complete answer to the question of how to create and maintain an efficient and effective organization. Since the 1970s, a new approach has emerged: strategic management theory (not to be confused with the strategic contingencies approach). Strategic management theory provides a way to integrate the prior perspectives and approaches into a more or less coherent whole.

The next section contains a brief description and critical assessment of the original four approaches. Then, six supplementary concepts are introduced that are useful to those who are applying theoretical concepts. Following this is a description of strategic management theory.

Open Versus Closed Systems and Rational Versus Natural Approaches

The basic assumptions underlying each of the four approaches are dramatically different. These assumptions are reflected in either a closed or open system perspective of organizations and, within each of these systems, a rational or natural approach. The closed versus open system perspective reflects the degree to which it is believed that the external environment of the organization must be taken into account when managers make decisions. The rational versus natural approach reflects the degree to which management is perceived to involve (rational) pre-planning of objectives and the means to achieve them, as opposed to a more (natural) dynamic process of ongoing adaptation to changing circumstances.

The result of these differences in basic assumptions is that each approach leads to dramatically different solutions. Table 10.1 shows how these four approaches affect seven key organizational issues. For example, both closed system perspectives (rational and natural) tend to support the idea that there is a "one best way" to manage, but this is largely the result of discounting or ignoring the impact that a wide variety of factors in the environment can have upon the organization. To illustrate this, *classical bureaucratic theory* may seem to be the best way to deal with cost and quality control in a situation where the management issues are complex and the consequences of error are severe. It is difficult to defend this position, however, if one recognizes that many employees have strong negative feelings about rigid authoritarianism because of attitudes they bring to the work situation from outside the organization. The *human relations school* recognizes that workers often prefer more participation in decision making (and therefore concludes that the one best way to manage is an approach that encourages worker involvement in decision making); it fails to recognize, however, that many workers do not wish to accept the responsibility that comes with participation because of commitments and interests they have outside of the organization.

By the early 1960s, the open system perspective had gained prominence because researchers began to recognize the undeniable importance of environmental variables. It was not long before a large number of *technical, political,* and *social factors* were considered to be potentially important to any given organization. These insights initially led to the idea of a *contingency approach* to dealing with organizational issues. This means that there is no one best way to manage, and the most appropriate management action is seen to be contingent upon the particular combination of environmental variables that act upon each specific organization at a given point in time. Within this open system perspective, proponents of the rational approach argue that one can assess the environment and develop a plan to cope with its effects.

In the early 1970s, the *open natural approach* emerged when some researchers came to believe that environmental complexity and rate of change are so great that the organization cannot plan for environmental changes and can only respond in an ad hoc fashion. There is a troubling aspect to this approach: the assumption that the environment dominates rather than shapes the organization can lead to a dysfunctional organization, as evidenced by the response to issues such as *effectiveness, conflict,* and *social integration* when using this approach (see Table 10.1). The approach can also be used by a dishonest or incompetent management team to justify otherwise unacceptable behaviour by allowing the managers to argue that the environment is too complex to be properly dealt with.

Needless to say, each approach has some degree of usefulness, depending on the circumstances. The rational, pre-planned, and centralized authority techniques of *scientific management* (a subset of classical bureaucratic theory) are often of great value when the work is highly repetitive and routine, as it is on an assembly line. At the same time, some aspects of *participative management* will almost always enhance employee morale, and some degree of contingency planning is necessary to protect the organization from sudden external changes (e.g., advances in robotic technology that rendered much of the assembly line obsolete, or a change in employee attitudes that caused them to begin resisting a tradition of highly centralized decision making).

Styles of Management and Management Theory

This "mix and match" approach to management provides many different options, depending on circumstances specific to the management situation. It is helpful to think of these options as falling on a continuum that extends from *mechanistic* to *organic*, with the intermediate range of the continuum being described as *ambidextrous*. A mechanistic style emphasizes rules, procedures, a clear hierarchy of authority, centralization, and a task-oriented approach to employee morale. It tends to

Table 10.1 Summary of Theoretical Perspectives on Organizational Issues

Organizatonal Issues	Closed System	
	Rational Approaches	**Natural Approaches**
	Classical bureaucratic theory (Taylor, 1911; Gulick & Urwick, 1937; Weber, 1947; Mooney, 1947; Gouldner, 1954)	The "human relations" school (Barnard, 1938; Roethlisberger & Dickson, 1939; McGregor, 1960; Argyris, 1966; Likert, 1967)
Efficiency	Classical/Bureaucratic Theory Position May be obtained through application of work-study methods and predetermined principles of "good" management. Maximized through a hierarchically ordered chain of positions and specified procedures for operation.	Human Relations Position Best brought about by integrating individual aspirations with organizational goals. Involve workers in their job through participatory decision making, job enlargement, job enrichment, etc.
Effectiveness	As above.	In addition to profit, growth, and quality, individual member satisfaction in the organization is viewed as a major goal in its own right.
Conflict	Should be avoided. This can be accomplished by constructing appropriate departmentalization, chains of command, and span of control. Minimize potential for conflict by having a rule or procedure for everything.	Is generally viewed as dysfunctional, but should be managed and confronted openly when it occurs.
Change (innovation)	Handle by means of rational accommodation and intervention, establishment of new rules and procedures.	Must be accommodated through changes in the informal structures of the organization as well as the formal structures.

Table 10.1 (Continued)

Open System	
Rational Approaches	**Natural Approaches**
(Burns & Stalker, 1961; Woodward, 1965; Lawrence & Lorsch, 1967; Thompson, 1967; Perrow, 1967; Katz & Kahn, 1966; Becker & Gordon, 1966; Hage, 1965, 1980; Khandwalla, 1974; Shortell, 1977; Simon, 1965; Cyert & March, 1963; Alexis & Wilson, 1967)	(Hickson et al., 1971; March & Olson, 1976; Meyer & Rowan, 1977; Hannan & Freeman, 1977; Pfeffer & Salancik, 1978; Tushman & Nadler, 1978; Aldrich, 1979)
Contingency/Decision Theory Position May be attained in several ways depending on the nature of the tasks involved, the people involved, and external circumstances. Depends on the quality of the decisions made under uncertainty.	Strategic Contingencies/Political Negotiation/Resource Dependence/ Population Ecology Position Overall objective is not efficiency per se but system survival. As such, political as well as economic transactions become important.
As above. In addition, one way that organizations survive is by expanding or changing their goals to meet new demands from the environment. Emphasis is on goal attainment.	As above. Emphasis is not on goal attainment but on obtaining resources and balancing internal political considerations of those vying for power in order to survive.
Not necessarily viewed as dysfunctional. Can promote creativity and innovation. The problem is to minimize disruptive conflict. Attending to different goals at different times may be helpful.	Viewed as a natural consequence of internal negotiations over power, given the strategic contingencies the organization faces.
Can occur either from within or without the organization. Again, depends on nature of tasks, people, and environment. Some evidence to indicate that more loosely structured organizations are more innovative in an "inventive" sense but that more tightly structured organizations may be better at implementing and diffusing the innovation. Ability to change or innovate is also a function of organizational learning over time.	Comes about both through external demands and internal political adjustments to those demands. Those who can most influence the type, pace, and direction of change at one point in time may not be most influential at another point in time as the organization's environment changes and its need for different kinds of expertise changes accordingly.

Table 10.1 (Continued)

Organizatonal Issues	Closed System	
	Rational Approaches	**Natural Approaches**
Social Integration/ Motivation	Can be attained through appropriate structural mechanisms (unity of command, span of control, etc.). Little attention given to the individual.	Achieved through the informal system of relationships among workers. Emphasis on nonpecuniary rewards, such as intrinsic job satisfaction and opportunities for personal expression and growth.
Coordination	A primary goal of the organization. May be achieved through appropriate departmentalization, hierarchy, and specification of rules and procedures.	Little attention given to it. Again, emphasis is on the informal work group as a coordinative mechanism.
Maintenance (adaptation to environment)	Essentially not considered.	Essentially not considered.
	Limitations 1. Incomplete motivational assumptions. 2. Little appreciation of nature or role of conflict. 3. No consideration of the limitations of individuals as information-processing beings. 4. Essentially no consideration of the environment in which organizations function. 5. A "one best way" approach: the "only way" to manage.	**Limitations** 1. Many of the studies upon which the theory is based have been poorly designed. 2. Limited view of human motivation—assumes all individuals want more participation and involvement. 3. Essentially no consideration of the environment. 4. A "one best way" approach.

Table 10.1 (Continued)

Open System	
Rational Approaches	**Natural Approaches**
May be achieved in a variety of ways including both intrinsic and extrinsic factors contributing to job satisfaction. The emphasis is on role—getting people to function in their role and understanding each other's roles.	Is achieved through internal accommodation among competing groups that agree to go along with the dominant coalition at the time because it is in their best interest to do so.
The more specialized the organization and the greater the degree to which tasks are interdependent, the greater the need for coordination. May be achieved through committees and task forces as well as informal organization.	Primary reliance is placed on informal and emergent processes rather than on formal rules, procedures, or committees. Coordination is achieved through negotiation and bargaining.
Crucial to understanding organizational behaviour. The organization must "negotiate" its environment by engaging in search procedures, dealing with uncertainty, and structuring itself to meet the demands of the environment.	Of primary importance. Those in leadership positions must manage the organization's environment as well as the internal structures and processes. Leaders must seek to "enact" their environments in addition to simply "reacting" to them.
Limitations A conceptually sound approach for the study of organizations, but requires much more research to replicate some of the early findings and define further the nature of the interaction between an organization and its environment. Problem of measuring the environment; perceptual versus nonperceptual measures.	**Limitations** There has been little empirical study to date of the open natural systems approach. The approach may also be somewhat of an overreaction to the rational contingency approaches. A middle ground would suggest that organizations survive in the long run through some degree of goal attainment in which certain kinds of organizational designs and processes provide a structural framework for channeling internal political negotiations. In brief, some degree of goal attainment would appear necessary in order for the organization to maintain sufficient credibility to continue to attract needed resources.

Source: From *Health Care Management: A Text in Organizational Theory and Behaviour* (pp. 26–29), by S. Shortell and A. Kaluzny, 1983, New York: John Wiley & Sons. Reprinted with permission of the authors.

incorporate many elements of the closed system orientation. An organic style emphasizes flexibility, individual initiative, decentralization, and encouragement of individual creativity. It tends to reflect many elements of the open system approach. Management styles found at or near the midpoint of the continuum incorporate elements of both approaches and are described as ambidextrous.

Recognition of the open system concept and the organic/mechanistic concept represented a breakthrough in the utility of management theory, but the price of this progress was complexity and ambiguity. In the open system, an enormous number of environmental variables potentially require analysis. There are also a large number of management options to consider. Furthermore, environmental variables keep changing, and this often changes the nature of a suitable management response. It became quite clear that good management decision making was much more complex, and had to be much more adaptable to changing circumstances, than had been previously recognized. By the early 1980s, it was evident that a new theoretical framework was necessary—one that would deal more effectively with the complexity and ambiguity of the new insights.

Strategic management theory is what emerged. Although it is based on the open system/rational approach, it allows a wide range of environmental and managerial options to be taken into account much more easily. It also provides a way to make selective use of all the prior perspectives and approaches in a more or less integrated fashion.

Factors Influencing Organization Design

Before examining the exciting new perspective of strategic management theory, it is useful to review six important peripheral concepts that have emerged from the research since the turn of the 20th century. These supplementary ideas are not central components of any perspective, approach, or theory; however, as with the concept of ambidexterity, they are useful rhetorical tools when it comes to applying theory.

History of an Organization and Personality of its Actors

The history of an organization and the personality of its members are the key influential factors to consider. Two important historical considerations are the size and life cycle of the organization. It is obvious that as an organization grows in size it will tend to develop more mechanistic characteristics in the form of rules, regulations, policies, impersonality, and so on. What is not quite so obvious is that organizations go through cycles of change depending on changes in the environment or on ways in which the organization undertakes to respond to environmental constraints and opportunities. For example, steady increase in the complexity and instability of the environment usually creates significant new challenges in maintaining an ambidextrous balance between mechanistic elements of management (which are necessary for effective coordination and control) and organic elements (which increase the speed with which the organization can adapt to a changing environment).

Changes in leadership and the personality of managers can also create a new cycle because different individuals assess the environment, and respond to it, in different ways. Some managers are highly skilled in this regard, and some are not; some learn and improve with experience, and some do not; and finally, some are emotionally stable people who can deal with ambiguity in a mature fashion, and some are not. All managers are not created equal.

Organizational Levels and Subsystems

One automatically thinks of the total organization as a system, but it is made up of many subsystems (work teams, units, departments, divisions, and so on) and is itself only a small part of larger systems (e.g., a hospital is a subset of the acute care system, which is a subset of the health care system). Organization design theory can be used with respect to any level (subsystem) of the organization, but the nature of the environmental factors bearing upon each subsystem is likely to be different; therefore, different management solutions may be appropriate at different levels of the organization. The technical, political, and cultural environments of importance to the manager of a pediatric ward, for example, are quite different from those of a geriatric ward, and both are different from the overall division of nursing. Accordingly, the best combination of organic and mechanistic components of a management solution may be quite different within and between different levels of the organization.

The Environment

This concept concerns summarizing data on the nature of the environment. This is most commonly done in terms of two dimensions, each of which is a continuum: *simplicity/complexity* and *stability/instability*. Generally speaking, the more simple and stable the environment, the more mechanistic the organization can be because the need for adaptability is less. Conversely, the more complex and unstable the environment, the more organic the organization can and should be. During the mid-1980s and early 1990s, for example, as the external environment of most health organizations became dramatically more complex and unstable, senior managers responded by trying to make their organizations more organic. It was assumed that this approach would enable health service organizations to adapt more quickly to change. A number of management innovations were advocated on the basis that they would decentralize authority for decision making and thereby encourage more participation in the decision process. Throughout this process, the boundaries and previously well-understood roles of health disciplines other than medicine were intentionally blurred. Changes in organizational structure, the redesign of work processes, the widespread introduction of quality circles, and promotion of the virtues of self-directed teams were among the management experiments of this period. More recently, as health services have been regionalized in most provinces, a return to more centralized decision making can be observed.

Technical Variables

Technical variables involve relatively tangible and inanimate factors such as money supply, number and types of workers, and types of knowledge, material, and equipment. The nature of relevant technology is an unusually important environmental variable because it frequently establishes rigid limitations on the options available to managers. Two subconcepts, *complexity* and *interdependence*, are basic to the idea. Technological complexity is defined by the number (variety) of exceptions to the "normal" case that is indicated by the technology and, given that technology, by how easy it is to define (analyze) an appropriate way to handle these exceptions. *High variety* (many exceptions) and *low analyzability* (difficulty in defining the best solution to the exceptions) are described as non-routine technology and tend to call for more organic forms of management. Low variety and high analyzability represent routine technologies and lend themselves to more mechanistic approaches. Looking only at this complexity aspect of technology, for example, one might well expect a relatively organic management style to be used in a psychiatric ward because the knowledge (theory) underlying psychotherapy allows for many exceptions to the normal case and many variations on how to treat each individual case. Conversely, a more mechanistic style might be appropriate on a ward dealing with uncomplicated surgery.

The other subconcept has to do with the degree of interdependence created as a result of the technology, especially with other work groups, professions, departments, and so on. Interdependence can range from *pooled* (very low, as between a nursing unit and the accounting office), to *sequential* (the output of one unit is input for another, such as admitting and nursing), to *reciprocal* (where outputs flow back and forth, such as a surgical ward and the surgical suite).

Nursing technology, for example, creates high levels of interdependence with a wide variety of diagnostic, clinical, and support groups or units. The higher the level of interdependence, the greater the need for attention to communication and coordination. Accordingly, the need for good communication and coordination techniques within nursing subsystems, and between them and other subsystems, is greater than in many other components of the hospital. This generally requires more organic styles of management so that rapid adaptability is easier. At the same time, many of the interdependencies of nursing are pooled or sequential so that both mechanistic and ambidextrous styles are also often appropriate.

Organizational Dilemmas

Many of the most important decisions in management involve balancing requirements that are in many ways incompatible but must be provided for if the organization is to survive. This is the concept of *organizational dilemmas*. For example, both coordination and communication are essential for an organization to survive. Communication is usually improved if hierarchy is minimized (which can be done, for example, by reducing the number of supervisors and decentralizing authority), but this measure will almost always make coordination more difficult because coordination is heavily dependent upon hierarchy, especially in larger organizations. Many other examples could be given, but they can be generally summarized in terms of an organic/mechanistic dilemma. Both styles have merit, and all organizations must have elements of each; therefore, the challenge is to achieve and maintain an ambidextrous style that creates an appropriate balance. These dilemmas cannot be avoided—they can only be endured. As a result, they are one of the major challenges, and one of the major responsibilities, facing managers.

Health organizations must deal with a number of unusual dilemmas. One of the more important is the need for *high reliability* in areas where the cost of error is so great that extraordinary means must be taken to minimize mistakes. The degree to which an organization must require high reliability varies within the organization, and within each subsystem, along a continuum. When a nurse is assisting with transplant surgery or injecting intravenous chemotherapy, for example, there is a need for high reliability. With many other nursing functions, the need may be much lower. High reliability creates a dilemma for the organization because, on the one hand, an organic style of management may encourage the sense of individual responsibility that is needed to minimize errors, but, on the other hand, a mechanistic style is more likely to ensure that controls are in place to prevent ill-informed or irresponsible behaviour. Professionalization of a work group, incidentally, is an expensive but effective way to increase reliability in work situations, such as nursing, where it is difficult to use mechanistic controls.

The growing emphasis on patient expectations has created a similar dilemma. It is important to be attentive to the preferences and personal satisfaction of the patient, and this is compatible with an organic style that allows front-line workers more flexibility in decision making. On the other hand, the organization as a whole has both a legal and a moral responsibility for the acts of its employees and agents, and this requires certain mechanistic elements to be in place if their behaviour is to be properly monitored and controlled.

Ethical Accountability

The last key concept relating to organization design theory concerns ethical implications of management decision making. It is unfortunate that this most important concept has yet to receive the attention it deserves from either organization design theorists or management practitioners. It is fortunate, however, that an open system/rational approach is well suited to deal with the complex problems presented by ethical issues in management. The open system orientation requires that management consider the ethical milieu of the organization in terms of both its impact on the organization and the impact the organization has on the environment. The rational approach requires that due and deliberate consideration be given to all relevant management variables, and there is no justification for arguing that ethical issues are not relevant in delivering health services. Furthermore, the organic/mechanistic concept facilitates analysis of the extremely important ethical issues related to determining how the organization can best fulfill its responsibility for the actions of its staff.

Strategic Management Theory

The problem of designing and implementing a management theory that was more able to deal with complexity and ambiguity led to the idea of strategic management. Strategic management involves four steps:

Step 1. Assess the environment.

Step 2. Devise an overall management strategy based on this assessment.

Step 3. Make day-to-day decisions based on the overall management strategy.

Step 4. Modify the management strategy on an ongoing basis in response to changes in the environment and feedback from the daily decision-making process.

It is important to note that this theory provides a way to integrate all of the earlier perspectives and concepts. Looking again at Table 10.1, for example, we can see that this approach incorporates the open system perspective (Step 1), including either of the rational or natural approaches (Steps 2 and 3), and recognizes the associated need for adaptability due to either a changing environment or to actual experience associated with implementing the strategy (Step 4). It similarly allows for easy accommodation of the ideas from the closed system perspective as well as peripheral concepts, such as the six outlined above.

There is no overall consensus about the details of strategic management theory, but a framework developed by Tichy (1983) is useful in addressing this problem. The Technical, Political, and Cultural (TPC) Model has been adapted for use in this chapter, as shown in Table 10.2. In the following discussion, the nine cells of the table will be referred to by number.

Tichy's framework incorporates four important assumptions. First, organizations are affected by three major categories of environmental variables: technical, political, and cultural. (Tichy's ideas are sometimes described as TPC theory.) Technical variables involve relatively tangible and inanimate factors such as money supply, number and types of workers, and different types of knowledge, material, and equipment. Political variables basically involve the distribution of power in the environment, such as that held by government, professional associations, unions, pressure groups, and even individuals. Cultural variables include the values and beliefs of individuals and groups, such as attitudes regarding women's rights, professionalism, and commitment to a work ethic. (It thus reflects an open system perspective.)

Second, in response to these environmental variables, organizations must develop three internal systems: technical, political, and cultural. The technical system deals with how managers plan for and organize the technical resources that are available from the environment (cells 1–3 of Table 10.2). The political system deals with how managers distribute power within the organization (cells 4–6), and the cultural system deals with how they manage attitudes and values, including both adjusting to the employee culture and attempting to change it (cells 7–9). In developing these systems, managers can draw on the entire range of ideas presented in Table 10.1 concerning how to respond to organizational issues, whether from the open or closed perspective.

Third, it is important that the three systems be aligned or, put another way, be mutually supportive. For example, if the political system emphasizes staff involvement and decentralization of authority, the technical system should place relatively less emphasis on detailed position descriptions and rules and regulations. If this is not done, there is system misalignment, and, in this case, employee cynicism could result from the discrepancy between how the work is actually done and how the work roles are formally defined.

Fourth, managers have three basic tools they can use to ensure alignment: mission and strategy (cells 1, 4, and 7), organizational structure (cells 2, 5, and 8), and human resource management, which is referred to in the table as "processes" (cells 3, 6, and 9). All of the ideas in Table 10.2 can be made part of this "toolkit."

The following brief example demonstrates how this theory can be applied to a real situation. Many health organizations have reduced their number of supervisors (a change in cell 2 of the technical system, and also a change in the organizational structure). Many of these organizations have also moved to change the cultural system by modifying their mission and strategy

Table 10.2 Managerial Tools for Strategic Management

Managerial Areas	Technical System	Organizational Structure	Processes
Technical System	(1) • Assessing environmental threats and opportunities. • Assessing organizational strengths and weaknesses. • Defining mission and fitting resources to accomplish it.	(2) • Differentiation: organization of work into roles (production, marketing, etc.). • Integration: recombining roles into departments, divisions, regions, etc. • Aligning structure to strategy.	(3) • Fitting people into roles. • Specifying performance criteria for roles. • Measuring performance. • Staffing and development to fill roles (present and future). • Matching management style with technical tasks.
Political System	(4) • Who gets to influence the mission and strategy. • Managing coalitional behaviour around strategic decisions.	(5) • Distribution of power across the role structure. • Balancing power across groups of roles (e.g., sales vs. marketing, production vs. research and development, etc.).	(6) • Managing succession politics (who gets ahead, how do they get ahead). • Decision and administration of reward system (who gets what and how). • Managing the politics of appraisal (who is appraised by whom and how). • Managing the politics of information control and the planning process.
Cultural System	(7) • Managing influence of values and philosophy on mission and strategy. • Developing culture aligned with mission and strategy.	(8) • Developing managerial style aligned with technical and political structure. • Development of subcultures to support roles (production culture, R&D culture, etc.). • Integration of subcultures to create company culture.	(9) • Selection of people to build or reinforce culture. • Development (socialization) to mould organizational culture. • Management of rewards to shape and reinforce the culture. • Management of information and planning systems to shape and reinforce the culture.

Source: Adapted from *Managing Strategic Change: Technical, Political and Cultural Dynamics* (p. 119), by N.M. Tichy, 1983, New York: John Wiley & Sons. Adapted with permission of John Wiley & Sons, Inc.

(cell 7) in such a way that staff are encouraged to exercise their own values, attitudes, and judgment regarding their work (in other words, decentralizing authority). These two changes can be described as a shift to a more organic and less mechanistic management process.

Unfortunately, the above changes often result in a misalignment with the political system. Encouraging staff autonomy tends to reduce the power of middle managers, and this is exaggerated by extra work demands imposed on supervisors as a result of their reduced numbers. This type of misalignment can create many problems, but one of the most dangerous is the blurring of accountability, particularly with regard to high reliability functions. One way to rectify the problem is to modify the policies and procedures (cell 2) in such a way that the parameters of supervisory authority are more clearly defined and there is less ambiguity about when participatory management techniques are acceptable for planning, coordination, and quality control, and when they are not. In other words, the solution involves moving the balance point toward the mechanistic side of the organic/mechanistic continuum. Achieving the correct balance, of course, can be difficult in this type of situation.

When used in the foregoing fashion, Tichy's model can help to substantially reduce the complexity of strategic management because it provides a relatively uncomplicated set of guidelines regarding what variables should be examined and how the interactions between them can be planned for. The steps in strategic management now become the following:

Step 1. Assess the environment in terms of technical, political, and cultural variables.

Step 2. Devise an overall management strategy that includes (a) planning and design of appropriate technical, political, and cultural systems in terms of the environmental variables; and (b) planning and implementation of management strategies involving goals, structure, and processes that will establish and maintain alignment.

Step 3. Establish a process whereby day-to-day management decision making is based on the above overall management strategy.

Step 4. Establish a process whereby management strategy can be modified on an ongoing basis in response to changes in the environment and feedback from daily decision-making experiences.

These steps can be used to describe or assess an existing organization and, as well, to develop a strategy for change.

Applying Strategic Management Theory

A critical assessment of some management changes that occurred in many Canadian nursing departments during the 1980s and 1990s illustrates how strategic management theory is used. Nursing departments in tertiary care hospitals are used as an example because this type of organization is among the most complex in modern society and, therefore, offers a larger variety and magnitude of strategic management problems for examination than any other health organization. Details of the discussion are based entirely on the personal observations and opinions of the author. Not all events happened in all hospitals, but the described events are representative of general developments in health care environments and in organizational responses across Canada during this time period.

The main purpose of the discussion is to show readers how to apply TPC theory to an analysis of their own personal experiences, their own knowledge of management theory and research, and the environmental and institutional realities of their own organizations. The case example provides an opportunity to define issues and management challenges that face acute care nursing and, through extension, other nursing and health services in Canada.

Step 1: Environmental Assessment

The first step in strategic management is to assess the environment in terms of technical, political, and cultural variables. The focus in this section is the nursing division in its totality as the "system." Therefore, the "environment" includes all relevant external variables whether they exist within or outside the hospital.

In the technical arena of the hypothetical hospital described in this example, there had been rapid and continuing growth in the variety and complexity of the knowledge, skills, and equipment related to hospital operations, especially to medical and nursing practice. The changes in nursing were particularly important because they reflected a rapid growth in the profession's foundation of research-based knowledge. The overall impact of these changes had been to increase costs, but, at the same time, external funding agencies had steadily become more determined to reduce the rate of increase of hospital funding. Technological change had in effect created a severe cost-revenue crisis.

This crisis was particularly acute in nursing for two related reasons. First, senior management (i.e., the chief executive officer and the board, who are ultimately responsible for all management policy and decisions) had not developed effective techniques for planning and controlling the acquisition and use of technology by physicians, which had a substantial impact on nursing budgets. Second, newer nursing workload and output-measurement technologies provided valuable information, but this was largely ignored by senior management because the data indicated the nursing budget was increasingly inadequate, and senior management did not wish, largely for political reasons, to divert funds away from the priorities of physicians.

In the political environment, there had been rapid growth in the influence of nursing unions, a parallel growth in the technical sophistication as well as the professional self-esteem of nurses, and a slow but steady erosion of traditional medical dominance. Nevertheless, nurses continued to have relatively low political credibility, inside or outside these hospitals, in great part because of the disunity caused by major differences in their education, work assignments, and career expectations and because of the much greater social prestige of physicians. This credibility was improving as the profession gained more experience in pressure-group tactics and became more highly educated, but a major constraint on this progress was the continuing strength of chauvinistic attitudes directed at nurses—the stubborn myth that nurses were physicians' handmaidens (fuelled by the fact that most nurses were female), and the mistaken belief that the nurturing elements of the nursing role are low-skill activities based more on maternal instinct than on professional expertise. A further constraint was the aforementioned rejection of the information system as a means of providing objective data about workload, output, and productivity.

The cultural environment of the hospital was dominated by changes in the attitudes of nurses toward work and the nature of their organizational commitment. The advent of the "me generation," feminism, single parenting, unionization, research-based professionalization, different patterns of entry-level education, two-income families, and extensive experience with staff cutbacks had dramatically reduced the traditional willingness of many nurses to accept an authoritarian work environment or to make a strong personal investment in a specific organization. These changes were further exaggerated by changing expectations of patients, who tended to be more knowledgeable and demanding, and the growing militancy of nursing union leaders, who were frustrated by the amount of effort required to move toward equity in pay and better work conditions.

The overall degree of environmental instability and complexity (turbulence) in the hospital had increased rapidly during the past few years and the rate of increase was continuing. The single most significant outcome was a growing cost-revenue crisis, to which nursing was particularly vulnerable because the main cause was utilization decisions made by physicians, and nursing was not able to influence these decisions.

Steps 2 and 3: Development and Implementation of a Management Strategy

These steps require nursing departments to describe and assess the development and implementation of a management strategy in terms of technical, political, and cultural systems.

Although the hospitals frequently had formal statements of mission and strategy (cell 1), these usually had been approved but never truly accepted by senior management. Senior management's mission, as opposed to the formal statement, was to respond to changes that were driven by the new technologies requested by physicians and approved in a relatively ad hoc decision-making process. Implementation of a management strategy depended on the resourcefulness of middle management nurses in nourishing the individual and collective commitment of nursing staff to the needs of patients and quality of care. The lack of comprehensive planning by senior management had precipitated a long series of "add-on" services, such as transplant services and trauma units, which dramatically increased operating costs and management complexity as well as workload and stress at all levels of the nursing hierarchy.

Technical structures (cell 2) usually reflected the foregoing pattern. A traditional hierarchy mainly based on clinical service units had been expanded over the years as new services were added. Absolute numbers of middle and senior managers and support staff (including educators and clinical specialists) had increased significantly in response to increasing environmental turbulence, exponential growth in research findings relevant to nursing practice, ad hoc expansion of services, and a myriad of problems associated with growing pressures on the budget. Although these nursing departments were well integrated internally, with extensive formal and informal mechanisms for planning and coordination, their cross-departmental linkages had not kept pace with their growing interdependence with other departments, particularly medicine. This was partly due to preoccupation with cost-revenue problems on the part of nursing managers, but most importantly, it was due to a lack of initiative and support from senior management, who did not understand the growing importance of nursing/physician liaison.

The technical aspect of processes (cell 3) was relatively ambidextrous but was under steady pressure to become more mechanistic. Selection criteria for middle managers emphasized leadership ability, teamwork skills, and commitment to quality care. There had been a tradition of extensive consultation with staff nurses, but in response to the cost-revenue pressures, the process was becoming increasingly centralized. The rapid rate of change and growth in technology, for example, had required the development of policy and procedure manuals, orientation programs, and in-service education activities; the sheer volume of this workload meant that the process had become more centralized. In response to the growing competition for funds, a nursing information system had been implemented in an effort to develop objective workload and output data. It included patient classification, quality assurance, various aspects of cost analysis, and in an effort to reduce costs, a variable staffing component that required some nurses to "float" between wards and services depending on the workload of the unit. These measures also increased the centralization of staffing decisions as well as the time spent on data collection activities at the unit level, which caused some morale problems among staff nurses and criticism from the union.

The political and cultural systems had been in reasonably good alignment with the technical system, but this was beginning to show signs of breakdown. Politically, there had been a tradition of wide involvement among department members in formulating strategy, and these dialogues resulted in effective coalition management and minimum conflict over the distribution and balancing of power within and between the nursing subsystems. The associated cohesive spirit within the nursing department, which had served in the past to enhance its shaky credibility, was rapidly deteriorating. As a result, there was unhappiness with the growing centralization, staff disenchantment with workload (caused by ad hoc expansion of services in the absence of adequate funding), and a consequent increase in the militancy of the union. Succession politics, appraisal, and reward systems were still strongly based on teamwork skills and commitment to quality care, but it was necessary for managers to put more and more emphasis on the formal union contract as a framework for relationships with their staff. The most important emerging misalignment, however, was the growing gap between the high technical need and the low political feasibility of a coalition with medicine for the planning of cost and quality control mechanisms.

Surmounting the challenges imposed by contradictory requirements of the technical and political systems had traditionally depended heavily on the professional commitments of nurses. These commitments were derived from the occupational socialization experiences of nurses and a cultural structure and process within the organization that supplemented and sustained these commitments. This too had begun to degenerate as differences in educational backgrounds, work assignments, and career expectations of nurses increased and the values of unionism became more influential. The relationships between nursing managers and staff nurses were steadily becoming more difficult at the very time when cohesion and commonality of purpose were of increasing importance.

Step 4: Modifying the Strategy

Although the problems facing nursing were the result of normal evolution in the face of a turbulent and hostile environment, they reached a point where corrective action was required. In general theoretical terms, these departments had been using an open system/rational approach to management, but the style of management, which had been highly ambidextrous, had slowly moved under the pressure of rapid change toward the mechanistic end of the continuum. In terms of the strategic management process, senior nursing management had been forced into a reactive posture by limited influence over the acquisition and use of new medical technology. Nursing management needed to move from this reactive strategy, which had been necessary during the period of rapid growth, to a proactive strategy, formulated and implemented in close cooperation with the medical department and oriented to restraint and cutbacks. Nursing management also needed to return to a more organic style of management and to reinvigorate the commitment of staff nurses to the professional values of nursing.

Based on the case evidence presented here, the necessary changes were quite clear. At least three were needed in the technical system. The first was the need for the nursing departments to develop a strong strategic management program with a major emphasis on mission definition and strategy formulation, and to do this in close cooperation with a comparable program in medicine and at all levels of the two departmental structures. This was the most important priority because until this rationalization of the management process was underway, the remaining two priorities could not be accomplished. The second priority was to streamline the structure of middle management and support personnel, which would allow some reduction in their numbers as a result of the rationalized strategy process. The third priority was to reduce the labour intensity of the information system, improve its reliability and validity, and better integrate it with operating cost data because this data would become especially important as the hospital moved toward more rational planning and increased budgetary restraint.

The highest priority changes in the political and cultural systems related to the top and middle managers in nursing. The remarkable complexity and turbulence of the environment, and of the organization itself, had vastly increased the importance of middle managers as technical experts, political actors, and cultural leaders. Politically, the most important issue was the need to strengthen their prestige and influence in the eyes of both their staff and the physicians. In terms of the cultural system, it was becoming increasingly urgent to re-emphasize their leadership role in demonstrating the validity of professional nursing values, reconciling these values with the complementary aspects of the union priorities, and establishing constructive ways of reconciling the differences. Implementing these changes would have required substantial initiative and support from senior management. In particular, changing the pattern of medical decision making and renewing the prestige and flexibility of middle managers, while simultaneously reducing their numbers, would require a great deal of creativity, courage, and skill on the part of the chief executive officer and the board.

Results of the Management Strategy

The cost-revenue problem reached crisis proportions for this typical hospital when senior management was impelled to implement massive cost reductions. Given the magnitude and persistence of government deficits, and the costs of medical technology, it had become quite clear that the two most important elements of a solution lay outside the nursing department: rationalization of both physician utilization decisions and interinstitutional competition for services and programs. This would require a major redefinition of the mission and goals of the hospital but would result in significant cost reductions and improved quality of care. Senior management was either unwilling or unable to directly confront either of these issues and chose to focus change on structure and process in other services and programs.

Nursing was poorly positioned for the ensuing interdepartmental competition for funds. The nursing department was accountable for the largest single component of the total hospital budget, and it was an area of rapid and continuing growth in costs. Because neither its strategic plan nor its information system had credibility at the senior levels of management, the perception had been created that nursing had little objective policy or data with which to justify its priorities and little ability to rectify the problem. Nursing lacked sufficient inherent political power to overcome these deficits and its weakness was compounded by the cultural divisions within the department, particularly the growing split between nursing management and the union, as well as the lack of active support from medicine.

In the above context, in many hospitals, senior management frequently took direct control of nursing. Typically, the head of the nursing department was replaced by an incumbent willing to represent senior management to nursing, rather than represent nursing to senior management. Mission and strategy decisions for nursing could then be controlled at the most senior level by persons who were not nurses. In many Canadian hospitals at this time, the senior executive nursing position was simply eliminated. Staff members responsible for the information system were disbanded, and variable staffing was terminated. Many middle management and support staff positions were eliminated, including evening and night supervisors, specialized clinical teams (such as those to administer IVs), and most nursing researchers and educators. A policy of decentralizing responsibility to the staff nurse level was instituted. This compromised the authority and stature of remaining managers so severely that many began to question the relevance of their roles. Those who questioned or who failed to actively support the management changes were dismissed; many of those let go were among the most experienced and professionally committed managers, and the threat implicit in these terminations was clearly understood by those who remained. Large reductions were also made in the staff nurse complement and this, in conjunction with the decentralization of responsibility for a good deal of day-to-day decision making to the staff nurse level, substantially increased nursing workloads. In such situations, senior management often undertook to introduce a "new" corporate culture and established a separate group of staff to initiate and maintain its acceptance.

Decisions relating to the technical system were now controlled by lay administrators who were unencumbered by objective data regarding quality or workload. Politically, the nursing department had been purged of its management leadership; the illusion that nursing power had been increased was created through decentralization, but in the absence of an effective nursing hierarchy, it meant that staff nurses and their immediate supervisors now had increased accountability but little authority and influence. It also meant that the union was now the main voice for nursing as a collectivity and that the power for all major policy decisions regarding nursing was vested with senior management. By introducing a new corporate culture, senior management also had undertaken to define what was considered appropriate in terms of values and philosophy. The litany of popular management buzz words that were introduced, such as empowerment, shared governance, coaching, customer (for patient), and total quality management, created the illusion that the new management strategy was more organic and that a new and better "vision" of institutional values had been created. In reality, the policy decision process for the department was more centralized and arbitrary than ever before. In addition, by discounting the inherent dependency of patients in a complex technological milieu, important moral and legal issues involved in determining how the organization and the individual professional should share their joint responsibility for each patient had been trivialized.

Analysis of the Management Strategy

The fourth step in strategic management, modifying the strategy, had been guided primarily by the open/natural approach rather than the open/rational approach. As a result, relatively few elements of a reasoned and responsible management strategy were evident. Nursing departments had been precluded from developing a proactive strategy guided by the requisites for maximizing quality of care. Close cooperation in strategic management between medicine and nursing had not been facilitated. The nursing information system had been abandoned. The move to a more organic style of management, through an exaggerated form of decentralization, had seriously compromised the remaining prestige and influence of middle managers. The new vision of cultural values was based more on superficial popular interpretations of management in Japanese automobile factories than on a science-based assessment of the complex professional realities of nursing in the Canadian cultural environment and in high tech–high touch health care organizations. In addition, the formal responsibility for professional leadership had been removed from middle managers in nursing, which further reduced their prestige and influence.

Senior management had misdiagnosed what was appropriate for the hospital and for nursing—and, most of all, for patients—and had failed to anticipate negative consequences of their decisions.

A serious error was committed when senior managers failed to focus on rationalizing physician decision making and interinstitutional competition. This was partly due to their failure to understand that the modern hospital had entered a new phase in its life cycle—one in which the environmental changes were so great that the basic mission and strategy of the organization had to be drastically changed if it was to cope adequately with its current and future cost-revenue problems. It was also due to a failure to acknowledge their moral responsibility to know, understand, and act on information that suggested traditional patterns of institutional autonomy and resource utilization by physicians resulted in grossly inefficient use of social resources and unnecessary levels of ineffective service.

Senior management also had failed to recognize that rapid advances in the technology of nursing, especially in educational levels and the profession's research base, had created a need for a stronger, not weaker, administrative presence on the part of the nursing department. It had failed to understand that a proactive nursing management strategy, not subordinate to, but in cooperation with the medical department, was essential if the hospital was to be assured that the benefits of the burgeoning professional expertise of nursing would be delivered to patients. Senior management had also dismissed the importance of an information system at a time of drastic restraint and cutbacks when objective data regarding nursing workload and output had reached a new level of importance.

In the political and cultural arenas, senior management had seriously underestimated the need to support strong professional and administrative leadership at the senior and middle levels of nursing management. As a result, it overreacted to the need for a more organic style of management and reduced the number and power of nursing managers and support staff to the point where they were dangerously limited in their ability to fulfill their responsibilities for political and cultural leadership.

At a more general level, senior managers failed to understand the concept of organizational dilemmas and the negative potentials associated with them. In many important ways, along with subscribing to the disadvantages of the open/natural approach, they had also incurred the disadvantages inherent in a "one best way" approach to management. In their rush to enhance communication by massive decentralization and management dismissals, they had seriously hampered coordination. In an effort to reduce traditionalism by introducing a "new" corporate culture, they had undermined important professional values and norms. In an effort to stimulate individual initiative by staff empowerment, they damaged the ability of the organization to properly fulfill its moral and legal responsibility for the acts of its employees and agents in delivering high-reliability services.

An additional important oversight was in the area of managerial ethics. Even though the clinical professions had been active in the definition and resolution of ethical issues involving patients, senior management had failed to grapple with the ethical issues surrounding development and implementation of management policy on budget restraint and cutback. Termination of life, the right to information, and the right to respect, for example, were now recognized as important patient issues that required careful assessment, but the same standards were not applied to employees. Careers were terminated with impunity, planning information was withheld from key actors, and little respect was shown for the integrity, judgment, or experience of middle managers when the time came for planning and implementing how budget reductions would be effected.

It is predictable from theory, that the management strategy described in this example will not persist; it creates too many problems. Inadequate utilization of nursing technology will result in increased patient complaints, more lawsuits, and lowered staff morale. The reduced number of middle managers and the increased degree of decentralization will lower administrative efficiency to unacceptable levels. The organization will be under great pressure to modify its approach in the direction of a more mechanistic style and to place more emphasis on professional values and norms.

Unfortunately, there are two major constraints on the degree and rate of change. First, until the mission of the institution is rationalized, there will be insufficient funds available for more than minor improvements. In nursing, as in other sectors of the health care system, optimizing the range and quality of service will be dependent on more progress in rationalizing physician decision making and interinstitutional competition. Second, change will be heavily dependent on the skill and vigour with which nurses pursue efforts to increase their power within the institution. Power is not a sufficient cause of sound management, but it is a necessary cause, and, in the final analysis, inadequate intraorganizational power is the root cause of the problems facing this nursing department.

Recent Developments

In the mid-1990s, one positive change began to emerge as the result of decisions by most provincial governments in Canada. They imposed institutional integration through various forms of regionalization, and these regional structures have begun the process of rationalizing physician decision making. It is too early to tell how successful this has been as, for the most part, the implementation process was rushed and the consequent problems of political unrest and sheer administrative logistics impeded adequate planning for these changes. There is now evidence that, at least where hospitals and hospital mergers are concerned, "bigger is not necessarily better" (Canadian Health Services Research Foundation, 2002). The Canadian Centre for the Analysis of Regionalization and Health has been established, and studies examining the effects of aggregating and consolidating health services have become a funding priority theme for national research agencies in Canada.

In the early 2000s, as the effects of current and future nursing shortages have begun to be widely publicized and appreciated by the public, there has been some attention to the need to reinvigorate the profile and involvement of nursing and nursing leaders in tertiary care centres and regional health organizations. Positions for well-qualified nurses at senior levels have been re-introduced in some organizations. These new positions, however, are often advisory in nature and do not include authority or responsibility for the day-to-day operation or evaluation of nursing services. Their mandate generally involves external liaison and communication, internal relations between disciplines and services, educational issues, and professional and clinical development, including the facilitation of nursing research. It remains to be seen whether these developments will serve to strengthen the technical core of nursing and improve the cultural integration of professional and union subgroups within the discipline, and whether they will achieve retention of expert practitioners and create the required organizational conditions to enable practitioners to apply their technical knowledge.

The introduction of program management models to organize clinical services has the potential to strengthen the alignment of political, technical, and cultural systems and bring about a more significant role for nurses in achieving efficient and effective health care services. Where program management is in use, clinical services are sometimes co-directed by nurse managers and physicians. However, the program management model was directly criticized in the report of the inquest into the deaths of babies at the Winnipeg Health Sciences Centre (Sinclair, 2001) because reporting and accountability relationships were unclear and ineffective. The overall mid- and long-term outcomes of program management models have yet to be evaluated with respect to their effects on patient safety and quality of care and their ability to deliver on the promises of improved efficiency, teamwork, and job satisfaction that accompanied its introduction.

Leadership Implications

In this chapter, a representative example of acute care nursing management problems in Canadian hospitals in the 1990s has been analyzed in the context of organization design theory. Insofar as this interpretation is valid, it is clear that the public has not been well served by those assigned stewardship for these hospitals; in particular, the vitally important contribution of nursing to efficient and effective care has been diminished, not enhanced.

This is a serious problem because nurses are engaged in one of the most complex, difficult, and important professional roles in society. Nurses provide their services when patients are highly vulnerable. Their relationship with patients is intimate, intense, and often continuous for long periods. They must be skilled in dealing with the physical, social, emotional, and spiritual needs of patients and, often, of relatives and friends as well, and they are responsible for keeping up with a knowledge base that is growing rapidly in all of these areas. They routinely deal with profound ethical problems. They function in a technical, political, and cultural environment that is one of the most complex in society, and one that is often hostile to both their personal and professional needs and potential.

It is not possible for registered nurses to realize their individual and collective potential for improving the efficiency and effectiveness of health services without support. There is strong theoretical justification that, because of its centrality to the mission of most health services, nursing requires superior and consistent organizational infrastructure and executive leadership support. Nurses must also accept and vigorously pursue new opportunities for leadership in health organizations, and they should be able to do so without feeling a need to leave behind their professional knowledge and disciplinary roots as they assume more senior corporate responsibilities.

Nursing has made substantial progress in enhancing the research foundation that underpins its professional status and in establishing a powerful union movement that protects the wages and work conditions of its members. The benefits of this progress to both the patient and the individual nurse will continue to be threatened, however, if nurses do not recognize the importance of nursing leadership roles and undertake to support them vigorously.

The situation presented in this chapter illustrates how theoretical concepts can be used to critically examine organizational structures, practices, and decisions. The application of this or other analytic frameworks can assist in raising and understanding issues to improve current decision making and can assist in interpreting the mid- to long-term consequences of leadership decisions. The theoretical perspective presented in this chapter, and others that might be applied, is an important tool for planning and interpreting research that is designed to understand the effects of, and to improve, leadership practices in health service organizations. The issues and intellectual challenges raised through the critical application of analytic frameworks and processes can help leaders at all levels to become reflective practitioners in their leadership roles.

Summary

- Open and closed systems represent two useful perspectives for understanding the development of organization design theory.

- Open versus closed perspectives reflect the degree to which it is thought that the external environment must be taken into account when making management decisions about an organization.

- Two distinct approaches within these perspectives (rational and natural) reflect the degree to which management is perceived to involve pre-planning of objectives and means, as opposed to a more dynamic process of ongoing adaptation to changing circumstances.

- The three categories of environmental variables identified by Tichy (1983) are assumed to play a critical role in the design of efficient and effective organizations; they are technical, political, and cultural factors. Corresponding subsystems in organizations must be developed and maintained in alignment with each other.

- A series of supplementary ideas need to be taken into account when applying theory (e.g., describing the organization's technology and recognizing inherent dilemmas in organization design).

- Managers have three basic tools to assist them in keeping the three subsystems of an agency in alignment: mission and strategy, organizational structure, and processes.

- A contingency perspective results in management styles that range on a continuum from mechanistic (i.e., rule-oriented), through ambidextrous, to organic (i.e., flexible).

- Strategic management theory provides a four-step process to assist managers in identifying the relevant variables to consider when designing organizations that can operate efficiently and effectively in an increasingly complex and ambiguous environment.

- Strategic management theory can be used to analyze and explain the dissolution of nursing organizations in large tertiary care hospitals in Canada during the 1980s and 1990s.

- For nursing to realize its potential for improving the efficiency and effectiveness of hospital services, it must have superior leadership and support from senior management.

- The application of analytical perspectives from organization design and management theory can contribute to reflective leadership practice and to the design and interpretation of research to improve management in the health system.

Applying the Knowledge in this Chapter

Exercise

Using an analytical process similar to the one presented in this chapter, select a specific health care agency (or clinical service) where you have worked or spent time as a student, and consider the following questions.

1. What role does the external environment play in the organization and management of this agency?

2. Is management a rational process involving systematic use of information and pre-planning, or is it a naturalistic process of dynamic adaptation to changing circumstances?

3. Would you describe this agency as a closed or open system?

4. Select one of the organizational issues listed in Table 10.1. Describe the theoretical approach to this issue and the role of nurses, if any, in addressing the issue.

5. Describe the technical, political, and cultural subsystems, and consider the extent to which they shape the organization of nurses' work in this agency.

6. Are the subconcepts of technical complexity and interdependence useful in analyzing the work of nurses in this agency? Given your analysis of nurses' work, what are the leadership implications for maximizing the contribution of nursing to the agency's mission and goals?

Resources

evolve Internet Resources

Canadian Health Services Research Foundation Mythbusters:
  www.chsrf.ca/mythbusters/
The Canadian Centre for the Analysis of Regionalization and Health:
  www.regionalization.org/Centre.html
The Canadian Centre for Policy Alternative:
  http://policyalternatives.ca/index.html

Further Reading

The following books and articles are good sources of information on formal organizations and structure and process in health care agencies. Some are more than 30 years old, but remain classics in their field.

Blau, P., & Meyer, M.W. (1987). *Bureaucracy in modern society.* New York: Random House.
  The first edition of this short book was published in 1956 by Peter Blau as sole author. As many of the traits of bureaucracy persist in today's social organizations, future leaders and administrators should be well grounded in the functional and dysfunctional aspects of bureaucracy, as well as its interrelationship with the principles of democracy.
Blau, P.M., & Scott, W.R. (1962). *Formal organizations.* San Francisco: Chandler Publishing.
  Blau and Scott synthesized a good deal of the existing research and contributed a number of valuable

interpretations and insights, including the concept of organizational dilemmas.

Daft, R.L. (2001). *Organization theory and design* (7th ed.). St. Paul, MN: West Publishing House.
There are many excellent introductory textbooks in organization design and this is one of them. It provides much more detail on theory and research than was possible in this chapter.

Growe, S.J. (1991). *Who cares: The crisis in Canadian nursing.* Toronto, ON: McClelland & Stewart.
This book provides a brilliant analysis of the problems and the promise facing Canadian nurses, especially those at the service delivery level. This is essential reading for anyone with an obligation to understand the nursing profession.

Juzwishin, D.W.M. (1993). *Ethical issues in health services administration: Canadian health care management.* Toronto, ON: MPL Communication.
Juzwishin was one of the first to recognize and write about ethical issues in management. This is an excellent overview of the existing literature and the major issues.

Perrow, C. (1973). The short and glorious history of organizational theory. *Organizational Dynamics, 2,* 2–15.
Written more than 30 years ago, this short article is still one of the best available critiques of modern organization theory. The annotated bibliography is also useful.

Rachlis, M., & Kushner, C. (1994). *Strong medicine: How to save Canada's health care system.* Toronto, ON: Harper Collins.
This is the second highly readable book from the authors of 1989's successful *Second Opinion: What's Wrong with Canada's Health Care System and How to Fix It.* The authors continue their critical appraisal of the system, conclude that fundamental structural reform is essential, and propose some radical changes.

Shortell, S.M., & Kaluzny, A.D. (1988). *Health care management: A text in organizational theory and behaviour* (2nd ed.). New York: John Wiley & Sons.
This is a collection of commissioned articles on core topics in both organization behaviour and design as applied to health organization. It is of unusually high quality, but is designed for expert readers.

Storch, J.L. (1982). *Patients' rights: Ethical and legal issues in health care and nursing.* Toronto, ON: McGraw-Hill Ryerson.
Storch was a pioneer in the area of ethical issues in health care, and this is still one of the best available overviews of the topic. The bibliography is also excellent.

Tichy, N.M. (1983). *Managing strategic change: Technical, political, and cultural dynamics.* New York: John Wiley & Sons.
This book provides a detailed exposition about the origins and substance of TPC Theory and is only recommended for the advanced reader.

Tichy, N.M., & Devanna, M.A. (1986). *The transformational leader.* New York: John Wiley & Sons.
The authors use the TPC framework to discuss the planning and implementation of organizational change. Examples and cases from American business management are used extensively to provide practical and realistic insights.

References

Canadian Health Services Research Foundation. (2002). *Myth: Bigger is always better when it comes to hospital mergers.* Retrieved March 19, 2004, from http://www.chsrf.ca/mythbusters/

Sinclair, C.M. (2001, May). *Report of the Manitoba pediatric cardiac surgery inquest: An inquiry into twelve deaths at the Winnipeg Health Sciences Centre in 1994.* (The Sinclair Inquiry). Winnipeg, MB: Provincial Court of Manitoba.

Tichy, N.M. (1983). *Managing strategic change: Technical, political, and cultural dynamics.* New York: John Wiley & Sons.

Acknowledgments

Although the content of this chapter is solely my responsibility, I wish to thank several people who provided invaluable assistance: Bruce Finkel, Felicity Hey, Don Juzwishin, Dave Reynolds, Ginette Rodger, and Janet Storch. A special thanks to my three favourite nurses: Beth, Dorothy, and Jacqueline.

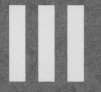

SECTION

III

STANDARDS AND ACCOUNTABILITY

Section III is devoted to a discussion of how various legal requirements and other types of standards impose structure upon health agencies and individual professionals who operate under organizational auspices. The authors of the chapters in this section include experts in health law, accounting, and national and international standards organizations that are outside of the traditional boundaries of the health system. The relationship of standards to accountability is emphasized, and the importance of senior leadership behaviour in the creation of both healthy and dysfunctional aspects of organizational culture is considered.

In Chapter 11, *The Legal Framework for Health Agencies and Services*, the legal requirements that influence or prescribe the responsibilities of health agencies and the leaders and employees who work in them are described. Readers should not expect to find detailed discussion of clinical situations with legal implications or detailed analyses of the law in this chapter as these can be found in textbooks and articles devoted exclusively to this topic. Rather, the vicarious liability of employing organizations for the actions of their employees is emphasized in keeping with the overall focus on leadership and management in this text.

Although the Canadian health system is not highly regulated from a legal standpoint, there are many different types of standards that influence the practice of individual health professionals and the health agencies in which they practice. Chapter 12, *Standards and Quality in the Canadian Health System*, contains descriptions of various types of standards and the sources of their authority. This discussion is relevant to all nurses in clinical practice because it explains why professional nursing associations are not able to directly influence health agencies in matters relating to the nursing practice environment that are within the legal jurisdiction of health agencies and not professional associations. Professional standards govern the individual practice of members of regulated professions, but in unregulated professions, such as health administration, there is no provision for discipline of an individual who acts unprofessionally, unless there is also a breach of the law. Professional standards have often had positive influence on policies and practice in health agencies, but the Canadian Nurses Association Standards for Nursing Administration that were widely accepted in the 1980s have been disregarded in recent years despite a growing body of evidence validating their content. Nurses' unions have been able to exert direct influence on work environments and organizational practices because health agencies, as employers, are required to honour legal standards in the form of collective agreements. All organizations, and particularly those that receive public funds, must ultimately meet the standards of the community. The growing importance of community standards and citizen expectations is reflected in the emergence of a focus on accountability in the health system as a major public policy issue in Canada.

In Chapter 13, *Accountability in the Canadian Health System*, the concept of accountability is explored from both conceptual and practical viewpoints. Although the individual accountability of corporate leaders in the health system has not generally been a matter emphasized by courts of law, there is growing evidence of citizens' expectations of personal accountability by senior executives in all areas of society. CEOs in the health system are increasingly expected to provide personal leadership that creates a culture of safety in which mistakes are acknowledged and employees' concerns documented without fear of reprisal. There is also a growing expectation that problems of incompetence or unacceptable behaviour of medical staff must be dealt with more decisively than in the past. Improving accountability in the Canadian health system has become a matter of key public concern and professional debate. Researchers in this area have emphasized the need for greater transparency in decision-making processes to complement the traditional emphasis on financial accountability and the achievement of positive health outcomes. The US National Institutes of Medicine also have recommended transparency in the health care system, advocating for patients to be fully informed participants in their own care. This conclusion validates the professional standards and individual efforts of nurses in all practice settings who have strived to advocate for clients in ambiguous and sometimes non-supportive organizational environments.

THE LEGAL FRAMEWORK FOR HEALTH AGENCIES AND SERVICES

Richard C. Fraser, QC and Leah Evans Parisi, JD

Learning Objectives

In this chapter, you will learn:

- That corporations and organizations are entities which have fiduciary and legal responsibilities to clients and staff

- The importance of the vicarious liability of health agencies for the actions of employees and professional staff

- The difference between public law and private law and the key elements of each

- The importance of the *Canadian Charter of Rights and Freedoms* to health care

- Lessons from a recent government inquiry

- The delegation of professional regulation from governments to professions

- Basic elements of malpractice liability, including the legal doctrine of informed consent

- The legal importance of health care records

- The importance of risk management

- The basics of employment law

It is the intent of this chapter to provide information that will enable nurses, especially those in management positions, to better understand public law, private law, and legal concepts such as fiduciary obligations negligence, informed consent, and vicarious liability. Unlike most discussions of nursing and the law, the emphasis here is on the general legal responsibilities of organizations and managers rather than on the individual responsibilities of clinical nurses, which are often emphasized in the nursing literature. The law provides a basis for organizational practices and processes such as risk management, quality assurance, and quality improvement measures. Each situation has specific characteristics, and because of this, nothing in this chapter is intended as legal advice or as a substitute for legal advice.

The Canadian Legal System

It is important for all nurses, especially those at the management level, to have a general understanding of the legal system in Canada and the areas of law that affect professional nursing in the organizational context where most nursing practice occurs. The Canadian legal system is not identical to that of the United States, but it is similar in following a cultural trend of emphasizing individual rights over the rights of the collective or the state. Judges on both sides of the border increasingly emphasize patient autonomy even when in conflict with resource allocation decisions. The two systems are different in the degree to which certain aspects of law are emphasized. For example, damage awards for medical malpractice are clearly much higher in the US, class actions are more prevalent, and individuals or corporations are more likely to be held accountable for wrongdoing, often as a result of legislatively protected whistle-blowers.

In Canada, as in most democracies, law can best be understood by separating it into public law and private law. *Public law* is the body of law that governs relations between and among governments (e.g., the *Canada Health Act*); it also governs relations between governments and the citizens subject to their power (e.g., criminal law as expressed in the *Criminal Code of Canada*). In certain cases, such as health information legislation, public law governs the relationships among citizens. *Private law* governs the relations and interactions between individuals or corporations without direction from the government, such as civil law and civil litigation. It is facilitated through the use of courts, arbitration, and professional regulatory bodies.

In public law, the *Constitution Act of Canada* (*Canada Act*, 1982) sets forth the respective rights and powers of the federal and provincial governments. The *Canada Health Act* (*Canada Health Act,* 1985) is federal legislation that, through the mechanism of financial penalties, encourages provinces to abide by the five principles of the legislation: universality, comprehensiveness, accessibility, portability, and public administration. In turn, in each of the provinces, municipal government legislation allows delegation of provincial constitutional power to municipalities.

Public law also allows governments to govern the conduct of individuals and provide rules that individuals can rely on when dealing with the state. Accordingly, the *Criminal Code* (1985) sets forth the rulebook for conduct in a civil society. The *Canadian Charter of Rights and Freedoms*[1]

---

[1] Part 1 of the *Constitution Act,* 1982, being Schedule B to the *Canada Act,* 1982 (UK) 1982.

grants citizens protection from unchecked state power. Through the section 15 "Equality" provision and other sections of the *Charter*, individuals and groups are able to influence and change government conduct. This can range from sexual discrimination in the workplace to the effect of legalization of small amounts of marijuana for medicinal use.

Public law can also govern relations between and among individuals. This is best seen in privacy legislation that sets forth rules on how private information, including individually identifying health care information, is collected, used, and disclosed. Public law also sets forth minimum standards in the health care field through various provincial hospital acts, including requirements for health records. As well, public law can provide for an investigatory or inquisitorial process to ascertain facts, come to conclusions, and make recommendations. This can be done through coroners' inquests, fatality inquiries, or special government inquiries, such as the Commission of Inquiry on the Blood System in Canada conducted in 1997 by the Honourable Mr. Justice Horace Krever.

Finally, public law can delegate functions to self-regulating professions. This model has been followed across Canada, and as a result, health care professionals regulate themselves. This is to be done in the public's interest and usually involves public representatives appointed by the government to provide a window on the profession.

Public law is pervasive, yet in the health care field, it does not seem to warrant as much attention as private law. This may be because private law often hits very close to home for health care professionals through disputes over employment contracts, collective bargaining difficulties, and the often-feared medical malpractice litigation. Most health care professionals have an ongoing concern about being involved in any way with civil malpractice litigation. This is understandable given that such litigation is based on an adversarial model of finding fault and assessing damages. Nevertheless, knowledge of this area and of the vicarious liability of employing organizations is helpful in reducing fear.

Public Law

Government to Government

The most recent and best example of government-to-government relations is seen in the ongoing federal and provincial discussions on the future of health care in Canada. The report of the Commission on the Future of Health Care in Canada (2002) conducted by Roy Romanow, QC (also called the Romanow Report) is based on the five principles found in the *Canada Health Act*. The Romanow Report recommended the establishment of a Canadian Health Care Council composed of representatives from governments, the professions, and the public. It is yet to be seen if the council will play an important role in shaping the future of health care in Canada.

Government to People

Of more immediate concern to nurse managers are a series of cases dealing with an individual or group's right to health care or equal access to health care. These court decisions are important because they may result in the need to change health care practices, policies, and procedures. Nurse managers should be at the forefront of shaping these changes to our health care system.

In October of 1997, the Supreme Court of Canada released its decision in *Eldridge* v. *British Columbia (Attorney General)* (*Eldridge,* 1997) that effectively required all hospitals and health care facilities to ensure that deaf patients are provided with funded interpreters when necessary for effective communication. One commentator noted that it is not a big leap to apply the reasoning in *Eldridge* to support the argument that funded interpretation services should be provided for any patient that does not speak English (or, in Quebec, that does not speak French) or that does not understand the language of the health care provider (Margo, 1999). From the day this decision was released in October 1997, it became the law of the land. It has the potential to impact hospital budgets and practices. At a minimum, it requires the re-examination of relevant policies and procedures, including those dealing with consent. Nurse managers need to be generally aware of such decisions and ask if relevant policies and procedures accord with the revised law.

Another important decision was *Cameron* v. *Attorney General of Nova Scotia,* given in 1999 by the Court of Appeal of Nova Scotia. In this case, the Court concluded that denying funding for a specialized form of in vitro fertilization infringed upon the section 15 "Equality" rights of the *Canadian Charter of Rights and Freedoms*, but under section 1, was a reasonable limit justified in Canadian democracy (Carver, 2003). It should be noted, however, that the claimants had received some prior government support for infertility treatments.

No government support was provided in the case of *Auton* v. *Attorney General of British Columbia,* decided by the British Columbia Court of Appeal in 2002 (*Auton,* 2002). In this case, parents of four preschool-aged children sued the government of British Columbia and the Medical Services Commission for their refusal to fund Lovas Autism treatment, which cost between $45,000 and $60,000 per child per year. Both the trial judge and the British Columbia Court of Appeal found in favour of the parents and ordered the authorities to provide the treatment. The British Columbia Court of Appeal characterized this case as an "issue of the right to treatment" rather than as a case of "equal access to treatment," which was the case in *Eldridge* at the time of the writing. In 2004, the *Auton* case was under appeal to the Supreme Court of Canada.

Finally, in the case of *Gosselin* v. *Quebec,* decided on December 19, 2002, the Supreme Court of Canada held that the Quebec government's decision to cut back welfare rates in the mid-1980s was not a breach of the section 7 Charter right that everyone "has the right to life, liberty and security of the person" (*Gosselin,* 2002). However, Chief Justice McLachlin, in speaking for the majority of the Court, stated, "I leave open the possibility that a positive obligation to sustain life, liberty or security of the person may be made out in special circumstances" (*Gosselin,* 2002, p. 83; see Carver, 2003).

A section 7 argument could apply to a claim for health care services if the government purported to exclude the private sector from ensuring and providing a necessary medical service which was not adequately provided for by the government. This issue was reviewed in a report by the Canadian Bar Association that stated, "It would likely be difficult for government to deny an individual access to medically necessary services when they are not being effectively provided by the government due to lack of funding, lack of cooperation between the federal and provincial governments or deliberate intention" (Canadian Bar Association, 1994, p. 94). Nurse managers who assist in shaping health care policies and procedures or risk management protocols need to be generally aware of these important court decisions.

Government Inquiries

Coroners' inquests, fatality inquiries, and special commissions can have an immediate and direct impact on nursing and organizational practices. At the time of this writing, this had been demonstrated most recently in the report of the Manitoba pediatric cardiac surgery inquest that conducted an inquiry into 12 infant deaths at the Winnipeg Health Sciences Centre in 1994. This inquiry was conducted by Associate Chief Judge Murray Sinclair.

The Sinclair Inquiry

A brief timeline of the Sinclair Inquiry is helpful. One commentator summarized the events as follows:

> To some staff involved in the program problems seemed evident very soon after Chief of Service Dr. Jonah Odim's arrival. Concerns about problems were expressed to those in authority by nurses and anesthetists between February and May 1994 but until the death of the fifth child in May no formal review took place. Following the twelfth death in December [1994] the program was suspended pending an external review which was done in January 1995. On February 14, 1995 members of the public and parents of children who died were informed through the media that the program was suspended for six months. Outrage and intense publicity surrounded this announcement. On March 15, 1995, the Chief Medical Examiner for Manitoba ordered an inquest into the twelve deaths. Thereafter, Judge Sinclair commenced the hearing in the summer of 1995. It concluded three years later in the fall of 1998. The report itself was released two years later on November 27, 2000 (Martens, 2002, pp. 66–67).

The Sinclair Inquiry found that "of the twelve deaths five were preventable, four were possibly preventable, two were uncertain and one was likely preventable" (Martens, 2002, p. 67). Judge Sinclair made 36 recommendations (Sinclair, 2001); those of particular relevance for nurses and all managers, senior executives, and governing boards of health agencies are highlighted in Box 11.1.

The recommendation relating to a patients' rights handbook has already been acted upon by another province. The government of New Brunswick in the spring of 2003 introduced legislation entitled the *Health Charter of Rights and Responsibilities Act* (*Health Charter*, 2003). After an introductory preamble that includes a reference to the five principles of the *Canada Health Act,* certain rights and responsibilities are stated, which include the following:

Rights

- A right to timely access to health care services (i.e., a right of access to primary health care services at all times in accordance with the plans established under the *Regional Health Authorities Act* as to time and place; it also includes timely referrals to other necessary health care services)

Box 11.1

Recommendation Highlights of the Sinclair Inquiry Report

Treatment of Nurses

1. Restructure the Health Sciences Nursing Council and allow nurses to select their own members.

2. In turn, the Nursing Council should be represented on the Health Sciences Centre governing body and should be responsible for monitoring, evaluating, and making recommendations about the nursing profession within the hospital.

Reporting Concerns about Risks to Patients

1. There is need for a policy that clearly states to whom all staff should report concerns and that ensures there is no risk to the person reporting.

2. The province should consider passing "whistle-blowing" legislation to protect health care professionals from reprisals when they disclose a genuine concern.

Risk Management

1. There should be legislation requiring hospitals to have appropriate quality assurance and risk management programs, including legislative protection to be granted to those discussions provided that the right of patients to full disclosure is not compromised.

2. The Health Sciences Centre and Winnipeg Regional Health Authority should develop quality assurance and risk management procedures that employ the principles from the report.

3. The Health Sciences Centre should exclude doctors involved in a case from participating in the decision-making processes relating to a standards committee review of the case.

Patients' Rights Handbook and the Right to Informed Consent

1. The Health Sciences Centre should review its policies on consent and communication with families.

2. Medical staff must be forthright and truthful in disclosing all relevant information, including the fact that a surgeon had not performed a particular surgical procedure on her/his own in an unsupervised setting.

3. A Patients' Rights Handbook should be produced that would clearly set out that patients and their families have rights, such as the right to be fully informed before giving consent to medical treatment, the right to information about a surgeon's experience, the right to a second opinion, and the right in certain circumstances to be referred out of province to have a procedure performed by a more experienced surgeon.

Source: Adapted from The Manitoba Pediatric Cardiac Surgery Inquest (p. 68), by C. Martens, 2002, *Risk Management in Canadian Health Care*, *3*(7), 65–73. Reprinted with permission of LexisNexis.

- A right to the investigation of complaints (i.e., a right of easy access to simple and clear complaints mechanisms, a right to have complaints investigated promptly with explanations given, and a right to the assistance of a Health and Wellness Advocate if needed)

  Responsibilities
- A responsibility to use health care services in a reasonable manner (which includes a responsibility to access those services appropriately)
- A responsibility to use complaints mechanisms appropriately and cooperatively (see Dykeman, 2003, p. 22)

Sections 5(1) and 5(2) of the Act are important qualifiers and read as follows:

1. Where a right or a responsibility in this Act is defined or specified elsewhere (e.g., under another Act or law or in a standard established under the Regional Health Authorities Act), it must be interpreted in accordance with the other instrument.
2. Subject to the rule above, the rights and responsibilities in the Health Charter are to be interpreted by reference to accepted standards of practice, having regard to available resources (financial, human, and material) and the expectations and demands that individuals and health care providers can reasonably make of each other (Dykeman, 2003).

These sections appear to allow the provincial government the ability to rely on resource allocation arguments to avoid the possibility of guaranteeing waiting-list times. Guarantees for waiting-list times were recommended by both the Kirby Report in 2002 and the Mazankowski Report in 2001. (See the Further Reading section at the end of the chapter for more information on these reports.)

Health care reform is likely to be advanced in the coming years by an increasingly informed public who embrace the principle of patient autonomy and individual rights when it comes to their health care. Nurse managers should be at the forefront of policy development in this area.

Government Delegation to Professional Regulatory Bodies

Provincial statutes and regulations govern nursing as one of the regulated professions. The primary purpose of professional regulation is public protection. The regulatory body is given the power by the provincial or territorial government to set registration requirements, practice standards, and criteria for continuing competence and discipline that apply to individual members. As a result, legislation includes procedures for entry into the profession and for the ability to continue to practice, methods of handling complaints, disciplinary procedures, and development of codes of ethics and practice standards. Each nurse practicing in a province or territory must be on the current register of the regulatory body and must meet all criteria set forth for continuing membership. In this way, the public is assured that each nurse is competent to practice nursing.

Regulatory bodies, often called colleges, act in the public interest and must be differentiated from professional associations, such as provincial associations or unions, which act in the interest of their members concerning issues like working conditions. Each provincial or territorial regulatory body has its own specific procedures for handling complaints against individual registrants as tested against the standards of professional practice. Nurse managers must be familiar with the requirements of their jurisdiction. Some jurisdictions impose specific reporting responsibilities on the employer or regulated professional. For example, in Ontario, the regulations in the 1991 *Nursing Act* provide that it is an act of professional misconduct for a nurse to fail to report an incident of unsafe practice or unethical conduct of a health professional to the individual's employer, or, where the health professional works independently, to the college to which the individual belongs (Spencer, 2002). It is important to emphasize that the responsibilities of the professional association are to assure public safety by holding individual members responsible for maintaining standards of practice set by the profession. As will be explained in Chapter 12, these professional standards may differ from the organizational standards and practices of health care agencies, and this sometimes creates dilemmas for individual practitioners.

Although jurisdictions vary as to specific procedures, the complaints received by professional regulatory bodies are all subject to similar general processes. Once a written complaint is filed, the named nurse is notified that a complaint was received, and details of the allegations should be provided to him or her. The nurse may be advised to seek legal counsel. A union may also provide assistance. An investigation then ensues. At this stage, there is usually no requirement that witnesses speak with investigators, but cooperation is generally encouraged. Witnesses should limit discussion to their personal knowledge of the facts. While issues are under investigation, or during a disciplinary proceeding, the issues should not be discussed apart from that required for the proceeding.

After the investigation, the appropriate body reviews the written report, and the action is dismissed, a warning is issued, or the complaint is referred for negotiated resolution or disciplinary hearing. If the complaint proceeds to a disciplinary hearing, the governing body must demonstrate that the nurse has committed an act that constitutes professional misconduct. Such proceedings are more informal than proceedings in a court of law and usually follow similar, but less stringent, rules of evidence. The investigative proceedings and findings of professional associations are increasingly open and available to the public.

If a nurse is found to have committed professional misconduct, penalties vary from revocation, limitation, or suspension of registration to a fine or reprimand. There may also be requirements imposed on continuing registration, such as successful completion of continuing education courses or treatment of a contributing health problem. The individual professional can appeal to a court of law following the disciplinary proceeding. Details regarding the appeal process vary with provincial legislation.

Employers should obtain evidence of valid licensure for all registered employees. Employers who do not document current registration, or who do not independently investigate claims of professional misconduct in their institution or agency, may be subject to claims of negligent hiring or employment if an unregistered care provider is hired and causes injury.

Private Law

Private law governs the relationships and interactions of private parties including patients, health care professionals, hospitals, and regional health authorities. It may even involve provincial governments if they are named as defendants in medical negligence litigation. An allegation of negligence in the health care sector is always troubling for health care professionals. After all, health care professionals are educated and trained to do good and not to do harm. When harm occurs, and negligence is alleged, health care professionals may quite naturally feel unease, concern, fear, and even guilt. Because no one is perfect and because negligence can result in serious harm and even death, health care professionals must pay constant attention to programs of quality improvement, quality assurance, and risk management. When harm does occur, it must be investigated and dealt with appropriately.

Vicarious Liability

Most nurse managers or staff nurses are employees of health care facilities. In law, if they are found to be negligent, their employer is also considered to be negligent. This occurs because of the legal concept of vicarious liability. This legal doctrine states that when an employee's act is done in "the course of employment," it is deemed to be an act of the employer. As well, "an employee's wrongful act will be deemed to have been done in the course of employment if it is authorized by the employer; or it is a wrongful and unauthorized mode of doing some act authorized by the employer" (Aranjo, 2001 p. 4).

Liability of employers has even been extended by the Supreme Court of Canada to include criminal acts of its employees. This is based on a new "enterprise risk" approach. This approach reflects the policy purposes of compensation and deterrence that also underlie vicarious liability. It is generally used in circumstances where an employer allows a vulnerable person such as a child or senior to be exposed to a "significantly increased risk of harm." For example, if an employer puts an employee in a position of trust and allows him or her to perform the assigned tasks, which are then wrongfully or criminally carried out, the employer may be found vicariously liable (Aranjo, 2001).

Accordingly, in the case of *Bazely* v. *Curry* (*Bazely*, 1999), the Supreme Court of Canada found the Children's Foundation of British Columbia liable for the acts of its facility counselor, Mr. Curry, in the sexual abuse of children. However, in a decision released at the same time in *Jacobi* v. *Griffiths*, the Court did not find the Vernon British Columbia Boys and Girls Club liable for the sexual assault acts of its program director, Mr. Griffiths. This was partly on the basis that non-profit employers "have no efficient mechanisms to transfer costs to society as a whole" (*Jacobi*, 1999, p. 83). Chief Justice McLachlin, who wrote the unanimous decision in the *Curry* case, wrote a strong dissent in the 6 to 3 decision in the *Griffiths* case. These cases are complex and fact specific.

In October 2003, the Supreme Court of Canada found two public authorities not liable for harm to children as a result of sexual abuse. The first case, *K.L.B.* v. *British Columbia* (*K.L.B.*, 2003) dealt with a claim that the Province of British Columbia was responsible for harm to children in foster care. While the Court said liability might have been found on the basis of negligence or vicarious liability, the claims were statute barred because they were not brought within two years as required by the provincial statute of limitations. In the second case, *E.D.G.* v. *Hammer* (*E.D.G.*, 2003), the Court found no liability on the part of a school board for the actions of its janitor in a residential school setting. While the specific outcomes of these last two cases may give some comfort to public authorities, the public increasingly expects that public, voluntary, and private organizations be vigilant in their attempt to ensure that children in their direct or indirect care are not exposed to harm.

From the employee's standpoint, the scope of vicarious liability for employers is wide and certainly includes acts of medical negligence. For this reason, employers carry malpractice insurance, and as a result, employees are generally protected by insurance coverage. Hospitals and their employees are covered by a variety of public and private insurance. Physicians for the most part will rely on the Canadian Medical Protective Association. Like physicians, nurses in private practice must get individual insurance coverage, which may be accessed through the Canadian Nurses Protective Society. In most instances, nurses who are employees are covered by the insurance held by their employing agency.

It is important for nurse managers to have a basic understanding of malpractice law that may expose them, staff nurses, or, more likely, their employers to liability. It is helpful in designing effective risk management policies and procedures to do so in a collaborative setting that involves all relevant members of the health care team.

Malpractice Liability

There are several areas of law that may result in liability for medical harm: negligence, lack of informed consent (a form of negligence), battery (a form of assault), and breach of a fiduciary relationship. A fiduciary relationship involves a duty of utmost good faith by a health care provider to a patient because of the imbalance of power and knowledge between the health provider and the patient. By far the most common liability is negligence, which includes actions based on a lack of informed consent. Where there is no consent, consent that is exceeded, or consent that is defective (perhaps because of fraud or misrepresentation), then the action is based on the intentional tort of battery. Finally, an action may be founded on the basis of a breach of a fiduciary relationship between the health care provider or facility and the individual patient. This is arguably wider than the scope for negligence, and the elements of this relationship can be seen in the *Curry, Griffiths, K.L.B.,* and *E.D.G.* cases previously discussed.

Negligence

There are four elements required to establish a negligence action:
1. A duty of care owed by one to another
2. A breach of that duty
3. Damages occurring
4. A causal connection between the damages and the breach (Morris, 1991)

This last element is usually the most difficult hurdle for a plaintiff to overcome in malpractice litigation founded on negligence. Of particular relevance to nurse managers are cases that find negligence based in part on a hospital's failure to implement policies and procedures or, more commonly, to ensure that policies and procedures are followed. This is an important area for nurse managers to focus on in relation to risk management activities.

As indicated in 1996 by Madame Justice Ellen Picard and Gerald Robertson in *Legal Liability of Doctors and Hospitals and Canada*, the most common duties of a hospital to a patient, and in which nursing managers are routinely involved, are the following:

1. To select competent staff and monitor their continued competence
2. To provide proper instruction and supervision
3. To provide proper facilities and equipment
4. To establish systems necessary for the safe operation of the hospital (as cited in Miller, 2001)

Examples of failing to provide a safe system were set forth in the case of *Yepremian* v. *Scarborough General Hospital* (1980) as follows:

1. Inadequate or improperly maintained equipment
2. The failure to provide proper measures for protecting a disturbed person from injuring himself and other patients
3. The failure to provide sufficient personnel to permit rotation of nurses without danger to patients (e.g., coffee breaks)
4. The failure to provide for proper record keeping and the effective transmission of information within the institution

Further examples of negligence from cases include the following:

1. The failure to have proper policies and procedures in place for an obstetrical nurse to follow when admitting a premature mother
2. The failure to ensure that doctors and staff are reasonably suited to do the work they might be expected to perform
3. The failure to ensure that proper coordination occurs between medical specialties and that the treatment program operates as a unified and cohesive whole
4. The failure to ensure that all reasonable medications are properly stocked in the hospital
5. The failure to ensure constant observation while a patient posed a high suicide risk, the failure to hold an intake conference, and poor charting.

As can be seen from these many examples, it is often the making of simple mistakes or simply not following existing policies and procedures that results in liability for hospitals. Nurse managers must use their best efforts in seeing that policies and procedures are followed. When they are not, this should be documented and reported in writing to the appropriate person in the administration of the organization.

In the case of *Braun Estate* v. *Vaughan* (*Braun,* 1997, 2000), a physician took a routine Pap smear to screen for the early detection of cancer. The laboratory report, dated some 10 days later, showed evidence of abnormal cells indicative of a precancerous condition. This type of cancer detected at an early stage has an almost 100% recovery rate. Unfortunately, the lab results were not given to Mrs. Braun until approximately 11 months later after she had sought further medical attention. This failure was due in part to the closure of the clinic where the original test was taken. Tragically, Mrs. Braun later died of cancer (Margo, 2001). Not surprisingly, the trial judge and the Manitoba Court of Appeal found the physician negligent for not ensuring that a reasonably effective "follow-up system" was in place for the timely review of test results. However, the Manitoba Court of Appeal also found the hospital 20% liable for not ensuring that such a system was in place. Chief Justice Scott stated, "It would have been a simple enough matter, for example, for the hospital to set its own policy and procedures to see that a safe system was in place. This could have been satisfied by ensuring that the physician in the clinic had an effective system" (Margo, 2001, p. 51).

The need to follow existing policies and procedures was also emphasized in the case of *Saint John Regional Hospital* v. *Comeau* (*Saint John Regional Hospital*, 2001). The family of a man who died of a ruptured aorta a few hours after discharge from the hospital's emergency department successfully sued the hospital and medical staff. Two doctors, a resident and a specialist in internal medicine to whom the patient had been referred, were found to have failed to consult the emergency room doctor (i.e., the first doctor to assess the patient) according to established policy, and the hospital was found to be directly liable for not taking appropriate steps to ensure compliance with that policy (for a case commentary, see Dimitriadis, 2002).

Informed Consent

The basis for the legal doctrine of informed consent is based on individuals' autonomy and right to decide what is done or not done to their physical person (Champion, 2001). Because of this, a doctor may be held liable for negligence regardless of the fact that the procedure itself may have been performed without negligence. What will be important is whether or not the patient consented to the procedure and, more importantly, that the consent was informed. However, Gerald B. Robertson, QC, Law Professor at the University of Alberta, notes the following:

> In informed consent litigation the plaintiff usually loses — in more than 80% of the cases. Even where (as is often the case) the plaintiff is able to prove that the doctor was negligent in failing to disclose material information (for example, information relating to the risks of treatments), causation is frequently an insurmountable obstacle. The test for causation in informed consent cases, according to the Supreme Court of Canada in *Reibl* v. *Hughes (1980)* is as follows: would a reasonable person in the patient's circumstances have declined treatment if the information had been disclosed? (Robertson, 1999, p. 11)

The standard of disclosure first set forth in the Supreme Court Canada decision in *Hopp* v. *Lepp* has been codified in the 1996 *Health Care Consent Act* of Ontario. Patients should be informed of

- all information that a reasonable person in the same circumstances would require pertaining to the nature of the treatment;
- the expected benefits of the treatment;
- the material risks of the treatment;
- the material effects of the treatment;
- alternative courses of action; and
- the likely consequences of not having the treatment (Champion, 2000).

Disclosure

The duty of informed consent requires health care providers, primarily physicians, to provide necessary disclosure to patients in order to obtain informed consent. Furthermore, there is a duty for health care providers to inform patients when errors occur. Professor Gerald Robertson notes there is a legal duty to do so. "It is now well-established that a doctor who makes an error in the course of treatment is under a legal duty to disclose this fact to the patient if it is something which a reasonable person in the patient's position would want to know" (Picard & Robertson, 1996, p. 170).

The duty of nurse managers and staff nurses concerning the disclosure of errors is also very important. In the case of *Shobridge* v. *Thomas* (*Shobridge*, 1999), an abdominal roll was not counted in the preoperative count as required by hospital policy. The physician did not remove the roll before completing the surgery. It was discovered during a second surgery and as one nurse testified, "the operating room fell silent so that you could hear a pin drop" (Patton, 2001, p. 52). The doctor did not encourage the reporting of this incident and initially the nurses did not file an incident report, which was contrary to hospital policy. A nurse eventually reported the incident and, thereafter, a member of administration spoke to the physician who informed the patient some two months after the discovery of the roll. The Court found both Dr. Thomas and the hospital liable. In commenting on the duty of the nurses, the Court stated: "Their duty was to complete an incident report in accordance with hospital policy. They knew it was Dr. Thomas's duty to inform his patient, not their duty. They were anxious that he do so. They gave him time to do the obviously right thing" (Patton, 2001, p. 54).

Finally, there is also a developing duty to warn third parties of harm. The case that captured many health care professionals' attention was the American case of *Tarasoff* v. *Regents of University of California,* decided in 1976, which held that "the privilege of confidentiality ends where public peril begins" (Ferris, 1999, p. 25). Most recently, the Supreme Court of Canada in the case of *Smith* v. *Jones* in 1999, in dealing with the case of solicitor client privilege, commented favourably on the Tarasoff case. The Supreme Court of Canada set forth factors that could justify breaching solicitor client privilege:

1. Is there a clear risk to an identifiable person or group?

2. Is there a risk of serious bodily harm or death?

3. Is the danger imminent?

In the case of *Pittman Estate* v. *Bain* in 1994, Justice Lang found "that it was reasonable for a hospital to rely on the treating physician to warn the patient of the risk of transfusion/associated AIDS" (Hoaken, 2001, p. 60) through the principle of the learned intermediary. However, the hospital, while not obliged to the patient directly, "was under an obligation to ensure that the physician had the necessary information with which to give an informed warning to the patient" (p. 60).

Battery

The duty of informed consent requires health care providers, primarily physicians, to provide necessary disclosure to patients in order that the consent is informed consent. As stated, if there is no consent or defective consent, then the action is founded on battery and not negligence. The leading case in this area is *Mallette* v. *Shulman,* decided in 1990; this case also sets forth the right to refuse treatment. In the *Mallette* case, a Jehovah's Witness was brought unconscious into a hospital after being involved in a motor vehicle accident. The patient had on her possession a card giving explicit instructions that there was to be no blood transfusion under any circumstances. Notwithstanding these clear instructions, the doctor administered a blood transfusion in order to save the patient's life. The Court held, in finding the doctor liable for battery, that the prior expressed wish by the patient must be respected provided that the wish is clear and unequivocal (*Mallette,* 1990). This case forms the basis for subsequent provincial legislation in dealing with advanced and personal directives and the role of substitute decision makers.

Documentation

Charting

Nurse managers are responsible for ensuring that proper nursing and other health records are maintained. Standards related to documentation requirements and how long records must be kept are derived from provincial statutes, professional standards, and local policy. Documentation must be carried out as an integral part of care. This facilitates communication between health care team members and assists with care continuity. In addition, records are used to demonstrate accountability, provide quality assurance, and facilitate research.

Forms used for documentation may incorporate many recognized approaches to charting. Charting must be consistent for each professional group, department, or procedure, and it must meet requirements of the standard of care. Forms should facilitate documentation by allowing care to be documented in an accurate, inclusive, and timely manner. To the extent possible, charting should be carried out immediately after care is provided, and notes should be made in chronological order. If it is necessary to make a late entry, it should be marked as such and the time of entry should be noted. Such entries should be limited to situations of absolute necessity.

In the Ontario case of *Kolesar* v. *Jeffries* (1976), a postoperative patient was found dead. The last nursing note had been made five hours previously. It was the routine that nurses charted near the end of the shift and assisted each other to recall the events to be recorded. In this instance, there was no proof that the patient had been assessed for five hours. Even if assessment had occurred, the practices of late charting and discussion with others called the accuracy of the records into question. The Court stated that one will always be suspicious of records that are made after the event (*Kolesar,* 1976). Therefore, the care provider who actually provides care, or who witnesses the event, should chart what was done, or seen, immediately or as soon as possible after the event.

This case emphasizes the need for nurses to chart in a timely manner, never alter records, and limit late entries to exceptional situations. It is recognized that in situations such as cardiac arrest or trauma care, care providers cannot both chart and care for the patient. Therefore, a recorder is designated to chart. In such cases, it is recommended that the recorder note the name of each caregiver involved and that each caregiver initial the documentation of his or her own actions at the conclusion of the procedure. By doing so, not only is an accurate record provided, but if a legal action should arise, each care provider can speak about the care they provided.

Charting should be clear, concise, and accurate. Opinions must be avoided unless related to nursing or medical diagnoses. Significant statements by the patient and family should be quoted accurately. The record of observations should state exactly what was observed and should include changes from previous assessments. A nurse should chart so that, if called to testify several years later, after reading the chart, the nurse can recall what events occurred and give credible evidence of the care provided. Legal cases may take five years or even longer to come to court. Because memory is likely to fade during that period, the record may provide the only evidence of the events. The records can be relied on during testimony and are admissible as evidence. Complete, accurate, precise, and timely charting will allow the nurse to convey information included in the record even if he or she has no direct memory of the case.

Nurses and others in management positions do not usually make entries in the patient record. Their managerial activities and decisions are recorded in other ways, such as memoranda, minutes of meetings, e-mail correspondence, and appointment diaries. Records of this nature may become evidence in legal proceedings. Managers often have a practice of writing "Notes to file" to record details of unusual situations.

Electronic Health Records

The movement toward the use of electronic health records is well under way in Canada and is supported by both the federal and provincial governments. Electronic health records promise greater efficiencies and a better quality of care in the health system. However, they also carry significant risks to patients in terms of maintaining the privacy and confidentiality of their personal health care information. This was noted by the United Kingdom's NHS Information Authority in a consultation document entitled *Caring for Information: Model for the Future*. Among other things, the document noted that even if "most GPs and hospitals now have some form of patient record on computer that can be shared among their own staff…information is relatively 'locked away' from anyone outside the particular hospital or surgery" (NHS Information Authority, 2002, p. 1).

Such will not be the case with electronic health records in which many health care providers and agencies may have access to personal health care information. The UK document attempted to strike a balance between allowing "informed patients…as much control as possible over who sees their health information" and not creating "impossible barriers to information sharing for good care" (NHS Information Authority, 2002, p. 6). The recommended solution was to allow patients the ability to restrict access to certain parts of their health care information through the use of electronic "sealed envelopes." This was based on principles found in the *Data Protection Act 1998* (UK), the *Human Rights Act 1998* (UK), and the common law duty of confidentiality.

Similar principles are less clearly defined in Canada. Authors McSherry and Somerville (1998) note that, at best, courts may support a qualified approach to a right to privacy grounded in reasonable expectation. The *Canadian Charter of Rights and Freedoms* is silent as to an express right to privacy. Privacy is not articulated as a fundamental right, although some judges of the Supreme Court of Canada have express sympathy for the view that the *Charter* guarantees a "reasonable expectation" of privacy. The courts, however, have been careful to talk about a "reasonable expectation" of privacy, rather than a "fundamental right of privacy *per se*" (Dykeman, 2001, p. 27).

Fortunately, Ontario, in its proposed *Health Information Protection Act* (2003), contains a type of "lock box" similar to the sealed envelope concept. Unfortunately, Alberta chose a different path. In February 2003, Bill 10 was passed which repealed section 59 of the *Health Information Act* (2000) and thereby removed the requirement to get patient consent before information could be shared by electronic means. This removal of patient consent was not replaced with any lock box or sealed envelope safeguard. Given that privacy law is developing in Canada, and given that consent is the cornerstone of any good privacy code, it will be interesting to see what ultimately transpires in Alberta.

The significance for nurse managers is that, with the introduction and use of electronic health records, it will be more important than ever to ensure that privacy laws and patients' privacy rights are protected. Only those with a clear and authorized need to know should be allowed access to personal health information contained in electronic health records.

Employment Contracts

Nurses, whether in independent practice or as employees, have employment contracts. A contract is defined as "an agreement between two or more persons which creates an obligation to do or not to do a particular thing" (Nolan & Connolly, 1979, p. 291). There are several requirements for a contract to exist: (a) each party entering the contract must be competent, (b) each party must understand the subject matter and obligations of the contract, (c) each party must have obligations and derive benefit from the contract, and (d) legal consideration must create the inducement to enter a contract. In the case of employment, the legal consideration that induces the contract may be that the employer provides work and the pay for that work, and the employee performs the work. At a minimum, all employment contracts must meet the standards set forth in provincial and federal labour standards and codes.

Employment contracts may be verbal, written, or implied. If an employer offers a position, either in writing or verbally, and the nurse accepts, there is a contract that may be enforced. If no union is involved, the nurse and the employer may negotiate an individual employment contract that sets forth the rights and obligations of each party. In an individual contract, terms and conditions may vary for each employee, although, in actual practice, hospitals and agencies tend to have similar contracts for all employees in a given job classification. Terms and conditions may be set forth in detail, or the contract may be simple with few conditions stated. In a unionized organization, the terms and conditions of employment are those of the union contract (collective agreement) with the employer.

Verbal employment contracts are often more difficult to enforce than written contracts because of the problem of providing proof of the terms negotiated. Thus, the nurse in a non-union position may be wise to have important terms put in writing. Such terms may include duration of the contract, issues regarding probation, negotiated time off, notice of termination, and job description.

Employment is regulated by federal and provincial employment statutes, common law, industry standards, accreditation standards, human rights legislation, and institutional policies, as well as by employment and union contracts. All contracts must meet legal conditions to be enforceable and must contain the basic elements of parties, property (services), and price (salary).

In all employment contracts, the employee has the expectation of reimbursement, and the employer has the expectation that the employee will perform the expected work and will follow professional standards and practice and any additional policies set by the institution. In a union environment, the terms and conditions of the contract are negotiated between the employer and the union and become the collective agreement. All employees within the given bargaining unit of the union are subject to the same terms and conditions of employment.

Discipline is subject to contractual, statutory, and common law requirements. The employee disciplinary procedure is usually progressive, consisting first of counselling, then a verbal warning, followed by a written warning that becomes part of the employment record, suspension with or without pay, and, finally, written notice that further discipline will lead to discharge, or actual discharge itself.

Performance appraisals may be used as a method of performance documentation and should often be supplemented by anecdotal notes that are discussed with the employee and kept as part of the employee record. The employee is usually required to sign the performance appraisal or anecdotal note as evidence that he or she has seen it and that discussion has taken place; however, the signature does not indicate the employee's agreement with the contents of the appraisal or note.

Nurse managers who are "out of scope" (out of the bargaining unit) are often involved in representing the employer in collective bargaining. In a union environment, discipline must follow labour relations laws, prior arbitration decisions, and the collective agreement grievance procedure. Arbitration is the binding means of determining the case, although few cases proceed that far. Both the employer and the union representing the employee must follow the terms of the collective agreement. In rare instances, particularly when mistakes are alleged in relation to the resolution procedure, the case may be appealed to the judicial system after an arbitration decision.

In a non-union environment, the employer may dismiss an employee at will subject to the statutory and common law principles of reasonable notice or, alternatively, subject to compensation for the required notice period. If there is just cause (e.g., theft from the employer), reasonable notice may not be necessary. The length of the notice period usually depends upon the length of employment and other factors.

The remedy in regard to wrongful dismissal is usually monetary damages based on what would have been earned during the notice period or for the period of the contract. The employee is usually expected to try to find new work, and the award may be reduced if new employment is found. Similarly, an employee is also expected to give the employer notice of termination pursuant to the employment contract and employment standards.

In a union environment, dismissal is governed by the collective agreement, which must meet the requirements of law and which usually sets forth specific procedures to be followed by each party. In times of downsizing, layoffs and terminations must follow the collective agreement, which usually means that seniority governs which union members retain employment. Each union agreement, however, may have specific terms, particularly in regard to specialty nursing.

Labour relations statutes protect employers from illegal strikes and from certain behaviours by employees or unions. These statutes require that notice and bargaining obligations be met prior to strike. Some also preclude strikes by essential employees such as nurses. Remedies for illegal work actions may include injunction, back to work orders, and fines (Morris, 1991).

Leadership Implications

It is important for nurse managers to have a general understanding of the law. A helpful way to do this is to know the difference between public and private law. Public law deals with interactions between governments and between governments and the public. A good example of this is the rights granted to Canadians under the *Canadian Charter of Rights and Freedoms*. Private law deals with interactions between citizens. A good example of this is medical malpractice litigation. With an understanding of the differences between public and private law, it is easier to follow past, present, and future legal developments.

The Sinclair Inquiry was a public law inquiry that reviewed issues surrounding the deaths of numerous infants in the cardiac unit of a major hospital. Justice Sinclair provided many thoughtful recommendations that should be implemented. In addition, parents whose infants died on the unit will have recourse through private law to sue public and private parties for damages. In so doing, they will have to prove that either there was lack of informed consent or that there was negligence.

The elements of negligence include a duty of care owed by one to another, a breach of that duty, damages that occurred, and a causal connection between the damages and a breach of care. If nurses are included in litigation, they should automatically be covered by their employer's insurance plan through the principle that the employer is vicariously liable for the actions of its employees. The employees themselves will have been originally employed through an employment agreement that may also be the subject of a collective agreement. The collective agreement itself and the original employment agreement are examples of private law.

In any litigation, great reliance will be placed on health records. For this reason and for purposes of risk management, it is essential that nurse managers ensure that accurate and timely records are maintained. It is also important that they protect the privacy and confidentiality of health care records, especially electronic health records.

Nurse managers enter the 21st century with more legal responsibility, more accountability, and more reliance placed on their skills than ever before. A general understanding of the law that forms the foundation of so many of their activities is essential.

Summary

- The broad area of public law provides the legal framework for relationships between the federal and provincial governments and between governments and individuals, including government inquiries and government delegation to provincial regulatory bodies.

- Professional regulatory bodies are established through provincial statutes and regulations and exist for the purpose of public protection. Health professions, including nursing, must set practice standards and criteria for registration, continuing competence, and discipline that apply to all individual members of the profession.

- Most nurses are employed by health agencies that are corporate entities or organizations, which have fiduciary duties and legal responsibilities to their clients and staff.

- The fiduciary relationship involves a duty of the utmost good faith by a health care provider to a patient because of the imbalance of power and knowledge between the health provider and the patient.

- Through the principle of vicarious liability, organizations are legally responsible for the actions of their employees or other agents of the organization, including those in the domain of private law, which includes malpractice liability, negligence, matters of informed consent, and battery.

- Organizational leaders and managers acting on behalf or their employing organizations must be conscious of fiduciary duties and vicarious liability as they establish organizational policies and standards and as they conduct their day-to-day activities.

- Organizational policies and the practices of individual professions are subject to legal requirements and precedents to provide patients with the information they need to give informed consent and to disclose information when an error has been made and it is something a reasonable person in the patient's position would want to know.

- Risk management, quality assurance, and quality improvement programs are some of the processes used to minimize errors and the liability of organizations.

- Documentation practices are critical to risk management for individual professionals and health agencies and have figured in many legal actions.

- Employment is regulated by federal and provincial employment statutes, common law, industry standards, accreditation standards, human rights legislation, and institutional policies as well as by employment and union contracts.

- Contracts may be either oral, written, or implied.

- Employee discipline is subject to contractual, statutory, and common law requirements and is usually a progressive process.

- Non-unionized employees, including nurse managers, may not have employment contracts, but they are entitled to the statutory and common law principles of reasonable notice of dismissal or compensation for a period of notice that customarily takes into account the length of service.

- Health care reform is likely to be advanced in the coming years by an increasingly informed public who embrace the principle of patient autonomy and individual rights when it comes to their health care. Nurse managers should be at the forefront of policy development in this area.

Applying the Knowledge in this Chapter

Exercise

Risk management has been defined as "the systematic process of identifying, evaluating and addressing (treating or preventing) potential and/or actual risks which are a source of injury or loss of money or reputation" (Mrazek, 1994, p. 555).

As the program manager of a clinical service, describe your risk management responsibilities in relation to the following: patients or clients, staff and co-workers, the physical environment, material and financial resources, and your employer.

Resources

evolve Internet Resources

Canadian Legal Information Institute:
www.canlii.org/index_en.html
This is Canada's main source of free access to primary legal material. It was created for the Federation of Law Societies at the University of Montreal's Public Law Research Centre. Details of many of the cases cited in this chapter can be found on this Web site.

Mazankowski Report:
www.premiersadvisory.com/reform.html

Further Reading

Cameron v. Nova Scotia (Attorney General) (1999), 177 DLR (4th) 611 (NSCA).
Commission of Inquiry on the Blood System in Canada. (1997). *Final report*. 3 vols. Commissioner: Mr. Justice H. Krever. Ottawa, ON: Government of Canada.
Hopp v. Lepp (1980), 112 DLR. (3d) 67 (SCC).
Picard, E.I., & Robertson, G.B. (1996). *Legal liability of doctors and hospitals in Canada* (3rd ed.). Toronto, ON: Carswell.
Pittman Estate v. Bain (1994), 112 DLR (4th) 257 (Ont. Gen. Div.).
Premier's Advisory Council on Health. (2001). *A framework for reform. Report of the Premier's Advisory Council on Health.* Chair: D. Mazankowski. Edmonton, AB: Government of Alberta.
Reibl v. Hughes (1980), 114 DLR (3d) 1 (SCC).
Risk Management in Canadian Health Care.
This is a newsletter published by LexisNexis Canada, Inc. approximately four times a year.
Standing Senate Committee on Social Affairs, Science and Technology. (2002). *The health of Canadians – The federal role. Final report on the state of the health care system in Canada. Volume 6, Recommendations for reform.* Chair: The Honorable M. J. L. Kirby. Ottawa, ON: Parliament of Canada.
Tarasoff v. Regents of University of California, [1976] 17 Cal. 3d 425, 131 Cal. Rptr. 14, 551 P. 2d 334.

References

Aranjo, E.M. (2001, April). Case comment: Update on employer liability for employee assaults. *Risk Management in Canadian Health Care, 3*(1), 3–7.

Auton (Guardian of) v. British Columbia (Attorney General) (2002), BCCA 538.

Bazley v. Curry, [1999] 2 SCR 534.

Braun Estate v. Vaughan, [1997] M.J. No. 616 (Man. Q.B.); *Braun Estate v. Vaughan,* [2000], 3 WWR 465 (Man. C.A.).

Canada Act 1982, (U.K.), 1982, c. 11.

Canada Health Act, RSC 1985, c. C-6.

Canadian Bar Association Task Force on Health Care. (1994). *What's law got to do with it? Health care reform in Canada*. Ottawa, ON: Canadian Bar Association.

Carver, P.J. (2003). Notes for a talk to the Constitutional Law Subsection of the Canadian Bar Association, February 10, 2003.

Champion, J.B. (2000, February). Informed consent or compromised consent? Walking the fine line. *Risk Management in Canadian Health Care, 1*(12), 89–100.

Champion, J.B. (2001, March). When "enough" may not be enough: Informed consent and patient communication. *Risk Management in Canadian Health Care, 2*(8), 81–88.

Commission on the Future of Health Care in Canada. (2002, November). *Building on values: The future of healthcare in Canada – Final report*. Commissioner: R. Romanow. Ottawa, ON: Parliament of Canada. Retrieved January 20, 2004, from http://www.hc-sc.gc.ca/english/care/romanow/index.html

Criminal Code, RSC 1985, c. C-46.

Dimitriadis, F. (2002, January). Case comment: Adoption and enforcement of hospital policies. *Risk Management in Canadian Health Care, 3*(7), 73–76.

Dykeman, M.J. (2001, July). Patient sexuality in institutional health settings. *Risk Management in Canadian Health Care, 3*(3), 25–29.

Dykeman, M.J. (2003, April). New Brunswick introduces patient charter. *Risk Management in Canadian Health Care, 5*(2), 21–24.

E.D.G. v. Hammer, [2003] SCC 52.

Eldridge v. British Columbia (Attorney General), [1997] 3 SCR 624.

Ferris, L.E. (1999, June). Duty to inform: Update for Canadian health care facilities. *Risk Management in Canadian Health Care, 1*(4), 25–30.

Gosselin v. Quebec (Attorney General), [2002] 4 SCR 429.

Health Charter of Rights and Responsibilities Act, 2003.

Health Information Act, RSA 2000, c. H-5.

Health Information Protection Act, 2003.

Hoaken, E. (2001, December). Duty to warn: The civil liability perspective, *Risk Management in Canadian Health Care, 3*(6), 57–64.

Jacobi v. Griffiths, [1999] 2 SCR 570.

K.L.B. v. British Columbia, [2003] SCC 51.

Kolesar v. Jeffries (1976), 59 DLR (3d) 367 at 373 (Ont. H.C.); varied 12 O.R. (2d) 142 (C.A.); aff'd (1978), 2 CCCLT 1970 (SCC).

Malette v. Shulman (1990), 67 DLR (4th) 321 (Ont. CA).

Margo, N. (1999, November). Supreme Court of Canada mandates deaf interpreter services. *Risk Management in Canadian Health Care, 1*(9), 68–70.

Margo, N. (2001, November). Case comment: Hospital liability for failure to create a test results review "system." *Risk Management in Canadian Health Care, 3*(5), 49–52.

Martens, C. (2002, January). The Manitoba pediatric cardiac surgery inquest. *Risk Management in Canadian Health Care, 3*(7), 65–73.

McSherry, B., & Somerville, M. (1998). *Sexual activity among institutionalized persons in need of special care*. Windsor Yearbook Access to Justice 90 at 105.

Miller, J.G. (2001, February 21/22). *Duties of care: Hospitals*. A paper prepared for the Legal Education Society of Alberta, Alberta, Canada.

Morris, J. (1991). *Canadian nurses and the law*. Toronto, ON: Butterworths.

Mrazek, M. (1994). Risk management. In J.M. Hibberd & M.E. Kyle (Eds.), *Nursing management in Canada* (pp. 554–573). Toronto, ON: W.B. Saunders.

NHS Information Authority. (2002, October). *Caring for information: Model for the future*. Retrieved February 18, 2004, from http://www.nhsia.nhs.uk/confidentiality

Nolan, J.R. & Connolly, M.J. (Eds.). (1979). *Black's law dictionary* (5th ed.). St. Paul, MN: West Publishing.

Patton, L.M. (2001, November). Case comment: Cause and effect—limiting liability in malpractice cases. *Risk Management in Canadian Health Care, 3*(5), 52–55.

Picard, E.I., & Robertson, G.B. (1996). Legal liability of doctors and hospitals in Canada (3rd ed.). Ottawa, ON: Carswell Thomson Canada.

Robertson, G. (1999, November). *Causation in medical malpractice cases*. A paper prepared for the Legal Education Society of Alberta, Alberta, Canada.

Saint John Regional Hospital v. *Comeau* (2001), NBCA 113.

Shobridge v. *Thomas,* [1999] BCJ No. 1747 (SC) (QL).

Sinclair, C.M. (2001, May). *Report of the Manitoba pediatric cardiac surgery inquest: An inquiry into twelve deaths at the Winnipeg Health Sciences Centre in 1994*. Winnipeg, MB: Provincial Court of Manitoba.

Spencer, P.C. (2002, December) Developing a hospital policy re: disclosure of adverse medical events. *Risk Management in Canadian Health Care, 4*(6), 65–72.

Yepremian v. *Scarborough General Hospital* (1980), 28 OR (2d), 494 (CA).

12

STANDARDS AND QUALITY IN THE CANADIAN HEALTH SYSTEM

Donna Lynn Smith, Leona Zboril-Benson, and Grant Gillis

Learning Objectives

In this chapter, you will learn:

- The importance of standards in assuring the quality and cost-effectiveness of health services

- The origins and evolution of interest in the concept of "quality" in health care

- Definitions of common terms associated with quality management

- Similarities and differences in various types of standards, including the sources for their authority

- About the educational standards and certification program of the Canadian College of Health Service Executives (CCHSE)

- Evidence-based standards for nursing services and administration and the accreditation of nursing services

- The role of the Canadian Council on Health Services Accreditation (CCHSA) and its approach to the development and measurement of standards

- The relevance of the Canadian Standards Association (CSA) and the International Organization for Standardization (ISO) to the Canadian health system and their approaches to developing and measuring standards

A professional education includes knowledge of the discipline, but also an awareness of the standards that are applicable to that discipline. The work of individual health professionals and health agencies is complex and highly visible. Mistakes are costly and can lead to iatrogenic illness or even death. Some are the result of errors on the part of individual professionals, but many are the result of dysfunctional processes, practices, or policies in departments, systems, or organizations. Efforts to prevent mistakes and to improve the quality of care are not new in health care. Florence Nightingale used statistical information and her knowledge of the relationship between cleanliness, poor nutrition, and health to recommend reform of the working and living conditions of enlisted British military personnel during the Crimean War. Since that time, and especially since the 1980s, efforts to improve quality in health care have created a multi-million dollar industry.

This chapter begins with an introduction to the some of the terminology used to describe standards and quality in health services as well as a discussion of contextual issues affecting quality management. A conceptual framework that is the foundation for many developments in this field is then presented. Various types of standards and the sources of their authority are discussed. The development of standards for nursing services and nursing administration is described in a historical perspective with current examples. The Canadian Council on Health Services Accreditation (CCHSA) has had a major influence on the development of standards for health services in Canada. The work of this important organization is described and compared to the approaches for developing and measuring standards used by two other organizations, the Canadian Standards Association (CSA) and the International Organization for Standardization (ISO). Managing risks and assuring or improving quality are related but different activities that must continually be in progress in health organizations. There can be serious consequences to patients, individual professionals, and health agencies when relevant standards are not met.

Quality Management

Concepts and Terminology

There have been many variations on the theme of quality since formal programs of quality assurance began in health organizations more than three decades ago. Table 12.1 is a glossary of terms that reflect past and current emphasis in the field that is now broadly defined as "quality management." Readers may wish to return to this table from time to time as they proceed through the chapter.

Contextual Issues

Quality management approaches originally emerged within specific disciplines, and nursing was at the forefront of these developments. More recently, developments in business, industry, and science have influenced approaches to quality management in health care. As the costs of health care have risen and neo-conservative economic viewpoints have gained popularity, a plethora of management

Table 12.1 Key Terms for Quality Management in Health Care

Accountability[1]

Answering for one's actions and the consequences of those actions; acting within the authority of one's position to accept responsibility for specifying standards, measuring performance against those standards, and making decisions as necessary to correct problems and improve quality.

Balanced Scorecard[2]

Originally developed by Kaplan and Norton in 1992, the balanced scorecard is one approach to organizational performance measurement, providing executives with a comprehensive framework to translate an organization's strategic objectives into performance measures. They urged organizations to go beyond financial measures of performance to develop a complementary set of measures based on a variety of dimensions. The balanced scorecard would provide answers to four basic questions: (a) How do customers see us? (customer perspective), (b) What must we excel at? (internal business perspective), (c) Can we continue to improve? (innovation and learning perspective), and (d) How do we look at funders? (financial perspective). Kaplan and Norton maintain that by creating measures in these four areas, health care organizations could obtain feedback, thus providing a balanced view of organizational performance.

Benchmark[1]

"A reference point signifying the highest mark of quality of certain goods, services, or processes used as a comparison point for quality in like organizations or situations."

Criteria[1]

Statements describing predetermined elements that clarify the intent of a standard and the degree to which that standard has been accomplished.

Clinical Practice Guidelines[3]

"Clinical practice guidelines are systematically developed statements to assist practitioner and patient decisions about appropriate health care for specific clinical circumstances."

Continuous Quality Improvement (CQI)[4]

"The philosophy of Continuous Quality Improvement, or CQI, is based upon using a team approach to examine and improve work processes using a problem-solving model making organizations more efficient." Key concepts of CQI include (a) customer satisfaction, (b) employee empowerment, and (c) continuous improvement.

Evidence-Based Management[5]

A management approach that focuses on basing decisions on evidence to help "define a problem, diagnose its causes, or evaluate interventions so that management action is judged reasonably 'accurate, precise, sufficient, representative, and authoritative' and is so perceived by stakeholders."

Table 12.1 Continued

Evidence-Based Management Cooperatives (EBMCs)[5]	"Evidence-based management cooperatives (EBCMs) exist to create organizations at the health system level that bring together managers, consultants, and researchers with a common mission of improving health care management, data bases, and organizational performance."
Evidence-Based Medicine[6]	Described as an approach to health care practice in which the clinician is aware of the evidence in support of his/her clinical practice, and the strength of that evidence and is "the conscientious, explicit, and judicious use of current best evidence in making decisions about the care of individual patients."
Guidelines[1]	"Authoritative statements describing recommended courses of action for specific clinical situations, technical conditions, or patient populations".
Indicators[1]	Observable and measurable dimensions that provide information on aspects of care.
Measurement[1]	The process of determining whether a standard has been met.
Outcome[1]	Any change that takes place in the client as a result of the inputs and interactions between client and provider, including changes in health status and client satisfaction.
Process[1]	Activities that occur between clients and care providers while care is taking place.
Quality[1]	Level of excellence, value or worth; conformance to standards that are either implicit or explicit. • An umbrella term encompassing all systematic approaches to the assessment and improvement of quality. • A systematic process wherein there is a data-based, judgmental appraisal of a selected element of care and subsequent improvement; a term that is gradually replacing the more traditional term "quality assurance" (QA). • A collaborative team process, usually interdisciplinary and statistically supported, used to respond systematically to discrete opportunities for improvement. • A leadership paradigm that subscribes to quality as a driving value for an organization; the value is operationalized by top-down total employee commitment and participation in consumer-focused continuous quality improvement of all work processes throughout an organization.

Table 12.1 Continued	
Standard[1]	A broad statement of agreed-upon quality for a given element of care.
Structures[1]	Human and material resources; organizational frameworks or systems. Sometimes referred to as "inputs."

Sources:

1. Adapted from *Quality Management in Nursing and Health Care* (pp. 25, 41, 61, 589), by J.A. Schmele, 1996, Albany, NY: Delmar.
2. A Balanced Scorecard for Canadian Hospitals, by G.R. Baker and G.H. Pink, 1995, *Healthcare Management Forum, 8*(4), p. 13.
3. *Clinical Practice Guidelines: Directions for a New Program* (p. 38), by Institute of Medicine, 1990, Washington, DC: National Academy Press.
4. *Mission and Vision for Continuous Quality Improvement,* by Hartford Health, 2003, Retrieved August 2003, from http://www.co.ha.md.us/health/cqi.htm
5. Evidence-Based Management, by A.R. Kovner, J.J. Elton, and J. Billings, 2000, *Frontiers of Health Services Management, 16*(4), pp. 10, 17.
6. Evidence-Based Medicine: What It Is and What It Isn't, by D.L. Sackett, W.M. Rosenberg, J.A. Gray, R.B. Haynes, and W.S. Richardson, 1996, *BMJ, 312*(7023), p. 71.

interventions have been successfully marketed by consultants. Many organizational experiments, some of which qualify as management "fads" or "fashions" (Abrahamson, 1991, 1996), have been adopted in response to rhetorical claims that they will improve quality and save money in the process. In this context, expert nursing knowledge, policies, procedures, and standards for assuring quality were sometimes disparaged as ritualistic "turf protection." Rondeau and Wagar (2004) note that "in the past decade, two of the most significant change initiatives witnessed by healthcare organizations have been the introduction of total QM/Continuous Quality Improvement (TQM/CQI) and organizational downsizing. In many settings these initiatives have been introduced at the same time, often with disastrous consequences" (p. 22). The mood of the day is illustrated by a Canadian book on quality improvement for hospitals, in which one chief executive officer (CEO) advocated fewer managers and self-directed teams as the way of the future, stating: "I'm damn sure that out of our $260 million budget, there's probably $75 to $80 million that should be dropping out of that budget without any compromise to quality of care" (Hassen & Lindenburger, 1993, p. 190).

The paradox of implementing total quality management (TQM) / continuous quality improvement (CQI) while reducing the workforce is discussed by Rondeau and Wagar. They note that while workforce reductions are directed to the short-term objective of cost-cutting, TQM/CQI initiatives are intended to achieve organizational efficiencies in the long term by improving organizational processes primarily by empowering the employees (who are the "process owners") to find better ways of serving the customer, thus leading to enhanced employee and customer satisfaction (Rondeau & Wagar, 2004, p. 23).

The issue of whether these two objectives are compatible has received limited attention by organizational scholars and although "some observers have suggested that the two processes work in a complementary fashion... a contrary body or argument suggests that downsizing poses a serious threat to the practice of TQM/CQI" (Rondeau & Wagar, 2004, p. 24). Reported effects of introducing TQM/CQI initiatives while downsizing and restructuring the workforce have included the alienation of workers whose support is needed to successfully implement the initiatives, disruption of teamwork, lowered commitment and motivation among surviving employees, and disruption of other change initiatives. In a survey of the perceptions of CEOs in 221 Canadian hospitals, Rondeau and Wagar (2004) found the hospitals that performed best were those with the lowest workforce reductions and the highest quality management (QM) orientation. They speculate that, through elevated levels of employee involvement, empowerment, and participation, quality obsessed hospitals are better able to withstand the adverse consequences of severe workforce reduction. An alternate explanation is suggested by Cummings and Estabrooks (2003). They conducted a systematic review of research literature to assess the effects of hospital restructuring, including layoffs, on the nurses who remained employed. The findings of their initial search yielded 1203 articles, of which 84 abstracts met the inclusion criteria for the review. These papers were then further screened against inclusion criteria, including requirements for rigorous research methodology and a reported relationship between the independent variable (e.g., a measure of hospital restructuring) and the dependent variable (e.g., nursing outcomes such as emotional exhaustion and changes in role or job satisfaction). Only 22 empirical papers met the criteria, and a detailed analysis led the authors to conclude that hospital restructuring that included layoffs led to significant deterioration in the health, well-being, and professional efficacy of the providers, in this case, the nurses who remained employed. The authors identified the need for further research to determine if negative effects are temporal or if they can be mitigated by individual or organizational strategies. Cummings and colleagues subsequently reported the results of a study that demonstrated, through structural equation modelling of a large data set, that emotionally intelligent nursing leadership was a significant factor in enabling the remaining nurses to cope with downsizing. This nursing leadership focused on building relational capital by investing energy into developing relationships and managing emotion in the turbulent workplace. Nurses were thereby enabled to construct new meaning about their work, contributing to improved well-being and ultimately achieving quality patient care (Cummings, Hayduk, & Estabrooks, in press).

The various organizational experiments undertaken as "quality solutions" have been costly to implement, and as one after another has occurred without evaluation or consolidation, former processes and accountability mechanisms have been disrupted or dispersed. In turn, these experiments have contributed to cynicism, the loss of specialized professional expertise, and low morale among the professional health workforce. Reviews of literature and recent studies in this area reveal that sustained positive effects of these organizational experiments have not been demonstrated.

Early in the 21st century, there is growing concern about issues of basic safety and accountability in the health system. In the United States, severe and costly regulatory mechanisms have been implemented in response to escalating liability claims by health care consumers who have suffered damages as a result of carelessness, malpractice, and even fraud. In Canada, both federal and provincial governments have been hesitant to impose and monitor standards, and although it is not widely recognized, regulatory requirements for health services in Canada are minimal in comparison to the US system. However, standards are required to guide the work of clinical professionals and organizational leaders and to assure public protection. In this context, the broad objective of this chapter is to provide information about various types of standards, their sources of authority, and the ways in which they are measured. The importance of transparency in the development of standards and the measurement and reporting of safety and quality is emphasized.

A Framework for Health Care Standards

A conceptual framework developed by Donabedian (1966) provides a foundation for understanding standards and quality in health care and the types of information needed for quality assessment. The framework is shown in Table 12.2.

Structure refers to the environment or setting for health services and includes material and human resources, the structure of the organization, policies and procedures, and documentation

Table 12.2 **Types of Information Required for Quality Assessment**	
Structure	The attributes of settings in which care occurs (physical and organizational tools and resources) Includes: • material resources (e.g., facilities, equipment, money) • human resources (e.g., number and qualifications of personnel) • organizational structure (e.g., medical staff organization, peer-review methods)
Process	What is actually done in giving and receiving care (the activities that occur between client and provider) Includes: • patient's activities in seeking care and carrying it out • practitioner's activities in making a diagnosis and recommending or implementing treatment
Outcomes	The effects of care on the health status of patients and populations (the changes in status attributable to antecedent health care) Includes: • improvements in a client's knowledge • changes in a client's behaviour • degree of client satisfaction with care

Source: Adapted from Evaluating the Quality of Medical Care, by A. Donabedian, 1996, *Milbank Quarterly*, *44*(Suppl 3), pp. 166–203.

requirements. An example of a structural standard is the requirement that all nurses employed in an agency be registered in their jurisdiction. Process standards are concerned with the activities involved in providing health services. These include clinical processes as well as the other processes and systems required to support clinical care. An example of a process standard is the requirement that all adverse occurrences be promptly and accurately reported in written incident reports. As can be seen from these examples, *structural standards* (sometimes called inputs) are the easiest to measure. *Process standards* are more challenging, and it is in the area of process that many total quality management programs or continuous quality improvement programs strive to make a difference (Mendez, 1999; Van Der Weile, Williams, & Dale, 2000; Kibbe, Kaluzny, & McLaughlin, 1994).

Outcome standards are concerned with the effects of health services and changes to the health status of individuals and populations. They are the most difficult to define and measure because there are many different kinds of outcomes, including some that are patient-focused, others that are provider-focused, and others that are "organization-focused" (Jennings, Staggers, & Brosch, 1999). Outcome indicators are often selected as proxy measures of outcome. For example, *diagnosis*, or *condition-specific*, *indicators* such as the rate of postoperative infection or the incidence of pressure sores are used to monitor the progress of an illness and the effects of treatment. But other, more holistic indicators such as functional status, mental status, quality of life, or satisfaction with care are also very important because they are *patient-focused outcomes*. For example, client satisfaction questionnaires may be used to determine whether people feel that they have been treated with kindness and respect by health care providers.

Prescription rates, the number of surgical infections per provider, the rate of medication errors, and caregiver burden are examples of *provider-focused outcomes*. A nursing-sensitive, provider-focused indicator might be the percentage of discharged patients who are readmitted to hospital because of problems in administering their medications. Familiar *organization-focused outcomes* include the quality and costs of care. Since quality is a multi-dimensional outcome, aggregate indicators such as the mortality or complication rate are measured and reported in order to compare health care organizations.

The selection of indicators to be monitored at the level of health organizations and the health system is a complex task and is often determined by the type of information that is readily available in administrative data sets. Unfortunately, this type of administrative data reflects the structure and priorities of the health system of the past, and outcomes valued by ordinary citizens, such as convenient access to health services, have not traditionally been measured (Kovner, Elton, & Billings, 2000; Davies et al., 1994).

Although it seems obvious that one must understand structure and process to appreciate the significance of outcomes, some leaders have advocated that only "results" should be measured. When only outcomes are measured (or, as usually happens, selected indicators assumed to represent outcomes), it can be difficult to understand and interpret why some outcomes are achieved while others are not. Without information about the context, structure, and processes in the delivery of health services, it is also difficult to interpret the effects of decisions made within the organization. In 1999, an entire issue of the *Journal of Health Services Research* (Volume 34, Issue 5) was devoted to a series of papers discussing the importance of qualitative information in understanding and interpreting quantitative findings. Without multi-dimensional information, there is a particular danger that outcome measurement will be superficially focused on easily quantifiable indicators.

Types of Health Care Standards

Safety and quality cannot be assessed or improved without reference to standards. In manufacturing and production, it is relatively easy to establish standards for the appearance, composition, functionality, and safety of a product. But, as the organizational theorist Charles Perrow (1979) has pointed out, complexity in organizations arises from differences in raw materials, structure, technology, and the environment. In manufacturing processes, rules can be "built into machines," whereas in "people-changing" organizations such as schools and health services, professional workers are employed because their education prepares them to engage in the "search behaviour" needed to define and solve complex problems. Health care organizations have been described as the most complex of all organizational types, sharing features with other knowledge-based industries but having "non-standard" raw materials (i.e., the people who receive and provide services). The broadly based education of health professionals prepares them to integrate knowledge, principles, and direct observation to make discretionary judgments in specific and often unique situations. For all of these reasons, determining standards for health services and measuring their achievement are complex tasks.

Understanding the sources of authority for standards is necessary to determine when and how the standards apply in specific situations. The sources of authority for educational professional, ethical, organizational, community, and legal standards are different. In Table 12.3, these various types of standards and their sources of authority are summarized. Each is now discussed in more detail.

Education and Credentialing Standards

Traditionally, professions have been defined by their educational standards and resulting credentials. Some professions, particularly medicine, continue to be defined in this manner and retain complete control of the educational processes and requirements for entry to practice in the profession. Although nursing is a self-governing profession, it does not have the legislated authority to prescribe the educational standards for its members. Wotherspoon (2002) has commented, "Since the nineteenth century, with the emergence of the well-known 'Nightingale system' prescient nurses and nursing supervisors have recognized the potential value of training to a distinct sphere of nursing activity within the overall health system. However, the nature of that training and role has been subject to varying, often conflicting, conceptions of groups within nursing and interests outside nursing" (p. 83). From a sociological perspective, he concludes that nursing education emerged as a compromise, arising from inadequate resources, struggles for control, and the nature of nursing as women's work and that it must be understood as part of a wider network of social, political, and economic realities. Over a number of decades, there has been strong resistance to efforts by professional nursing associations to require a baccalaureate degree as the entry qualification to practice as a registered nurse (RN). This

Table 12.3 Types of Standards

Standards	Source of Authority
Educational	• Scientific knowledge/formal learning • Membership or certification requirements in professional organizations • Legislation and government regulations
Professional	• Scientific knowledge/formal learning • Professional expertise • Experience in the "art" of the profession • Legislation for self-governing professions
Ethical	• Moral principles
Organizational	• Governing board and officials of the employing organization • Leads to policies, procedures, culture
Information	• Professional expectations and legal requirements for clinical record-keeping and accounting • Structure and organization of the health system and corresponding management reporting requirements • Organizational policy in relation to clinical and management records • Database structure and data definitions for national, provincial, and regional reporting requirements
Legal	• Legislation and government regulations
Community	• Commonly held values and expectations of ordinary people

position is now being adopted in some Canadian provinces as other changes in legislation have broadened the scope of practice for licensed practical nurses (LPNs). Some decision makers have been persuaded that LPNs can substitute for RNs in many areas of health care or provide the same level of care at lower cost. Currently, despite a growing body of strong research evidence for the efficacy of advanced practice nursing roles, the introduction of legislation and policy to establish and fund these roles in the health system continues to meet ideological resistance (Burl, Bonner, Rao, & Khan, 1998; Chiarella, 2003; Hanucharurnkul et al., 2002; Hooke, Bennett, Dwyer, van Beek, & Martin, 2001; Larkin, 2003; Lindberg, Ahlner, Ekström, Jonsson, & Möller, 2002; MacLellan, Gardner, & Gardner, 2002; Olmsted & DeMint, 1997; Vincent & Mackey, 2000).

Credentialing and education standards for health service administrators have also been advocated and advanced through education programs and professional associations. Conferences on the education of health service administrators were funded by the Kellogg Foundation in 1974 in the US and in 1977 in Canada. A fundamental premise of these conferences was that health services administration is an "educational specialty" and that "the need for highly educated executives to provide leadership for the system becomes more evident every day" (Canadian College of Health Service Executives, 1978, p. 3). Subsequently, a number of major universities in Canada developed accredited graduate programs in this area. Professional associations of health administrators were formed with the objective of raising standards. The Canadian College of Health Service Executives (CCHSE) is one such organization, and like its US counterpart, it has established criteria for membership and continuing education requirements. The college conducts and sponsors various educational activities. Key among these is a certification program organized around a set of defined competencies in the areas of leadership, conceptual skills, communication, resource management, responsiveness to consumers and the community, and compliance to ethical and legal standards. Members of the college who pass the certification examination may use the designation Certified Health Executive (CHE). The college also sponsors and promotes continuing education activities in an attempt to ensure the continuing competence of all its members.

There is no legislated requirement that health service administrators in Canada be licensed or have particular credentials, so specific education requirements and membership in professional associations of health administrators are not mandatory. Although some health care administrators assume positions of leadership after being credentialed in a regulated health profession, others acquire their positions without exposure to the requirements and standards of licensed professionals and, sometimes, without any formal education or experience in the health system. Since health services administration is not a regulated profession, the only disciplinary penalty that can be enforced by CCHSE is withdrawal of membership in the association. This penalty is ineffectual since membership in the association is not a requirement to be employed as a senior executive in the Canadian health system.

Professional Standards

The sources of authority for professional standards are scientific knowledge, professional expertise arising from science and formal learning, and experience in the art of the profession. The knowledge base for professional practice continues to evolve rapidly, creating challenges for members of all health professions in maintaining standards of practice. To meet the expectation of public accountability, professional associations with licensing and regulatory responsibilities now generally include public representatives on their governing boards and disciplinary tribunals. They also publish information about members who have received significant disciplinary penalties, and they are required to implement mechanisms through which members must demonstrate continuing competence in order to remain licensed.

Competence is one key dimension of professional standards and embodies the idea that practitioners will have and maintain the knowledge necessary for competent practice. In the past, expectations of clinical competence were developed through a consensus of expert professional opinion as to what constituted acceptable or "best practice" in a particular area. Expert opinion as communicated through textbooks, peer-reviewed literature, and other forms of formal learning continues to be important in the development of standards. However, as described in Chapter 17 on evidence-based practice, RNs and other health professionals now seek to base their clinical practice on scientific evidence to the greatest extent possible. Confirmed research evidence can and should dictate changes in practice. For example, the treatment for stomach ulcers has changed after repeated studies confirmed that ulcers are caused by a bacterium and not, as was previously thought, by stress. Ideally, in clinical practice, a series of replicated randomized clinical trials or the equivalent must be conducted and provide unequivocal results before an evidence-based standard is established or changed. This ideal is not always achievable, particularly when interventions are complex (Whittemore & Grey, 2002; Morse, Penrod, & Hupcey, 2000; Rosswurm & Larrabee, 1999; Kelly, Gardner, Johnson, McCloskey, & Maas, 1994).

Most professional standards contain statements of expectation that professionals will be familiar with broadly accepted knowledge pertinent to their work. Professionals can find themselves in compromising positions when organizational policies are at odds with accepted professional knowledge. For example, organizational policies that require or permit the re-sterilization of supplies that were designed to be disposable may not be evidence-based, yet care providers may have no choice about whether to use the re-sterilized materials. Such situations are particularly problematic for employed professionals such as nurses. Some professional standards do acknowledge the influence of organizational variables on the ability of professionals to carry out their responsibilities. For example, the standards of the Alberta Association of Registered Nurses (AARN) contain an appendix that describes the organizational supports needed to support nursing practice. These include an appropriate number and mix of human resources, educational supports, quality improvement programs, and an environment conducive to the development of therapeutic relationships. Other organizational supports required to support professional nursing practice include appropriate systems for health records management and communicating information and resolving conflicts, appropriate facilities and equipment, appropriate nursing leadership, and opportunities for professional development (AARN, 1999, pp. 24–25). Professional standards also often include a requirement that individual professionals act as advocates for clients and for changes in the practice environment that may be needed to assure competent and appropriate care. The Standards of the CCHSA (discussed in more detail later in this chapter) now specify that health service organizations must have processes that "make it easy" for staff members to bring forward concerns they may have about clinical or other aspects of their work life. Unfortunately, when there is no legislated protection for whistle-blowers, employed professionals may become personally vulnerable when they attempt to act upon these professional requirements. This issue is discussed in greater detail in Chapter 13.

Behavioural expectations are a fundamental feature of most professional standards. Professionals are required to represent their credentials and knowledge truthfully and to identify areas in which their knowledge may not be sufficient for particular responsibilities. The behavioural expectations in professional standards provide the basis for professional disciplinary processes that limit the practice of individuals who are found to have engaged in criminal activities such as theft or fraud, who have problems of substance abuse, or who display violent or other seriously inappropriate behaviour.

Ethical Standards

The authority for ethical standards is derived from moral principles. The ethical standards of health professions affirm the obligation to provide competent, safe, and respectful care. However, ethical codes have traditionally had some differences in emphasis. For example, codes of ethics for physicians have traditionally placed a strong emphasis on loyalty and collegiality among physicians, whereas the nursing codes of the past emphasized obedience to authority. The influence of these historical values can still be seen in the cultures and relationships of these professional groups today.

The Canadian College of Health Service Executives (CCHSE) has also adopted standards of ethical conduct. These state that health executives are expected to serve as moral agents whose management decisions and actions must be assessed for their consequences on individuals, organizations, and communities and that health service executives must accept responsibility for the results of these decisions and actions. Furthermore, the standards affirm that health executives have responsibilities to their profession and that they must ensure their decisions are not compromised by conflict of interest (CCHSE, 1993). Health service administration is not a regulated profession, and membership in the CCHSE is not a prerequisite to employment as a health service administrator. Therefore, the CCHSE code of ethics has no regulatory authority, although it undoubtedly has educational and persuasive value.

In recent years, individuals whose experience is limited to industrial or business organizations, and who have no credentials in a health discipline or in health services administration, have sometimes been hired into CEO positions in health ministries or agencies. A prominent organizational theorist and researcher has directly challenged this practice, emphasizing the complexities of the health system and the expert knowledge needed to manage it (Mintzberg, 1997). Clinical professionals and first-line or middle managers must be prepared to explain to senior leaders educated in non-regulated disciplines the importance of professional standards in the workplace and the consequences of not being able to meet them.

Organizational Standards

The source of authority for organizational standards in a legally autonomous health care organization is the organization's governing board. The board is morally and legally accountable for the actions of all employees, medical staff, volunteers, and officials appointed or hired directly by the board. Organizational standards usually take the form of policies and procedures developed to guide predictable aspects of operations. They also provide guidance for complicated or high-risk situations, for example, what to do when emergency departments are overburdened and ambulances need to be diverted from one hospital to another. Some organizational standards are formally documented; others, such as the dress code for senior managers or the style for written communication in memoranda, are expressed less formally through the norms of the corporate culture.

Standards in health organizations have both administrative and clinical dimensions. Administrative policies and procedures range from staff recruitment and hiring practices to board policies regarding the investment of reserve funds. Most organizations conduct their operations through various committees, and the memberships and terms of reference for the main decision-making committees (whether written or unwritten) are also a matter of administrative policy. The graphic representation of organizational structure in the form of an organizational chart reflects administrative policy, illustrating how authority and responsibility are vested in various positions and to whom organizational officials are required to report.

There is sometimes conflict at the point where administrative and clinical policies intersect in health service organizations. Ideally, clinical policies and procedures are evidence-based and provide guidelines that encourage and enable clinical staff to use best practices in their work. Health professionals often feel that the administrative perspective does not adequately acknowledge the complexities and demands of clinical care. Professional associations may express concerns about certain types of organizational policies on behalf of their members who feel compromised in their ability to provide safe and accountable care. For example, many professional nursing associations have been critical of decisions to employ increasing numbers of multi-skilled, non-licensed or ancillary workers and to delegate tasks to them that were formerly the responsibility of licensed professionals or paraprofessionals. Such decisions have often been touted as a way of improving service through teamwork, but it is obvious that many have been implemented as cost containment measures. Although professional associations may express concern and disapproval of such organizational policies, they are unable to exert any direct influence because the governing board of an organization, and not the professional association, is the source of authority for organizational policy.

Nurses and other health professionals often experience a sense of conflict between the expectations of their employing organizations and the standards and ethical obligations of their professions. This problem has been exacerbated as traditional positions of leadership in clinical departments, such as vice president of nursing, director of rehabilitation medicine, and manager of social work, disappeared from most large health care organizations in the mid-1990s. Individuals in these positions were able to interpret and reconcile professional practice standards with the demands of the organization and inform administrative colleagues with non-clinical backgrounds of the facts, issues, risks, and benefits of various courses of action. Significantly, medical staff organizations tend to be constituted much as they always have been, and most major hospitals or health regions have continued to have a medical executive position at the level of vice-president. However, other professionally distinct departmental structures have been dissolved in many health agencies. In some cases, new positions of *professional practice leaders* have been introduced for nursing and other non-medical disciplines. As explained in Chapters 8 and 9, these positions tend not to have operational authority and are often positioned at the middle management level where there is limited opportunity to interpret and advocate for professional nursing standards or to provide professional advice as organizational standards are being developed.

Information Standards

The authority for health information standards is not the responsibility of any single agency or profession. Yet standards for health information are vitally important to the ability to assess clinical performance, health outcomes for individuals, and performance of health agencies and the health system. Valid and reliable information is necessary to manage risks and improve quality in the health system. Current performance must be compared to previous performance and analyzed in the context of historical trends. Comprehensive information about the health system is needed to support decision making by clinicians, managers, and policy makers. Over the past several decades, information technology has become more convenient to use and more universally available. Some settings, such as large acute care hospitals, have introduced a variety of management and clinical applications. Other settings, such as rural hospitals, stand-alone continuing care centres, and smaller community health programs, may have some standardized and automated processes. However, in general, it is still problematic to record, track, and aggregate the information needed for quality improvement and other purposes within and between various care settings and across provincial jurisdictions.

Information systems may yield three types of content: data, information, and knowledge. According to Blum (1986), *data* refers to discrete entities described objectively without interpretation. *Information* describes data that are interpreted, organized, and structured. *Knowledge* refers to information that has been synthesized so that the interrelationships are identified and formalized. It is obvious that data do not automatically become information or knowledge. Information management, including the processes of information systems planning, is required to structure data so that they become useable. Everyone who has a personal computer will appreciate how important it is to be able to structure data in ways that facilitate convenient and timely retrieval. The catch phrase "garbage in, garbage out" applies to large data sets and information systems as well as those used by individuals.

In making decisions about how to structure health information, the following factors need to be considered:

• What information is needed, when, by whom, and for what purposes?

• How can this information be best structured; in what format should it be collected and displayed; who should collect it; how often should it be updated?

• Who is the custodian of the information? That is, who has access to the information, and who is responsible for monitoring and maintaining the accuracy and integrity of the databases that will be created as information is collected?

• What information needs to be "online" for frequent and interactive use, and what information can be stored for periodic "batch" production and reporting?

• How will the information be retrieved, and by whom?

• How much will the system be relied on when it is functioning normally?

• What regular reports will be produced using the information? What will be required to produce extraordinary reports for special purposes?

The answers to these questions must be known before it is possible to determine whether a particular technical platform or software application will meet the needs for supporting clinical or organizational decision making. Unfortunately, in the acquisition and implementation of information systems, preoccupation with technology often obscures these fundamental issues.

Traditionally, clinical and management information systems have been distinct from one another in health service organizations. Structures for clinical information originated in the foundational disciplines of medicine and nursing as clinicians developed standard approaches for the content, sequence, and quality of their handwritten histories and notes. Accurate and complete records are required to manage care and communicate among disciplines. It is also important to be able to follow the pathways of individuals who receive care in more than one service setting. These needs have driven the development of large-scale initiatives to create and implement an electronic health record. This, in turn, will intensify the need for information standards that ensure privacy and confidentiality of individually identifiable health information.

Management information systems are designed to improve the accuracy and efficiency of statistical record keeping and reporting and to make this information widely available for management decision making, resource allocation, and outcome measurement at the organizational, regional, and system levels. These systems were the first to be automated as computers were initially introduced to health care organizations. Each individual clinical record is specific to one person. To improve managerial and organizational decision making and outcomes, it is necessary to be able to standardize and aggregate client-specific information into larger data sets. It is now recognized that the client-specific electronic health record is needed as the basis for all health information systems, to enable appropriate comparisons to be made between different clinical services, client populations, costs, and outcomes.

To be of value for clinical and management decision making, information must be reliable, valid, and comparable. This is achieved through the development and implementation of information standards and definitions. Once individual data elements have been identified as important, a standard data definition for each element must be agreed upon. Ideally, data definitions are mutually exclusive; that is, the meaning of each item is distinct from all others so that there is reliability in the initial recording or entry of information into the data set. Clinical professionals or managers who use information systems and the data generated from them may be unaware of these underlying structures until they realize that unfounded or incorrect comparisons are being made. The everyday expression "comparing apples with oranges" reflects the problem that arises when data elements and data definitions are not standardized and distinct.

Generally speaking, information systems are designed so that data elements can be added and definitions refined. Individual elements of data are aggregated and reported through the use of classifications or coding systems. Some of these have evolved from the traditions of professional disciplines or from previously separate sectors of the health system and can be difficult to change. Clinicians and managers can observe and critique the structure and standards of the health information being collected in their work settings as they use forms and records and read daily reports.

Nurse managers are often involved in the entry, use, retrieval, and disclosure of health information and in using and interpreting reports produced by various information systems. They are in a position to observe how health information is structured and protected and can contribute to the integrity of health information by knowing and correctly using protocols and data definitions. Nurse managers may also participate as implementers and agents of change as new approaches to the structuring of health information are introduced. In Canada, the Canadian Institute for Health Information (CIHI) plays a national leadership role in standardizing, structuring, and reporting health information. Readers can learn more about the CIHI by visiting their Web site, listed in the Internet Resources at the end of the chapter.

Community Standards

The sources of authority for community standards are the commonly held values and expectations of the community. John Raulston Saul (2001) has drawn attention to the importance of "common sense," defined more specifically in terms of two key elements: "shared knowledge and plain language." As our society becomes more pluralistic, it is sometimes difficult to know what the standards of the community are at any given time. The emergence of social consensus has led governments to enact legislation over the last few decades to protect the rights of workers, establish standards for occupational health and safety, protect civil and human rights, and prevent discrimination. Many community values remain implicit and unlegislated until a specific instance of extreme behaviour by an individual or organization calls forth a strong public response to the human tragedy, atrocity, or crime. Box 12.1 describes a case example in which community standards and common sense were expressed through the leadership of an ordinary citizen in an everyday situation.

Box 12.1

Community Standards in Action

What, Then, Must I Do?

We live in such an entertainment culture that it is sometimes startling when real life walks up and knocks on our forehead. So comfortable with being an audience, no one expects to be dragged onto the main stage as a live actor. Last month, a rare moment arrived when the curtain went up on a drama of sharp edges. It evolved before our eyes on a steamy August flight from the East. The plane was packed. As if on cue, the aircraft's air conditioning sputtered and quit. Humidity rose, patience fell as the captain chirped that we'd just have to get up to cruising altitude for things to cool down.

The plane was taxiing to the runway slowly. A few rows ahead, I could hear a young child crying. Then, during a pause in the white noise, the father's stern voice carried back, "Shut up kid!" This admonition was followed by several whacks from what must have been a rolled-up newspaper. Predictably, this brought more crying and whining from the child. The mother, who was holding an infant, tried to calm dad down, but he was not to be put off his tantrum. His biting language cut into the crying child and spilled over onto the baby. The cabin became deathly still. The abuse was obvious, and it was equally clear that this fellow was oblivious to the damage he was inflicting on his family.

"What, then, must I do?" That's what we were all thinking as we buried our doubts in the flight magazine. It's the keystone ethical question. All our faithful action depends on how we answer it.

My initial reaction was to hide behind Hollywood optimism. Maybe the troublesome man will just go away or offer a public apology. Could he be calmed by the in-flight movie? Where are the Promise Keepers when you need them?

Eventually the abusive father took himself to the washroom. Immediately, a woman who was sitting in front of the family turned to the young mother and explained how her husband was being very cruel. "You don't have to take this treatment. Don't let him speak like that to your children." When the man returned to his seat, the woman confronted him about his behaviour, telling him to get help and stop exacting the price of his anger from his children. The man smiled through his teeth and sulked in his seat.

I thought it was a noble attempt to name the injustice, and my heart applauded this woman's courage—a prophet in our midst. Having been alerted by the other passengers, the purser also came back and repeated a similar message.

Alas, these interventions didn't seem to alter the fellow's temper. When it flared again, at the small child, another passenger in front of the couple turned and quietly said, "Look, it's a hard flight for all of us. How about I take the youngster for a walk down the aisle?" No rebuke, no angry muttering, just an offer to help relieve the strain.

A saint was on that plane. This older gentleman (the best and noble label to give him) kept the child happy and laughing for three hours as he walked in the aisle with him, taking a pass or two through the first-class cabin to visit the flight deck. After the plane landed, the language began again. The gentleman quietly spoke to the father. "I guess we've all had a long night, haven't we? The little guy is doing his best." This seemed to cool down the hot flares in the father's eyes.

Thank you to the saint and the prophet. You've taught me again that it's not enough to have ethical thoughts—eventually they have to get out into the light of day, casting out the shadows that would otherwise overtake us.

–Chris Levan

"What, then, must I do?" by C. Levan, 1997, *The Edmonton Journal*, September 20. Reprinted with permission of the author.

Citizens can use their knowledge, experience, and their power as stakeholders to make demands on businesses and public sector organizations. They expect value for their money and increasingly demand that products or services are safe and dependable. Manufacturers can be held liable by the public for promoting and selling products that result in egregious consequences. For example, tobacco companies have been held legally liable for health problems and costs incurred by people who became addicted to smoking.

Public organizations and governments are not immune to the effects of evolving community standards. For example, the forced sterilization of people with mental and physical handicaps, once legal, is now abhorred. Growing expectations of accountability by public officials can be seen in widespread support for such initiatives as the prosecution of war criminals and investigations into the contamination of the blood supply in Canada. Public officials are increasingly held accountable for knowing what is available to be known, and acting responsibly with the best information at hand to make decisions that protect public safety.

Legal Standards

The authority for legal standards comes from legislation and regulation enacted by federal and provincial legislatures and from judicial or quasi-judicial tribunals. For example, health care providers were required through court decisions to change policies and practices for obtaining and ensuring informed consent. As explained in Chapter 11, numerous legal requirements must be met by individual professionals and health service organizations. These requirements, expressed in the form of criminal law, civil law, and government regulations, arise from the expectations and values of the community or from professional organizations (Feeny, Guyatt, & Tugwell, 1986; Rozovsky & Rozovsky, 1987). Not all community standards become law since legislative and legal processes are complex and time-consuming. Governments sometimes enact laws or regulations as a last resort in response to citizen demands and expectations.

Standards for Nursing Services and Nursing Administration

Nursing as a profession has a proud history of attending to issues of quality. Standards for nursing services and nursing administration are a subset of professional standards that are of particular interest to readers of this textbook on nursing leadership and management. The development and impact of these standards in the US and Canada are discussed in more detail below.

American Nurses' Credentialing Center and the Magnet Recognition Program

During a national nursing shortage in the 1980s, a group of nurse fellows from the American Academy of Nursing (AAN) established a task force to study what nurses found satisfying about their work and work environments in hospitals that appeared to have fewer problems recruiting or retaining professional nursing staff. These hospitals were termed magnet hospitals (McClure, Poulin, Sovie, & Wandelt, 1983; Havens & Aiken, 1999; Scott, Sochalski, & Aiken, 1999). It was expected that understanding the characteristics or conditions of the nursing work environments in these magnet hospitals would enable other hospitals to develop similar nursing workplace characteristics and become more successful in recruiting and retaining a professional nursing workforce.

The initial study carried out by the task force was a descriptive study of 41 magnet hospitals (McClure et al., 1983). Drawing upon the perceptions of directors of nursing and staff nurses, researchers identified several important characteristics that were present in all of the hospitals. For example, management style, nursing autonomy, quality of leadership, organizational structure, professional practice, career development, and quality of patient care and were believed to influence job satisfaction and low turnover rates among nurses within the magnet hospital setting (Havens & Aiken, 1999; McClure et al., 1983; Scott et al., 1999). Three broad categories of organizational characteristics were consistently identified in association with the ability to recruit and retain RNs. These broad categories were (a) leadership qualities of the nursing administration, (b) professional practice attributes of the staff nurses, and (c) an environment that supported professional development.

Nursing Administration

Interviews with the directors of nursing and staff nurses from each magnet hospital revealed that these hospitals were perceived to have highly visible, accessible, and responsive nursing leaders who practiced a form of participative management that was termed "management by walking around" (Havens & Aiken, 1999; McClure et al., 1983; Scott et al., 1999). In these hospitals, it was not uncommon for the CEO or chief nurse to make visits to the patient care areas. There was an administrative commitment to the free flow of communication between staff and management. The open lines of communication eliminated the need for excessive meetings which, in turn, enabled nursing administrators to spend time in the patient care areas and engage staff nurses in discussions of professional matters.

Nurse leaders in magnet hospitals were described as visionary, enthusiastic, and able to create an empowered environment for the RNs (Havens & Aiken, 1999; McClure et al., 1983; Scott et al., 1999). These leaders were described as knowledgeable and highly qualified within their respective clinical area and as possessing a patient-centred care philosophy. The existence of a clear philosophy, made explicit in the daily operations of the nursing department, resulted in high standards and high staff performance expectations.

The nursing leaders in magnet hospitals were perceived to hold positions of power and status within the organization. Nursing directors regularly attended board meetings and were involved on board committees. One perceived benefit of this was that nursing had a voice at the top decision-making level. Another was that the governing board was provided with insight into the value of nurses' contributions to patient care and thus to the overall reputation of the organization (McClure et al., 1983). In most of these magnet hospitals, senior nursing administrators had educational preparation at the graduate level, and several had earned doctorate degrees. Many of these nurse executives were also actively involved in state and national professional organizations.

Professional Nursing Practice

Another important characteristic of the magnet hospitals was a decentralized decision-making structure that provided specific nursing units and individual RNs with professional autonomy and control over their work environments (Havens & Aiken, 1999; McClure et al., 1983; Scott et al., 1999). Nurses were perceived to have had both clinical and organizational autonomy. Clinical autonomy meant that the nurses had control over decisions regarding patient care within their scope of practice and would be supported in their decision making by management. Organizational autonomy meant that clinical nurses had input into the decisions that affected their work unit and the organization. In the magnet hospitals, the perception of RN autonomy was frequently associated with job satisfaction and productivity (Kramer & Hafner, 1989; McClure et al., 1983).

Other factors perceived to enhance professional practice in magnet hospitals were the use of primary nursing as the nursing care delivery model and collaborative relationships between nurses and doctors. Positive patient outcomes (e.g., low mortality rates, high patient satisfaction) and positive nurse outcomes (e.g., low reported rates of needlestick injuries and emotional exhaustion) also characterized the magnet hospitals (Havens & Aiken, 1999; McClure et al., 1983; Scott et al., 1999; Aiken, Havens, & Sloane, 2000; Aiken & Sloane, 1997a; Aiken, Sloane, & Klocinski, 1997; Kramer & Schmalenberg, 1988a, 1988b).

Professional Development for Nurses

In the magnet hospitals there was evidence of a high emphasis on professional growth and development of the nursing workforce (McClure et al., 1983). The focus on education, both formal and informal, demonstrated the commitment to improving the quality of patient care and appeared to be extremely important to the nurses interviewed. A number of educational opportunities were available, including a structured orientation for new RNs, inservice and continuing education, and opportunities for formal education.

Career progression for RNs was facilitated in the magnet hospitals through formal mechanisms such as clinical laddering (Havens & Aiken, 1999; McClure et al., 1983; Scott et al., 1999). Study participants reported that clinical ladders were based on competency with specific requirements for each level. Opportunities for career advancement existed in either a clinical or management track and included planned continuing education leading to certification. Clinical ladders provided nurses with the opportunity to grow as individuals and as professionals through recognition and rewards in the form of salary and title changes (McClure et al., 1983).

The original magnet hospital study by McClure and colleagues was the result of intuitive ideas of the leaders of the AAN regarding the importance of nursing leadership and management in the context of the nursing shortage that existed in the US at that time. The original magnet hospital research was descriptive, and further studies were needed to confirm the generalizability of the original findings. A growing body of research now demonstrates the significance of magnet hospital characteristics and their relationship to patient outcomes, such as lower complication and mortality rates (Aiken, Clarke, & Sloane, 2000; Aiken et al., 2001; Aiken, Clarke, Sloane, Sochalski, & Silber, 2002; Aiken, Havens, & Sloane, 2000; Aiken & Sloane, 1997a, 1997b; Aiken, Sloane, & Klocinski, 1997; Aiken, Sloane, & Lake, 1997; Aiken, Sloane, Lake, Sochalski, & Weber, 1999; Aiken, Sloane, & Sochalski, 1998; Aiken, Smith, & Lake, 1994; Blegen, Goode, & Reed, 1998; Cummings, 2003; Needleman, Buerhaus, Mattke, Stewart, & Zelevinsky, 2002; Sochalski, 2001; Tourangeau, Giovannetti, Tu, & Wood, 2002).

In the US, the American Nurses Association (ANA) provided leadership in consolidating and communicating the findings of the magnet hospital research to the public and to policy and decision makers in the health system. The US has a national program for the accreditation of hospitals that operates under the auspices of the Joint Commission on Accreditation of Healthcare Organizations (JCAHO), which is similar to that operated by the Canadian Council on Health Services Accreditation (CCHSA) in Canada. Professionals and the public see accreditation status as an indicator of high-quality hospital care (Aiken, Havens, & Sloane, 2000). The ANA established its own national accreditation process for the assessment and accreditation of nursing services through the American Nurses' Credentialing Center (ANCC), which is a subsidiary of the ANA. The overall goal of the program is to identify excellence in the provision of nursing services and to recognize those institutions that act as a "magnets" by creating a work environment that recognizes and rewards professional nursing (ANA, 2003a). As the program evolved, the factors identified in the original magnet hospital study were combined with quality indicators from the standards of nursing practice as defined in the ANA's Scope and Standards for Nurse Administrators, thereby utilizing both quantitative and qualitative methodologies to evaluate nursing services and quality patient care.

Accreditation through the Magnet Nursing Services Recognition Program is a voluntary process. Hospitals applying for this recognition must demonstrate how they implement the Scope and Standards for Nurse Administrators within the organization's structure, leadership, and management philosophy, as well as how the standards are incorporated within the policies and procedures of nursing services. Accreditation through the program is valid for a four-year period, after which the organization must reapply.

The Magnet Nursing Services Recognition Program was expanded in 2000 in response to international interest (ANA, 2003b). The program was renamed the Magnet Recognition Program in 2002, and it has been adapted for universal application in other countries and in all types of health care settings ranging from acute and long-term care facilities to community services. The first pilot site outside the US was Rochdale Infirmary and Birch Hill Hospital of Rochdale, Lancashire, England. Rochdale successfully achieved magnet accreditation in March 2002.

The ANA has also been active in communicating the characteristics of an accredited nursing service to the public and to political leaders through publication of a nursing report card (ANA, 1997, 1999, 2000) and through political action. The Magnet Recognition Program provides a powerful example of how an initial descriptive study of 41 hospitals provided the impetus for development of a body of evidence with significant public policy impact.

Canadian Standards for Nursing Services and Administration

Canada was affected by the same nursing shortage that gave rise to the magnet hospital research in the 1980s. This shortage was of sufficient concern to prompt the release of a joint statement approved by five national organizations in October of 1986 (Canadian Nurses Association, 1986). These organizations were the Canadian Association of University Schools of Nursing, the Canadian College of Health Services Executives, the Canadian Hospital Association, the Canadian Nurses Association (CNA), and the Canadian Public Health Association. At that time, there was consensus among these associations that nursing administrators had an important impact on the delivery of health care in Canada through their contributions to health policy, their responsibilities for ensuring an appropriate nursing practice environment, and their ability to attract and retain nursing professionals. The joint statement emphasized the need for graduate-prepared nursing managers and continuing education opportunities as these would have a positive impact not only on nursing administration, but also on the health care system as a whole.

The organizations supported the development of a position paper on the role of the nurse administrator, and this, in turn, provided impetus to the development and publication of a document entitled *The Role of the Nurse Administrator and Standards for Nursing*

Administration (CNA, 1988). These standards were intended to address nursing administration in all settings, and they began with the premise that nursing administration is concerned with knowledge of systems, organizations, and groups as it relates to the environment, health, and nursing. The various levels of nursing administration are depicted conceptually on a continuum that distinguishes between the professional and corporate dimensions of nursing management. In the *professional dimension*, the nurse administrator demonstrates knowledge and expertise with respect to professional nursing, exerts leadership in relation to the discipline, and acts as an advisor on nursing matters. In the *corporate dimension*, the nurse executive participates in the organization's senior administrative team for the purpose of determining policies, priorities, allocation of resources, and general management issues. Highlights from the seven standards in this document are summarized in Table 12.4 and illustrate the influence of the magnet hospital research.

Recent findings from an international study on patient and nurse outcomes have reported reductions in front-line and middle management nursing positions and the elimination of executive-level nursing management positions in many hospitals (Aiken et al., 2001). Canadian statistics confirm this trend (Au, 2003). The position statements and nursing standards developed in response to the nursing shortage of the mid-1980s have been withdrawn from circulation and are no longer available except in library archives. Provincial nursing associations and

Table 12.4 Standards for Nursing Administration in Canada

Standard 1	Nursing administration plans for and implements effective and efficient delivery of nursing services.
Standard 2	Nursing administration participates in setting and achieving of organizational goals, priorities, and strategies.
Standard 3	Nursing administration provides for allocation, optimum use, and evaluation of resources such that the standards of nursing practice can be met.
Standard 4	Nursing administration maintains information systems appropriate for planning, budgeting, implementing, and monitoring the quality of nursing services.
Standard 5	Nursing administration promotes the advancement of nursing knowledge and the utilization of nursing findings.
Standard 6	Nursing administration provides leadership that is visible and proactive.
Standard 7	Nursing administration evaluates the effectiveness and efficiency of nursing services.

Source: *The Role of the Nurse Administrator and Standards for Nursing Administration* (p. 10), by Canadian Nurses Association, 1988, Ottawa, ON: CNA.

the Canadian Nurses Association did not adopt the accreditation approach or the nursing report card concept that were implemented by the ANA in the US, and which have now been extended to other sectors and settings of care. In not doing so, they missed an opportunity to inform the Canadian public about the relationship between magnet characteristics and health outcomes and about the ability of health care organizations to recruit and retain RNs. As this book goes to press, there is still no equivalent in Canada to the ANA's American Nurses' Credentialing Center or the Magnet Recognition Program. Decreases in the number of nursing leaders in Canada may help to account for this situation, which deserves thoughtful consideration by all RNs and professional nursing associations. The number of nurses who reported being employed in senior leadership positions fell from a total of 4,116 positions in 1992 to 1,754 positions in 2002 (CIHI, n.d.). When all levels of nursing management positions are combined, there has been a decrease from 25,458 positions to 16,681 positions in this 10-year period.

As Buchan (1999) observed, the magnet concepts have a universal relevance and applicability. This has been recognized by Canadian policy analysts from outside the nursing profession who have commented on the matter (Canadian Health Services Research Foundation, 2004; Rachlis, 2004). In this context, the development of The Quality Practice Settings Attribute Model by the College of Nurses of Ontario (Mackay & Risk, 2001) represents an important step forward by professional nursing associations in Canada.

The importance of the magnet hospital research and subsequent studies is also acknowledged in the many citations and references to this work in the policy documents of provincial nursing associations, the CNA, the federal Office of Nursing Policy, and in several broadly based policy consultations and task force reports that have predicted or sought to address the shortage of RNs. In response to national attention to the issue of the quality of nurses' work life, organizational attributes of health care institutions have recently been incorporated into the accreditation program of the Canadian Council on Health Services Accreditation, where they appear as standards that are equally applicable to all disciplines and employees. Between 1999 and 2001, the CCHSA introduced a new dimension in the accreditation process to assess quality of work life in health care environments (CCHSA, 2000). More recently, the CNA approved eight quality of work life indicators for nurses in Canada and has recommended that these indicators be incorporated into the 2004 AIM Standards of the CCHSA (CNA, 2003).

Measuring and Certifying the Quality of Health Services in Canada

The traditional approach to the development of standards and accreditation processes for the health care industry in Canada has its roots in the culture of the health professions and the broad area of professional standards. Two approaches to the development and measurement of standards are now described and compared. The first is the program of the CCHSA. The second is the program of the Canadian Standards Association (CSA) and the International Organization for Standardization (ISO).

The Canadian Council on Health Services Accreditation

Efforts to develop standards for Canadian hospitals began in 1917 in association with American organizations. In 1952, the CCHSA was formed to create an independent, non-profit, non-governmental Canadian program for hospital accreditation. The founding board of the new organization included the Canadian Hospital Association, the Canadian Medical Association, and the College of Physicians and Surgeons of Canada. The Canadian Long-Term Care Association joined the board in 1980 and the Canadian Nurses Association, in 1981. Since that time, the board has expanded to include other organizations and representatives of consumer and customer organizations. The scope and process of accreditation has been broadened to include all sectors of the health system. The CCHSA receives operating revenue from annual fees paid by health service organizations that voluntarily seek accreditation status. Individual health organizations or health regions can be accredited. CCHSA reported that in 2002, 327 accreditation surveys were conducted in 992 different sites in the provinces and territories of Canada (CCHSA, 2003).

The CCHSA standards that are in effect as this book goes to press are entitled Achieving Improved Measurement, or AIM (CCHSA, 2002). They were developed by university researchers based on current evidence and best practices and with the consensus of health professionals brought together in working groups across Canada. Since the accreditation and survey is a peer-review process, only individuals who are currently senior managers in health service organizations are considered eligible to be surveyors. They must go through a formal application process and, if selected, participate in an extensive orientation program. They signify their compliance to a Code of Ethics for surveyors by personal signature. In 2002, there were 377 surveyors representing the disciplines of administrator (37%), chiropractor (0.2%), lab scientist (0.8%), medical doctor (19%), occupational therapist (0.8%), physical therapist (0.8%), psychologist (0.8%), registered nurse (37%), respiratory therapist (1.8%), and social worker (1.8%) (CCHSA, 2003).

As accreditation surveys are conducted, two kinds of information are considered. In the self-assessment phase, teams of organizational representatives rate their own organization on each applicable standard and related criteria. This phase is followed by a peer-review phase in which an interdisciplinary team of surveyors make site visits to the organization and conduct team interviews and focus groups with representatives from the board, senior management, support departments, and clinical staff. Surveyors visit clinical areas, examine patient records, and interview patients at each site. In addition, they conduct separate focus groups with users of the health system, community members, and staff. Members of the survey team record and compare their individual ratings to reach consensus on the results that will be communicated to the organization.

There are several possible levels of outcome of the accreditation process. Full accreditation was achieved by 154 (47.1%) of the health organizations surveyed in 2002. Non-accreditation is a possible outcome, but this is rare; only three organizations (0.9%) of those surveyed in 2002 received this rating. Between full and non-accreditation, there are several levels of conditional accreditation. CCHSA reported that 170 (52%) of all organizations surveyed in 2002 received the status of "Accreditation with Condition." CCHSA has reported on the areas of its standards that are most frequently associated with conditional accreditation (CCHSA, 2003). To obtain full accreditation, organizations in these conditional categories are advised to do the following:

1. Implement organization-wide quality improvement plan and processes.

2. Complete and test all aspects of disaster/emergency plans.

3. Provide a safe environment (e.g., safe storage, security, infection control, regularly tested equipment, space utilization).

4. Improve patient/client charting (e.g., chart completion, integrated charting, access, security).

5. Ensure availability of appropriate staff training and/or orientation.

6. Develop board/governance accountability and improve strategic planning.

7. Conduct evacuation exercises and practice fire prevention.

8. Improve care processes (e.g., consents, needs assessments, care plans, integrated planning).

9. Improve medication system.

10. Implement organization-wide risk management.

Once the results of an accreditation survey are reported by CCHSA to a region or organization, the responsibility for informing the public of the results rests with the board of the organization being accredited. When an organization or region achieves full accreditation status, this is usually communicated to the public by display of the accreditation certificate in a prominent place. Some regions have set a new benchmark for transparency by reporting the recommendations of an accreditation survey on their regional Web site for public viewing. However, organizations or regions that have not achieved full accreditation status may not be identifiable to the public, and citizens would not be able to readily obtain information about the areas of deficiency cited in the report of a CCHSA survey.

The Canadian Standards Association and the International Organization for Standardization

The Canadian Standards Association (CSA) is a member-based organization governed by a multidisciplinary board of directors. The majority of directors are elected by the voting membership. There are over 9,000 members from all walks of life, including 7,500 volunteer committee members and 1,500 sustaining and corporate sustaining members. Over 290 consumer volunteers are involved through standards development committees or through surveys, forums, and other outreach activities.

The process for standards development is intentionally designed to balance the vested interests of various stakeholders in order to achieve integrity and technical credibility. Anyone can come forward and request a standard. The process for selection and prioritization of standards development is inclusive of individual stakeholders, including users, health care providers, consumers, manufacturers, and other groups. Standards are developed using a balanced matrix approach in which individual stakeholders, committees of technical experts, and governments and regulatory authorities participate by considering information from publications, data bases, and other sources. The balanced matrix approach is structured to capitalize on the combined strengths and expertise of participants, with no single group dominating the process. There are several consultations with stakeholders during the process of standards development, including a formal enquiry stage in which the draft standard is offered for public review and comment for a period of 60 days (CSA, 2003).

While developing national standards, the CSA follows the policy of harmonizing these standards with North American and international requirements. This harmonization may be stipulated if required by regional or international standards development agreements. It may be advantageous to harmonize standards in response to prevailing business or consumer conditions. The CSA is a member of the International Organization for Standardization (ISO). Certification to CSA or ISO standards is a mark of recognition that is nationally and internationally appreciated. The ISO now has a single standard that specifies the requirements of a quality management system (American Society for Quality, 2001). Audits and reviews are regularly conducted in order to achieve and maintain a particular certification or registration. The Misericordia Hospital (part of the Caritas Health Group in Edmonton, Alberta) was the first Canadian health organization to achieve ISO certification for one of its programs—the Cranial, Osseointegration and Maxillofacial Prosthetic Rehabilitation Unit (COMPRU). This program is described in Box 12.2.

Comparison of Approaches and Emerging Issues

As can be seen from the discussion above, there are some interesting differences in these organizations and their approaches to developing standards and assuring safety and quality. Whereas the CCHSA began and has continued as an organization of health care providers and administrators, the CSA is a member-driven organization that includes individual members as well as health care providers and administrators among its categories of membership. The approach to developing, assessing, and reporting compliance to standards reflects these basic differences.

The standards developed by both organizations result from a consensus development process that includes consideration of factual and scientific information as well as expert professional opinion. Although representatives of consumer organizations and the public have been added to the board of the CCHSA in recent years, there is limited provision for public participation in the development of the CCHSA standards. In contrast, CSA standards (even those of a highly technical nature) are developed through a transparent process in which many members of the public actively participate along with technical and professional experts. The need to assure "neutrality" in the standards development process and to separate the processes of assessment and certification from other processes are goals that are formally recognized in the structure of CSA and ISO certification and registration regimens.

Whereas CCHSA assessment focuses on self-report and focus groups of selected individuals, the CSA and ISO particularly emphasize the external audit of processes and the independence of the assessment or auditing function. This means that the documentation of standard operating procedures (SOPs) is reviewed and the processes themselves directly and independently observed. Processes for identifying and correcting mistakes are among those scrutinized in this way. The linkage between results and quality improvement efforts is also a distinguishing feature of the CSA and ISO approach. Increasingly, this approach to quality is required for business purposes in a global economy. If and when Canadian consumers begin to pay more out of

Box 12.2

ISO 9000 Certification of a Canadian Hospital Program

The COMPRU Program

In 1998, the Cranial, Osseointegration and Maxillofacial Prosthetic Rehabilitation Unit (COMPRU) at the Misericordia Hospital in Edmonton was awarded the first publicly funded health care program in Canada to receive ISO 9000 registration. Preparation for the ISO 9000 assessment was carried out under the umbrella of the overall total quality improvement program within the corporate organization of the Caritas Health Group, of which the Misericordia Hospital is a member.

The business leader responsible for the COMPRU program explained that extensive staff education was required to prepare for the rigourous assessment and to achieve the "buy in" necessary for the team to commit to the process and be successful. The certification process gave the staff pride in the quality of its program.

Practices in the program are consistent; when practice does not conform to the established standard operating procedures, the reasons why are documented to provide a basis for continuous improvement. Records are current, and each member of the team is familiar with the responsibilities of other team members. These requirements facilitate continuity of service, enhance the satisfaction of patient and care providers, and support achievement of the clinical outcomes of the program.

The reference materials available to the staff (and for examination by ISO auditors) include standards and expectations related to the unit's operations. One section, for example, outlines the roles, responsibilities, and training requirements of all personnel in the program (structure), while another describes how staff will behave in relation to patients and to each other (process).

The process standards empower individuals at all levels and in all roles of the COMPRU program to accept personal and professional accountability for acting when they believe something has gone wrong or may be about to go wrong. If the actions of the person who identified the problem are not able to prevent or correct it, that person is expected to take it to a higher authority. These process standards, reinforced by the structural standards that describe accountability and responsibility, support the identification and correction of problems in care that could lead to unsuccessful outcomes for patients. In fact, the standards for the program specify the desired patient outcomes and are "service-oriented" towards patient satisfaction.

Although quality, rather than risk management, is emphasized in the ISO 9000 standards system, the example of the COMPRU program illustrates how risks can be mitigated through compliance to structure, process, and outcome standards. When supported by the corporate culture, the involvement of individuals at all levels of the program, and the appropriate training, standards that are in compliance with ISO 9000 can help to increase patient and caregiver satisfaction and improve treatment outcomes.

pocket for health services, or become more aware of safety issues in the health system, there will be pressure from the public and from international customers to reach this level of quality assurance in the Canadian health system.

In general, it can be seen that the standards development process of the CSA has the broadest public input, involving and directly communicating with many individual members who are consumers and with their target market audience—the organizations wishing to achieve certification. In contrast, the CCHSA is focused entirely on health services. Since fees for its accreditation services and products are the major source of corporate revenue, this organization has the challenge of making the accreditation standards, process, and results reporting acceptable to its customers, that is, the organizations being evaluated. This is less of a problem for the CSA and the ISO because their funding and revenues come from more diverse sources; therefore, the neutrality of the processes of developing, measuring, and reporting standards is of paramount importance to all the participants. This explains why so many CSA and ISO standards have become part of regulations and legislation. In some provinces, public hospital acts recognize CCHSA standards.

Transparency in the processes of standards development and reporting of assessment outcomes is a key feature of the CSA and ISO approaches. The CCHSA has published a National Health Accreditation Report in which the accreditation standards and process are described in broad terms, and aggregate information about the number and types of accreditation surveys is summarized. However, information about the accreditation status or areas of deficiency of individual health organizations and regions is not readily available to the public. This is significant because 52% of the organizations surveyed in 2002 received a conditional accreditation and were deficient in one or more important areas. To make an informed decision about whether to obtain care in these health organizations or regions, and ultimately in the electoral process, citizens need easy access to specific information about the accreditation status, areas of deficiency, and corrective measures being taken by the health regions or organizations in their communities and provinces.

There has been growing concern about issues of patient safety in the health systems of Western countries, particularly since the publication of the Institute of Medicine's report *To Err is Human* (Kohn, Corrigan, & Donaldson, 1999), which estimated that between 44,000 and 98,000 patients die each year in the US due to medical errors. Despite high participation in the CCHSA accreditation process, this concern has now been recognized in Canada. Information about the rate of adverse events in health care in Canada has been limited. One study on a general surgery service found that 39% (75 of 192) of patients suffered complications. Of these, 18% (26 of 144) were attributable to human error (National Steering Committee on Patient Safety, 2002; Wanzel, Jamieson, & Bohnen, 2000). A different study by Forster and colleagues (2004) reported that 76 of the 328 patients discharged from a general internal medicine unit experienced at least one adverse event, and in half of the patients (38 of 76), the adverse events were either preventable or ameliorable. Most recently, results of the first Canadian study to determine the types and frequency of adverse events that occur in Canadian hospitals were published in May 2004. The overall adverse event rate in Canadian hospitals was found to be 7.5%, which translates to approximately 185,000 of the almost 2.5 million adult hospital admissions in Canada per year (Baker et al, 2004). Almost 37% of the adverse events were potentially preventable. These results are expected to provide a baseline reference against which to measure subsequent efforts to improve patient safety. As the researchers were developing the adverse events study, a National Steering Committee on Patient Safety was initiated with support from Health Canada, provincial/territorial ministries of health, and 26 Canadian health care organizations. The committee reported in September 2002, recommending that a new Canadian Patient Safety Institute be established. This recommendation was promptly acted upon by the federal government and the new institute, to be located in Edmonton, Alberta, was announced in December 2003.

Patient safety has now become a prominent public policy concern. Growing public awareness and broader concerns about organizational and political accountability will create pressures for increased transparency in the development of standards and the independent assessment and public reporting of safety and quality in the Canadian health system. There is evidence that health care organizations and senior leaders are becoming more aware of their personal and organizational accountability in this area.

Leadership Implications

Members of the public expect that health professionals will know and practice the standards of their disciplines and that health services will conform to community and legal standards. There can be serious individual consequences for members of regulated professions who breach professional standards. Some executive level leaders in the health system are members of regulated professions, and some have voluntarily met requirements for membership and certification with the Canadian College of Health Service Executives. However, nursing managers cannot assume that all senior managers understand the knowledge or support the values that are the basis for professional standards in nursing or other health disciplines.

Organizational standards, expressed through policies, procedures, the structure of the organization and its information systems, can sometimes be at odds with professional and community standards. In fact, one key role of nursing managers is to present and interpret the standards of the nursing discipline within their workplaces and to advocate for changes that enable RNs to practice in accordance with professional requirements and community expectations. A growing body of research evidence links magnet hospital characteristics (and the ability to recruit and retain a workforce of RNs) with lower complication and death rates for patients (CHSRF, 2004; Rachlis, 2004). Professional nursing associations and individual nurses who hold leadership positions have a responsibility to bring this evidence to the attention of organizational decision makers and policy makers and apply it in their operational decision making.

Legal standards are an ultimate expression of community standards and apply to all individuals and organizations. Whereas quality improvement objectives are oriented to the achievement of excellence or best practices, risk management is undertaken to reduce organizational liability for errors. When decisions and practices in professions and health service organizations fall behind community standards, it is predictable that there will be public pressure to strengthen regulatory requirements and protect whistle-blowers. An example of this can be seen in the nursing home and home care sectors of the US health system, where an elaborate regulatory framework has been instituted in response to public outrage about safety issues and poor business practices of organizations that receive public funds to serve vulnerable populations.

Nursing leaders need to be familiar with the broadly based standards of the Canadian Council on Health Services Accreditation and will have opportunities through their management practice to participate in this voluntary accreditation process. In the context of a global economy, and as consumers are faced with the prospect of paying out-of-pocket money for health and human services, there will be pressure on Canadian health service organizations to meet other national and international standards that incorporate consumer expectations for quality of service. Safety and quality must be evident in all aspects and at all levels of health service organizations. Achieving quality requires high levels of professional and organizational commitment and investments in infrastructure. The report of the National Steering Committee on Patient Safety has underscored the need for a "culture of safety" in health care organizations. It is the responsibility of senior leaders to create and exemplify this culture. One key element of this culture is the prompt and truthful disclosure of errors and adverse effects to those affected by them. As a result of several court decisions, this is now a legal requirement in Canada.

Many different approaches to quality improvement in health care have been advocated. Other objectives such as cost reductions have sometimes been bundled with quality improvement initiatives, and this has made it problematic to assess the relative value of the various approaches, some of which have been called "fads and fashions" by management scholars (Abrahamson, 1996, 1991). The concept and value of continuous quality improvement are widely accepted and many health organizations are implementing this through use of a balanced scorecard approach. This approach, which combines risk management and quality improvement, is discussed in more depth in the following chapter on accountability.

The nursing profession was at the forefront of historical developments in quality assurance and improvement. The high level of trust that members of the public place in RNs requires particular attentiveness by nursing leaders to patient- or person-centred issues that relate to standards and quality of health services.

Summary

- Standards are needed to provide benchmarks against which to measure the quality of service provided by individual professionals and the quality and cost-effectiveness of services provided in health agencies.

- A foundational framework developed by Donabedian identified the dimensions of structure, process, and outcome as areas in which information for quality assessment is needed.

- Standards originate and derive their authority from a variety of sources. An understanding of the sources of authority is needed to understand how, or if, certain standards can be enforced in a particular instance or setting.

- *Educational standards* derive their authority from scientific knowledge, formal learning, and, in some cases, from legislation and government regulation.

- *Professional standards* derive their authority from scientific knowledge, formal learning, professional expertise and legislation for self-governing professions.

- *Ethics standards* derive their authority from moral principles. When incorporated into the standards for self-governing professions, ethics standards carry the authority of professional regulation, and individuals breaching these standards can be subject to disciplinary penalties, including withdrawal of the licence to practice.

- Health service administration is not a self-governing profession, and senior health service executives are not required to have specific credentials in Canada. Therefore, the educational and ethical standards of the Canadian College of Health Service Executives (CCHSE) have persuasive, rather than regulatory, authority.

- *Organizational standards* are established under the authority of governing boards and officials of health agencies, giving rise to organizational policies, procedures, structure, and culture.

- *Standards for health information* have no single source of authority. Standardized information is needed to assess and improve the quality of health care and the organizational performance of health agencies and to compare agencies and their outcomes with one another. The Canadian Institute for Health Information (CIHI) has a national leadership role in standardizing, structuring, and reporting health information.

- *Legal standards* derive authority from legislation and regulation at various levels of government.

- *Community standards* are the commonly held values and expectations of ordinary citizens that result in social consensus on particular issues. The emergence of strong social consensus on particular issues has influenced governments to introduce legislation in a number of important areas of relevance to the health system.

- In Canada, the Canadian Council on Health Services Accreditation (CCHSA) has played a leadership role in developing standards for health services. Standards are developed through a consensual interdisciplinary process and with consideration of scientific evidence and expert professional opinion. There has been limited citizen engagement in the CCHSA process of standards development, and citizens do not have access to detailed reports of accreditation surveys for the health agencies in their communities.

- The Canadian Standards Association (CSA) and the International Organization for Standardization (ISO) have developed processes for the development and review of standards that provide for citizen engagement. Compliance with CSA and ISO standards is assessed through an independent external audit of standard operating procedures and processes. This approach is now increasingly required in business and industry and can be expected to influence developments in the health system as citizens' demands for greater inclusiveness, transparency, quality, and accountability in health services continue to be expressed.

- *Standards for nursing services administration* are a matter of particular interest to readers of this book. They are a specialized type of professional standards supported by evidence from the magnet hospital research and many subsequent studies.

- Magnet hospitals were originally defined through descriptive research in the early 1980s. Since that time, a substantial body of research has linked magnet characteristics to patient outcomes such as lower complication and death rates, and to a variety of nurse outcomes such as less burnout and improved retention.

- In the United States, the American Nurses Association (ANA) established its own national accreditation process based on the Magnet Nursing Services Recognition Program. Hospitals voluntarily apply for recognition under this program and, to receive accreditation, must demonstrate how they implement ANA magnet standards for nurse administrators and nursing workplaces within their organizational environments.

- In Canada, a joint position statement confirming the importance of nursing administration to health and nursing outcomes was developed and published in 1986. This precipitated the development of a document entitled *The Role of the Nurse Administrator and Standards for Nursing Administration*, which was published by the Canadian Nurses Association (CNA) in 1988.

- Between 1992 and 2002, the number of nursing administrators in Canada fell as organizational downsizing and restructuring took place. Management initiatives to implement total quality management and continuous quality improvement programs were often introduced in parallel with downsizing and layoffs that affected clinical nurses and nursing administrators, particularly those at senior levels. During this period, the CNA Standards for Nursing Administration were withdrawn from publication.

- The CNA has advocated for the inclusion of indicators to assess the quality of nursing work life in the standards of the CCHSA and in the information structures of the CIHI.

- The Ontario College of Nurses has developed a Workplace Attributes Model, but there is no Canadian equivalent to the ANA's Magnet Nursing Services Recognition Program.

- At the beginning of the 21st century, issues of safety and quality of health services have become high priority public policy issues, and there is now an explicit expectation that senior health executives will provide leadership for the development of a culture of safety to address the root causes of adverse occurrences in their organizations.

Applying the Knowledge in this Chapter

Exercise

1. Visit the Web site of CCHSA (see Internet Resources). Examine the information about how to become a surveyor and the application form and process. Do you know anyone who is, or has been, a surveyor? Would you be eligible to be a surveyor? If you think so, complete and send in the application form.

2. Visit the Web sites of the CCHSA, CSA, and ISO. As a member of the public, can you see how these organizations represent your interests? Can you see how you can have an influence on standards development?

3. Find out the following information about the CCHSA accreditation status of health services in your vicinity.
   - Are the services accredited by CCHSA?
   - When was the last accreditation survey done?
   - If the organization or some services were not fully accredited, is there information available to the public about the areas of deficiency and what is being done to address them?
   - If not readily available to the public, how could this information be obtained?

4. Find out whether any health services in your organization or region have been certified by CSA or registered with ISO.
   - Which services were they?
   - How are members of the public informed about the CSA or ISO certification?
   - Since these types of accreditation are not obligatory, find out who lead the initiative to achieve these certifications and obtain information about their positions and professional training.

Resources

evolve Internet Resources

Alberta Association for Registered Nurses:
www.nurses.ab.ca

Nursing Practice Standards:
www.nurses.ab.ca/pdf/NursingPracticeStandards.pdf

American Nurses Credentialing Center:
http://nursingworld.org/ancc/index.html

The Magnet Recognition Program:
http://nursingworld.org/ancc/magnet.html

Canadian College of Health Service Executives (CCHSE):
www.cchse.org/

Canadian Council on Health Services Accreditation (CCHSA):
www.cchsa.ca/

Canadian Institute for Health Information (CIHI):
http://secure.cihi.ca/cihiweb/splash.html

Canadian Nurses Association (CNA):
www.cna-nurses.ca/_frames/welcome/frameindex.html

Code of Ethics for Registered Nurses:
www.cna-nurses.ca/pages/ethics/ethicsframe.htm

Standards from Registered Nursing Associations across Canada:
www.cna-nurses.ca/pages/whats_new/standards/standards.htm
Nursing Education:
www.cna-nurses.ca/pages/education/educationframe.htm
Canadian Standards Association (CSA):
www.csa.ca/
College of Nurses of Ontario (CNO):
www.cno.org/
Hartford Health: Mission and Vision for Continuous Quality Improvement:
www.co.ha.md.us/health/cqi.htm
International Organization for Standardization (ISO):
www.iso.ch/iso/en/ISOOnline.openerpage
Quality Digest: Performance Measurement in Health Care:
www.qualitydigest.com/may99/html/body_health.html
Workplace Attributes Model:
www.cno.org/qa/pscp/ismywork.html

The Workplace Attributes Model developed by the Ontario College of Nurses represents an important Canadian milestone in the dissemination of publicly accessible information about evidence-based standards for nursing services and nursing service administration. The seven attributes of a quality practice setting (based on the *Quality Practice Settings Attributes Model*™) are outlined in an online article by E. Doucette, "Is my workplace a quality practice setting?" Readers are encouraged to review the published article and monitor ongoing developments in its use.

References

Abrahamson, E. (1991). Managerial fads and fashion: The diffusion and rejection of innovations. *Academy of Management Review, 16,* 586–612.

Abrahamson, E. (1996). Management fashion. *Academy of Management Review, 21*(1), 254–285.

Aiken, L.H., Clarke, S.P., & Sloane, D.M. (2000). Hospital restructuring: Does it adversely affect care and outcomes? *Journal of Nursing Administration, 30*(10), 457–465.

Aiken, L.H., Clarke, S.P., Sloane, D.M., Sochalski, J., Busse, R., Clarke, H., et al. (2001). Nurses' reports on hospital care in five countries. *Health Affairs, 20*(3), 43–53.

Aiken, L.H., Clarke, S.P., Sloane, D.M., Sochalski, J., & Silber, J.H. (2002). Hospital nurse staffing and patient mortality, nurse burnout, and job dissatisfaction. *Journal of the American Medical Association, 288*(16), 1987–1993.

Aiken, L.H., Havens, D.S., & Sloane, D.M. (2000). The magnet nursing services recognition program: A comparison of two groups of magnet hospitals. *American Journal of Nursing, 100*(3), 26–35.

Aiken, L.H., & Sloane, D.M. (1997a). Effects of organizational innovations in AIDS care on burnout among hospital nurses. *Work and Occupations, 24*(4), 453–477.

Aiken, L.H., & Sloane, D.M. (1997b). Effects of specialization and client differentiation on the status of nurses: The case of AIDS. *Journal of Health and Social Behavior, 38*(3), 203–222.

Aiken, L.H., Sloane, D.M., & Klocinski, J.L. (1997). Hospital nurses' risk of occupational exposure to blood: Prospective, retrospective, and institutional reports. *American Journal of Public Health, 87*(1), 103–107.

Aiken, L.H., Sloane, D.M., & Lake, E.T. (1997). Satisfaction with inpatient acquired immunodeficiency syndrome care: A national comparison of dedicated and scattered-bed units. *Medical Care, 35*(9), 948–962.

Aiken, L.H., Sloane, D.M., Lake, E.T., Sochalski, J., & Weber, A.L. (1999). Organization and outcomes of inpatient AIDS care. *Medical Care, 37*(8), 760–772.

Aiken, L.H., Sloane, D.M., & Sochalski, J. (1998). Hospital organization and outcomes. *Quality in Health Care, 7*(4), 222–226.

Aiken, L.H., Smith, H.L., & Lake, E.T. (1994). Lower Medicare mortality among a set of hospitals known for good nursing care. *Medical Care, 32*(8), 771–787.

Alberta Association of Registered Nurses. (1999). *Nursing practice standards.* Edmonton, AB: Author.

American Nurses Association. (1997). *Implementing nursing's report card: A survey of RN staffing, length of stay and patient outcomes.* Washington, DC: American Nurses Publishing.

American Nurses Association. (1999). *Nursing sensitive quality indicators for acute care settings and ANA's safety & quality initiative.* Retrieved June 15, 2004, from http://www.nursingworld.org/readroom/fssafe99.htm

American Nurses Association. (2000). *Nurse staffing and patient outcomes in the inpatient hospital setting.* Retrieved June 15, 2004, from http://www.nursingworld.org/pressrel/2000/st0504.htm

American Nurses Association. (2003a, November). *American Nurses Credentialing Center, magnet recognition program.* Retrieved June 11, 2004, from http://www.nursingworld.org/ancc/magnet.html

American Nurses Association. (2003b, November). *Credentialing international.* Retrieved June 15, 2004, from http://www.nursingworld.org/ancc/inside/about/aboutCI.html

American Society for Quality. (2001). *IWA 1: Quality management systems: Guidelines for process improvements in health service organizations.* Milwaukee, WI: ASQ Quality Press.

Au, A. (2003). *Roles and responsibilities of directors of nursing in continuing care in Alberta and Canada.* Unpublished report of Nursing 900 Project presented to complete requirements for the MN degree, Faculty of Nursing, University of Alberta, Edmonton, Alberta, Canada.

Baker, G.R., Norton, P.G., Flintoft, V., Blais, R., Adalsteinn, B., Cox, J., et al. (2004). The Canadian adverse events study: The incidence of adverse events among hospital patients in Canada. *Canadian Medical Association Journal, 170*(11), 1678–1686.

Baker, G.R., & Pink, G.H. (1995). A balanced scorecard for Canadian hospitals *Healthcare Management Forum, 8*(4), xxx–xxx.

Blegen, M.A., Goode, C.J., & Reed, L. (1998). Nurse staffing and patient outcomes. *Nursing Research, 47*(1), 43–50.

Blum, B.I. (1986). *Clinical information systems.* New York: Springer-Verlag.

Buchan, J. (1999). Still attractive after all these years? Magnet hospitals in a changing health care environment. *Journal of Advanced Nursing, 30*(1), 100–108.

Burl, J.B., Bonner, A., Rao, M., & Khan, A.M. (1998). Geriatric nurse practitioners in long-term care: Demonstration of effectiveness in managed care. *Journal of the American Geriatrics Society, 46*(4), 506–510.

Canadian College of Health Service Executives (CCHSE). (1978). *Unmet needs: Education for health services administration in Canada.* Ottawa, ON: CCHSE.

Canadian College of Health Service Executives. (1993). *Standards of ethical conduct for health service executives.* [Mimeograph]. Ottawa, ON: CCHSE.

Canadian Council on Health Services Accreditation (CCHSA). (2000, November). *A summary of the findings of the 1999 CCHSA accreditation surveys.* Retrieved January 20, 2004, from http://www.cchsa.ca/riskreport/summary.html

Canadian Council on Health Services Accreditation. (2002). *AIM standards.* Retrieved January 20, 2004, from http://www.cchsa.ca/site/pt_link.php?query=KeyCompon&plain=1

Canadian Council on Health Services Accreditation. (2003). *2002 National health accreditation report.* Retrieved January 20, 2004, from http://www.cchsa.ca/pdf/2002report.pdf

Canadian Health Services Research Foundation (CHSRF). (2004, Spring). Nurses' role in patient safety. *Links, 7*(1), 1.

Canadian Nurses Association (CNA). (1986). *Joint statement on nursing administration.* Ottawa, ON: CNA.

Canadian Nurses Association. (1988). *The role of nurse administrator and standards for nursing administration.* Ottawa, ON: CNA.

Canadian Nurses Association. (2003). *Quality of worklife indicators for nurses in Canada.* Retrieved June 18, 2004, from http://www.cna-nurses.ca/pages/resources/quality_workplace_indicators.pdf

Canadian Standards Association (CSA). (2003). *About CSA.* Retrieved August, 20, 2003, from http://www.csa.ca/about/Default.asp?language=english

Chiarella, M. (2003). Nurse practitioner roles: An exercise in professionalism, safety and quality. [Guest editorial]. *Australian Critical Care, 16*(1), 4–5.

Cummings, G. (2003). *The effects of hospital restructuring on nurses: How emotionally intelligent leadership mitigates these effects.* Unpublished doctoral dissertation. University of Alberta, Edmonton, Alberta, Canada.

Cummings, G., & Estabrooks, C. (2003). The effects of hospital restructuring that included layoffs on individual nurses who remained employed: A systematic review of impact. *International Journal of Sociology and Social Policy, 23*(8/9), 8–53.

Cummings, G.G., Hayduk, L., & Estabrooks, C. (in press). Mitigating the effects of hospital restructuring on nurses: The responsibility of emotionally intelligent leadership. *Nursing Research.*

Davies, A.R., Doyle, M.A.T., Lansky, D., Rutt, W., Stevic, M.O., & Doyle, J.B. (1994). Outcomes assessment in clinical settings: A consensus statement on principles and best practices in project management. *Journal on Quality Improvement, 20*(1), 6–16.

Donabedian, A. (1966). Evaluating the quality of medical care. *Milbank Quarterly, 44* (Suppl 3), 166–203.

Feeny, D., Guyatt, G., & Tugwell, P. (1986). *Health care technology: Effectiveness, efficiency and public policy.* Montreal, QC: Institute for Research on Public Policy.

Forster, A.J., Clark, H.D., Menard, A., Dupuis, N., Chernish, R., Chandok, N., et al. (2004). Adverse events among medical patients after discharge from hospital. *Canadian Medical Association Journal, 170*(3), 345–352.

Hanucharurnkul, S., Leucha, Y., Chutungkorn, P., Chantraprasert, S., Athaseri, S., & Noonill, N. (2002). Cost-effectiveness of primary care services provided by nurses' private clinics in Thailand. *Contemporary Nurse, 13*(2), 259–270.

Hartford Health. (2003). *Mission and vision for contiuous quality impprovement.* Retreived August 2003, from http://www.co.ha.md.us/health/cqi.htm.

Hassen, P., & Lindenburger, S. (1993). *Rx for hospitals: New hope for Medicare in the nineties.* Toronto, ON: Stoddart Publishing.

Havens, D.S., & Aiken, L.H. (1999). Shaping systems to promote desired outcomes. *Journal of Nursing Administration, 29*(2), 14–20.

Hooke, E., Bennett, L., Dwyer, R., van Beek, I., & Martin, C. (2001). Nurse practitioners: An evaluation of the extended role of nurses at the Kirketon Road Centre in Sydney, Australia. *Australian Journal of Advanced Nursing, 18*(3), 20–27.

Institute of Medicine. (1990). *Clinical Practice Guidelines: Directions for a New Program.* Washington, DC: National Academy Press.

Jennings, B.M., Staggers, N., & Brosch, L.R. (1999). A classification scheme for outcome indicators. *Journal of Nursing Scholarship, 31*(4), 381–388.

Kelly, K.C., Gardner, D.H., Johnson, M., McCloskey, J.C., & Maas, M. (1994). The medical outcomes study: A nursing perspective. *Journal of Professional Nursing, 10*(4), 209–216.

Kibbe, D.C., Kaluzny, A.D., & McLaughlin, C.P. (1994). Integrating guidelines with continuous quality improvement: Doing the right thing the right way to achieve the right goals. *Journal on Quality Improvement, 20*(4), 181–191.

Kohn, L.T., Corrigan, J.M., & Donaldson, M.S. (Eds). (2000) *To err is human: Building a safer health system.* Washington, DC: National Academy Press.

Kovner, A.R., Elton, J.J., & Billings. J. (2000). Evidence-based management. *Frontiers of Health Services Management, 16*(4), 3–24.

Kramer, M., & Hafner, L.P. (1989). Shared values: Impact on staff nurse job satisfaction and perceived productivity. *Nursing Research, 38*(3), 172–177.

Kramer, M., & Schmalenberg, C. (1988a). Magnet hospitals: Institutions of excellence. Part I. *Journal of Nursing Administration, 18*(1), 13–24.

Kramer, M., & Schmalenberg, C. (1988b). Magnet hospitals: Institutions of excellence. Part II. *Journal of Nursing Administration, 18*(2), 11–19.

Larkin, L. (2003). The case for nurse practitioners. *Hospitals & Health Networks, 77*(8), 54–56.

Levan, C. (1997, September 20). What, then, must I do? *The Edmonton Journal,* xxx–xxx.

Lindberg, M., Ahlner, J., Ekström, T., Jonsson, D., & Möller, M. (2002). Asthma nurse practice improves outcomes and reduces costs in primary health care. *Scandinavian Journal of Caring Sciences, 16*(1), 73–80.

Mackay, G., & Risk, M. (2001). Building quality practice settings: An attributes model. *Canadian Journal of Nursing Leadership, 14*(3), 19–27.

MacLellan, L., Gardner, G., & Gardner, A. (2002). Designing the future in wound care: The role of the nurse practitioner. *Primary Intention, 10*(3), 97–110.

McClure, M.L., Poulin, M.A., Sovie, M.D., & Wandelt, M.A. (1983). *Magnet hospitals: Attraction and retention of professional nurses.* Kansas City, MO: American Academy of Nursing.

Mendez, K.C. (1999). *Performance measurement in health care.* Retrieved August 21, 2003, from http://www.qualitydigest.com/may99/html/body_health.html

Morse, J.M., Penrod, J., & Hupcey, J.E. (2000). Qualitative outcome analysis: Evaluating nursing interventions for complex clinical phenomena. *Journal of Nursing Scholarship, 32*(2), 125–130.

Mintzberg, H. (1997). Toward healthier hospitals. *Health Care Management Review, 22*(4), 9–18.

National Steering Committee on Patient Safety. (2002). *Building a safer system: A national integrated strategy for improving patient safety in Canadian health care.* Ottawa, ON: Author.

Needleman, J., Buerhaus, P., Mattke, S., Stewart, M., & Zelevinsky, K. (2002). Nurse staffing levels and the quality of care in hospitals. *New England Journal of Medicine, 346*(22), 1715–1722.

Olmsted, K.L., & DeMint, S. (1997). Integrated delivery systems: Nurse practitioner center expands access to primary care. *Healthcare Financial Management, 51*(2), 30–33.

Perrow, C. (1979). *Complex organizations: A critical essay* (2nd ed.). Glenview, IL: Scott, Foresman and Company.

Rachlis, M. (2004). *Prescription for excellence: How innovation is saving Canada's health care system.* Toronto, ON: Harper Collins.

Rondeau, K.V., & Wagar, T.H. (2004). Implementing CQI while reducing the workforce: How does it influence hospital performance? *Healthcare Management Forum, 17*(2), 22–29.

Rosswurm, M.A., & Larrabee, J.H. (1999). A model for change to evidence-based practice. *Journal of Nursing Scholarship, 31*(4), 317–322.

Rozovsky, L.E., & Rozovsky, F.A. (1987). How CCHA guidelines have evolved into law. *Health Care, 29*(8), 62.

Sackett, D.L., Rosenberg, W.M., Gray, J.A., Haynes, R.B., & Richardson, W.S. (1996). Evidence-based Management. *BMJ, 312*(7023), xxx–xxx.

Saul, J.R. (2001). *On equilibrium.* Toronto, ON: Penguin Canada.

Scott, J.G., Sochalski, J., & Aiken, L. (1999). Review of magnet hospital research: Findings and implications for professional nursing practice. *Journal of Nursing Administration, 29*(1), 9–19.

Schmele, J.A. *Quality managment in nursing and health care.* Albany, NY: Delmar.

Sochalski, J. (2001). Quality of care, nurse staffing, and patient outcomes. *Policy, Politics and Nursing Practice, 2*(1), 9–18.

Tourangeau, A.E., Giovannetti, P., Tu, J.V., & Wood, M. (2002). Nursing-related determinants of 30-day mortality for hospitalized patients. *Canadian Journal of Nursing Research, 33*(4), 71–88.

Van Der Wiele, A., Williams, A.R.T., & Dale, B.G. (2000). Total quality management: Is it a fad, fashion, or fit? *Quality Management Journal, 7*(2), 65–79.

Vincent, D., & Mackey, T. (2000). Cost analysis: A tool for measuring the value of nurse practitioner practice. *Nurse Practitioner Forum, 11*(2), 149–153.

Wanzel, K.R., Jamieson, C.G., & Bohnen, J.M.A. (2000). Complications on a general surgery service: Incidence and reporting. *Canadian Journal of Surgery, 43*(2), 113–117.

Whittemore, R., & Grey, M. (2002). The systematic development of nursing interventions. *Journal of Nursing Scholarship, 34*(2), 115–120.

Wotherspoon, T. (2002). Nursing education: Professionalism and control. In B.S. Bolaria & H.D. Dickinson (Eds.), *Health, illness, and health care in Canada* (3rd ed., pp. 82–101). Scarborough, ON: Nelson Thomson Learning.

ACCOUNTABILITY IN THE CANADIAN HEALTH SYSTEM

Donna Lynn Smith, Richard Fraser, QC, Allan Heyhurst, CA,
Margaret Mrazek, QC, and Noela Inions, LLM

Learning Objectives

In this chapter, you will learn:

- Definitions and perspectives of accountability
- The history, structure, and processes of risk management
- Basic concepts about the management of financial risk
- The balanced scorecard approach for coordinating and reporting risk management and quality outcomes
- Differences in the requirements for managing predictable and unconventional emergencies
- Expert views of what constitutes executive competency and mistakes
- About the accountability of executive leaders for organizational culture and its consequences, including root causes of adverse events
- The causes, consequences, and prevention of the groupthink phenomenon in organizational decision making
- Why experts have recommended that whistle-blowers and dissenters in health service organizations need procedural protection

As this book goes to press, a series of studies on accountability in the Canadian health system is being conducted by the Canadian Policy Research Networks. Fooks and Maslove (2004) point out that accountability has become a common term used in health care reform discussion in Canada. They believe this is because "it conjures up processes in which citizens might come to understand where their tax dollars go, why certain policy decisions are made, or where they can turn if they are dissatisfied with the care they received. It hints at an environment in which a health care system might take responsibility for improving the health of the population" (p. 3). These authors identify the following elements that underpin various definitions of accountability:

- *Establishment of a relationship* between those making decisions and those affected by them
- *Agreed upon responsibility* for an individual or organization
- *Authority delegated or conferred* by governments to individuals and organizations
- *Answerability* for decisions made and actions taken
- Judgments about *performance*
- Processes for *sanction or correction*

There are four mechanisms of accountability. A *legal* approach provides recourse to legislation, government regulations, contracts, agreements, and processes for redress of disputes through the courts. In the *public reporting* approach, citizens receive selective information from the authority. The *citizen governance* approach is commonly seen in the roles of boards and provides a direct accountability relationship between the board and citizens.

The fourth element, *citizen engagement,* is less common and requires governments and organizations to go beyond traditional approaches to consultation or public participation to engage citizens in the agenda-setting dimensions of policy making. The merits of this approach are discussed in detail by Abelson and Gauvin (2004). They point out that in the traditional view of accountability, sanction is considered the strongest mechanism for assuring accountability, as illustrated in Figure 13.1.

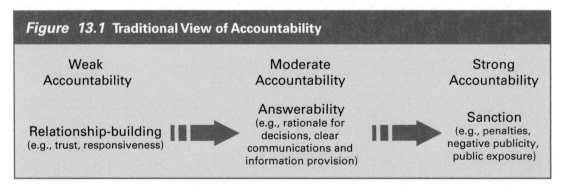

Figure 13.1 Traditional View of Accountability

Weak Accountability	Moderate Accountability	Strong Accountability
Relationship-building (e.g., trust, responsiveness)	Answerability (e.g., rationale for decisions, clear communications and information provision)	Sanction (e.g., penalties, negative publicity, public exposure)

Source: From Engaging Citizens: One Route to Health Care Accountability, by J. Abelson and F.P. Gauvin, 2004, *Health Care Accountability Papers, 2,* p. 16. Ottawa, ON: Canadian Policy Research Networks. Retrieved May 6, 2004, from http://www.cprn.com/en/doc.cfm?doc=560

However, since sanctions tend to be invoked as a last resort and only after problems have arisen, building relationships and developing processes for involving citizens in health policy and decision making are more likely to produce meaningful results. This is illustrated in Figure 13.2.

Abelson and Gauvin (2000) have pointed out that public involvement, in the form of surveys and highly structured consultation processes, is not the same as citizen engagement, in which there is transparency of processes and citizens have opportunities for meaningful and consistent participation in decision-making processes. They conclude that "the use of citizen engagement in the Canadian health system is in its infancy," and a major barrier to its acceptance is the fact that it "presents major challenges to the long-standing power relations that characterize health system decision-making in Canada" (p. vii).

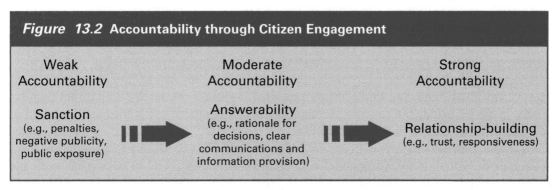

Figure 13.2 **Accountability through Citizen Engagement**

Weak Accountability	Moderate Accountability	Strong Accountability
Sanction (e.g., penalties, negative publicity, public exposure)	Answerability (e.g., rationale for decisions, clear communications and information provision)	Relationship-building (e.g., trust, responsiveness)

Source: From Engaging Citizens: One Route to Health Care Accountability, by J. Abelson and F.P. Gauvin, 2004, *Health Care Accountability Papers, 2*, p. 16. Ottawa, ON: Canadian Policy Research Networks. Retrieved May 6, 2004, from http://www.cprn.com/en/doc.cfm?doc=560

Leadership Responsibility and Accountabilty

A professional education includes not only the knowledge specific to the discipline, but also awareness of the standards that are applicable to that discipline. Professionals are expected to use discretionary judgment in the application of their specific knowledge to particular situations, and the public holds them accountable for informed ethical practice in which the well-being of clients is a priority. Senior leaders in health service organizations have accepted responsibilities that go beyond those associated with their original professions or occupations. Through the authority vested in their positions, they become accountable for safeguarding the well-being of both patients and staff in units, programs, or entire organizations. They are held accountable for the stewardship of funds and other resources provided by the community, and they are in a position to directly influence the health of the community. Executives typically earn higher than average incomes and also receive perquisites (sometimes referred to as "perks"), such as greater discretionary use of their time, a company vehicle, or discretionary allowances. In return, it is expected that they will behave with integrity and will not abuse their positions of privilege. As Friedman (2002) has noted, health service executives and organizations are particularly likely to attract criticism if they fail to live up to public expectations because they "have been granted a special standing in society. Even within the well-known and widely publicized managed care backlash, people still generally trust their personal doctor and local hospitals to do the right thing and to be available in times of need. By virtue of this extraordinary level of trust, healthcare executives must continually strive to do their work and make decisions using the highest possible ethical and moral judgments" (p. 2). Citizens have grown intolerant of mistakes made by health professionals and health care managers. They will no longer accept discourteous or paternalistic behaviour, and they expect that deficiencies and inefficiencies in service and management will be prevented or promptly corrected.

Ideally, standards are available to provide guidance to leaders as to when and why they should take action and to whom they are accountable. But standards are not available in every situation, and leadership offers and requires opportunities for discretionary judgment. When individuals choose to be responsible, reasonable, and responsive, they accept accountability (Gardner & Russell, 1989). Responsibility can be seen in the action taken. A "responsible" individual or corporate entity is trustworthy, reliable, able to tell right from wrong, and able to think and act reasonably. We may not know at the time what is reasonable, so the accountability relationship has to include the concept of responsiveness. Responsiveness is the quality evident in activities that are undertaken to receive and search out relevant information. It implies an awareness of and sensitivity to factors in the environment that affect the ability to accomplish a task (Gardner & Russell, 1989). Campbell (2002) points out that an unwillingness to acknowledge mistakes reflects an abdication of responsibility since it is not possible to be a responsible executive in the moral sense without first being willing to acknowledge one's role in a decision, plan, or action that has gone awry.

Risk Management

Risk management is a dimension of accountability that is related to, but different from, quality assurance and quality management. Quality management focuses on patient care and requires persons with requisite clinical or professional expertise to establish standards and then determine whether the care provided meets those standards. These processes and various types of standards are discussed in Chapter 12. Risk management, on the other hand, is concerned with minimizing the liability of an organization by preventing mistakes or minimizing their consequences.

Risk management is defined as "the systematic process of identifying, evaluating and addressing (treating or preventing) potential and/or actual risks which are a source of injury or loss of money or reputation" (Mrazek, 1994, p. 555). Since there are risks of some form in almost every aspect of health service delivery, everyone has a role to play in a risk management program. Although the processes of risk management and quality assurance are different, there is a surprising degree of overlap in the processes needed to achieve both objectives. However, risk management is primarily a management responsibility.

Risk management is important because the boards of health agencies are either directly or vicariously accountable to the patient through the actions of hospital medical staff or employees. Legal liability extends to labour, contract, tort, real estate, corporate, environmental, administrative, intellectually property, and even criminal law concerns. Tort liability, for negligence in care, has traditionally been the major area of risk.

Liability arises out of the duties owed to the patient. These duties include:

- selecting competent staff;
- instructing and supervising agency personnel;
- reviewing and monitoring the qualifications and competence of professionals performing services within the hospital (i.e., physicians); and
- establishing and applying policies and procedures so that facilities and equipment are utilized and maintained so as to provide reasonable care to patients.

Risk Management in Historical Context

The concept of risk management is well known and well developed in industry. For example, the insurance industry has a particularly rich history of risk management. The application to the health care field is relatively new and arose in the United States as a response to the proliferation of malpractice and negligence claims in the 1970s. To control escalating insurance costs, companies insisted that health care facilities covered by their plans have risk management programs. As an incentive to introduce such programs, some insurance companies offered reduced premiums.

In the Canadian health system, litigation was not the initial impetus for the development of risk management programs, which were promoted by the Canadian Council on Health Facilities Accreditation Program in the 1980s (Dickens, 1993; Picard & Robertson, 1996; Stock & Lefroy, 1988). In this context, hospitals were advised to develop coordinated risk management systems that included the following elements (Allen, 1986):

- Appointment or designation of a risk manager who has authority and responsibility for developing, implementing, and coordinating the risk management system
- Establishment of a multidisciplinary risk management committee to support and advise the risk manager
- Development of a risk management policy statement endorsed by the board to provide support and accountability for the risk management program
- These elements were seen as necessary to coordinate individual loss control programs and centralize responsibility for a risk management system.

During the 1990s, the Canadian health system was restructured, downsized, and destabilized. A rhetoric that emphasized teamwork was used to rationalize management innovations with claims that they would create improved quality through better coordination and thus control costs. As these changes occurred, many traditional approaches and processes for monitoring standards and assuring quality were abandoned, fragmented, or displaced. Infrastructure such as nursing procedure committees, which had traditionally been the mechanism for introducing new research evidence into clinical nursing practice and assessing the appropriateness of equipment and supplies, were dismantled. In this process, nurses' expectations that nursing work would be managed by members of the nursing profession were discounted, and standard operating procedures taught and traditionally used by nurses to manage procedural integrity were sometimes disparaged as ritualistic and costly "turf protection." In this context, risk management was often handled one issue at a time and without the infrastructure that coordinated clinical risk management activities or linked them with other organizational process.

During this period, a prominent management theorist conducted observational research in hospitals in England and Canada. In the Canadian teaching hospital observed over a period of several months, the author noted a lack of coordination between the care activities of nurses, which were described as continuous and organized around workflow, and the cure activities of physicians, which were described as intermittent, specialized, and occurring in chimneys or silos (Mintzberg, 1997). Fragmentation and a lack of coordination were observed in 19 different hospital committees. The problem of overcrowding in the emergency department came up repeatedly—in eight meetings of medical committees, in three committees involving board members, and in other management meetings as well—but discussion was circular and ineffectual, lacking a systems perspective of the problem or possible solutions. Nurses or nursing managers participated in only a few of the committees observed. Mintzberg noted that "everyone could benefit from more productive meetings, and in hospitals, that means ones that are less representative of the narrow specialties and more representative of the collective problems" (p. 14). Difficulties arising from the intrinsic structure of hospitals (described as the hospital administration triad in Chapter 8) were described, and deal making and a lack of transparency in process were noted as two problematic factors. Mintzberg (1997) concluded the following:

> A good rule of thumb on deals should be that if anyone would feel embarrassed were the deal made public, then it should not be made. Better still, all deals should be made public as policy. That way the bad ones would not pass and there would be less need for gossip and rumours in the corridors, not to mention counter-deals to cope with the fall out of deals. We are brought back to the dangers of fragmentation, and brought forward to a popular word these days – transparency of process. In the building up of an excellent institution, which can only be a long slow process, there is no substitute for openness of procedure (p. 8).

In the early 21st century, accountability of leaders and governing boards in all sectors has become a prominent public policy concern. Policy, leadership, and organizational culture in health service organizations have been recognized as system-level factors that create the conditions in which clinical mistakes occur. Patient safety has become a pressing public policy issue, and risk management has re-emerged as a leadership priority. A newsletter entitled *Risk Management in Canadian Health Care* is published eight times a year by Butterworths Canada and deals with timely issues. Statements issued by national organizations, including the Canadian College of Health Service Executives (CCHSE, 2003) emphasize the role of health system executives in creating a "culture of safety" in which it is a priority to prevent errors and respond appropriately when errors occur.

Structural Elements of Risk Management

Effective risk management requires an infrastructure of structure and processes. *Organizational standards* in the form of *policies and procedures* are key structural elements in risk management. Where policies or procedures exist, courts are likely to look upon them as setting out the organization's position. It is therefore important that organizations regularly review and update policies and procedures and inform all staff about what is expected of them. If a policy exists but is not followed, the position of the organization and the actions of its employees or staff are put into question. If an employee or physician does not follow an established policy, that person would be acting as an individual in contravention of the action expected by the organization. When employed staff disregard policies, disciplinary action may result. In instances where a policy does not exist, and an injury occurs, the knowledge and discretionary decision making of professionals will be evaluated against community standards or common sense. The case example in Box 13.1 illustrates an instance in which a physician was held liable even though the established hospital policy was adhered to.

Box 13.1

Case Example: Discretionary Judgment by Professionals

A generally accepted legal standard is that "approved practice" must be met in the clinical setting. However, meeting this standard may not be sufficient to defend an allegation of negligence. In 1949, an example arose in the case of *Anderson v. Chasney* (*Anderson*, 1949). Approved practice was met when cherry swabs were used, and not counted, during a tonsillectomy and adenoidectomy procedure. The child subsequently suffocated and died from a cherry swab left in the lower part of his throat.

A lawsuit by the parents was successful. The court recognized that "approved practice" (i.e., not to count cherry swabs) had been met in the circumstances, but ruled that this practice did not meet a reasonable standard of care and therefore was insufficient to exonerate the defendants. The message in this case is that, where a precaution could be used that would entail little expenditure of time and money, and where a person with no professional training in the area would judge the precaution to be reasonable, the failure to take the precaution may be found to be negligent, even where other professionals also fail to take care. The lesson to be learned is that a court may, in rare circumstances, disagree with the adequacy of a professionally agreed upon "approved practice" and impose a higher standard. It is clear from this case that blind adherence to generally accepted practices, even when these practices have been professionally approved, is not a substitute for professional diligence and thoughtful judgment.

It is interesting to note that in this case only the surgeon was found negligent. The court held that the surgeon has the duty to check and remove all sponges. In this case, the surgeon had access to string swabs as well as to nurses who could have counted the cherry swabs, but did not request either of these precautions as this was not the usual practice of this surgeon or of this hospital. It should be noted that this case was heard almost 50 years ago; a court today would likely make a finding of negligence against the hospital staff and the hospital as well as the surgeon due to changes in the standard of care for organizations and professional staff.

Traditionally, policies and procedures that apply to employed staff have not been applied to physicians, and performance problems of physicians have not been addressed in a timely manner. This has had significant financial consequences for health service organizations and for the companies that insure physicians. In 1993, the Federation of Medical Licensing Authorities of Canada launched a project to address the issues necessary to ensure that physicians in practice maintain an appropriate level of performance for the duration of their professional lives. Four major areas of physician performance were identified in this project. These were competence, behaviour, health and fitness to practice, and use of resources (National Steering Committee on Patient Safety, 2002). The recognition of potential risks in these areas and the development of remediation programs sponsored by medical licensing bodies are hopeful initiatives. Unions have had an important influence on the development of organization-wide policies that require respectful treatment of all patients and staff, and, although resisted by management at the bargaining table, these policies (once implemented and consistently enforced) can be expected to reduce corporate risk and liability arising from instances of harassment, intimidation, abuse, and assault.

Documentation practices and standards are another structural way of managing and minimizing risk. Requirements for documentation are reflected in professional and organizational standards. Some organizational policies, such as charting by exception, disregard professional standards and legal precedent. From a risk management point of view, accurate, complete, and contemporaneous notes can assist in reducing risks in the provision of care by ensuring that anyone having contact with a patient is aware of that patient's condition and the care and treatment provided. This can prevent mistakes and duplication in treatment. Courts have sometimes viewed the absence of documentation as evidence that no treatment has been provided (*Meyer*, 1981; Picard & Robertson, 1996).

Processes for Risk Management

Effective processes are a key requirement for effective risk management programs. Processes are required to identify and prevent risks and to assess and respond to specific risks when they occur.

Identifying and Preventing Risks

Loss and liability can be minimized through proactive processes that involve collecting and compiling information from program reports, unusual incident or occurrence reports, departmental surveys, and external reports.

Program reporting involves the regular compilation of information from specific programs, such as occupational health and safety, clinical programs, security and fire prevention, and human resources, in a format that can be regularly reviewed for risk management purposes.

Generic reports are generated across all programs and departments. Critical or *unusual incident reports* are the most common example. Typically, an organizational policy specifies that all staff are required to complete an unusual incident report under certain circumstances. Unusual incident reports are carefully structured to restrict reporting to factual information because they can be called into evidence in court. Reporting may be obligatory for certain types of incidents such as patient falls, medication errors, staff incidents, and environmental incidents; however, there is often an expectation that staff will use discretion and complete incident reports for unusual incidents that do not fall into predetermined categories. *Occurrence reporting* is typically narrower in focus but broader in coverage than incident reporting, which is sometimes confined to incidents directly associated with patient care. Occurrence reporting focuses on incidents identified as carrying high risk and is typically required of all staff. Work-related injuries, cardiac arrests, and fires are common examples of incidences requiring occurrence reporting.

Departmental surveys may be conducted to enable or encourage managers or staff to identify risks in their departments or units. Total quality management programs often incorporate data collection processes to enable staff and managers to identify and respond to potential risks in their immediate work environments.

External reports include individual letters of complaint or notification from patients, family members, or lawyers as well as formal reports from accreditation surveys, municipal fire authorities, or regulatory bodies.

Assessing and Responding to Specific Risks

When an event or outcome is identified as a specific risk, the following actions usually take place:
1. Evidence is gathered to determine the facts. The incident is reviewed with the individuals involved, who are often requested to prepare written statements. The patient's health record or other pertinent documents are reviewed to determine how the occurrence and responses to it were documented.
2. The insurer and/or legal counsel are notified of the incident by a designated official of the organization who inquires about coverage and seeks advice as necessary.
3. Immediate responses are made to patients and family to communicate good intention and thereby discourage claims.
4. A detailed and objective investigation is conducted.
5. Preparations are made for legal defense or for arranging out-of-court settlements.

Registered nurses (RNs) and nurse managers may find themselves in the position of having to appear in legal proceedings involving risks and liability. When employees, including managers, become personally involved in a situation at issue while carrying out the responsibilities of their position, the organization will normally be vicariously liable for their actions provided that they were working within the scope of their employment. The health organization as an employer may pursue an action against a negligent employee to recover monies paid on behalf of the employee in legal action. A nurse manager should take the necessary steps to assess the potential for individual liability.

During their professional education, RNs typically learn principles and standard operating procedures that minimize risk. Aseptic technique, proper techniques for lifting and moving patients, and protocols for checking and administering medication and treatment and for informing patients and obtaining their consent are examples. Nursing textbooks may be used as reference points in evaluating whether the practices of individual professionals or organizational standards and management practices are prudent. Nurses and nursing managers may also be called as expert witnesses when matters of nursing knowledge are at issue.

Managing Financial Risk

Proper stewardship of financial resources is a concern of all organizations. Professional, organizational, and legal standards provide a framework for the management of financial risk in health agencies.

The Accounting Profession and Standards

In Canada, there are three recognized accounting designations: Chartered Accountant (CA), Certified Management Accountant (CMA), and Certified General Accountant (CGA). Significant training and professional exams are required before a designation may be achieved. The CA and CMA programs have a university degree entrance requirement. Accountants must also meet requirements for continuing professional development. Professional accounting associations are self-governing and have standards and codes of ethical conduct. One key requirement is that external auditors must be independent of the organizations they are auditing. Breaches of standards or ethics can result in disciplinary action, up to and including the loss of designation.

Once qualified, an accountant can choose to work in private practice, for an accounting firm, or for a particular business or public organization. Accountants are also employed in the finance departments of health departments and organizations. In most organizations, the chief financial officer (CFO) is a member of the executive management team.

General Principles of Financial Management

Financial management includes the responsibility of establishing processes to assure financial accountability in organizations. It also includes the management of the finance department, which has its own staff of accountants and administrative support personnel. The finance department coordinates the process of budget development and the financial aspects of business planning. Once approved by the governing board, the budget provides a benchmark for the assessment of financial performance, which is accomplished through the accounting function. Regular financial reports are provided to managers at all levels of the organization on a monthly basis. Ideally, unit, department, and program managers work with personnel in the finance department early in the budget process. This input and participation enables them to feel ownership and accountability for the budget and to knowledgeably monitor and interpret variances.

Generally Accepted Accounting Principles

Generally accepted accounting principles (GAAP) are guidelines that the accounting professions must follow when reporting financial results. These guidelines are published by the Auditing and Assurance Standards Oversight Council; further information about these standards and the processes for their development are available from the Canadian Institute of Chartered Accountants. (See Internet Resources at the end of the chapter.) These standards ensure that financial statements for all organizations are reported consistently. In addition to GAAP, many provinces also issue financial directives through their respective health departments. Such directives can be thought of as policies and procedures to guide health organizations in the content, format, and frequency of financial and organizational reporting.

Organization of Accounts

Within each organization, a chart of accounts sets the framework for financial reporting. Within the Canadian health system, a standardized approach to financial reporting has been adopted to ensure that each health organization reports results consistently. The chart of accounts for health organizations is contained within management information systems (MIS) guidelines. These guidelines have developed over time by provincial ministries of health in conjunction with the Canadian Institute for Health Information (CIHI). Budgets and accounting costs are organized around specific cost centres. For example, the cost centre for the emergency room (ER) is always 7131-00-000. Drugs are always coded to 4655000. Therefore, drugs consumed in the ER are coded to 71310000-4655000 no matter where the hospital is located in Canada. The extra zeros can be used internally to further analyze costs that may be appropriate for the organization. The extra two zeros in the department code may be further determined by the MIS guidelines. For example, the general code for the operating room is 7126-00-000, and the urology operating room code is 7126-08-000. The last three zeros are unique to each organization. Procedures and standards of this sort enable systematic analysis and comparison of financial transactions across organizations.

Organizational Policies and Practices

Every organization develops internal policies and practices governing financial management. Within the organization, strategic direction and policy for financial decision making are the responsibility of the board of directors. Administrative policies are developed by senior management and would include such policies as approval levels on expenditures, travel guidelines, or purchasing practices.

Nurse managers need to know what policies and procedures apply to their units or programs and must be alert to any potential conflict of interest for themselves as they hire staff, order supplies, or approve expenditures. The principle of division of duties provides one fundamental type of internal control designed to prevent unauthorized or inappropriate expenditures and the possibility of fraud. This principle is operationalized through policies and procedures that require one-over-one approval of expenditures. When followed, such policies prevent even senior officials from approving their own travel or personal expenses. They are intended to assure that no single individual is able to authorize contracts or order, receive, or pay for supplies and services on behalf of the organization without an appropriate mandate.

Auditing

Auditing is an independent review of financial results, internal controls, and management practices. Provincial and federal Auditors General scrutinize the financial practices of public institutions and the government itself, reporting to the legislature. All health organizations must have an external auditor, and some larger organizations create the position of internal auditor. Accounting firms are engaged to perform external audits of organizations such as regional health authorities and hospitals. Through generally accepted auditing standards, auditors perform appropriate tests, review internal controls, and form opinions on the financial statements prepared by the organization. An external auditor only performs enough tests to form an opinion and does not review all transactions; therefore, an external audit may not detect fraud.

To provide an objective opinion, auditors must be completely independent of the organization, function, or process being audited. Internal auditors are in a particularly sensitive position within the organizations where they are employed. For this reason, they are usually positioned to report directly to the CEO and/or the board of directors to ensure that they cannot be influenced by the finance department. The role and scope of practice of internal auditors is typically broad in order to enable them to go beyond an examination of accounting processes and investigate and report on all processes with potential for financial risk or poor accountability in all areas of the organization.

It is of paramount importance that auditors are not in a position of conflict of interest. Prior to the Enron scandal in the United States, it had become a common practice for the consulting arms of accounting firms to do other business with the companies they were auditing, and such was the case of the auditors from the international firm of Arthur Anderson Consulting and the Enron Corporation. In the aftermath of the Enron scandal and other similar occurrences, regulatory mechanisms in the US and around the world have been closely scrutinized. An audit of leading auditors suggests that the situation with Arthur Anderson Consulting was not unique (*How bad was Anderson?* 2003; Eisenberg & Macey, 2003).

The Canadian Comprehensive Auditing Foundation (CCAF) has developed a framework organized around 12 attributes of effectiveness: management direction, appropriateness, achievement of intended results, secondary impacts, costs, productivity, responsiveness, financial results, working environment, protection of assets, monitoring, and reporting. The framework is intended to be used by senior management to analyze and report to the governing board on the performance of the organization so that it can "exact accountability from management in the exercise of its [overall] responsibilities" (CCAF, 1992, p. 11). The standards go beyond the customary focus on financial and operational data, which is most readily available and easily interpreted, to incorporate the board's responsibility for monitoring quality of care issues and the results achieved through health programs and services where information is much more limited. The Effectiveness Reporting Framework was first applied in a health organization in a pilot project at the Queen Elizabeth Hospital in Toronto, Ontario. A booklet and videotape about this project became resources to assist other health organizations in implementing the framework.

Nurse Managers and Financial Accountability

As custodians of organizational resources, nurse managers have financial as well as clinical accountability. Their role in the preparation of budgets is discussed in Chapter 29. They must monitor and interpret financial reports and identify areas where change in the type or volume of activities is likely to have an effect on expenditures. The compensation budget is created from the staffing mix and patterns and is determined to a considerable extent by collective agreements. Supply budgets are often created from past patterns and projected activity levels. Nursing managers are in a position to identify priorities for the replacement or acquisition of capital equipment, which is usually funded from a different source. Colleagues in the finance department usually provide information about inflation, price trends, and the interpretation of financial reports; however, they are not knowledgeable about clinical requirements and risks. Therefore, accounting professionals and nursing managers must cultivate respectful relationships that combine the knowledge of both disciplines to achieve broad organizational goals, including all aspects of risk management.

Balanced Scorecard

The balanced scorecard approach integrates risk prevention and management activities with other organizational processes. The balanced scorecard is a comprehensive framework that incorporates the strategic objectives of an organization into a coherent set of performance measures (Kaplan & Norton, 1992 as cited in Baker & Pink, 1995). The balanced scorecard incorporates four perspectives. The *customer perspective* measures how the organization is perceived by those it serves. The *internal business perspective* measures performance in areas of excellence. The *innovation and learning perspective* focuses on quality improvement. When indicators and measures in these areas are integrated with the *financial perspective*, the organization can obtain feedback that gives a balanced view of organizational performance.

The Chinook Health Region (CHR) in southern Alberta has adopted and reported on this approach (Oliver, 2002). CHR was created in 1995 when the provincial government dissolved all existing health boards and created regional health authority (RHA) boards for 17 regions. The CHR is the fourth largest in Alberta, serving a rural and urban population of about of 150,000 people. The boundaries of this region remained unchanged when a second phase of regionalization took place in Alberta in 2002 and 2003.

In 2002, a corporate planning and support department was created to coordinate the provincially legislated business planning processes, manage preparation for the accreditation surveys by the Canadian Council on Health Services Accreditation (CCHSA), and create a regional quality management program. The resulting program incorporated the philosophy and systems features of total quality management (TQM), including elements of risk management and utilization management. The balanced scorecard approach recommended by Kaplan and Norton was modified to align the business planning goals of the region with the quality dimensions of the CCHSA process. Figure 13.3 illustrates the elements of this program.

To implement the program, a *Quality Council* was created as a new committee of the regional board. *Reporting structures and templates* were designed to facilitate ease of reporting and to provide the council with meaningful summary information. Specific *quality indicators* are regularly reported and monitored. *Indicators of service delivery responsiveness,* such as waiting times for specific procedures and services, surgical cancellation rates, and occupancy rates, are regularly monitored. *Patient/client/community focus* is measured through indicators that include immunization rates, unusual incident rates, nosocomial infection rates, and eating facility inspection results. *Work-life indicators* include the number of workers' compensation claims, filed grievances, sick days, and disability claims.

Figure 13.3 Use of the Balanced Scorecard in the Chinook Health Region

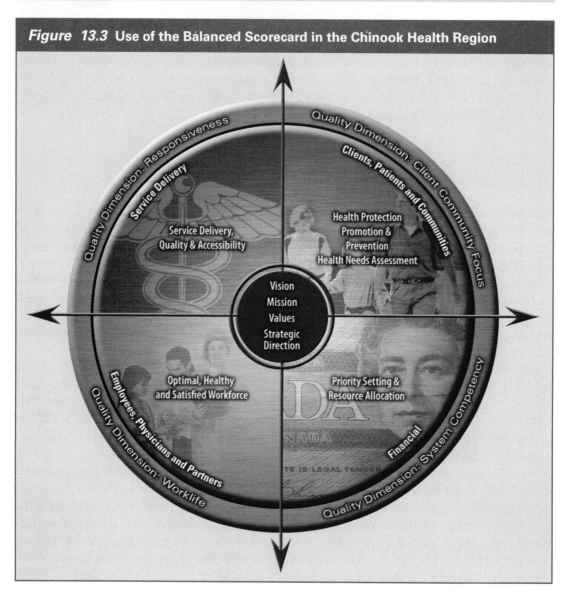

Source: From *Use of the Balanced Scorecard as a Framework for a Total Quality Management Program,* by K. Oliver, 2002. Paper presented at the Improving Performance Measurement in Healthcare Conference, Canadian Institute, Toronto, Ontario, Canada. Used with permission.

Targets or *goals* are specified for each indicator. After being reviewed through administrative channels, business plans and reports from clinical and administrative departments are presented to the Quality Council. The *Board Quality Indicators Report* enables the board to examine and compare the same indicators against regional targets for all sites and services in the region.

Managing Emergencies and Crises

Situations of emergency or crisis present particular management challenges, and risk management is an integral part of emergency preparedness (Lynch & Cox, 2003). The interface between risk management and crisis management is a process whereby the decision to activate an emergency plan is made. Crisis management is then concerned with managing the emergency response (Lynch & Cox, 2003). Conventional disasters such as hurricanes, earthquakes, fires, and plane crashes are relatively easy to plan for, and plans for this type of disaster can be formulated in advance and tested periodically through table-top exercises or simulations. However, when the magnitude or type of disaster is unprecedented (as was the case in the Quebec ice storm in 1998, the 9/11 terrorist attack in the US, the power blackout of 2003 that affected the eastern seaboard, and the 2003 SARS outbreak), it is not clear at the outset what the extent and nature of the disaster will be or what caused it. This situation of not knowing critical information while having to manage an evolving emergency situation is described as managing within a knowledge vacuum (Lynch & Cox, 2003).

In unconventional emergencies where a knowledge vacuum exists, the command and control paradigm that works well in conventional emergencies is not adequate. To manage within the knowledge vacuum typical of unconventional emergencies and crises, leaders must be able to create learning and discovery processes that can address highly specific issues very rapidly. In discussing how the SARS issue was managed in the British Columbia Centre for Disease Control (BCCDC), Lynch and Cox (2003) make the case that a state of emergency preparedness must be part of an existing cultural acceptance of "best practices" in normal times. To effectively manage unprecedented emergencies that develop in an ad hoc fashion, there must be a pre-existing culture of shared learning characterized by creative thought, collegial relationships, and organic leadership. Creating this type of organizational environment requires a long-term investment of values and leadership by the CEO because "the reality is that structures, personal linkages and resources need to be in place prior to any emergency happening, and such protocols should be subject to periodic review" (p. 70).

Individual Accountability of Health System Leaders

Administrative and leadership behaviour is a broad area of study in programs of business and public administration. In Canada, as in other Western countries, there is a growing public concern about leadership accountability for errors of judgment and conduct. Three high profile case examples in the Canadian health system have been reported extensively in the media and are summarized here. The first case example, described in Box 13.2, is the well-known situation of contamination of the Canadian blood supply. The second case (Box 13.3) deals with conflict

Box 13.2

Case Example: Contamination of the Canadian Blood Supply

Leadership decisions that allowed the Canadian blood supply to become contaminated were illuminated through a public inquiry conducted by Justice Krever (www.hc-sc.gc.ca/english/protection/krever/). In this instance, leaders in the Canadian Red Cross were found to have ignored scientific evidence and to have allowed contaminated blood to be put into inventory and distributed to hospitals.

The public inquiry led to structural changes in the management of the Canadian blood supply, compensation to individuals who had received contaminated blood, and eventually criminal charges. However, the process of pursuing accountability by means of legal action in the criminal justice system is costly and protracted.

Readers interested in learning more about this case may refer to the resources listed in the Further Reading section at the end of the chapter.

Box 13.3

Case Example: Conflicts of Interest between a Medical Scientist and a Drug Company

Conflict of interest between governing officials of a major Canadian university and senior hospital leaders is illustrated in the case of Dr. Nancy Olivieri, who stopped a clinical trial when she observed that children receiving the drug were developing dangerous side effects. The trial was funded by a drug company through a research contract involving the university and the hospital. This case was reported widely in the press (news@UofT, 2002; Valpy, 1998) and has since been described in publications in the peer-reviewed literature (Viens & Savulescu, 2004).

The drug company, hospital, and university applied pressure to prevent Dr. Olivieri from stopping the trial and disclosing her observations about the side effects to the parents of the children being treated and through the scientific literature. An initial investigation was conducted on behalf of the hospital's research ethics board and chaired by a prominent Canadian scientist and concluded that hospital staff and executives did not act improperly (MedicalEthics.ca, 2001). However, this report documents instances of false and misleading testimony to hospital and university committees and failures by hospital administrators and committees to provide due process (Canada's Voice for Academic Staff, 2001).

Subsequently, an independent panel considered more complete information (Thompson, Baird, & Downie, 2001) and found that the drug company and certain senior hospital and university staff had incorrectly accused Dr. Olivieri of misconduct and had used these allegations as the basis for serious public actions against her. Although discredited, the hospital's actions in making these complaints were subsequently used by the drug company in defending the reputation of its drug.

The final conclusion of this independent panel was that the university did not do enough to protect Dr. Olivieri's academic freedom and to help her after it had been alleged that she was "constructively dismissed." The hospital made a complaint against Dr. Olivieri to the College of Physicians and Surgeons of Ontario. The hospital's complaint was dismissed, and instead the review by the College concluded that Dr. Olivieri had acted correctly and in the best interest of her patients. Subsequently, a settlement was reached among Dr. Olivieri, the hospital, university, and the faculty association (a union representing university teachers), which had supported her.

In a published commentary in a medical ethics journal, a number of experts discussed this case in a broader international context. One concluded that the institutional design of academic medicine systematically ignores serious ethical problems and regards whistle-blowers as enemies of the institution and punishes them (MedicalEthics.ca, 2001). A national newspaper reported that the Olivieri case was "Canada's worst academic and research scandal in decades" and that Dr. Olivieri had been demoted, harassed, and "smeared with allegations attacking her competence, integrity, sanity and personality" (Wente, 1999).

This case attracted international attention to the potential for conflict of interest in financial and research funding arrangements between universities, hospitals, and drug companies, and it has provided impetus for major changes to the requirements for ethics review and monitoring of drug trials in Canada.

of interest and the professional obligations of a medical scientist, and the third (Box 13.4) illustrates a lack of responsiveness in the behaviour of administrative officials in the case of unexpected infant deaths at the Winnipeg Health Sciences Centre.

In the sections that follow, expert views are presented on the competencies expected of health service executives and the executive mistakes they make. These perspectives provide a framework for analysis of the administrative behaviour and errors in the case examples described above. The interim report of the commission headed by Justice Campbell to inquire into SARS and public health in Ontario provides a more recent case example that could be similarly evaluated (Campbell, 2004).

Executive Competencies

The CEO and executive management team express and communicate the values of the organization through the organization's structure and through their individual and group behaviour. Competency is an important dimension of accountability. Nine administrative competencies identified and examined by the Canadian College of Health Service Executives (CCHSE) are listed in Table 13.1.

Box 13.4

Case Example: Unexpected Infant Deaths at the Winnipeg Health Sciences Centre

The need for policy procedures to protect internal whistle-blowers was a prominent recommendation in the findings of Justice Sinclair, who presided over a lengthy inquest into the deaths of neonates and young children at the Winnipeg Health Sciences Centre Children's Hospital (www.pediatriccardiacinquest.mb.ca/).

In this case, over a nine- to 10-month period, clinical nurses repeatedly reported concerns to various administrative officials, including medical and nursing leaders, about their observations of the performance of an inexperienced cardiovascular surgeon and their perceptions of the relationship of his actions to deaths and complications in children. Although at one point during this period, the program had been suspended while an internal review was conducted, senior executives of the hospital gave evidence to the inquest that they were unaware of the problems in the program.

In his extensive report, Justice Sinclair commented on the lack of respect for female professionals (nurses and anesthesiologists) and for nursing knowledge that was prevalent in the organizational culture. He criticized the lack of leadership accountability and, more specifically, was critical of the program management structure in which there was no executive-level representation of the nursing discipline or voice for nursing concerns. He commented on the failures of the medical peer-review process and the absence of any written documentation, including incident reports. He also noted specific incidents in which administrative representatives gave incorrect information, deceived parents, or concealed information from them. Recommendations of this inquiry can be found in Chapter 10 of the report (Sinclair, 2001).

A comparative case study of this case at the Winnipeg Health Sciences Centre and an earlier case of unexpected infant deaths at the Toronto Hospital for Sick Children identified a number of similarities in context and administrative behaviour (Paras, 2004).

Executive Mistakes

In 2002, a leading American journal of health care administration *(Frontiers of Health Services Management)* devoted an entire issue to the subject of "Morally Managing Executive Mistakes." The reasons for focusing on this topic were explained in the editorial as follows:

> Although clinical errors have been the focus of attention in the national media, administrative errors are just as important. An individual's life may not be hanging in the balance, but numerous errors made by health care managers have had a significant effect on the health and well-being of their organizations and on the many stakeholders within. Mistakes relative to decisions to start, change, or stop a strategic service unit can have an

Table 13.1 Canadian College of Health Service Executives: Executive Competencies	
Leadership	Vision Team building Flexibility Stress management Commitment
Communication	Verbal communication Listening Written communication
Lifelong Learning	Self-directed learning Teaching/Mentoring
Consumer/Community Relations	Public relations Responsiveness
Political and Health Environment Awareness and Sensitivity	Political awareness and sensitivity Health environment
Conceptual Skills	Analysis and synthesis Implementation Systems thinking
Results Management	Planning Implementation Monitoring/Evaluation
Resource Management	Human resources Financial resources Capital/Material assets Information
Compliance with Standards	Accreditation Ethical standards Legal standards

Source: Excerpted from Professional Competencies. Canadian College of Health Service Executives. Retrieved November 14, 2003, from http://www.cchse.org/c_procom.htm

important impact on a community. Staff can find themselves out of work when mistakes are made in the planning of mergers and acquisitions. Shareholders and investors are placed at risk when the mistakes made by executives and governing boards result in poor financial performance (Friedman, 2002, p. 1).

Executive mistakes may involve errors of omission or commission. A typology of executive mistakes is presented in Table 13.2.

Table 13.2 Executive Mistakes of Omission and Commission

Omission	Commission
Failure to anticipate significant factors affecting decisions	Permitting decisions to be made without adequate analysis
Failure to act promptly on changed conditions	Choosing political, not business solutions
Failure to consider all options	Making economic decisions that harm clinical care and outcomes
Failure to delegate and hold subordinates accountable	Allocating limited resources without applying objective criteria
Failure to balance power interests	Withholding negative information from individuals with the right to know
Failure to keep patient and corporate needs paramount	Making selective use of facts with different audiences
Failure to follow the law, economic principles, or prudent person rule	Showing favoritism among the board, management, medical staff, and employees
Failure to anticipate likely consequences	Signing contracts that are not achievable
Failure to fulfill contractual commitments and obligations to employees	Condoning discrimination among patient types on the basis of source of payment, ethnicity, gender, or other inappropriate or illegal factors
Failure to protect the assets of the corporation	Allowing a climate of male dominance to harm relationships between doctors and nurses, thus accelerating nurse turnover and poor patient care
Failure to lead where there are opportunities to improve the health of patients or the community	Making high technology investments without addressing access problems

Source: From Morally Managing Executive Mistakes, by P.B. Hofmann, 2002, *Frontiers of Health Services Management*, *18*(3), pp. 3–38. Used with permission.

Executives are also responsible for creating a culture in which staff are encouraged to report errors and are protected when they do so. This would include the reporting of mistakes that have been consciously suppressed by the person responsible for the error. Hofmann (2002a) recommends that executives regularly obtain employee perceptions on the following matters:

- Does the organization allow, within reasonable limits, the administrative freedom to fail or is the fear of potential criticism so great that managers rarely exercise initiative?
- Do individuals feel comfortable disclosing management mistakes? What will these individuals do if certain errors are made? What have they done in the past?
- Are identifiable resources available to provide constructive advice when mistakes are made? Who can staff members consult if they are uncertain of what to do?
- Is there an external entity they can turn to if internal lines are blocked?
- Have respondents encountered retributions when mistakes have been reported or disclosed?

In each of the case examples described in Boxes 13.2, 13.3, and 13.4, there was insularity in decision-making processes. In contrast, Hofmann (2002a) suggests that a mature ethical reasoning process is characterized by collaboration and a systematic methodology.

Accountability for Organizational Culture

The CEO and executive management team express and communicate the organization's values through their individual and group behaviour as well as through policies and decisions. The National Steering Committee on Patient Safety, established in 2001, confirmed the relationship between leadership, management, and patient safety and identified the following requirements:

- Place patient safety at the top of the leadership and management priority list.
- Promote a culture of patient safety in health care.
- Create an accountability framework for patient safety.

The committee was supported by Health Canada, eight provincial/territorial ministries of health, and 26 Canadian health care organizations. Its report, published in September 2002, acknowledges that the health care system is a highly complex, integrated and interdependent environment in which the elements of structure, process, and outcomes all play a role in achieving patient safety. Five categories of adverse events are described: (a) medications, (b) medical devices, (c) nosocomial infections, (d) medical interventions, and (e) broader systems issues. A model is presented to illustrate how broader systems issues, termed "blunt end or underlying causes," influence adverse events. The model is reproduced in Figure 13.4.

This model incorporates the *sharp and blunt end* theory that has been accepted and broadly applied in various industries and in health care. At the *sharp end* of the continuum of adverse events are the activities and interactions of practitioners with patients; the search for fault is often conducted here. The demands, resources, and constraints that create the

Figure 13.4. Sharp- and Blunt-End Influences on Adverse Events

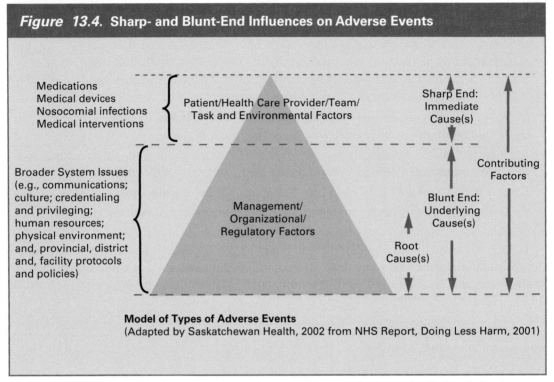

Model of Types of Adverse Events
(Adapted by Saskatchewan Health, 2002 from NHS Report, Doing Less Harm, 2001)

Source: From *Building a Safer System: A National Integrated Strategy for Improving Patient Safety in Canadian Health Care,* by the National Steering Committee on Patient Safety, 2002. Used with permission. Retrieved January 10, 2004, from http://rcpsc.medical.org/publications/building_a_safer_system_e.pdf.

work environment where clinicians work originate at the *blunt end,* which is the domain of regulators, administrators, policy makers, and technology suppliers and is remote from clinical care. Human factor engineers make the point that "the ability of sharp-end practitioners to avoid adverse events or near misses in which a patient has a narrow escape from injury or death depends directly or indirectly on a host of blunt-end factors rather than on the isolated error of human practitioners" (National Steering Committee on Patient Safety, 2002, p. 8).

There are many different ways that these broader systems issues can affect the number and types of adverse events associated with the delivery of health care. Fourteen issues are discussed in the report. Several of the issues are the direct result of decisions by senior health system leaders about the structure and culture of their organizations, as exemplified below:

- Continual restructuring and non-stop change compromise the organizational ability to identify issues and implement timely and appropriate strategies to address deficiencies in a coordinated manner.

- A culture of blame and many traditional and hierarchical organizational structures stifle the reporting of adverse events and any follow-up quality improvement discussions.

The committee concluded that broader system support and leadership is needed to conduct analyses of the root causes of adverse events, to identify the latent conditions and contributing factors that underlie variations in the performance of health organizations, and to develop and implement recommendations that will minimize the likelihood of recurrence. This will require that health system leaders acknowledge principles and recommendations for improving safety in the health care system. As individuals, leaders are responsible for creating a "culture of safety." This necessitates learning from what is already known in other sectors, such as the airline industry, and promoting appropriate disclosure of safety issues to patients, the public, health care personnel, and government. Leaders are also responsible for encouraging partnerships among all consumers and providers of care, which will require that the health care system become more flexible and less hierarchical in its structure.

The extent of renewed focus on issues of patient safety and leadership accountability was illustrated by the program of the National Conference of the Canadian College of Health Service Executives in 2003 (Devitt & McLellan, 2003; Etchells & O'Neill, 2003; Leape, 2003; Major, O'Callahan, & Donaldson, 2003; Nicklin, et al., 2004; Norton & Baker, 2003; Saxe-Braithwaite & Kopetsky, 2003; Smith, Rowe, & Clive, 2003). Of particular interest was a paper by Postl (2003) that specifically addressed actions in progress at the Winnipeg Health Sciences Centre to implement Justice Sinclair's recommendations for procedural protection for whistle-blowers. It has become obvious that specific leadership actions and organizational processes, including protection for individuals who dissent or who identify and report concerns, are necessary to achieve accountability and safety in the health system.

Anticipative, consultative, and participative qualities are needed to improve the quality of organizational decision making. Greenspan (2002) pointed out that failures can occur in performance, judgment, or ethics. He noted that

> Weighing risks and rewards openly is the hallmark of a culture that encourages good judgment and does not punish mistakes that are engendered within the participatory management process. Actions that are taken in response to judgment failures should first assess the environment and culture of decision-making within the organization (p. 38).

The key to minimizing the frequency and magnitude of executive mistakes is to create and sustain an organizational culture that encourages genuine candor and timely disclosure (Hofmann, 2002b). When individual executives and their organizations make mistakes there is a clear ethical obligation to disclose them. Hofmann points out that at the macro level, where the CEO (guided by the board) manages the organization's priorities, relations with the outside world, and strategic opportunities, the CEO's ego and lack of objectivity may interfere with the ability to recognize and evaluate a major error. At the micro, or operating level, at which the CEO establishes the organizational climate, makes decisions, and influences and monitors the decisions made by others, there is less excuse exist for failing to acknowledge and disclose mistakes (Hofmann, 2002a). A key principle of disclosure is that those in authority should promptly disclose mistakes to the people most affected by them. Such disclosure can increase organizational credibility and reduce financial risk.

Overcoming Insular Decision Making in Health Service Organizations

The Groupthink Phenomenon

The examples, research, and expert sources cited in this chapter highlight a persistent lack of transparency in the decision-making and administrative processes of health service organizations. Although understandable in terms of history and tradition, this problem exposes patients, individual health professionals, and health service organizations to risk, as illustrated by the three case examples in Boxes 13.2, 13.3, and 13.4. In each case, the actions or inactions of administrative authorities led to intense public criticism and outrage, the maltreatment of individuals and groups, and costly government inquiries. These outcomes are predictable when considered in light of the *groupthink* phenomenon.

Groupthink was originally conceptualized by Janis in 1972 to illuminate and explain certain historical fiascos in US foreign policy. The theory suggests that decision makers fell victim to the groupthink syndrome—they constituted highly cohesive groups that displayed a forceful tendency toward concurrence that led the group to uncritically decide upon faulty courses of action. The groupthink phenomenon was extensively re-examined from an interdisciplinary perspective by t'Hart in 1994. Groupthink theory helps to explain why the problem of insularity is so serious and how it can be prevented. Table 13.3 summarizes the predictable symptoms and consequences of groupthink.

Groupthink is not usually a problem in situations of routine decision making or in predictable emergencies. Rather, it occurs in situations where the stakes are high and standard solutions are lacking. In unconventional emergencies, where there is a knowledge vacuum, cohesiveness and insularity in a decision-making group may increase efficiency but also presents a particular danger (t'Hart, 1994, p. 19).

Where conditions of insularity and groupthink prevail, individuals who continue to ask questions, raise issues of evidence or ethics, or who express dissenting opinions or moral reservations are often subjected to accusations of disloyalty and to punishment. This is usually referred to as whistle-blowing, defined more specifically as a warning issued by a member or former member of an organization to the public about a serious danger created or concealed within the organization that the individual reporting the danger has unsuccessfully tried to correct using all appropriate channels within the organization (Fletcher, Sorrell, & Ciprano Silva, 1998). The historical record of the health system in dealing with internally reported concerns and dissent is an unfortunate one (Anderson, 1990; Fletcher et al., 1998; Rohland, 2002; Ahern & McDonald, 2002). There will continue to be social concern about this issue.

Table 13.3 Groupthink: Symptoms and Consequences

Symptoms	Consequences
Incomplete survey of alternatives and objectives	Overestimation of the group
	Illusion of invulnerability
Failure to examine risks of the preferred choice	Belief in inherent morality of the group
	Collective rationalizations
Failure to re-appraise initially rejected alternatives	Stereotypes of out groups
	Pressures toward uniformity
Poor information search	Self-censorship
Selective bias in processing information	Direct pressure on dissenters
Failure to work out contingency plans	Self-appointed mind guards
	Low probability of successful outcome

Source: Adapted from *Groupthink in Government: A Study of Small Groups and Policy Failure* (pp. 21–22), by P. t'Hart, 1994, Baltimore, MD: John Hopkins University Press.

Preventing Groupthink

Experts have suggested specific ways of preventing groupthink. Leaders of groups must establish and reinforce an open climate for giving and accepting criticism of ideas. At the outset of a group discussion, leaders can establish a climate of impartiality and open inquiry by refraining from stating their personal preferences. They can also set up parallel groups or subgroups to work under different leaders and report back. Bringing in outside experts to present new information or to challenge the views of the core members can also improve the quality of decision making. Leaders can establish and exemplify decision-making norms in which each member of the group is expected to privately discuss current issues and options with trusted associates outside the group and report back on their reactions. Decision making can be improved if each member of a group is expected to act as a critical evaluator of the group's course of action. Procedural protection of the right to say no for "motivated dissenters" and protection for whistle-blowers are two other ways of preventing groupthink. The difficulty of implementing such measures was acknowledged by t'Hart (1994), who stated the following:

> There is no easy way to streamline the processes of organizational and inter-organizational problem-sensing, information processing, and choice. There is no simple, if any method to get individual officials to enact well-trained skills and professional and ethical norms, to escape the logic of collective action, and to manage bureaucratic complexity to make organizational behavior more morally responsible. The best one can do is to continue to try and understand the conditions of success and failure, to rethink standards of evaluating the quality of government, and to produce policy-relevant theories to make improvements (p. 295).

CEOs are responsible for the quality and outcomes of organizational decision making and their leadership behaviour is a key determinant of the quality of decisions. Quality management reviews and audits can provide some reassurance to the CEO that "best practices" for decision making are being followed. Critical tasks illustrating best practices for high-quality decision making are summarized in Box 13.5.

Box 13.5

Critical Tasks for High-Quality Decision Making

(a) Canvass a wide range of available courses of action.

(b) Survey the full range of objectives to be fulfilled and the values implicated by the choice.

(c) Carefully weigh the risks, costs, and benefits of each alternative.

(d) Search intensively for new relevant information to enable further evaluation of each alternative.

(e) Seriously consider and assimilate new information or expert judgment, even if it is critical of the initially preferred course of action.

(f) Re-examine the positive and negative consequences of all known alternatives before making a final choice.

(g) Make detailed provisions for implementing the chosen option.

(h) Make contingency plans to be used if various known risks materialize.

Source: Adapted from *Groupthink in Government: A Study of Small Groups and Policy Failure* (p. 8), by P. t'Hart, 1994, Baltimore, MD: John Hopkins University Press.

Leadership Implications

Certain structural characteristics of an organization increase the likelihood of groupthink. These characteristics include (a) insulation of the decision-making group, (b) absence of a tradition or culture of impartial leadership, (c) absence of norms requiring methodological procedures for decision making, and (d) lack of diversity in the social background and ideology within the decision-making group (t'Hart, 1994). When a decision-making group has these characteristics, it may be unable to make high-quality decisions.

Experts agree on a number of issues about how accountability in the health system can and must be improved. Prompt and appropriate disclosure of mistakes, including executive mistakes, is among the actions needed. Because organizations often take punitive action toward whistle-blowers, there is a growing consensus that confirms the need to protect the rights of individuals employed within the health system who express concerns or who internally dissent.

There is also growing social pressure to improve accountability at what is called the "blunt end" of the health system, where administrative policies, decisions, and behaviour affect the ability of clinicians to safely care for patients and which ultimately carries financial and reputational risk for the organization and the health system as a whole. While licensed professionals can be held individually accountable through the disciplinary processes of their professions, senior executives and many others who participate in the delivery of health services are not similarly regulated or obligated. However, experts have recommended that mistakes, including executive mistakes, must be promptly disclosed and that individual executives must be held accountable for incompetence, deceit, abusive behaviour, or other unsanctioned activity.

The case examples, research, and expert sources cited in this chapter highlight the problem of insularity, or lack of transparency, in the decision-making and administrative processes of health service organizations. This problem exposes patients, health professionals, and health service organizations to risk. In general, errors are best prevented and dealt with when there is not a culture of blame. However, there is growing public consensus that senior executives and boards of governors must be held accountable for their actions and decisions.

Power, status, and information differentials have made it particularly difficult for nurses' observations, concerns, and expertise to be included in corporate decision making (Picard, 2000; Kritek, 1995; Nicklin, 2003; Tremblay, 2003; Weir, 2003; Shamian, Laschinger, & O'Brien-Pallas, 2003). The need to overcome these barriers in order to improve the quality of organizational decision making is confirmed specifically in the public reports of the three cases described in this chapter and more broadly (Benveniste, 1977; Campbell, 2002; Chaleff, 1995; Greenspan, 2002). A study conducted to assess how citizen engagement can contribute to improved accountability in the Canadian health system concluded that public expectations of improving the accountability of the system are high, but that "information exchange, power sharing and partnership are threatening to a policy sector dominated by professional expertise, in the clinical and management domain" (Abelson & Gauvin, 2004, p. 41). Hofmann (2002b) concluded that

the key to minimizing both the frequency and magnitude of executive mistakes is to create and sustain an organizational culture that encourages genuine candor and timely disclosure, along with clearly established decision-making processes and performance standards (p. 48).

Summary

- Accountability for health services and the health system has been identified as an issue of high priority and urgency in Canadian public policy discourse.
- Various definitions of accountability include the following elements: establishment of a relationship, agreed upon responsibility, answerability, judgments about performance, and processes for sanction or correction.
- Four mechanisms of accountability are a legal approach, a public reporting approach, a citizen governance approach, and citizen engagement.

- Leaders of health agencies have been granted a special standing in society, and by virtue of this extraordinary level of trust, they are expected to make decisions using the highest possible ethical and moral judgments.

- Risk management is concerned with minimizing the liability of an organization by preventing mistakes or minimizing their consequences. While everyone has a role to play in risk management, it is a management responsibility to create structures and processes for risk management. Documentation practices and standards are an important mechanism for minimizing risk. Loss and liability can be minimized through proactive and comprehensive reporting processes.

- Processes for managing the financial resources and minimizing financial risk originate in the professional standards of the accounting profession. General principles of financial management, general accounting principles, and standardized practices for organizing accounts are mechanisms for achieving financial accountability. Financial risk is minimized by organizational policies based on the principle of division of duties and designed to prevent unauthorized or inappropriate expenditures and the possibility of fraud. One-over-one approval of financial transactions and various levels of auditing are other standard mechanisms for financial risk management.

- The balanced scorecard approach integrates risk prevention and management activities with other organizational processes by incorporating four perspectives: (a) customer perspective, (b) internal business perspective, (c) innovation and learning perspective, and (d) the financial perspective.

- Situations of emergency and crisis carry high levels of risk and require planning for emergency preparedness in conventional disasters. In unconventional emergencies, such as the initial SARS outbreak, leaders must manage the emergency within a knowledge vacuum. A pre-existing culture of best decision-making practices in normal times enhances the likelihood of good decision-making in unconventional emergencies.

- Individual health system leaders are expected to be competent and accountable. Benchmarks for assessing executive competence and accountability are found in the administrative competencies identified and examined by the Canadian College of Health Service Executives and a typology of executive mistakes published in a leading journal of health care administration.

- Senior executives are responsible for the culture of the health agencies they lead, particularly for creating the conditions that enable a culture of safety. "Blunt-end" or underlying causes that arise from the demands, resources, constraints, and policies in the domain of administration and organizational policy and culture influence the clinical work environment and the occurrence of adverse events.

- Insularity and lack of transparency have been identified as common features in the decision making within hospitals and the health system in general. Whistle-blowers have usually been dealt with punitively. These structural conditions predict the likelihood that the quality of decision making will be compromised by the groupthink phenomenon which can lead cohesive and insulated decision-making groups to decide upon faulty courses of action.

- Many experts agree on the need for greater inclusiveness and transparency of process in health care policy and decision making. Since traditional practices, vested interests, and power relations make this difficult to achieve, experts have also identified the need to protect whistle-blowers.

- There is growing social pressure for accountability at what is called the "blunt end" of the health system, where administrative policies, decisions, and behaviour affect the ability of clinicians to safely care for patients and may create financial and reputational risk for the organization and the health system as a whole.

- Citizen engagement as a mechanism of accountability presents challenges to the long-standing power relations that characterize health system decision making in Canada; so far, it has not been widely used. This can be expected to change and will require that individual leaders and health agencies adopt more inclusive and transparent decision-making processes.

Applying the Knowledge in this Chapter

Exercise

1. Review the policies for unusual incident or occurrence reporting within your workplace or a health service organization in your community, and answer the following questions:
   a) Are all staff and physicians expected to report unusual incidents when they occur? If not, which categories of staff are exempt from reporting?
   b) Are other health professionals and staff expected to report incidents involving physicians? If not, how are unusual incidents or safety concerns involving physicians dealt with?

2. Chose a health service organization in your community. Find out whether the organization has a policy to protect whistle-blowers. If so, review the policy. If not, find out what channels should be used by a registered nurse who feels obligated to report a patient safety concern.

3. Obtain information about the committee structure of the organization where you work or another health service organization. Answer the following questions:
   a) Are there opportunities for participation of external stakeholders (i.e., processes for meaningful citizen engagement)?
   b) What avenues are available for internal stakeholder participation within the organizational and committee structure?
   c) What opportunities are available for discussing issues of concern to registered nurses?

4. Consider the cases presented in Boxes 13.2, 13.3, and 13.4. For each case, answer the following questions:
   a) Refer to the executive competencies summarized in Table 13.1. Which of the competencies are most relevant to the case?
   b) Refer to the executive mistakes summarized in Table 13.2. Were any of these mistakes made in the case?

Resources

evolve Internet Resources

Canadian Comprehensive Auditing Foundation (CCAF):
  www.ccaf-fcvi.com/english/
CCAF Mission and Strategic Profile:
  www.ccaf-fcvi.com/english/visitors/about/index.html
Canadian Institute of Chartered Accountants:
  www.cica.ca/index.cfm/ci_id/17150/la_id/1.htm
Auditing and Assurance Standards Oversight:
  www.cica.ca/index.cfm/ci_id/204/la_id/1.htm
Public Sector Accounting Standards:
  www.cica.ca/index.cfm/ci_id/225/la_id/1.htm
New technology standard to enhance corporate reporting transparency:
  www.cica.ca/index.cfm/ci_id/20172/la_id/1.htm

Further Reading

References related to the cases presented in Boxes 13.2 and 13.3 are provided here for readers who are interested in learning more about these real-life examples.

Contamination of the Canadian Blood Supply

Anthony, L. & Oziewicz, E. (2002, November 21). Victims hope for justice and expanded compensation. The *Globe and Mail*, p. A4.

Austen, I. (1996, November/December). Blood bath. *Elm Street*, pp. 23-28.

Kennedy, M. (2002, November 21). Accused face decade in prison. *Edmonton Journal*, pp. A1, A2.

Makin, K. (2002, November 21). Why Crown's prosecution may be long, expensive and complex. *The Globe and Mail*, p. A4.

McCarthy, S. & Laghi, B. (2002, November 21). Ottawa rejects Tory call to reconsider package. *The Globe and Mail*, p. A4.

Picard, A. (2002, November 21a). A painful step in Canada's healing process. *The Globe and Mail*, pp. A1, A6.

Picard, A. (2002, November 21b). RCMP lay 32 charges in tainted-blood case. *The Globe and Mail*, pp. A1, A6.

Thorne, D. (2002, November 21). It's time charges were laid: Hep C victims. *Edmonton Journal*, p. A2.

Tibbetts, J. (2002, November 21). No further aid for blood victims. *Edmonton Journal*, p. A2.

Conflicts of Interest between a Medical Scientist and a Drug Company

Canada's Voice for Academic Staff (CAUT). (2001, November 21). Report vindicates Dr. Nancy Olivieri. *Bulletin Online, 48*(9). Retrieved January 16, 2004, from http://www.caut.ca/english/bulletin/2001_nov/default.asp

MedicalEthics.ca. (2001). Patient safety, conflict of interest, and academic integrity: The Olivieri affair. Retrieved January 16, 2004, from http://www.medicalethics.ca/olivieri/

news@UofT. (2002, November 12). Joint statement concerning Dr. Nancy Olivieri, Sick Kids Hospital, and U of T. Retrieved January 16, 2004, from http://www.newsandevents.utoronto.ca/misc/olivieri.htm

Thompson, J., Baird, P., & Downie, J. (2001). Report of the Committee of Inquiry on the case involving Dr. Nancy Olivieri, the Hospital for Sick Children, the University of Toronto, and Apotex Inc. Retrieved January 16, 2004, from http://www.caut.ca/english/issues/acadfreedom/olivieri.asp

Valpy, M. (1998, Holiday). Science friction: Dr. Nancy Olivieri discovered that mixing business and medicine can be dangerous. *Elm Street,* 26–39.

Viens, A.M., & Savulescu, J. (2004, February). Introduction to the Olivieri symposium. *Journal of Medical Ethics, 30*(1), 1–7. Retrieved January 16, 2004, from http://jme.bmjjournals.com/cgi/reprint/30/1/1.pdf

Wente, M. (1999, December 23). Medicine, morals and money. *The Globe and Mail.*

References

Abelson, J. & Gauvin, F.P. (2004, April). Engaging citizens: One route to health care accountability. *Health Care Accountability Papers* (2). Ottawa, ON: Canadian Policy Research Networks.

Ahern, K., & McDonald, S. (2002). The beliefs of nurses who were involved in a whistle-blowing event. *Journal of Advanced Nursing, 38*(3), 303–309.

Allen, P. (1986). *The development of a risk management program.* Ottawa, ON: Canadian Hospital Association.

Anderson v. Chasney [1949], 57 Man. R 343; (1949), 4 DLR 71 (C.A.); aff'd (1950), 4 DLR 223 (SCC).

Andersen, S. (1990). Patient advocacy and whistle-blowing in nursing: Help for the helpers. *Nursing Forum, 25*(3), 5–13.

Baker, R.G., & Pink, G.H. (1995). A balanced scorecard for Canadian hospitals. *Healthcare Management Forum, 8*(4), 7–13.

Benveniste, G. (1977). *The politics of expertise* (2nd ed.). San Francisco: Boyd & Fraser.

Brown, P. (2004). Not documented! Not done! *ASBN Update, 8*(1), 7, 27.

Campbell, C.S. (2002). Preventive ethics and cultivating integrity. *Frontiers of Health Services Management, 18*(3), 41–46.

Campbell, J.A. (2004, April 15). *The SARS Commission interim report: SARS and public health in Toronto.* Toronto, ON: Government of Ontario, Minister of Health. Retrieved April 22, 2004, from http://www.sarscommission.ca/report/Interim_Report.pdf

Canada's Voice for Academic Staff (CAUT). (2001, November 21). Report vindicates Dr. Nancy Olivieri. *Bulletin Online, 48*(9). Retrieved January 16, 2004, from http://www.caut.ca/english/bulletin/2001_nov/default.asp

Canadian College of Health Service Executives (CCHSE). (2003). *Proffesional Competencies,* Ottawa, ON: CCHSE. Retrived November 14, 2003, from http://www.cchse.org/c_procom.htm.

Canadian College of Health Service Executives (CCHSE). (2003). *Position statement on the health executive's role in patient safety.* Ottawa, ON: CCHSE. Retrieved January 6, 2004, from http://www.cchse.org/PositionStatement-PatientSafety.pdf

Canadian Comprehensive Auditing Foundation (CCAF). (1992). *Reporting on effectiveness: The experience of the Queen Elizabeth Hospital.* Ottawa, ON: CCAF.

Chaleff, I. (1995). *The courageous follower: Standing up to and for our leaders.* San Francisco: Berrett-Koehler Publishers, Inc.

Devitt, R. & McLellan, B.A. (2003, February 13). *Improved patient safety through lessons learned.* Paper presented at the 5th Joint National Conference on Quality in Health Care, Canadian College of Health Service Executives, Toronto, Ontario, Canada.

Dickens, B. (1993). Implications for health professionals' legal liability. *Health Law Journal, 1,* 1–12.

Eisenberg, T. & Macey, J.R. (2003). Was Arthur Andersen different? An empirical examination of major accounting firms' audits of large clients. Working paper, Yale Law School, Center for Law, Economics and Public Policy Research Paper No. 287.

Etchells, E., & O'Neill, C. (2003, February 13). *Implementing a patient safety service.* Paper presented at the 5th Joint National Conference on Quality in Health Care, Canadian College of Health Service Executives, Toronto, Ontario, Canada.

Fletcher, J., Sorrell, J., & Cipriano Silva, M. (1998). Whistleblowing as a failure of organizational ethics. *Online Journal of Issues in Nursing.* Retrieved January 10, 2004, from http://www.nursingworld.org/ojin/topic8/topic8_3.htm

Fooks, C. & Maslove, L. (2004, March). Rhetoric, fallacy or dream? Accountability to citizens in Canadian health care. *Health Care Accountability Papers.* (1). Ottawa, ON: Canadian Policy Research Networks.

Friedman, L.H. (2002). [Editorial]. *Frontiers of Health Services Management, 18*(3), 1–2.

Gardner, L., & Russell, A. (1989). *The concept of accountability: A discussion paper.* [Mimeograph]. Edmonton, AB: Policy Development Division, Alberta Health.

Greenspan, B. (2002). Protecting the community's trust: Coping with executive mistakes. *Frontiers of Health Services Management, 18*(3), 35–40.

Hofmann, P.B. (2002a). Morally managing executive mistakes. *Frontiers of Health Services Management, 18*(3), 3–38.

Hofmann, P.B. (2002b). Reply: Reconciling different approaches to addressing executive mistakes. *Frontiers of Health Services Management, 18*(3), 47-49.

How bad was Andersen? An audit of leading auditors suggests that Arthur Andersen was not unique. (2003, December 6). *The Economist, 369*(8353), 68-69.

Kritek, P.B. (1995). Nursing: Negotiating at an uneven table. In L.J. Marcus, B.C. Dorn, et al. (Eds.), *Renegotiating health care: Resolving conflict to build collaboration* (pp. 207–236). Toronto, ON: W.B. Saunders.

Leape, L.L. (2003, February 13). *Accountability: The new imperative for leaders in quality care.* Paper presented at the 5th Joint National Conference on Quality in Health Care, Canadian College of Health Service Executives, Toronto, Ontario, Canada.

Lynch, T., & Cox, P. (2003). Emergency management of SARS: A quantum leap or a paradigm shift? *Risk Management in Canadian Health Care, 5*(6), 65–76.

Major, M., O'Callahan, T., & Donaldson, C. (2003, February 13). *Medication management: Toward a better system.* Paper presented at the 5th Joint National Conference on Quality in Health Care, Canadian College of Health Service Executives, Toronto, Ontario, Canada.

MedicalEthics.ca. (2001). *Patient safety, conflict of interest, and academic integrity: The Olivieri affair.* Retrieved January 16, 2004, from http://www.medicalethics.ca/olivieri/

Meyer v. Gordon (1981), 17 CCLT 1 (BCSC).

Mintzberg, H. (1997). Toward healthier hospitals. *Health Care Management Review, 22*(4), 9–18.

Mrazek, M. (1994). Risk management. In J. Hibberd & D. Smith (Eds.), *Nursing management in Canada* (pp. 554–573). Toronto, ON: W.B. Saunders.

National Steering Committee on Patient Safety. (2002, September). *Building a safer system: A national integrated strategy for improving patient safety in Canadian health care.* Retrieved January 10, 2004, from http://rcpsc.medical.org/publications/building_a_safer_system_e.pdf

news@UofT. (2002, November 12). *Joint statement concerning Dr. Nancy Olivieri, Sick Kids Hospital, and U of T.* Retrieved January 16, 2004, from http://www.newsandevents.utoronto.ca/misc/olivieri.htm

Nicklin, W. (2003, February 13). *Canadian nurses describe their perceptions of patient safety in teaching hospitals: Wake up call!* Paper presented at the 5th Joint National Conference on Quality in Health Care, Canadian College of Health Service Executives, Toronto, Ontario, Canada.

Nicklin, W., Mass, H., Affonso, D.D., O'Connor, P., Ferguson-Paré, M., Jeffs, L., et al. (2004). Patient safety culture and leadership within Canada's academic health science centres: Towards the development of a collaborative position paper. *Nursing Leadership, 17*(1), 22–34.

Norton, P.G., & Baker, G.R. (2003, February 14). *Creating a safer future for Canadian health care*. Paper presented at the 5th Joint National Conference on Quality in Health Care, Canadian College of Health Service Executives, Toronto, Ontario, Canada.

Oliver, K. (2002, December). *Use of the balanced scorecard as a framework for a total quality management program*. Paper presented at the Improving Performance Measurement in Healthcare Conference, Canadian Institute, Toronto, Ontario, Canada.

Paras, A. (2004). *Administrative behavior in two cases of unexpected children's deaths*. Unpublished master's thesis, University of Alberta, Edmonton, Alberta, Canada.

Picard, A. (2000). *Critical care: Canadian nurses speak for change*. Toronto, ON: Harper Collins.

Picard, E.I., & Robertson, G.B. (1996). Medical records. In E.I. Picard & G.B. Robertson (Eds.), *Legal liability of doctors and hospitals in Canada* (3rd ed., pp. 399–419). Toronto, ON: Carswell Thomson Professional.

Postl, B. (2003, February 13). *Learning from our experiences*. Paper presented at the 5th Joint National Conference on Quality in Health Care, Canadian College of Health Service Executives, Toronto, Ontario, Canada.

Rohland, P. (2002). Code language: What student nurses are taught about whistleblowing. *Revolution, 3*(6), 26–29.

Saxe-Braithwaite, M., & Kopetsky, D. (2003, February 13). *Walking the walk: Practical tools for a culture of safety*. Paper presented at the 5th Joint National Conference on Quality in Health Care, Canadian College of Health Service Executives, Toronto, Ontario, Canada.

Shamian, J., Laschinger, H., & O'Brien-Pallas, L. (2003, February 13). *An international examination of the cost and impact of turnover on patient safety and nurse outcomes*. Paper presented at the 5th Joint National Conference on Quality in Health Care, Canadian College of Health Service Executives, Toronto, Ontario, Canada.

Sinclair, C.M. (2001, May). *Report of the Manitoba pediatric cardiac surgery inquest: An inquiry into twelve deaths at the Winnipeg Health Sciences Centre in 1994*. Winnipeg, MB: Provincial Court of Manitoba.

Smith, L., Rowe, D., & Clive, B. (2003, February 13). *Patient safety: It's our business*. Paper presented at the 5th Joint National Conference on Quality in Health Care, Canadian College of Health Service Executives, Toronto, Ontario, Canada.

Stock, R.G., & Lefroy, S.E. (1988). *Risk management: A practical framework for Canadian health care facilities*. Ottawa, ON: Canadian Hospital Association.

t'Hart, P. (1994). *Groupthink in government: A study of small groups and policy failure*. Baltimore, MD: John Hopkins University Press.

Thompson, J., Baird, P., & Downie, J. (2001). Report of the Committee of Inquiry on the case involving Dr. Nancy Olivieri, the Hospital for Sick Children, the University of Toronto, and Apotex Inc. Retrieved September 10, 2002, from http://www.caut.ca/english/issues/acadfreedom/olivieri.asp

Tremblay, L. (2003, February 13). *Caring for the elderly: Esther's voice*. Paper presented at the 5th Joint National Conference on Quality in Health Care, Canadian College of Health Service Executives, Toronto, Ontario, Canada.

Valpy, M. (1998, Holiday). Science friction: Dr. Nancy Olivieri discovered that mixing business and medicine can be dangerous. *Elm Street*, pp. 26-39.

Viens, A.M., & Savulescu, J. (2004, February). Introduction to the Olivieri symposium. *Journal of Medical Ethics, 30*(1), 1–7. Retrieved March 1, 2004, from http://jme.bmjjournals.com/cgi/reprint/30/1/1.pdf

Weir, C. (2003, February 13). *Esther's voice: A story of a health system failure and hope for the future*. Paper presented at the 5th Joint National Conference on Quality in Health Care, Canadian College of Health Service Executives, Toronto, Ontario, Canada.

Wente, M. (1999, December 23). Medicine, morals and money. *The Globe and Mail*.

In Section IV, the discussion focuses on leadership and its impact on the nursing profession. Professions depend on their leaders for vision and intelligence in identifying critical issues and for resourcefulness in ensuring the development and maintenance of the discipline and responsible service to the public. The chapters dedicated to leadership theory will be of interest to all nurses because nurses engage in leadership activities wherever they practice. It is important for undergraduate students to identify their leadership potential as they will undoubtedly find themselves in leadership positions as they enter the profession as registered nurses.

This section also includes other topics of importance to the delivery of nursing services, namely professional practice governance, evidence-based practice, nursing information and outcomes, and nursing administration research. Undergraduate nurses should have a general knowledge of these topics as they will be exposed to them from time to time in their working lives and will be expected to have a grasp of the issues and, indeed, to contribute to the continuing development of these professional activities. Other readers, such as experienced registered nurses, graduate students, and managers, who already have an understanding of these areas, may find the content a baseline resource for further reading and development of more in-depth knowledge.

Chapter 14, *Leadership and Leaders*, contains an overview of the history of the development of leadership theory. The principal characteristics of leadership are compared to those of management because it is important to understand the distinction between these two concepts. Skilled leaders are not necessarily good managers, and managers are not necessarily effective leaders. However, both leadership and management can be learned and developed. The profiles of six contemporary nurse leaders in Canada are presented throughout the chapter to illustrate the career paths, values, and achievements of successful leaders. Nurses in these and other strategic positions can serve as advocates and role models and contribute to the improvement of the health system as well as the advancement of the nursing profession.

In Chapter 15, *Ethical Dimensions of Leadership*, Storch notes that almost every action a manager takes involves ethics. She discusses the scope of ethical responsibility and provides four case examples of typical situations that might arise in the workplace. Nurses who deal with such situations will undoubtedly want to reflect on her analysis of ethical theories as well as the concepts of ethical fitness and the building of a moral community in the workplace.

Chapter 16 focuses on the complex relationship between *Health Agencies and Self-Governing Professions*, illustrating how these professions are accommodated within bureaucracies administered by boards of trustees. The discussion is purposely limited to physicians and nurses in acute care hospitals because decision-making structures and processes in these settings are more complex than in other agencies. There are significant differences in the organizational arrangements and autonomy of physicians and nurses. Models of professional practice of both medicine and nursing are presented, and concepts such as medical privileges and shared governance are discussed. This information will enable nurses at all levels to understand why and how it is possible for decisions made by hospital-based physicians to have a direct impact on the practice of nursing. If medical decisions and practices do not enable safe nursing practice, clinical nurses and nursing leaders must know how to work within organizational structures and processes to assure that patients' needs are met and their safety protected.

The application of new knowledge to clinical and administrative practice is now a concern of all health professionals and leaders. Chapter 17, *Promoting Evidence-Based Practice,* deals with the professional imperative that decisions about nursing interventions be based on scientific evidence and an established body of knowledge. Clinicians must be knowledgeable and skilled in the use of research findings, and the environments in which nurses work must support a spirit of inquiry and be receptive to change, including the adoption of proven best practices in patient care. Leaders in the work setting are responsible for creating an environment that allows research and its dissemination to flourish.

The problem of invisible nursing work is discussed in Chapter 18, *Nursing Information and Outcomes.* Tourangeau explains that much of what nurses do has not been recorded in systematic ways that support the study of nursing outcomes. Although clinical nursing responsibilities include recording patient data and charting, only limited information about nursing care is ultimately recorded in the permanent health records. Much discussion in the literature has been devoted to questions of what nursing information should be collected, who should collect it, where to store it, and who should maintain it. When changes are proposed in nursing services that will have a known impact on outcomes of care, leaders in the profession must have access to accurate sources of nursing and health information in order to inform policy decision makers.

Nursing Administration Research, addressed in Chapter 19, may not seem relevant to undergraduate nursing students, but it is of great significance to the efficient and effective deployment of their services once they enter the workforce. Heather K. Spence Laschinger, PhD, explains the importance of basing administrative decisions on the best available evidence, including research findings. She holds a number of nationally funded research grants and leads a major program of nursing administration research at the University of Western Ontario. Studies in this field can be grouped into the following areas: nursing productivity, quality of care, work environment quality, patient outcomes, and studies of the relations between these factors. This chapter will be of interest to nurses in advocacy positions and senior administrative roles who are interested in identifying the best practices in the deployment of nursing human resources.

This section concludes with Chapter 20, *Leadership Challenges and Directions*, written by one of Canada's most prominent nursing leaders and recipient of the prestigious 2004 Jeanne Mance Award from the Canadian Nurses Association. Ginette Lemire Rodger maintains a global perspective in her discussion of nursing leadership, and she suggests that for the 21st century we need leaders at all levels, international, national, provincial and local, who have four important characteristics: vision, knowledge, confidence, and visibility.

14 LEADERSHIP AND LEADERS

Judith M. Hibberd, Donna Lynn Smith, and Dorothy M. Wylie

Learning Objectives

In this chapter, you will learn:

- Definitions of leadership and management and how these two processes are related
- The development of leadership theory and some well-known schools of thought on leadership
- The importance of visible and effective leadership in the nursing profession
- Issues in leadership research and educational preparation for leadership roles
- Career paths of eight Canadian nurses currently occupying strategic leadership positions in the health care system

The study of leadership and leaders reveals that in almost every field of endeavour, the search for effective and successful leaders is a constant concern. The immense body of research in this area continues to grow as social scientists attempt to understand the complexities of leadership and determine the characteristics required of individuals to succeed as leaders. The issue of leadership in health care becomes increasingly important in light of reforms and structural innovations in the Canadian health care system during the past decade. Financial constraints and changing organizational structures have placed additional strain on middle-and first-level managers, who must contend with advances on the clinical, technical, and information fronts, as well as emerging workforce issues such as shortages of physicians and professional nurses. It has been argued that a new kind of leadership in nursing is required for these turbulent times, but it is difficult to recruit people into leadership positions that may not be considered attractive to potential leaders (Tamlyn & Reilly, 2003; Ferguson-Paré, Mitchell, Perkin, & Stevenson, 2002).

Nursing is professional work that requires a basic understanding of leadership because leadership skills are exercised not only in daily interactions with clients, patients, and co-workers, but also in positions traditionally assumed to require managerial or executive expertise. Therefore, the aim of this chapter is to provide a general introduction to the topic of leadership.

Throughout the chapter, portraits of Canadian nurses occupying positions of strategic importance to health care are presented as exemplars of successful professional leadership. Their careers illustrate many of the concepts and ideas expressed in the literature on the individual criteria necessary for success as leaders. These leaders have agreed to describe the nature of their work, their educational preparation and career choices, and their major accomplishments. They have identified some of the people and circumstances that have influenced their careers as well as their values and thoughts about leadership itself.

What is Leadership?

Leadership is described and defined in many ways. Tannenbaum, Weschler, and Massarik (1961) describe it as "interpersonal influence, exercised in situation and directed, through the communication process, toward the attainment of a specified goal or goals" (p. 24). Burns (1978) states, "Leadership over human beings is exercised when persons with certain motives and purposes mobilize, in competition or conflict with others, institutional, political, psychological, and other resources so as to arouse, engage, and satisfy the motives of followers" (p. 18). Leaders are characterized by Nanus (1992) as those who "take charge, make things happen, dream dreams and then translate them into reality" (p. 10).

Regardless of the definition one might choose, essential to leadership is a process of involving people, gaining their commitment, and energizing them to participate in the tasks related to achieving mutual goals.

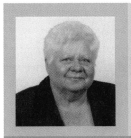

LEADERSHIP PROFILE *14.1*

Dorothy M. Wylie

Former Vice-President, Nursing
Toronto General Hospital

Dorothy Wylie is the Canadian nurse leader for whom a nursing leadership institute has been named. The Dorothy M. Wylie Nursing Leadership Institute was established in recognition of her innovative leadership in several senior positions in Ontario and her pioneering work in different facets of nursing leadership while she was a professor in the Faculty of Nursing at the University of Toronto (Simpson, Skelton-Green, Scott, & O'Brien-Pallas, 2002). Reflecting on her career, Dorothy writes:

> I have been retired from an active nursing career for nine years, although I don't believe you ever truly leave nursing. For me, the apex of my career was in 1987 when I started my own consulting business. In 1985, I completed a graduate program in Human Resource Development at the American University, Washington, DC. I was anxious to put my new skills into practice. This new career path at the age of 57 took a fair amount of courage; however, it turned out to be a rewarding and fulfilling experience.
>
> My leadership career began as a head nurse at New York Hospital, Cornell Medical Centre, New York, where I had the benefit of a wonderful supervisor as a mentor. While in New York, I also completed my baccalaureate degree and master's degree. It was a far cry from my "training days" at St. Michael's Hospital in Toronto. On return to Canada in 1969, there were few nurses prepared at the graduate level in nursing administration, so opportunities were endless. My first senior position was Director of Nursing at Sunnybrook Medical Centre. As a novice, the challenges were many, and I learnt along the way; fortunately, I had supportive senior management colleagues. Upgrading the staff and the establishment of the clinical nurse specialist role were highlights for me.
>
> The next career move was to Vice-President, Nursing at The Toronto General Hospital, an even more demanding and complex situation. There, I assembled a talented team of nursing directors who were mutually supportive and provided the strength to initiate change and influence practice. Leadership is not a one-man show—teamwork and the development of a critical mass of followers are essential to initiate and sustain change. My philosophy has always been to keep quality patient care at the forefront and to support the nurses in carrying out professional practice. To this end, mentoring and counselling nurses were important aspects of my role that provided much satisfaction during my career.
>
> I believe that nursing leaders need to participate in a wide range of activities beyond their place of employment. This led to my involvement with teaching activities at various universities, being past President of the Council of the College of Nurses of Ontario, and being past editor of the *Canadian Journal of Nursing Leadership*. I'm proud to have received the designation Fellow from Ryerson Polytechnic Institute, to be an Honourary Life Member of the Registered Nurses Association of Ontario, and to have my colleagues name a nursing leadership institute after me to prepare future nurse leaders.

Managers Versus Leaders

A manager's position is a designated organizational role carrying formal power within the hierarchy of the organization, but a leader's role can be assumed by anyone and does not require formal power or status. Therefore, managers and leaders are not one and the same; however, the effective manager is usually one who exercises effective leadership behaviour. Bennis (1989) identified 12 major differences between managers and leaders:

- The manager administers; the leader innovates.
- The manager is a copy; the leader is an original.
- The manager maintains; the leader develops.
- The manager focuses on systems and structure; the leader focuses on people.
- The manager relies on control; the leader inspires trust.
- The manager has a short-range view; the leader has a long-range perspective.
- The manager asks how and when; the leader asks what and why.
- The manager always has an eye on the bottom line; the leader has an eye on the horizon.
- The manager imitates; the leader originates.
- The manager accepts the status quo; the leader challenges it.
- The manager is the classic "good soldier"; the leader is his or her own person.
- The manager does things right; the leader does the right thing (p. 45).

It is important to keep in mind that Bennis's somewhat "black and white" distinction between leaders and managers is an analytical tool for understanding the differences between these two roles. In reality, there is no such a clear distinction. Successful managers use and apply leadership strategies, and effective leaders are mindful of the managerial implications of their initiatives and activities. The differences can be further illuminated in terms of focus and primary responsibility. According to Drucker (1996), management involves an obligation to achieve organizational goals, and increasingly those goals must be achieved through prudent use of human, material, and fiscal resources. Leadership, on the other hand, is about relationships with followers and influencing the process by which they jointly achieve organizational goals while striving for higher levels of quality and effectiveness.

In recent years, it has become politically popular to disparage the roles and contributions of managers. There have also been many well-publicized instances in which leaders in both private and public sector organizations have failed to exercise sound managerial judgment and skills, resulting in losses for stockholders and citizens. Leaders who are not effective managers sometimes become known within their organizations as "loose cannons" or "unguided missiles." Without the support of effective managers, leaders have difficulty fulfilling the obligations of leadership. If they ignore or become immersed in immediate and operational issues and problems, they will be unable to achieve strategic objectives successfully.

Effective leaders are constantly aware of strategic opportunities, and thus good leadership is often associated with change and development. Senge (1990) describes leaders as "designers, stewards and teachers" (p. 340). Leaders create a learning environment for themselves and others. The skills and competencies of both management and leadership can be learned, and, as will be seen later, this has implications for leadership development.

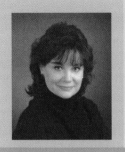

LEADERSHIP PROFILE *14.2*
Anne Sutherland Boal
Chief Nurse Executive
Assistant Deputy Minister
Clinical Innovation and Integration
Ministry of Health Planning, Government of British Columbia

As Chief Nurse Executive for the Ministry of Health Services in British Columbia, Anne Sutherland Boal provides executive leadership, strategic advice, and nursing expertise on a wide range of provincial health policy and program-specific issues related to nursing in BC, and also related to the interests of registered nurses (RNs), registered psychiatric nurses, and licensed practical nurses. One of her first accomplishments in this role was to work with a team of people from inside and outside government to provide information to the BC government that resulted in the government advancing the entry-to-practice competencies for new RN graduates. This means that there will be a transition to baccalaureate preparation for all nursing graduates by the year 2005. In addition to her role as Chief Nurse Executive, Anne is also Assistant Deputy Minister of Clinical Innovation and Integration, which involves review and redesign of selected clinical services.

Anne is a graduate of the Foothills Hospital School of Nursing, Calgary, Alberta. She holds a BA with distinction from Brock University, St. Catharine's, Ontario; an MHSA from the University of Alberta; and is currently Adjunct Professor, School of Nursing at the University of British Columbia. Her clinical background is in surgery and pediatrics. She developed an interest in administration and health services and chose an interdisciplinary master's program because it combined both these areas. She found the perspectives of students from a variety of social science backgrounds to be stimulating and valuable. Completion of her graduate studies in health services administration led ultimately to a series of increasingly responsible and senior administrative positions in Alberta and BC. At the British Columbia Children's Hospital, she held positions as Vice-President, Nursing; Vice-President, Programs and Services; and Interim President. She has served overseas as Director, Patient Care Services at the International Hospital in Beijing, China, and later as Director of the Canadian Education Centre and as clinic nurse at the Canadian Embassy in Beijing.

Two highly supportive mentors influenced her career. In academia, Dr. Shirley Stinson demanded critical thinking and first-rate work; and at the Calgary General Hospital, Marlene Meyers, RN, Vice-President, Patient Services, encouraged her to take on new challenges and was always ready to listen and provide advice and guidance.

In discussing her leadership style, Anne writes:

> With any leadership position I have found that you can't be successful by yourself. You require a team to work with and you have to have a shared vision of what you are trying to accomplish. Also, success to me means that all members of the team succeed and that those of us in leadership positions have to encourage people working for us to take on new and more responsible roles. I get enormous satisfaction following the advancing careers of nurses who have worked with me over the years. Finally, leadership is all about accountability, whether it is for the care that we provide or the decisions that we make.

And her advice to potential leaders in nursing is first to recognize the skills and abilities that as a nurse you bring to the workplace, and second, to seek out new opportunities—there are many—and set your sights on where you want to be and work towards that goal.

Leadership/Followership

Followers are essential to the leadership process; gaining commitment and involvement of others is vital to an effective leadership role. Burns (1978) believes leaders "induce" followers to act where the wants, needs, and expectations of both are similar.

Leadership occurs between people and is a reciprocal process. In fact, it is the followers who determine whether the leader is effective or not. Kouzes and Posner (1989) found that followers want leaders who are honest, competent, forward-looking, and credible. Followership becomes more important in the examination of different leadership styles. Transformational leadership and superleadership recognize the importance of followers and the need to develop their potential. Leaders need to establish a style and a climate that permit all members of the group to contribute to the achievement of group goals and to the maintenance and growth of the individuals and group. Followers flourish and develop in a supportive climate of trust and respect. Leaders with high standards who coach and assist their followers in meeting those expectations are more successful in influencing the group. The type of leadership behaviour required to support and empower followers will be described later in the chapter.

Overview of Early Leadership Theories

Early examinations of leaders and early research into leadership identified five theoretical perspectives for classifying characteristics or behaviours associated with leaders. Each of these is now examined further.

Personality Trait Theories

Early leadership theory focused on personal characteristics of the leader, often looking at persons who were prominent in a historical or political sense. The idea was that leaders were born, not made, and factors such as height, weight, intelligence, and energy level were thought to be significant. The social elite and the monarchy were described as "natural" leaders.

Such characteristics as self-confidence, emotional control, dominance, and independence were thought to be related to leadership. Charisma and public image were also important. Eventually, it was concluded that thinking in terms of personality characteristics and assuming all leaders were "born leaders" were not useful approaches. Researchers then began to look toward examining the behaviours that leaders displayed.

Behavioural Theories

Studies at Ohio State University and the University of Michigan in the 1940s strongly influenced the development of leadership theory. The Ohio study identified two dimensions of leadership behaviour and called them "consideration" and "initiating structure." The Michigan study identified similar concepts and labelled them "employee orientation" and "production orientation." Consideration (employee orientation) dealt with the extent to which a leader showed concern about an employee's welfare and job satisfaction. Initiating structure (production orientation)

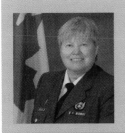

LEADERSHIP PROFILE *14.3*

Beverley E. Anderson, OMM, CD

Senior Principal
Chief Review Services
National Defence Headquarters

Colonel Beverley Anderson assumed her role as a senior evalulator with the Chief Review Services in the Department of National Defence in June 2004. She was formerly the Deputy Commander and Chief of Staff of the Canadian Forces Medical Group and she was the first officer with a nursing background to hold that position. In her current role with the Chief Review Services, she is responsible for departmental evaluation review services on behalf of the Deputy Minister of National Defence and the Chief of the Defence Staff of the Canadian Forces. The Chief Review Services is the Department of National Defence's focal point for ethics awareness and assistance.

Following graduation from the Toronto East General and Orthopedic Hospital in 1973, Beverley began her military career as a General Duty Nursing Officer on a surgical unit at the Canadian Forces Hospital in Kingston, Ontario. During her career, she has pursued two parallel continuing education paths—one focusing on her profession after earning a bachelor's and a master's degree in nursing, and the other focusing on military service, including flight nursing, flight nursing instruction, classroom instruction, and, later, graduating from the Canadian Forces Command Staff College, Toronto, in 1995. These courses prepared her for increasingly senior ranks and various leadership positions, including Regional Senior Nurse of Medical Units in BC and Assistant Director of Nursing at the National Defence Medical Centre in Ottawa. In 1996, she was promoted to the rank of Lieutenant Colonel and assigned as Project Director of a Defence Services Project to organize and equip a deployable field hospital. At the same time, she was posted to the Canadian Forces Base Petawawa as the Commanding Officer of 1 Canadian Field Hospital. Following promotion to the rank of Colonel, she was posted to establish and fill the position of Deputy Commander of the Canadian Forces Medical Group, responsible for the day-to-day management of all Canadian Forces Medical Group Units. In March of 2003, Beverley was posted to her present position.

Of the many accomplishments in her varied military career, Beverley feels most proud of putting the Canadian Field Hospital on the map as one of the most modern, sophisticated, and well-equipped field units within Canada's military and Allied Forces. Beverley was instrumental in having the garrison facility—built to accommodate field unit personnel and equipment—named after Captain Marion Sarah Barr, a WWII Nursing Sister who served with great distinction. As part of Beverley's efforts to build morale and pride among the staff of the Field Hospital and Medical Field Units, she initiated the long process of designing and obtaining approval from National Defence Directorate of History and Heritage for a camp flag, which they now proudly fly.

Colonel Anderson refers to her leadership philosophy and style as "servant leadership" because she believes that if you take care of your people, they will take care of business. Her philosophy is based on the concept of caring, which springs from her nursing background. From family and friends, she learned strong humanistic values and the importance of honesty, maintaining a sense of humour, perseverance, and hard work. She is confident in the support of her troops in looking after organizational needs because she cares about their needs. In appreciation of her leadership, Colonel Anderson's subordinates at 1 Canadian Field Hospital nominated her for induction as Officer of the Order of Military Merit for her career-long contribution to the military—an honour that was endorsed by senior military personnel.

dealt with the tasks of the group and how the leader organized and defined the work roles to achieve goals. One other significant finding was that leader effectiveness did not depend solely on the style of the leader, but was dependent upon the situation in which the style was used.

A classic study by Lewin, Lippitt, and White (1939) used a group of young boys to examine how three types of leadership style affected group productivity. The styles tested were democratic, autocratic, and laissez-faire. Democratic leaders gave information, encouraged group participation in decisions, and were flexible about how things were done. Autocratic leaders made all the decisions and supervised closely, giving more precise direction about what to do and how to do it. Laissez-faire leaders gave no direction and were extremely flexible. The researchers found that the style of leadership affected the productivity of the group. Productivity was highest in the autocratic-led group, but only when the leader was present. The democratic-led group showed greater cohesiveness and satisfaction than the other two groups and had the least absenteeism. The study suggests there is a continuum of leadership behaviours, ranging from autocratic through democratic to laissez-faire. Each style of behaviour has a different effect on group members' performance and level of satisfaction.

Tannenbaum, Weschler, and Massarik (1961) described a range of patterns of leadership behaviour across a continuum from autocratic to democratic in relation to task orientation and relationship orientation. Actions taken by the leader are related to the degree of authority used by the leader and the amount of freedom given to the followers to make decisions. The behaviours on one end of the continuum are those of a leader who wishes to *maintain* a high degree of control. Behaviours on the opposite end of the continuum are those of a leader who *releases* a high degree of control to the followers. Whichever style is chosen along the continuum, it is important that the leader clearly communicates to the group the style being used. Both parties need to understand and be clear about the degree of authority the leader wishes to keep and the degree of authority being given to the followers. Misunderstanding the division of authority frequently results in conflict.

The authors concluded that the type of leadership chosen is based on three factors: the leader, the followers, and the situation. The leader's behaviour is influenced by a value system, the degree of confidence in the followers, the comfort with the style chosen, and the level of security in an uncertain situation or tolerance of ambiguity. The followers also have a value system, and each has expectations of the leader and may wish for varying degrees of independence to make decisions. The situational forces include the values and traditions of the organization, the nature and urgency of the problem, and the overall effectiveness of the group in its ability to make decisions. The successful leader knows his or her own self, understands the individuals in the group, knows the context of the environment in which they operate, and clearly states any expectations of the followers.

Contingency Theory

A contingency approach to leadership matches the style of the leader with the characteristics of the situation. Fiedler (1967) believed that leadership styles are relatively inflexible. He found that certain types of leaders succeed in particular organizations and that this could be related to interests, personality, and the nature of the situation. Therefore, a leader may succeed in one

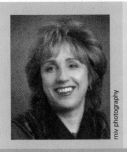

miv photography

LEADERSHIP PROFILE *14.4*
Deborah Tamlyn
President
Canadian Nurses Association

In June 2004, Deborah Tamlyn assumed the presidency of the Canadian Nurses Association, having served for the two previous years as President-Elect. She is also President of Tamlyn @ Associates Consulting in her hometown of Halifax, Nova Scotia. She has held a series of leadership positions in the past, including President of the Canadian Association of University Schools of Nursing; Dean of Nursing at Dalhousie University, Nova Scotia; and Dean of Nursing at University of Calgary, Alberta, where she continues her association as Professor Emeritus. She says that her involvement in nursing education keeps her immersed in the critical issues facing current and future nursing. In her role as consultant, she specializes in health and education projects related to research and leadership enhancement.

Deborah holds a diploma in nursing from Victoria General Hospital, Halifax; a Bachelor of Nursing (BN) from McGill University; a Master's in Education from Ottawa University; and a PhD from Dalhousie University. She considers her main accomplishments to be those that result in new programs and initiatives, for example, the establishment of the BN degree as entry to practice (in partnership with her alma mater Victoria General Hospital School of Nursing, Halifax Infirmary, and Dalhousie University). Similarly, her faculty at Dalhousie has worked with colleagues in Tanzania to launch a BN program in that country.

During her term as Dean of Nursing at the University of Calgary, new programs were initiated, including distance PhD, nurse practitioner, second-degree BN, and collaborative BN programs. Also during her tenure, the Southern Alberta Nursing and Health Resource Unit was opened to further the research activities of faculty and nurses in the Calgary Health Region. For her achievements in nursing education, she was awarded a YMCA Women of Distinction Award, and she is the recipient of a Governor General Medal. She has published extensively on topics in the field of nursing education and leadership.

In describing her leadership philosophy, Deborah draws on the field of human relations and the principles of social justice. She considers that success is achieved when one believes in and recognizes the potential that lies within people. She notes that it is not what the leader wants that is important, but what the group is willing to put its energy into. She identifies her mother as having taught her the importance of relationships, and the people she worked with in the mental health and palliative care fields further reinforced that concept for her.

She says she has an insatiable appetite for learning from every situation. Accordingly, her advice to nurses with leadership potential is to build knowledge and competency in the areas of communication, research, cultural and global diversity, and resource management. Finding a balance between work, family, and other pursuits will contribute to self-actualization and generate the energy required for leadership challenges. Ultimately, the goal of leadership is the good that it can bring to patients, families, and communities.

situation and not in another. The leader seeks to satisfy personal goals as well as those of the organization, and the ability to do so depends upon the leader's control and influence in the situation.

Fiedler identified three factors that lead to effective leadership. According to him, the most important factor is leader-member relations. When the relationship is one of mutual trust, respect, and admiration, there is little need to use formal authority. The second factor is task structure, which describes how rigidly the group's tasks are structured and affects the power of the leader. In high task structure, people are clear about what they have to do. Conversely, in low task structure, group and member roles are unclear, and the power of the leader is ambiguous. The final factor, position power, is the perceived authority of the leader. Where there is high position power, it is simple for the leader to influence followers, but in situations where there is low position power, it is more difficult for the leader to exert influence.

Fiedler contrasted leadership styles on the two dimensions of task-oriented and relationship-oriented style. He measured leadership style on the least preferred co-worker (LPC) scale, in which the leader identifies the person he or she would be least able to work well with. Those leaders with a high LPC rating are more people- and relationship-oriented; those with a low LPC rating are more task-oriented and less concerned with human relations.

Effective leadership is exercised when the leader's style, whether task-oriented or relationship-oriented, fits "favourably" with the situation.

Tri-dimensional Leader Effectiveness Model

Hersey and Blanchard (1982) developed a leadership model based on the concepts of consideration and initiating structure identified in the Ohio State studies. They described leadership style as the behaviour pattern of the individual, as perceived by others, when the person is attempting to influence the group.

The leader's own perception of his or her behaviour (self-perception) may be very different from that of the follower. Leadership style is determined by the combination of two factors—task behaviours and relationship behaviours. Task behaviours are defined as those in which the leader organizes the group and establishes channels of communication and ways of getting the task done. Relationship behaviours are those that facilitate relationships between the leader and the group members, open up communication, and provide socioemotional support.

Based on work by Reddin (1970), an effectiveness dimension was added to the Ohio State model. This third dimension, called the environment, integrates the style of the leader with the specific needs of the situation. The effectiveness of a leadership style is determined by the appropriateness of the style for the environment in which it is being used.

Situational Leadership

The Situational Leadership® model (Figure 14.1) arose from the development of the tri-dimensional leadership effectiveness model. This model emphasizes the behaviour of the leader in relation to the followers and is based on the interaction of three factors: (a) the amount of guidance and direction a leader gives, (b) the amount of socioemotional support the leader provides, and (c) the readiness of the followers to perform a task.

Figure 14.1 The Situational Leadership Model®

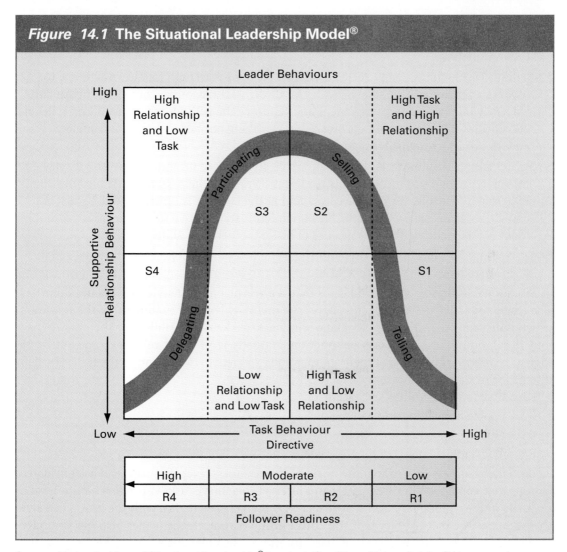

Source: Abstracted from *Situational Leadership® handout (San Diego University), by P. Hersey and K. Blanchard, 1988, Escondido, CA: Leadership Studies Inc. Used with permission of Leadership Studies Inc., Escondido, CA.
*Situational Leadership® is a registered trademark of the Center for Leadership Studies. All rights reserved.

   The model depicts the styles of leadership on a bell-shaped curve that passes through quadrants related to the task and relationship behaviours of the leader. The concept of follower readiness is portrayed on a continuum of low readiness (R1) to high readiness (R4). The four styles of leadership are indicated by the abbreviations S1 to S4 and are described as follows:

S1-Telling. This high task, low relationship style is to be used with followers who exhibit low readiness. This is a directive style for followers who are insecure or inexperienced in their task or function.

S2-Selling. This high task, high relationship style is to be used with followers with low to moderate readiness. This style provides for directive behaviour accompanied by supportive behaviour to give encouragement and reinforce the willingness of the follower. People classified as R2 followers are considered to be willing but not able (or not confident enough) to take responsibility for their skills.

S3-Participating. This low task, high relationship style is used for individuals who display moderate to high readiness. At this readiness level (R3), the person is able but unwilling to perform. The follower may be competent at the task but is unwilling due to lack of confidence (insecurity). A supportive nondirective style is used to give positive reinforcement and to facilitate the person's use of his or her personal ability.

S4-Delegating. This low task, low relationship style is used with followers who have a high level of readiness (R4) and are able and willing to take responsibility for their own efforts.

Situational leadership theory indicates that there is no one best style to influence followers. The leadership style chosen depends upon the maturity level, or readiness, of the followers, which is determined by their ability and willingness to take responsibility for their own behaviour in relation to a specific task or function. Maturity level is not related to age but to the individual followers in terms of their abilities and experiences in relation to the task. The definitions for readiness levels are described as follows:

- R1 = Unable and unwilling or insecure
- R2 = Unable but willing and confident
- R3 = Able but unwilling or insecure
- R4 = Able/competent and willing/confident

Both the readiness level of an individual and the readiness level of a group can be considered. Groups that come together frequently and interact to achieve tasks can reach a high level of maturity in their group function. The leader may then choose to deal with the group in a style that matches the maturity level of the entire group. However, the leader also has to understand that there are differing levels of maturity among the individuals who make up the group. Therefore, different leadership styles may be chosen when interacting on an individual level with the various members of the group (Wylie, 1994).

Recent Theoretical Concepts

The early concepts of leadership behaviour have been developed extensively in recent years and have led to different ways of describing leaders. All build on the previous notions of initiating structure and consideration. Later theories, such as transactional and transformational theory, strongly emphasize the consideration or relationship aspect between leader and follower.

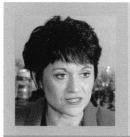

LEADERSHIP PROFILE *14.5*
Francine Girard

**Vice-President, Professional Practice & Research
and Chief Nursing Officer
Calgary Health Region**

Francine Girard was recruited from within the Calgary Health Region's nursing workforce to undertake the recently created position of Vice-President, Professional Practice & Research, and Chief Nursing Officer. Her mandate is to bring a unified voice and viewpoint for more than 9,500 nurses to the Calgary Health Region's decision-making process. She advises the executive and senior management on all issues affecting nursing practice and is responsible for developing a professional nursing practice environment in the region. She promotes the development and implementation of policy, practice models, and quality of work life measures that contribute to the retention of nursing staff, teamwork, and collaboration among other professionals in the region.

Francine also is responsible for the Primary Care Initiative, Calgary Health Link, and diagnostic and treatment centres. Under her guidance, a representative nursing council provides leadership in professional nursing practice. A research unit, established in 2001, is addressing such projects as scope of practice and skill mix, and the implementation and evaluation of community-based service delivery models.

The pattern that emerges in Francine's professional career is one of increasing responsibility coupled with continuous study. Her career began with a diploma in nursing from the CEGEP of Mantane, Quebec, after which she worked as a staff nurse in intensive care units in Quebec and Ontario. She moved out west to the Foothills Hospital in Calgary, Alberta, where she continued working in intensive care and coronary care. She has occupied several leadership roles, moving from team leader, to assistant head nurse, to patient care manager in the Cardiac Intensive Care Unit at the Foothills Hospital—a position she held for 15 years. During those years, she continued her professional studies, earning a Bachelor of Nursing, a Master's of Nursing, and a PhD in nursing from the University of Calgary.

Prior to her current position, she was the Director of the Southern Alberta Renal Program. She holds academic appointments in the Faculty of Nursing and in the Department of Community Health Sciences in the Faculty of Medicine, University of Calgary. She identifies Jeanette Pick, former senior nurse executive in the region, as having influenced her career in providing leadership and support.

Francine brings a passion and commitment to nursing and to teamwork. Besides being an excellent nurse and administrator, she respects people and strongly believes in fairness for all. On the recommendation of nurses in the Cardiac Intensive Care Unit, the Alberta Association of Registered Nurses honoured her with a Heritage of Service Award in 1999 for lifelong commitment and dedication to the nursing profession and to the health and well-being of others. In 2001, she was the recipient of the Canadian Council of Cardiovascular Nurses Baxter Leadership Award for excellence in that nursing specialty. She describes her leadership style as participatory and transformative and attributes her success to resilience. She believes that leaders must be committed to nursing and have a clear vision and strong communication skills, including listening. She also believes leaders must practice teamwork in order to be successful.

Transactional/Transformational Leadership

Transactional leadership is based on an exchange or transaction between the leader and the follower. Burns (1978) noted that such leadership "occurs when one person takes the initiative in making contact with others for the purpose of an exchange of valued things" (p. 19). The purposes of the exchange for each person are related, and each is aware of the power of the other. However, there is not a binding relationship, and each individual may go her or his own way after the transaction. Burns likened the transactional leadership style to that used by the traditional manager who concentrates on daily operational activities just to keep things going. Such a manager may institute first-level change at the operational level but is not as concerned with second-level change at the system level.

In contrast, transformational leadership occurs "when one or more persons *engage* with others in such a way that leaders and followers raise one another to higher levels of motivation and morality" (Burns, 1978, p. 20). The leader takes the initiative to develop the connection with the follower, and the dynamics of the relationship have a transforming effect. Burns cited the example of Gandhi, who elevated the hopes and expectations of the Indian population and personally enhanced the lives of millions.

Burns viewed leadership as a process of morality because the engagement between leader and follower is based on shared motives, values, and goals. The leader's first task is to encourage followers to recognize their own self-identities by being aware of their needs, values, and purposes. In this way, the leader arouses a sense of dissatisfaction in the follower, which then can become a source of energy to undergo change that the leader can influence.

Tichy and Devanna (1986) described transformational leadership in organizations as a three-act play. The first act is recognizing the need for revitalization; the second act is creating a vision; and the third is institutionalizing change. Characteristically, transformational leaders are described as follows:

- Identify themselves clearly as agents of change who want to make a difference
- Are courageous, but take prudent risks
- Believe in people and work toward empowerment of the individual
- Are able to describe their values and demonstrate them in their behaviours
- Are lifelong learners
- Have the ability to cope well with complexity, ambiguity, and uncertainty
- Are visionaries who can translate dreams and images to others.

Emotional Intelligence

In the 1990s, the concept of emotional intelligence and its implications for leadership emerged as a subject for research, particularly in neurology, psychology, and the business world. Goleman (1995) explained that there are two fundamentally different ways of knowing, which interact to construct our mental life. "One, the rational mind, is the mode of comprehension we are typically conscious of: more prominent in awareness, thoughtful, able to ponder and reflect. But alongside that there is another system of knowing: impulsive and powerful, if sometimes illogical—the emotional mind" (p. 8). The emotional mind is quicker than the rational mind and

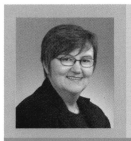

LEADERSHIP PROFILE *14.6*
Jean Morrison
**Senior Vice-President, Nursing and Health Services
Saskatoon Health Region, Saskatchewan**

In her current position as Senior Vice-President, Nursing and Health Services, Jean Morrison is responsible for 3,000 health and ancillary professionals. She provides strategic direction and leadership in the delivery of health services in Saskatchewan's largest health region. The Saskatoon Health Region serves a large rural population and is the major referral centre for the northern part of the province.

Jean's nursing career began at the University of Saskatchewan in 1983, where she earned a bachelor's degree in nursing. Following three and a half years of clinical practice in the field of public health, she attended Dalhousie University. In keeping with her clinical experience and interests, she focused her graduate studies on community health and evaluation. In 1989, she was awarded master's degrees in nursing and in health services administration. Her administrative career began in the remote Canadian North as Regional Nursing Officer and Executive Director for the Kitikmeot Health Board in the Northwest Territories. She provided leadership in the development and delivery of effective and efficient health programs in the central Arctic.

In 1995, Jean returned to Saskatchewan as Chief Executive Officer in the Parkland Health District. Key achievements included completion of the integration of a full spectrum of health services previously under separate governance structures; the implementation of primary and secondary prevention programs; the development of advanced and collaborative nursing practice roles; and the development of intersectoral partnerships with neighbouring health districts, boards of education, and not-for-profit community partners.

Jean was appointed to her present position in the Saskatoon Health Region in 2001. She is responsible for providing strategic direction and leadership to strengthen and support nursing practice, education, and research across the entire organization. She currently is building capacity in the area of nursing research, emphasizing the evaluation of outcomes and facilitating the development of innovative relationships with external partners to advance nursing education. She attributes her success in being appointed to this position to her varied experiences in the health field and to the contributions of many valued mentors. She has learned from these mentors and from her experiences that you must focus on treating people with respect, on collaborating with partners, and, most importantly, on valuing and supporting the application of the wealth of knowledge to be found within the members of health care teams.

may interfere with the deliberate and analytic reflection typical of the thinking mind. Goleman argued that intelligence alone is not enough to explain why some highly intelligent people fail and others of moderate intelligence succeed. The concept of emotional intelligence includes self-awareness, impulse control, persistence, zeal and self-motivation, empathy, and social deftness. When this theory is applied to leadership, the focus is on the leader and his or her relationship with followers.

According to Goleman, Boyatzis, and McKee (2003), leaders with high emotional intelligence demonstrate the following competencies:

- *Self-awareness,* including emotional self-awareness, accurate self-assessment, self-confidence
- *Self-management,* including self-control, transparency, adaptability, achievement
- *Social awareness,* including empathy, organizational awareness, service
- *Relational management,* including inspiration, influence, developing others, change catalyst, conflict management, teamwork, and collaboration

These authors describe two types of leadership based on the extent to which the leaders exhibit emotional intelligence and associated competencies. *Resonant leadership* refers to a leader who is attuned to the people being led, moving them in a positive emotional direction. Such leaders are visionary, affiliative, coaching, and democratic. The leader "resonates" with followers, and they in turn feel energized, enthusiastic, focused on their mission, supported, collaborative, willing, and able to get things done. *Dissonant leadership*, on the other hand, is pace setting and commanding, and these leaders resonate negatively, neither listening nor caring about followers, and being out of touch with their mood and feelings. This is the type of leader few respect and many dread.

According to this theory, dissonant leadership produces feelings of emotional discordance and being off balance, resulting in poor performance. The long-term effects of working with dissonant leadership include burnout and stress derived from a "toxic" or unhealthy workplace. The concept of resonant leadership is useful as it is likely to fit with the values and aspirations of health care workers and to produce professionally rewarding workplaces. Moreover, according to Goleman and colleagues (2003), the competencies of emotionally intelligent leadership can be learned and developed.

Recently, Cummings (2003) applied the concept of emotional intelligence in a secondary analysis of survey data collected from over 6,000 nurses in Alberta to determine the effects of hospital restructuring in that province. Layoffs, bumping, relocation, and other disruptions in nurses' work lives accompanied the restructuring. The objective of Cummings' study was to determine the extent to which the styles of nursing leaders (founded on emotional intelligence as perceived by the nurses) mitigated the effects of hospital restructuring on the nurses who remained employed. She concluded from her findings that resonant leadership styles tend to mitigate the effects of hospital restructuring on nurses, while dissonant styles tend to intensify those effects.

In conclusion, theories of leadership are still evolving as a result of a huge body of research and a continuing fascination with this important phenomenon among social scientists. Knowledge of leadership theory provides a foundation for developing individual styles of leadership and for identifying potential professional leaders for future clinical and managerial positions. Leadership theory also can serve as a guide for planning educational programs for both new and experienced managers. Theory is an integral part of research, whether deductive or inductive, and assists in the formulation of research questions.

Nursing Leadership Research and Education

Leadership Research

In a recent review of the research literature on leadership in business and health care, Vance and Larson (2002) concluded that studies of leadership are primarily descriptive. Of the 6,628 articles reviewed, only 4.4% (290) were reports of research based on data, and only two from the health care literature included data on the relationship between leadership and changes in the status of patients. Assuming that effective leadership is measured in part by its success in furthering the mission of organizations, its impact on staff performance, and its effect on patient outcomes, this is a disappointing finding. But as these authors note, the ability to measure meaningful outcomes is not only very difficult, it also is limited by imprecise definitions of leadership and a lack of sensitive and specific measurement instruments. Accordingly, they recommend that leadership research extend beyond examining the leader (and the led) to identifying specific outcomes for clients and the delivery of care.

Leaders and leadership in nursing have been the subject of much research by nurses and others, but again, these studies are predominantly descriptive and are often qualitative in design, using small convenient samples of subjects. Consequently, it is difficult to generalize from the findings of such studies. Nevertheless, they do offer useful insights into the nature of leadership in the nursing profession when viewed together with leadership research findings in other fields. For example, in a study of 205 nurse managers who responded to a survey, mentorship was identified as a major factor fostering their entry into management positions and their development of leadership characteristics (Moran et al., 2002).

The literature on mentorship in nursing suggests that the profession has been slow to realize the benefits of mentoring as a means of developing leadership ability, career advancement, and job satisfaction. It is not surprising then, that in the study by Moran and colleagues (2002), only one-third of the participants indicated that becoming a nurse manager was a conscious career decision, and most appeared not to have engaged in structured career planning at all. Only five of the respondents acknowledged higher education as a positive influence on their leadership development. This raises the questions of how future leaders should be prepared and what educational resources are available to assist them.

Leadership Education

Undergraduate programs in nursing can be expected to offer opportunities for individuals to acquire a beginning understanding of structure and process in organizations and the basic principles of management and leadership. Such preparation is essential for application to clinical practice and clinical leadership roles such as team leader or "in-charge" responsibilities for an area or shift. However, in today's complex environments, it is not sufficient preparation for first-level or middle management positions in health care. Broadly focused graduate programs in nursing and health services provide valuable preparation for people who will undertake senior clinical and executive roles; however, these programs may not address specific leadership knowledge and competencies or provide the contextual insights needed for successful leadership

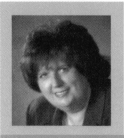

LEADERSHIP PROFILE *14.7*

Judith Shamian
President and Chief Executive Officer
Victorian Order of Nurses Canada

Judith Shamian assumed her position as President and Chief Executive Officer of the Victorian Order of Nurses Canada in June 2004. Prior to this, she served as the first Executive Director of the National Office of Nursing Policy from 1999 to 2004. In this role, she participated in national committees and working groups and provided advice and support to the policy work of Health Canada. She represented Health Canada as the former Co-Chair of the Advisory Committee on Health Human Resources and the Canadian Nursing Advisory Committee, making policy recommendations to the federal, provincial, and territorial Ministers of Health on health human resources issues.

Prior to 1999, Judith held several strategic leadership positions in nursing, including Vice-President, Nursing at Mount Sinai Hospital, Toronto; Director, Department of Nursing Research and Development at Sunnybrook Hospital, Toronto; and an elected position as President, Registered Nurses Association of Ontario.

While at Mount Sinai Hospital, one of her major accomplishments was the development of the first hospital-based World Health Organization Collaborating Centre. As head of this centre, she provided leadership for overseas projects in parts of the world such as South America, Africa, Eastern Europe, and the Caribbean. She is internationally recognized as a health care and nursing leader, serving on advisory groups for the World Health Organization and as a consultant to health organizations in Hungary, Israel, and China.

Judith's professional education began with a nursing diploma from Shaare Zedek Hospital, Jerusalem, Israel. She went on to earn a BA from Concordia University, Montreal in Community Nursing; a Master's of Public Health from New York University, New York in International Health and Education; and a PhD from Case Western Reserve University, Cleveland in the Nurse Executive track. Her clinical experience includes working as a nurse practitioner in a kibbutz and as a neurosurgical nurse. In addition to her many accomplishments, she is trilingual, speaking English, Hungarian, and Hebrew.

As a professor in the Faculty of Nursing, University of Toronto, Judith teaches and supervises graduate students and maintains an active research portfolio as a principal co-investigator and decision maker. She had a role in three research projects that were funded by the Nurse Effectiveness, Utilization, and Outcomes Research Unit at University of Toronto. Her research interests and publications have focused on healthy working environments, nursing workforce issues, management information, nursing informatics, health system outcomes, leadership and management, and primary health care. She is an accomplished public speaker and has travelled widely throughout Canada and the US as an invited keynote speaker and presenter at professional conferences.

In recognition of her many professional attributes and accomplishments, Judith has received numerous awards, including: Excellence in Leadership Award from Iota Omicron Chapter, Sigma Theta Tau, University of Western Ontario in 1992; Excellence in Nursing Administration Award from Lambda Pi Chapter, Sigma Theta Tau, University of Toronto in 1993; Most Distinguished Nurse Ross Award for Nursing Leadership from the Canadian Nurses Foundation, Ottawa, in 1995; Distinguished Alumni Award from Frances Payne Bolton School of Nursing, Case Western Reserve University, Cleveland, Ohio, in 2002; and a Queen's Golden Jubilee Medal. She is listed in *WHO'S WHO of Canadian Women* (1995, 1996, 1997) and in *WHO'S WHO of Canadian Jewry* (2000).

careers. For this reason, the Canadian Nurses Association (2002) has taken the position that quality professional practice environments depend on many circumstances; one of these is that nurses in leadership positions and potential leaders have access not only to graduate nursing programs, but also to *additional* management education.

The team of leaders whose combined vision resulted in the establishment of The Dorothy M. Wylie Nursing Leadership Institute in the Faculty of Nursing, University of Toronto, recognized the need for additional programming in leadership at many levels of health care organizations. They noted that:

> Few programs exist for nurses in leadership roles to better understand and utilize leadership concepts such as engaging and motivating professionals, developing human capacity, building learning communities, leading self-managed work teams, and managing practice change. Leadership development is seen by many nursing leaders both as an investment in the present—by helping the system adapt quickly to new requirements and challenges, as well as an investment in the future—by providing for necessary leadership succession (Simpson, Skelton-Green, Scott, & O'Brien-Pallas, 2002, p. 22).

The Institute offered an inaugural five-day residential program in 2001 for nurses from across the country who registered in dyads (i.e., an up-and-coming leader and an experienced leader attending together). Planning was preceded by the development of a conceptual framework and a set of principles to identify the content and design of the learning activities. The principles emphasized that learning would be experiential and collaborative, that theory would be linked with practice, and that all activities would challenge, stimulate, and deliver value. The participants were enthusiastic in their assessment of the course, suggesting that it was indeed meeting their leadership development needs.

Most health care managers learn their leadership skills and habits on the job, and approaches to leadership development have tended to be ad hoc and informal. Typical approaches to leadership development include short courses offered in-house by employers, temporary "stretch" programs (e.g., special assignments for skill development), external workshops or certificate courses, job rotations, and mentorship (Leatt & Porter, 2003). In nursing, preceptorship has been widely used in undergraduate and graduate programs. For example, undergraduate courses in management often assigned students to first-level leaders and managers for periods of one-on-one experiential learning and individual coaching, until the classes became too numerous and the managers too scarce. Opportunities for role modelling and recruitment of potential leaders were then lost.

Most of the current leadership development programs in health care are designed to assist individuals in acquiring additional knowledge, skills, and competencies. Important though these programs are, the benefits are mainly for the individual participant, while the benefits for the health care organization as a whole may not be clear or realized.

Leatt & Porter (2003) suggest a new approach to leadership development, particularly for senior health care leaders, based on a 10-point model. One of their most interesting points in this model is that, given the importance of teamwork and interdisciplinary collaboration in health care organizations, consideration should be given to whole teams undertaking leadership development together. They argue that the return on investment for health agencies is likely to be greater this way (i.e., have a greater impact on organizational effectiveness and quality improvement). Many of their suggestions for senior health care leaders in general are applicable for first- and middle-level leaders in nursing. For example, they advocate lifelong learning, the provision of competency-based courses, the use of adult education methods, the employment of quality improvement as a framework, and the provision of opportunities to learn through experiential teamwork (e.g., interdisciplinary learning about group process, not just completing group assignments).

The idea that health care professionals should learn together recently led to the establishment of a mandatory fourth year interdisciplinary course for all undergraduates enrolled in the health disciplines at the University of Alberta. The learning groups are made up of representatives from several health disciplines, including medicine, and students are required to deal with clinical issues and problems using context-based learning methods.

Leadership Profiles

The eight nurses profiled in this chapter agreed to answer questions about their professional education and work experiences and to talk about the people who influenced them, their greatest accomplishments as leaders, and their thoughts on leadership. They all previously held or currently hold senior administrative or advisory roles in which they are in a position to influence policies affecting the delivery of health care and the professional practice environments of nurses. Seven of the eight leaders began their professional careers in hospital diploma schools of nursing (the eighth began in a university school of nursing), and all went to university to obtain bachelor's degrees in nursing or the arts. Seven went on to graduate studies in nursing or health services administration, and three studied successfully at the doctoral level. Every one of these nurses practiced nursing for several years following graduation, some in public health or long-term care, and others in active treatment settings including intensive care.

Each nurse describes a career of increasing responsibility and continuous learning. Some chose teaching positions and private consulting, but all ultimately rose to senior positions in administration (either in education or service) or in advisory roles and policy development. Two of these leaders have held elected positions, one as president of a provincial nurses' association, and one as president of the Canadian Nurses Association.

The majority of the leaders identify mentors, parents, or both as having the greatest influence on their successful careers. Several mention that families and friends inspired them to acquire their strong work ethic, concern for social justice, and such qualities as respect, fairness, and belief in self and others. Four name previous supervisors as mentors who taught them about collaboration, accountability, transformative leadership, vision, teamwork, caring, the desire to improve the status quo, and about looking for the potential in people for whom they were responsible.

Their greatest accomplishments include new programs and successful projects in education, administration, or practice that were often achieved under difficult circumstances. Four of these leaders were appointed into newly created positions, and two others are in positions that were

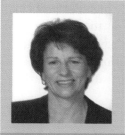

LEADERSHIP PROFILE *14.8*

Sheila Christine Weatherill

President and Chief Executive Officer
Capital Health, Alberta

Sheila Weatherill is President and Chief Executive Officer of Capital Health, one of Canada's largest integrated academic health regions. Capital Health provides comprehensive health services across the continuum of care to the Edmonton and surrounding area's 980,000 residents. Capital Health also provides specialized services to 1.6 million people across northern British Columbia, central and northern Alberta, Saskatchewan, Manitoba, the Northwest Territories, and Nunavut. These specialized services include trauma and burn treatment, pediatric cardiac surgery, organ transplantation, and high-risk obstetrics. Capital Health has over 20,000 staff, more than 2,300 physicians, and a budget of $2 billion. It was ranked as the top academic health centre in Canada from 1999–2002, and as the top health system in Canada in 2003 by *Maclean's* magazine and the Canadian Institute for Health Information. Sheila works with a 13-member board and is responsible for the budget and all operations of the region.

In identifying influential people and circumstances during her career, she says she has been fortunate enough to work with great people and to have excellent role models. From her father, she learned the importance of hard work and to believe in herself and others. She notes, "As a nurse in the continuing care and acute care sector and as an administrator in continuing care services, I had a strong vision of how community and hospital care could work together to improve patient care."

The call for health reform during the 1990s in Alberta and across Canada had a significant influence on her career. With the shift in emphasis from hospital to community care, the new focus on health promotion and disease prevention, and the establishment of regional health authorities in Alberta, Sheila welcomed the prospect of developing a new health care system based on collaboration and the integration of health services. She recognized that the emphasis on increasing accountability and efficiency and improving quality and patient safety would serve as a vehicle for innovation. These evolving areas presented new opportunities for her, including new models of leadership and an environment receptive to new directions and new ideas.

Sheila has a professional nursing background, having graduated from the post-RN baccalaureate program of the Faculty of Nursing, University of Alberta. Currently, she is an Associate Faculty Member in the Faculty of Nursing and an Adjunct Professor, Faculty of Medicine and Dentistry at the University of Alberta. She was past President of the Association of Canadian Academic Healthcare Organizations and is a member of Sigma Theta Tau International Honor Society of Nursing. She also serves on three boards of directors.

Commenting on her principal accomplishments, she says, "As a nurse, I was taught to think analytically, to be creative, and to respect others. Leading Capital Health's development over the last six years from a fledgling region to a strong vibrant organization has been a wonderful opportunity to effect change. Together with the Board, staff, and physicians, we have developed many innovative programs that have improved patient care and increased accountability and efficiency."

The values and beliefs that govern her leadership style include the need to have a vision and a desire to make things better, the willingness to work hard and to believe in one's self and in others, the ability to be positive and proactive, and the need to work together because collaboration is stronger than competition. She believes that being able to see opportunity and respond to it creates success. She also believes that nurses with potential for leadership and who share these values and beliefs will find wonderful opportunities today in health care services, administration, education, and research.

never previously held by a nurse. Their comments on leadership invariably included participation, working together, teamwork, support for colleagues, being willing to innovate, and resilience. As a clinical role model, one expressed her passion for nursing by advocating for nursing and nurses. Clearly, transformative leadership, consultation, participation, and respect for others have been significant considerations in the development of these nurses' leadership styles.

Leadership Implications

The Canadian Nursing Advisory Committee (CNAC) was established by the federal Minister of Health to recommend policy directions as a framework for provinces and territories to improve the quality of nurses' work life. The committee was made up of representatives from a broad range of health system stakeholders, including government, employers, nurses' associations, educators, and researchers from across Canada. They reviewed literature, consulted with experts, and conducted a series of studies. The findings with respect to leadership in nursing are contained in recommendations 21 to 23 of the report (CNAC, 2002).

In making their recommendations, the CNAC noted the shortages of nurses across the country and the need to improve their working environments in order to attract, support, and retain them in the system. They believe that nurses must have reasonable contact with first-line managers. Furthermore, in work settings where the majority of staff are nurses, first-line managers should be experienced nurses with strong leadership abilities and should be supported by adequate human and technical resources. The committee also observed that not enough nurses are moving into leadership positions and that it is necessary for employers, educators, and governments to work with nurses to institute succession planning and provide experiences to facilitate the movement of nurses into leadership positions.

The Academy of Canadian Executive Nurses believes that leadership resides in all nurses but that in a rapidly changing and turbulent environment, leadership must be cultivated at all levels. It notes that all health disciplines are dealing with how to lead their professions in today's evolving health care organizations and suggest that there is a need to put in place a shared leadership model. The academy believes that it is possible to cultivate leadership, management, and teamwork among all the disciplines while simultaneously working within each discipline to support and advance its own work (Ferguson-Paré et al., 2002).

Succession planning for leadership may well be organized on an interdisciplinary basis in the future. Provision for ensuring the continuity of strong effective leadership in nursing should include the following components:

- The identification of nurses with potential leadership abilities who demonstrate a willingness to undertake leadership roles and to commit themselves to continuous learning
- The establishment of a variety of learning opportunities, including short-term experiential assignments
- The establishment of a mentoring system for novice managers
- Access to career counselling

- Support for short-term and long-term educational programming with access to financial resources
- The establishment of policies governing conditions for educational leave of absence without loss of employment benefits

Nurses in senior administrative and clinical leadership roles are in a position to advocate for such programs in the interests of promoting healthy working environments for professional nurses and the highest standards of care to patients and clients.

Summary

- Theories of leaders and leadership have been developing over the years, focusing initially on leader traits, personality, and behaviour, then subsequently on followers, the relationship between leaders and followers, the goals of the group, the nature of the tasks, the situation, and the context within which leadership occurs. Leadership theory continues to evolve.
- The concept of leadership often is compared and contrasted with the concept of management. Management focuses on the efficient and effective achievement of organization goals and requires leadership ability to be successful. Leadership focuses on relationships with followers to achieve existing and future organizational goals and is mindful of the management implications of its innovations. Both leadership and managerial skills are necessary to achieve effective and lasting organizational outcomes.
- Knowledge of leadership theory is important for developing individual styles of leadership, recognizing potential leadership competencies in others, planning educational programs, and raising relevant research questions.
- Studies in nursing leadership are predominantly descriptive and use qualitative methods with small samples of participants, thus making generalizations difficult.
- A review of the careers of eight senior Canadian nurses in strategic leadership positions demonstrates a pattern of continuous learning (including graduate studies), progressive appointments to leadership positions with increasing scope and responsibility, innovative accomplishments, and leadership styles that reflect the influence of mentors and family members.
- There is a need for succession planning at all levels of health care agencies to attract sufficient numbers of nurses to fill leadership positions.
- Nursing requires strong knowledgeable leaders who can inspire others, who are visible, and who can support professional practice environments and high standards of care for patients and clients.

Applying the Knowledge in this Chapter

Exercise

Discuss the following questions with others in your class:

1. Think of a leader whom you admire. Who is it? Why do you admire this person? How has her or his behaviour or example influenced you?

2. Describe a workplace situation in which you observed leadership in action. What competencies did the leader exhibit? Who were the followers? What were the goals of the leader and group? What was the style of this leader and was it effective? If it was not effective, what were the reasons?

3. Consider the theories of leadership described in this chapter and assess your own leadership potential. What kind of a leader do you think you are now? What leadership skills would you like to develop?

Complete the following exercises individually:

1. Read the recommendations in the final report of the Canadian Nursing Advisory Committee, *Our Health, Our Future: Creating Quality Work Places for Canadian Nurses*. This report is available at http://www.hc-sc.gc.ca/english/for_you/nursing/cnac.htm.

2. Select one of the recommendations.

3. Develop a plan for implementing this recommendation in your current workplace or a workplace with which you are familiar.

Resources

evolve Internet Resources

Canadian Journal of Nursing Leadership:
   www.acen-cjonl.org
Canadian Nurses Association Position Statements: "Nursing Leadership" (2002):
   www.cna_aiic.ca/_frames/policies/policiesmainframe.htm
"Succession Planning for Nursing Leadership" (2003):
   www.cna-nurses.ca/_frames/search/ searchframe.htm
Journal of Advanced Nursing (UK):
   www.journalofadvancednursing.com
Ministry of Health Planning, Government of British Columbia:
   www.healthplanning.gov.bc.ca/ndirect/chief_nurse.html

Nursing Strategy for Canada (2000):

    www.hc-sc.gc.ca/english/pdf/nursing.pdf

Report of the Canadian Nursing Advisory Committee (CNAC):

    www.hc-sc.gc.ca/english/for_you/nursing/cnac.htm

The National Office on Nursing Policy:

    www.hc-gc.ca/onp-bpsi/english/about_us/index_e.html

References

Bennis, W. (1989). *On becoming a leader*. Reading, MA: Addison-Wesley.

Burns, J.M. (1978). *Leadership*. New York: Harper & Row.

Canadian Nurses Association. (2002). *Position statement: Nursing leadership*. Ottawa, ON: CNA.

Canadian Nursing Advisory Committee (CNAC). (2002). *Our health, our future: Creating quality work places for Canadian nurses*. Final Report. Retrieved November 12, 2003, from http://www.hc-sc.gc/english/for_you/nursing/cnac_report/index.html

Cummings, G. (2003). *An examination of the effects of hospital restructuring on nurses and how leadership styles mitigate these effects*. Unpublished doctoral dissertation, University of Alberta, Edmonton, Alberta, Canada.

Drucker, P.F. (1996). Foreword: Not enough generals were killed. In F. Hesselbein, M. Goldsmith, & R. Beckhard (Eds.), *The leader of the future: New visions, strategies, and practices for the next era* (pp. xi–xv). San Francisco: Jossey-Bass.

Ferguson-Paré, M., Mitchell, G., Perkin, K., & Stevenson, L. (2002). Academy of Canadian Executive Nurses (ACEN) background paper on leadership. *Canadian Journal of Nursing Leadership, 15*(3), 4–8.

Fiedler, R.E. (1967). *A theory of leadership effectiveness*. New York: McGraw-Hill.

Goleman, D. (1995). *Emotional intelligence: Why it can matter more than IQ*. New York: Bantam Books.

Goleman, D., Boyatzis, R., & McKee, A. (2003). *Primal leadership: Realizing the power of emotional intelligence*. Boston: Harvard Business School.

Hersey, P., & Blanchard, K.H. (1982). *Management of organizational behavior: Utilizing human resources* (4th ed.). Englewood Cliffs, NJ: Prentice-Hall.

Hersey, P., & Blanchard, K. (1988). Situational Leadership® handout (San Diego University). Escondido, CA: Leadership Studies Inc.

Kouzes, J.M., & Posner, B.Z. (1989). Leadership is in the eye of the follower. In J. William Pfeiffer (Ed.), *The 1989 annual: Developing human resources* (pp. 233–239). San Diego, CA: University Associates.

Leatt, P., & Porter, J. (2003). Where are the health care leaders? The need for investment in leadership development. *HealthcarePapers, 4*(1), 15–31. Retrieved November 12, 2003, from http://www.longwoods.com/hp/4-1Leaders/HP41PLeattJPorter.pdf

Lewin, K., Lippitt, R., & White, R. (1939). Patterns of aggressive behavior in experimentally created social climates. *Journal of Social Psychology, 10,* 271–299.

Moran, P., Duffield, C., Beutel, J., Bunt, S., Thornton, A., Wills, J., et al. (2002). Nurse managers in Australia: Mentoring, leadership and career progression. *Canadian Journal of Nursing Leadership, 15*(2), 14–20.

Nanus, B. (1992). *Visionary leadership*. San Francisco: Jossey-Bass.

Reddin, W.J. (1970). *Managerial effectiveness*. New York: McGraw-Hill.

Senge, P. (1990). *The fifth discipline: The art and practice of the learning organization*. New York: Doubleday/Currency.

Simpson, B., Skelton-Green, J., Scott, J., & O'Brien-Pallas, L. (2002). Building capacity in nursing: Creating a leadership institute. *Canadian Journal of Nursing Leadership, 15*(3), 22–27.

Tamlyn, D., & Reilly, S. (2003). Innovation and contemporary nursing leadership. In M. McIntyre & E. Thomlinson (Eds.), *Realities of Canadian nursing: Professional, practice, and power issues* (pp. 494–515). Philadelphia: Lippincott, Williams & Wilkins.

Tannenbaum, R., Weschler, I.R., & Massarik, F. (1961). *Leadership and organization: A behavioral science approach.* New York: McGraw-Hill.

Tichy, N.M., & Devanna, M.A. (1986). *The transformational leader.* New York: Wiley & Sons.

Vance, C., & Larson, E. (2002). Leadership research in business and health care. *Journal of Nursing Scholarship, 34*(2), 165–171.

Wylie, D.M. (1994). Leadership theory and practice. In Hibberd, J.M. & Smith, D.L. (Eds.), *Nursing management in Canada* (2nd ed., pp. 175–190). Toronto: W.B. Saunders Canada.

ETHICAL DIMENSIONS OF LEADERSHIP

Janet L. Storch

Learning Objectives

In this chapter, you will learn:

- Common ethical situations confronting nurse leaders and managers
- The scope of ethical responsibilities in health care management
- Common ethical theories and principles applied to health care
- Recent theoretical thinking in ethics applied to management
- Constraints on nurses' and nurse managers' moral agency
- Situations that create ethical conflict for leaders and managers
- Ways in which first-level managers can work toward building a moral community

The purpose of this chapter is to encourage reflection on the ethical dimensions of leading and managing. Although the content is geared towards first-level nurse managers, the considerations included are common to non-nursing first-line managers as well. The chapter includes examples of ethical problems that involve ethical or moral distress, moral uncertainty, and moral choices that require sound ethical thinking and decision making. It reviews principles and theories that can be used as approaches to ethical understanding and reasoning and elaborates on their relevance to ethical leadership and decision making in management. The chapter concludes with a discussion of the ways in which leaders and first-level managers can support and reinforce values-based practice.

Increased recognition of the leadership role of first-level managers and the return to greater consideration of everyday ethics in health care, along with the more global issue of biomedical ethics, have paved the way for a broader appreciation of ethics as both a managerial responsibility and a leadership imperative. There is little doubt that the excursion into moral philosophy and biomedical ethics that began in the 1960s (Pellegrino, 1993) has contributed significantly to enhanced understanding of ethics in health care. However, there is uneven, and often limited, attention paid to understanding the ethical comportment and obligations in relationships between health professionals and their patients/clients, health professionals and their communities, leaders/managers and health professionals, and leaders/managers and their senior executives and boards.

Leadership and Ethics

Theories of management and leadership have tended to focus on managing people through direction and control. This is true from the classical bureaucratic theories (including time and motion studies) to theories that recognize the human factor in management, including those supporting the notion that leadership in management is contingent upon setting. The concept of transformational leadership draws our attention to the reality that people, and particularly health care professionals, cannot be managed, but they can be led. Transformational leadership is leadership that appeals to higher ideals and moral values, such as humanitarianism, liberty, equality, solidarity, and justice. It is leadership that commits people to action.

The concept of transformational leadership highlights the manager as a leader who motivates the group of workers by integrating personal and organizational values in such a way as to influence commitment, rather than attempting to motivate through direction and control (Marriner-Tomey, 1993). This requires us to examine the nature and potential of management from entirely new perspectives. It means that almost every action by a manager involves ethical considerations because attempting to influence the commitment of others means placing one's values squarely before them. It follows that if first-level managers in health care are expected to convey values and influence nurses and other health care professionals to commit to those values, then those managers will require a broadened perspective on the meanings of, and the requirements for, ethical leadership.

Being an ethical leader requires at least three foci of being and doing (Mitchell, 1996). The first is to be a person of moral character; the second is to demonstrate moral behaviour (i.e., engaging in and modelling appropriate moral behaviour); the third is to work to establish a moral community, "a workplace where ethical values are made explicit and shared, where ethical values direct action, and where individuals feel safe to be heard" (Rodney & Street, 2004, p. 217). This requires that the leader ask the question, "How can I enable my staff to be committed to right and good action?"

Ethical Situations Confronting Leaders and Managers

Our understanding about ethical problems confronting health care professionals and their leaders and managers continues to grow. From viewing these problems as mainly ethical dilemmas, we have begun to explore the complexity of health ethics, particularly nursing ethics and nursing management ethics (Gaudine & Beaton, 2002; Johnstone, 1999; Rodney et al., 2002; Storch, Rodney, & Starzomski, 2004; Storch, Rodney, Pauly, Brown, & Starzomski, 2002). The limitations of bioethics and the marginalization of nurses within it have been more widely recognized in recent years (Chambliss, 1996; Johnstone, 1999; Storch, Rodney, & Starzomski, 2002). Furthermore, the types of ethical problems have been more distinctly identified, moving beyond ethical violations and dilemmas to ethical or moral distress, moral uncertainty, moral residue, and other types of moral and ethical situations affecting nursing today (Webster & Baylis, 2000). This is a very positive move because it allows us to communicate our ethical concerns more clearly and, in so doing, engage in more meaningful dialogue about the situations we are facing.

The Canadian Nurses Association (CNA) *Code of Ethics for Registered Nurses* acknowledged this development in health and nursing ethics by enlarging its focus to six types of ethical situations: everyday ethics, ethical violations, ethical dilemmas, ethical distress, moral residue, and ethical uncertainty (CNA, 2002, p. 5–6). In highlighting *everyday ethics* as a key ethical situation faced by nurses, the CNA (2002) sought to underscore "the way nurses approach their practice and reflect on their ethical commitment to the people they serve" (p. 1). Because this involves attention to common ethical events, many nurses would understand everyday ethics as a way of being in relationship to their nursing practice.

Ethical violations are clear to most registered nurses (RNs) and their managers. *Ethical dilemmas* often have been considered to be situations in which a difficult choice must be made between competitive and equally compelling arguments for opposing positions and actions. What has become clearer is that the choice is not necessarily a choice of right or wrong, nor does it only involve two options; rather, it may well be a choice between two or more good options, only one of which can be undertaken. For nurse managers, this ethical situation is common in decisions about best use of resources.

The situation of *ethical or moral distress* is one in which health professionals and their managers have little choice except to act, even though an action does not "seem right." (Corley, 1995;

CNA, 1997, 2002; Fenton, 1988; Jameton, 1984; Rodney, 1988; Rodney & Starzomski, 1993; Wilkinson, 1987/88). This may involve a situation in which individuals have difficulty exercising their moral agency (their self-determining or self-expressive ethical choice); that is, they are required to act against their sense of what is right because those in positions of greater authority have already decided a course of action.

Situations of *moral residue* involve a buildup of occasions in which nurses and others know they have continued to compromise themselves and their values. Situations of *moral or ethical uncertainty* arise when nurses are unsure what ethical principles or values should apply to a moral problem they are facing (CNA, 2002).

Codes of ethics can provide guidance for appropriate actions in dealing with ethical violations. Codes also serve as a shared reference point to clarify for professionals and the public the commitments they should expect (Kidder, 1995; Storch & Nield, 2003). For example, the CNA *Code of Ethics for Registered Nurses* includes eight statements of values, with guidance for RNs in fulfilling their major responsibilities in each area. These include values of safe, competent, and ethical care; health and well-being; choice; dignity; confidentiality; justice; accountability; and quality practice environments. A code of ethics also can serve as a powerful and meaningful political tool.

Moral action in situations of ethical dilemma and ethical distress defies easy prescription, as illustrated by the four case examples provided in Box 15.1. An understanding of ethics is important to reflect critically upon these situations. The cases involving nurse managers in Box 15.1 will be used to illustrate how ethical theories and principles might be applied to the practice of moral management and ethical leadership. These case examples raise the kinds of ethical problems that nurse managers may face at any time. How they deal with these situations depends upon their moral sensitivity to the fact that their decisions involve ethical choices and upon their overall ability to deal with ethical issues. Kidder (1995), an educational ethicist, emphasizes the importance of "ethical fitness." This seems an apt term to underscore the importance of preparation for the ethical leadership role the nurse manager must provide.

Being Ethically Fit

To be ethically fit is to be mentally engaged in the human activity of ethical reflection and justification. Such fitness requires a certain degree of knowledge and skill in ethical problem solving. It involves being and becoming a person of good moral character, engaging in ethical conduct, and building a moral community.

In the following section, an overview of the substance of these requirements is provided, with liberal use of references to take the nurse manager or other first-level manager further along the path towards ethical fitness.

Being and Becoming a Person of Good Moral Character

The idea that the source of good moral choice resides in moral character is based upon the theory of virtue ethics. According to the theory of virtue ethics, virtuous people have moral character

Box 15.1

Managerial Problems Involving Ethics: Four Case Examples

The Case of Angela Antonovsky

Angela Antonovsky has worked in long-term care for over 20 years. Five years ago, she was appointed to the Assessment and Placement Service in the health region. Up until the past year, her position involved assessing people for long-term care, explaining to them and their families the options available in various care facilities in the region, and tracking their names on a wait list for their choice of long-term care facility. One year ago, the provincial government ruled that there would no longer be choices offered in terms of facility placements and that entry to any long-term care facility was based upon need alone. Angela finds this policy difficult to apply, particularly when it means that a resident's spouse or family and friends are no longer able to visit him or her due to the geographic distance. She has worked to apply the policy, but she experiences ongoing ethical conflict in doing so. Nurses in the long-term care facilities that Angela works with have become increasingly distressed that residents are feeling abandoned by their families and friends, and some of the residents are not able to understand why. The nurses have begun to question Angela's leadership and values, suggesting that she is compromising the quality of life of these residents. Angela has tried to interpret the government policy to the nursing staff, explaining that all placements need to be fair and equitable, but she is troubled by her staff's conviction that current residents are suffering. How can Angela help her clients, her staff, and herself? To what degree does senior management face a moral problem in this situation?

The Case of Beth Wallace

Beth Wallace is nurse manager of an adult hospital-to-home care unit that is currently operating as a demonstration project. Upon her return from a two-week vacation, she learns that, due to a nursing medication error, a client's recovery has been delayed by approximately a week. Mrs. P., the client, will experience no long-term negative effects; however, Mrs. P. happens to be the wife of a local journalist who has been highly critical of the hospital's operation of the demonstration unit, alleging that it provides substandard care. Beth has checked out all of the journalist's allegations and found them to be without substance. Further, a recent visit from the health agency's accrediting body has commended the unit's operation and its client outcomes. Mrs. P. and her family have been informed that her setback was due to an unanticipated drug reaction, and Beth is informed that they seem satisfied with that explanation. She knows that any adverse publicity for the unit could be damaging at this point. She thinks about the effects on present and future clients if further negative reporting by the journalist should lead to closure of the unit. She also thinks about the fact that the staff has not told Mrs. P. and her family the real reasons for her setback. What should Beth do? Why? What responsibility does senior management have in this situation?

The Case of Claude DeChamplain

Claude DeChamplain was recently appointed supervisor of the Critical Care Unit (CCU) in a community hospital. He had considered it fortunate that the Sudden Acute Respiratory Syndrome (SARS) outbreak did not impact his hospital or any neighbouring hospitals. Despite the fact that the city in which his hospital is located is quite distant from the hospitals that experienced SARS admissions, he worked diligently to prepare the nursing staff for an eventual SARS admission. Two nights ago, a patient was admitted to the CCU through the emergency room (ER) with flu-like symptoms, and many ER nurses believed the patient might have SARS. One day after admission, nurses in both the ER and CCU were distraught about having to put themselves at risk in looking after this patient. Their fears escalated when it was learned that no adequate protective masks were available in the hospital. This morning, two RNs phoned in sick, and two others indicated that they wished to decline to care for this patient. Claude knows that the CNA Code and other professional documents indicate that there must be no discrimination when caring for patients. He also lived through the early years of HIV/AIDS admissions and realizes the fears and misinformation in this outbreak are much the same. How might he proceed to ensure the patient is cared for? Should he allow RNs a right to refuse to look after this patient? What responsibility does senior management have in this situation? Is this a moral problem?

The Case of Anju Kuwait

Anju Kuwait is administrator of several acute surgical units within three amalgamated hospitals. These are busy units, and she does not have sufficient time to spend on any one unit to feel she fully understands the unique pressures of each. At the Senior Executive Conference early in the week, nursing administrators were told that within the coming week they must cut back the overtime hours being claimed by nurses on their units. Anju takes a day or two to investigate her unit's overtime hours compared to other units and determines that all three units seem to be running excessive overtime hours. Further, compared to the previous year, she discovers that most nurses are claiming all their overtime rather than claiming only occasional overtime. Because she is under pressure to reduce this overtime within the week, she prepares a memo for nursing staff on all three units and simply asks them to stop or reduce requests for their overtime hours. She also provides the units with the data relative to overtime hours because she assumes the nurses will see the wisdom of her request once they see the figures. Nursing staff on all the units involved are extremely upset with the request made in the memo. They confront Anju, telling her she does not understand what those overtime hours represent. They tell her that their overtime hours are spent charting and/or assisting nurses on the entering shift to turn and care for two-person patients. A number of nurses threaten to resign, stating that Anju is devaluing the work they do by suggesting they should not ask for overtime pay for it, that she is jeopardizing patient care by demanding they cut overtime without addressing the problem of inadequate staff, and that she does not represent their plight to senior management. Is Anju Kuwait's problem an ethical problem? Why? What should she do? What responsibility does senior management have in this situation?

and choose ethical actions because their deeply held values direct them to wise and informed ethical deliberation, leading to good choices. Such values develop during early socialization and can be cultivated throughout a lifetime.

Our understanding of *virtue* in the Western world originated with Greek philosophers, particularly Aristotle, who emphasized that it is the disposition "an agent habitually brings to his acts…that make a person good and enable him to do well" (Aristotle, trans. 1962, p. 38). Virtue ethics has been restored to an important place in ethical decision making only during the past decade. Johnstone (1999) suggests this restoration has occurred because of dissatisfaction with mainstream theories that have failed to provide an adequate account of the moral life. Particular virtues considered worthy of respect and emulation include trust, compassion, prudence, justice, fortitude, temperance, integrity, and self-effacement (Box 15.2).

Box 15.2

Virtues Applied to Health Managers and Professionals

THE FIDELITY TO TRUST involves a relationship with a client or a fellow worker, such as mutual planning of care, which is characterized by sensitivity to the needs of the other person but also maintains intellectual honesty and humility.

THE VIRTUE OF COMPASSION is the ability to co-experience the suffering of another person to the extent that one is able to employ one's professional knowledge and competence to attend to that suffering.

THE VIRTUE OF PRUDENCE is the combination of intellectual virtue (theoretical wisdom and understanding) and moral virtue (e.g., self-control, beneficence) that leads to good judgment in dealing with clinical and ethical problems.

THE VIRTUE OF MORAL JUSTICE is the "strict habit of rendering what is due to others" (p. 92) as an extension of the love or charity we should show to others.

THE VIRTUE OF FORTITUDE is the moral courage that makes a person willing to suffer personal harm for the sake of a moral good (e.g., advocating for the vulnerable in health care despite a potential risk to one's own status or position).

THE VIRTUE OF TEMPERANCE is the responsible use of power for the good of patients and the control of excesses in the use of science and technology.

THE VIRTUE OF INTEGRITY is being "predictable about responses to specific situations" (p. 127) and being able to integrate all virtues into the whole. It involves wise judgment as to the relative importance of principles, rules, and guidelines in reaching a decision to act.

THE VIRTUE OF SELF-EFFACEMENT is the ability to accept responsibility for moral malaise and to seek to restore health and healing practices to be a moral enterprise.

To suggest that managers and leaders must be people of sound moral character is to say that it matters a good deal that nurse managers and other health care managers are people who intend to do good, who are good people, and who have a "deep core of ethical values" (Kidder, 1995, p. 13). Being a professional is to profess to have knowledge that will be used to benefit others (Hughes, 1963). The combination of nursing knowledge and managerial knowledge creates a powerful potential for good if the manager is a virtuous person, that is, a person who has certain moral traits of character that are embedded in an intention to do good.

Virtues form the basis of the intent to do good, which is crucial to making good choices and executing right actions. For example, consider the case studies in Box 15.1. In the case of Angela Antonovsky, virtues of trust, compassion, justice, and temperance are required; in the cases of Beth Wallace and Claude DeChamplain, trust, compassion, prudence, and integrity are needed; and in the case of Anju Kuwait, there is a need for compassion, justice, fortitude, and self-efface-ment. Understanding the significance of these virtues to the commitments of the health care enterprise is critical for first-level managers. Recent literature has turned attention to the devel-opment of a moral identity as a way to consider how one might adopt nursing's ethical values and virtues and commit to the "good" in practice (see, for example, Doane, 2002).

Most theorists suggest that moral character alone is insufficient for moral action but that knowledge and application of general principles and theories are also required to guide ethical conduct in nursing and managerial practice (Pellegrino & Thomasma, 1993, pp. 14–15).

Engaging in Ethical Behaviour: Knowing Ethical Theories and Principles

Because moral virtues (i.e., the disposition to do what is ethically right) are not by themselves sufficient for engaging in ethical conduct (i.e., making and acting on ethical decisions), knowl-edge of theories and principles is considered an essential tool for health professionals and their managers. Such knowledge enables a manager to understand ethical quandaries of manageri-al life and to come to terms with ethical problems by finding the terminology that gives mean-ing to these situations.

Ethic of Utility

One of the main theories derived from moral philosophy that has dominated bioethical think-ing is the *ethic of utility* (utilitarianism or ends-based thinking), which continues to be employed as strong justification for many managerial actions in health care. This is increasingly manifest in the current turbulent and fiscally restrained health care environment. Essentially, the ethic of utility is based upon the premise that choices of actions can be considered good if those choices lead to good outcomes. Generally, good outcomes are those that lead to the greatest number of people experiencing the greatest good, whether that good is happiness, access to health care, or general economic good. Jeremy Bentham and John Stuart Mill are regarded as the architects of this approach. In raw form, a utilitarian ethicist might argue that a good outcome for a size-able number of individuals justifies the ways in which the outcomes are achieved. That is why this theoretical approach is often described as one in which "the end justifies the means."

Using ends-based thinking in the case of Angela Antonovsky, a utilitarian would argue that, while it is a shame that people cannot be placed in long-term care facilities close to their home and suffer as a result, providing equitable access to the long-term care justifies the lack of choice about where people will spend their final months or years. In the case of Beth Wallace, a utilitarian argument might be that the deception about the medication should not have occurred, but continuity of the unit depends upon public confidence in the unit. Because of this assumption, maintaining public confidence outweighs the principle of honesty. In effect, because closure of the unit could result from negative media attention, the needs of many older patients for the services of the unit outweigh the importance of telling the truth to one patient and her family.

Ethic of Duty

The second main theory of moral philosophy is the *ethic of duty* (deontological theory or rule-based thinking). The theory of the ethic of duty is based upon duties or obligations derived from several sources, including theological sources. Secular ethics in our society, however, is mainly derived from the work of Immanuel Kant, a German philosopher who held that obligations or duties should be the basis of moral choices, irrespective of the consequences of such actions. Kant (1948) suggested that there ought to be an imperative that one would never act unless she or he believed that such an action should become the rule of conduct for all.

In the case of Angela Antonovsky, therefore, an ethic of duty theorist might argue that the duty to alleviate the social and psychological suffering of people placed in long-term care distant from their loved ones takes priority over the potential harm that might be caused to others who may not have equal access to long-term care as a result. In the case of Beth Wallace, a duty-based argument might hold that individuals have a duty to be honest with one another, regardless of the consequences, because this is a sound general rule for all to follow. Such honesty takes priority over whatever outcomes may result from the revelation of the medication error "cover-up" because of the overbearing importance of honesty.

Bioethical Principles

In order to provide a more accessible means of ethical decision making for health care professionals and managers, bioethics emerged as an applied discipline, with theories and principles that were mostly developed in the late 1970s and early 1980s. *Bioethical principles* were introduced into the mainstream of health care scholarship and practice mainly through rediscovery of the writings of W. D. Ross in 1930 and the work of Beauchamp and Childress in their popular text *Principles of Biomedical Ethics* (2001), first published in 1979. The four-principle approach set out by Beauchamp and Childress is now quite well known and widely used. The four bioethical principles are autonomy, beneficence, non-maleficence, and justice (Box 15.3).

Numerous textbooks of nursing ethics, medical ethics, and health care ethics have employed these principles as a means of enabling health professionals to become more ethically fit (Kidder, 1995) and thereby to make sound ethical choices. The principles assist in clarifying ethical dilemmas and situations of ethical distress and serve as a set of counterpoints in ethical decision making. In the case of Angela Antonovsky, for example, the principle of justice for many must be weighed against the principle of beneficence for many others; in the case of Beth Wallace, the principle of truthfulness (as part of beneficence) must be weighed against the principle of

Box 15.3

Ethical Principles

AUTONOMY: The principle of autonomy is the right to choose for oneself what one believes to be in one's best interests. It is the concept of self-determination, of being in charge of one's person. From this principle of autonomy comes our commitment to respect patients' treatment choices and their need to make informed choices about matters of life and death. The rights to privacy, honesty, confidentiality, and refusal of treatment are also duties that evolve from this principle.

BENEFICENCE: The principle of beneficence is the duty to benefit others. A central belief reflected in this principle is the duty or obligation to assist others, to contribute to their welfare, and in doing so, to always act in the best interests of the patient or client.

NON-MALEFICENCE: The principle of non-maleficence is the duty to do no harm and to protect others from harm. Non-maleficence includes minimizing harms that may be necessary in the course of treatment, anticipating harms that may occur, and avoiding harm. Such harms are not restricted to physical harms, but also include feelings of helplessness, isolation, and powerlessness, to name just a few of the many important considerations for all health professionals.

DISTRIBUTIVE JUSTICE: The principle of distributive justice has as its underlying value fairness that is based on the equal worth of individuals. While there are several criteria that may be applied to determine fairness (e.g., to each according to worth, to each according to need, to each according to contribution), equity is a value commonly held in Canada. Equity is fairness according to need.

Source: From *Ethical Decision-Making for Registered Nurses in Alberta: Guidelines and Recommendations* (pp. 7–8), by Alberta Association of Registered Nurses, 1996, Edmonton, AB: Author. Copyright 1996 by AARN. Reprinted with permission.

justice; in the case of Claude DeChamplain, the principle of beneficence and justice for patients must be weighed against the principle of fairness (justice) for the individual employee; and in the case of Anju Kuwait, the principles of non-maleficence to those in care and of fairness to the nurses who are overworked predominate. A good working understanding of these principles assists nurse managers to consider what is at stake in ethical situations.

Ethic of Care and Relational Ethics

Partly in reaction to the fact that these bioethical principles appear to be simpler than they are, making them susceptible to misuse, scholars of ethics (among them, nurse ethicists) have proposed different approaches to ethical decision making. Gilligan (1982) criticized these principles (or "principlism") as based too solidly in a justice perspective (or rights-based ethic) rather than an ethic of responsibility, which she described as an *ethic of care*.

Others suggest that the bioethical principles have too often have been employed in a non-contextualized reductionalist manner and that, while the principles are necessary, they are not sufficient for determining ethical conduct (Bergum, 1994; Johnstone, 1999; Rodney, Burgess, McPherson, & Brown, 2004). Many nurse ethicists, educators, and practitioners have found the ethic of care appealing in that it is a theory that takes into account the context of care (e.g., the setting, the patient's significant others, the patient's history) as well as the health professional's obligations in relation to patients and their care.

Bergum (1994), a nurse ethicist, suggested that the "kind of knowledge needed for ethical care must be constructed in the relationship between professional and patient" (p. 72). In that relationship, the nurse seeks to understand the patient's experience of disease and illness and to explore with the patient the meaning of the condition for that individual. Bergum also focused on developing a theory of *relational ethics*, which incorporates bioethical principles (a justice-based approach) and an ethic of care (an approach to caring that focuses on context, person, and relationship). Relational ethics consider the context and the lived experience of those in situations of health care. It also considers the bioethical principles only in the context of those relationships (Austin, Bergum, & Dossetor, 2003a; Bergum, 1994, 2004).

Applying an ethic of care and relational ethics to the case of Claude DeChamplain would focus the nurse manager's attention on the context in which health care is being provided (e.g., fiscal restraints, insufficient material resources, inadequate supports for nurses potentially risking their own lives), as well as on the duty of safe care. Using an ethic of care (i.e., an ethic of responsibility), a nurse manager like Angela Antonovsky, who was forced to consider the duties owed to both present and future residents, might be motivated to involve the staff in identifying important dimensions of care for these residents. She might work with staff to develop a petition (or proposal) to senior management for approaches that might mitigate the circumstances of the residents while documenting evidence of the harms they are experiencing. In the case of Beth Wallace, the nurse manager applying a relational ethic would attempt to consider all individuals involved—client, family, nurse, and relative—and seek ways to be faithful to the needs of all while upholding the fundamental value of honesty.

Contextualism

It bears repeating that nurse managers must recognize the ease with which it is possible to slide into models of ethical decision making that are too simple and too comfortable and do not always force full clarification and consideration of the ethical dimensions of difficult situations. In some cases, the use of bioethical principles alone, however helpful they may be, can produce a result that approximates a "medical work-up," a "nursing process," or some other scientific problem-solving approach. When used in linear thinking models, principles may even obscure the meaning of the ethical situation for everyone involved. As one practitioner noted, when we make ethical decisions regarding clients in care, we too frequently take a snapshot rather than consider the mural of the patient's life (Moss, 1994).

To that end, Winkler advocated for *contextualism*, which he described as appraising a moral situation from "the bottom up." One form of contextualism is Bergum's relational ethics, whereby principles or theories are applied only after the context of the situation is understood. Winkler elaborated on the parameters of the context, stating that moral problems "must be resolved within concrete circumstances, in their interpretive complexity, by appeal to relevant historical and cultural traditions, with reference to critical institutional and professional norms and virtues, and by utilizing the primary method of comparative case analysis" (Winkler, 1993, p. 344).

Cultural and Feminist Ethics

Rodney and colleagues support this approach and add to it *cultural ethics* and *feminist ethics*. Cultural ethics involves attention to individualized as well as shared values, beliefs, and systems of meaning. Feminist ethics "draws attention to the quality of the relationship—particularly the power in those relationships—at individual, organizational, and societal levels" (Rodney, Pauly, & Burgess, 2004, p. 84). Cultural ethics and feminist ethics direct us to focus on the particular aspects of an ethical situation, while bioethical principles and theories keep us mindful of more universal values. Further, broader organizational contexts that may have created situations of ethical distress are taken into account, rather than being discounted or overlooked. Senior management and governing boards often bear significant responsibility for creating serious ethical problems for front-line managers and their staff; these individuals, too, need to become ethically fit.

Alternate Approaches to Guide Ethical Decision Making

Over the past decade, numerous models have been proposed for ethical thinking and problem solving within the health care literature. A wide range of models has been summarized in the CNA booklet *Everyday Ethics: Putting the Code into Practice*. Many such models or ethics decision frameworks are principle-based, often utilizing the four principles or some variation of them. Silva (1990) offers examples of numerous decision-making models in her text, *Ethical Decision-Making in Nursing Administration*, and she provides case studies with step-by-step comments that address the ethical dilemmas inherent in the cases. First-level managers will find her text most helpful.

A relatively neglected resource in health care ethics is the work of Kidder (1995), whose approach seems particularly applicable to ethical issues facing health care managers. Kidder emphasizes the reality that ethical dilemmas are usually right-versus-right situations and urges those who would be ethical to seek middle ground in such dilemmas whenever possible. He suggests a dilemma might be examined in the context of the following four choices: justice versus mercy, short-term versus long-term, individual versus community, and truth versus loyalty.

No single "fixed" approach to ethical thinking can suit all nurses or health professionals. Nurse managers must discover individually the approaches that work best for them and that enable them to lead in a way that encourages staff to ask questions, identify issues, and pursue ethically justifiable choices. Thus, in addition to continued development of moral character, nurse managers need to choose models for ethical decision making that are meaningful and helpful to them.

Building a Moral Community

Working to build a moral community is a third critical element of the leadership role of the nurse manager. By way of their example and by sharing their vision with a team of workers, transformational leaders can significantly influence moral behaviour within their units or programs and within agencies. In fostering a moral community, nurse managers share information and their own interpretation of that information among and between their staff and demonstrate how ideals can be translated into conduct (Biordi, 1993).

Nurse managers' task of building moral communities with their staff goes beyond obligations to others and incorporates thoughtful reflection about the kind of nursing practice life they consider to be important and worthwhile. Such considerations are critical when choosing the type of a society we want to be and to become. These issues are particularly significant in contemporary Canadian health care settings (Yeo, 1993). Although such reflections may seem remote from the everyday world of the first-line manager, it is through the daily use of moral action and formal and informal ethical decision making that a moral community is ultimately realized.

Obstacles to Building a Moral Community

Within the world of managerial practice, there are numerous obstacles to building a moral community. A primary obstacle may be the nurse manager's own understanding and response to the perceived value of the objectivity of management science and medical science. This matters because the theories of management (or of medicine, health, and healing) determine what we treat as facts (Astley, 1985). There are no "bare facts." Facts depend upon and are defined by the manager's theories. Theories are comprised of certain terms and specific language, that is, a particular vocabulary. Each of these languages or vocabularies incorporates certain assumptions about values: these values are not normally made explicit.

Nowhere is this more apparent than in the confusing and often misleading vocabulary of health care management, including nursing management. Through the magic of language, it is possible to diminish the nature of a moral community by redefining client or agency problems. In doing so, meaning can be extracted from client experiences of health and illness and from the health professional's experience of ethical distress. A common example of this phenomenon is the way in which nursing advocacy for better staffing in order to ensure safe and competent client care often is reduced by politicians or senior executives to "whining by nurses" or to accusations of "staff protecting their jobs." For first-level managers caught between opposing positions, exercising ethical fitness is a way to remain true to oneself and one's values in everyday work life.

Nurse managers are cautioned to remember that even such commonly used terms as *quality*, *total quality management*, *clinical practice guidelines*, and *evidence-based care* are based on value-laden concepts. Within health care agencies, these conceptual models can determine what counts as important information for planning and evaluation. Many times, the supposedly objective facts of numbers and statistics are given priority over the more subjective aspects of client care and progress. It is not that any of these concepts are inherently wrong, but in building a moral community, they must be understood for what they are, tools to be used by health care managers, nurse managers, and health professionals. Unfortunately, in practice, these tools are too often used as ends in themselves rather than as means to an end. Unless the tools are appropriately used and take into account consideration of broader issues, such as what patients consider important, they miss the mark (Redman, 1996).

Over the past decade and more, serious cutbacks to health services, and particularly to nursing, have left a residue of unmet needs in nursing care (Rodney & Street, 2004; Storch, 2003). "Each cost constraint measure has had a direct impact on nursing practice, creating more work, more uncertainty, and less control over how nursing time is spent" (Varcoe & Rodney, 2002, p. 104). Varcoe and Rodney (2002), basing their analysis on separate research in two hospital acute medical units (Rodney) and two emergency rooms (Varcoe), demonstrated how an ideology of scarcity drives nursing practice to emphasize streamlining and efficiencies. They suggested that the media, senior executives, politicians, and others promote this talk of scarcity to the point where it is taken for granted as fact and is considered both inevitable and justifiable. For nurses, this has at least two implications: They continue their daily experiences of discrepancies between the care they value and the care they provide, a cause of great moral distress; and they spend time accommodating the efficiencies of others, leaving them even less opportunity to give patients the care that is needed.

Varcoe and Rodney (2002) maintain that cost efficiency exacts both a professional and personal toll on nurses, allowing them no time to think through or talk about their moral distress and other moral situations. Their sense of anguish and powerlessness often leads to moral resistance, where they feel forced to work around the system (guerilla tactics) to get their patients what they need. This is because, too often, the rules are developed by others who are removed from day-to-day care.

The findings of Austin, Bergum, and Dossetor (2003b), in their phenomenological study of mental health practitioners, provide further evidence of constrained moral agency and the moral distress of nurses. In such a climate of practice, the work of the nurse leaders and managers to develop a moral community becomes extremely challenging. Research has shown that this climate has a serious effect on nurse leaders and managers. In a study of nursing ethics in practice (Storch, Rodney, Pauly, et al., 2002), advanced practice nurses noted they often had to "pick their battles" when representing nursing staff at senior level meetings. Often their voices were not heard and sometimes they felt discouraged from raising issues of understaffing, unmet needs, and so on.

A study by Gaudine and Beaton (2002) reported similar findings. They found that the difficult budget decisions that nurse managers had to make put them at risk for ethical conflict. The nurse managers in this study reported four main types of ethical conflict: (a) "voicelessness (limited collaborative opportunities), (b) where to spend the money, (c) the rights of the individual versus the needs of the organization, and (d) unjust practices on the part of senior administration and/or the organization" (Gaudine & Beaon, 2002, p. 21).

Some particularly disturbing findings in this study were that several nurse managers stated they did not believe that their administrators wanted to understand nurses and had no intention of addressing their needs and that, due to poor receptivity, nurse managers seldom shared information with their hospital administrators or board members (Gaudine & Beaon, 2002, p. 23). Gaudine and Beaton noted how demeaning it would be for nurse managers to feel they are not supposed to speak out about the decisions being made around them (p. 29). Similarly, in another study, advanced practice nurses stated that if they spoke up too much, they were no longer invited to meetings at which important decisions were being made about nursing (Storch, Rodney, Pauly, et al., 2002).

In 2000, Andre Picard, a journalist with *The Globe and Mail*, published a book entitled *Critical Care: Canadian Nurses Speak for Change.* In it, he presented the findings of his observations and interviews with nurses in all types of nursing work across Canada. Among those interviewed was a nurse administrator, Mary Ferguson-Paré, who stated:

With full respect, I have to say that people in positions of power like mine often find themselves in politically [and presumably, ethically] compromising positions that are not good for nursing. Unfortunately, many nurses have taken an ecumenical approach when they get to the management level. That disappoints nurses who count on them to carry the day on every issue. But when you're in a position like mine, you have to decide: "What hill am I going to die on?" (Picard, 2002, p. 223).

Leadership Implications

In the introduction to this chapter, three main dimensions of ethical leadership were noted, namely, being a person of moral character, being a person who engages in moral behaviour, and being someone who builds a moral community. Values are critical to moral leadership. Nurse managers must be clear about the values that are important to them and recognize that commitment to these values will place demands on them.

A critical element in ethical leadership is the way in which important values are communicated to staff as a vision of care and service. To gain commitment and involvement in working toward those ends, the manager/leader must work to establish a culture in which attention to ethics plays a pivotal role. It must be a culture in which staff are encouraged to observe ethical problems in the workplace, are free to challenge the standards and practices they consider unethical (Longest, 1996), are encouraged to keep themselves ethically fit, are assisted in addressing ethical concerns, and are supported in being a moral agent who is attentive to everyday ethics and dealing well with tough ethical choices.

Such support can be provided through formal structures or informal means. As long as a climate of openness to ethics and ethical discussion exists on a unit or set of units, questions about ethical practice or the application of the CNA *Code of Ethics for Registered Nurses* can arise as an integral part of nurses' dialogue during the provision of care. Based upon ethically troublesome and recurring situations with agency-wide implications, nurses can be encouraged to initiate discussion and to draft proposals for agency ethics statements or policies.

Ethics committees also can be an important structure to promote ethical practice. Such committees bring visibility to the priority of ethics in the health agency and also serve as a useful learning forum for managers and staff. Many health agencies have ethics committees. Unfortunately, too often the nursing staff is unaware of these committees and of their work (Storch & Griener, 1992; Storch, Rodney, & Starzomski, 2002). The nurse manager can do much to raise awareness of ethics committees among staff members and encourage them to use and be involved with these committees. The manager can encourage staff to take everyday ethical problems to such committees for consideration.

Some nurses feel intimidated at the prospect of being involved in an agency ethics committee; some are uncomfortable even with the idea of submitting a problem case or issue to such a committee. Nevertheless, these same nurses often experience ethical distress on a daily basis and convey a deep commitment to ethics and ethical practice. Nurse managers can encourage the creation of formal or informal ethics committees or discussion groups within nursing departments or units, where nurses can share their concerns with colleagues. Such dialogue can be a way to enhance the comfort level of staff toward full participation in agency ethics committees and ethics education. If no agency ethics committee exists, the nursing ethics committee or the interdisciplinary ethics committee within a unit may well become the embryo for development of a committee that meets to reflect and consult on ethical problems in the health agency as a whole.

Liberal use of opportunities for ethics education for the nurse manager and staff is yet another way to stimulate reflection and discussion. This approach is particularly important as health regions, health agencies, and units within agencies grapple with such issues as advance treatment directives, research involving patients with dementia, privatizing health programs, and the apparent erosion of standards of confidentiality in occupational health services.

All these types of initiatives not only bring greater visibility to the priority of ethics among staff, but also serve as useful forums for mutual learning for managers and staff. At the same time, nurse leaders and managers need the ethical commitment of their senior management and boards. Without their commitment to organizational ethics, realizing safe, competent, and ethical care in practice will become an elusive goal; the level of moral distress amongst nursing staff will escalate, and the exodus from nursing will continue. As Rodney and Street (2004) observe, "Perhaps the first step to improve the moral climate...is to *name* it as a goal" (p. 217).

Summary

- Ethical leadership demands that managers be people of moral character and behaviour who are intent on building moral communities.
- Managers can provide ethical leadership by helping staff develop a commitment to moral values and ethical reflection.
- Tools for ethical fitness include knowledge of theories and principles and how these can be used to clarify ethical problems and make good choices.
- Ethical dilemmas can arise on a daily basis in a health care setting. It is imperative that managers reflect on the values that are important to them and that their actions reflect their ethical leadership.
- Nurse managers manage by leading, not by direction and control.
- Leadership commits staff to action by appealing to higher ideals and moral values.
- Almost every action a manager takes involves ethics.
- The Canadian Nurses Association *Code of Ethics for Registered Nurses* (2002) offers guidance for nurse managers and nursing staff.
- Being ethically fit means being engaged in ethical reflection and justification.

- Ethical fitness involves being and becoming a person of sound moral character, engaging in ethical behaviour by knowing and applying ethical theories and principles, and building a moral community.
- A person of moral character intends to do good and has a deep core of ethical values and particular moral traits (or virtues).
- Ends-based thinking, rule-based thinking, and relational-based thinking are three theoretical approaches to ethics, while principles help to illuminate ethical understanding and decision making.
- Building a moral community involves establishing a culture wherein ethics play a pivotal role.
- Informal ethics discussions, formalized ethics statements or policies, and ethics committees are structures that support a moral community.

Applying the Knowledge in this Chapter

Exercise

As a member of an informal ethics committee, you decide to discuss the four case examples presented in this chapter as a learning exercise. Keeping the concepts of ethical fitness and the responsibility for building a moral community in mind, what actions do you think the manager should have taken in each of these cases? How would you respond to the questions posed in each case?

Resources

evolve Internet Resources

Code of Ethics for Registered Nurses:

www.cna-aiic.ca

The "Ethics in Practice Papers" and CNA Position Papers (among the position papers are ones on ethical nurse recruitment, privacy of personal information, and many others pertinent to nursing leadership, including conflict resolution on the health care team) can be found on this Web site.

International Council of Nurses (ICN) Code of Ethics:

www.icn@icn.ch

Numerous position papers and other guideline documents related to nursing ethics, including the ICN Code of Ethics, are available here.

Further Reading

Beauchamp, T.L., & Childress, J.F. (2001). *Principles of biomedical ethics.* (5th ed.). New York: Oxford University Press.

This is a classic text because it provides a comprehensive discussion of the ethical principles of respect for autonomy, beneficence, non-maleficence, and justice, with liberal use of examples to illustrate the application of these principles in health care practice. Also included is a discussion of moral norms and moral character, professional-patient relationships, and an overview of types of moral theories.

Canadian Nurses Association. (1998). *Everyday ethics: Putting the code into practice.* Ottawa, ON: Canadian Nurses Association.

This book was first published in 1998 following the release of the 1997 CNA Code. It is currently under revision to conform to the 2002 Code. It contains basic values of the Code, cases for each value, values clarification exercises, and models for decision making.

Pellegrino, E.D., & Thomasma, D.C. (1992). *The virtues in medical practice.* New York: Oxford University Press.

Virtue theory and the virtues of medicine (appropriate to all health professionals) are given comprehensive treatment in this text. The authors have been able to provide a counter-balancing theory to the principle-based approach, while emphasizing the merits of principles and theories.

Silva, M.C. (1990). *Ethical decision-making in nursing administration.* Norwalk, CT: Appleton and Lange.

In addition to providing a fine overview of classical ethical theories and principles, Silva offers a wide range of applications for a decision-making model. Included in her text are six case studies that are thoroughly analyzed, plus an additional six ethical dilemmas involving nursing administrators. This is a very useful text for nurse managers and administrators.

Storch, J.L., Rodney, P., & Starzomski, R. (Eds.). (2004). *Toward a moral horizon: Nursing ethics for leadership and practice.* Don Mills, ON: Pearson Education.

This book was specifically written to support the teaching of a course in advanced nursing practice. It is directed to graduate students and nurse leaders and practitioners. Its focus is on the development of nursing ethics as an emerging field of ethics, and its contributed chapters are from nurses and others in different disciplines from across Canada and other countries. The focus of the work is on everyday ethics and ethics in practice. Early chapters provide a thorough review of nursing ethics history and current development. Later chapters address ethical concerns extending to the future.

Tschudin, V. (1994). *Deciding ethically: A practical approach to nursing challenges.* London: Baillière-Tindall.

Although there are numerous fine nursing ethics texts written in North America, this small book authored in the United Kingdom is suggested here because it offers some novel perspectives on ethics. Tschudin provides a practical approach to nursing challenges by covering theories, principles, and virtues, with liberal use of illustrations from nursing practice.

References

Alberta Association of Registered Nurses. (1996). *Ethical decision making for registered nurses in Alberta: Guidelines and reccomommendations.* Edmonton, AB: AARN.

Aristotle. (1962). *Nicomachean ethics.* (M. Ostwald, Trans.). Englewood Cliffs, NJ: Prentice Hall.

Astley, W.G. (1985). Administrative science as socially constructed truth. *Administrative Science Quarterly, 30,* 497–513.

Austin, W., Bergum, V., & Dossetor, J. (2003a). Relational ethics: An action ethic as foundation for health care. In V. Tschudin (Ed.), *Approaches to ethics: Nursing beyond boundaries* (pp. 45–52). Woburn, MA: Butterworth-Heinemann.

Austin, W., Bergum, V., & Dosssetor, J. (2003b). Unable to answer the call of our patients: Mental health nurses' experience of moral distress. *Nursing Inquiry, 10,* 177–183.

Beauchamp, T.L., & Childress, J.F. (2001). *Principles of biomedical ethics* (5th ed.). New York: Oxford University Press.

Bergum, V. (1994). Knowledge for ethical care. *Nursing Ethics, 1*(2), 71–79.

Bergum, V. (2004). Relational ethics in nursing. In J.L. Storch, P. Rodney, & R. Starzomski (Eds.), *Toward a moral horizon: Nursing ethics for leadership and practice* (pp. 485–503). Don Mills, ON: Pearson Education.

Biordi, D.L. (1993). Ethical leadership. In A. Marriner-Tomey (Ed.), *Transformational leadership in nursing* (pp. 51–68). St. Louis, MO: Mosby.

Canadian Nurses Association. (1997). *Code of ethics for registered nurses*. Ottawa, ON: CNA.

Canadian Nurses Association. (2002). *Code of ethics for registered nurses*. Ottawa, ON: CNA.

Chambliss, D.F. (1996). *Beyond caring: Hospitals, nurses, and the social organization of ethics*. Chicago: The University of Chicago Press.

Corley, M.C. (1995). Moral distress in critical care nurses. *American Journal of Critical Care, 4*(4), 280–285.

Doane, G.H. (2002). Am I still ethical? The socially-mediated process of nurses' moral identity. *Nursing Ethics, 9*(6), 623–635.

Fenton, M. (1988). Moral distress in clinical practice: Implications for the nurse administrator. *Canadian Journal of Nursing Administration, 1*(1), 8–11.

Gaudine, A.P., & Beaton, M.R. (2002). Employed to go against one's values: Nurse managers' accounts of ethical conflict with their organizations. *Canadian Journal of Nursing Research, 34*(2), 17–34.

Gilligan, C. (1982). *In a different voice*. Cambridge, MA: Harvard University Press.

Hughes, E.C. (1963, Fall). Professions. *Daedalus, 92,* 655–668.

Jameton, A. (1984). *Nursing practice: The ethical issues*. Englewood Cliffs, NJ: Prentice Hall Inc.

Johnstone, M.J. (1999). *Bioethics: A nursing perspective* (3rd ed.). Sydney, Australia: Harcourt.

Kant, I. (1948). *Groundwork of the metaphysic of morals* (H. J. Paton, Trans.). New York: Harper and Row.

Kidder, R.M. (1995). *How good people make tough choices*. New York: Fireside.

Longest, B.B. (1996). *Health professionals in management*. Stamford, CT: Appleton and Lange.

Marriner-Tomey, A. (1993). *Transformational leadership in nursing*. St. Louis, MO: Mosby.

Mitchell, C. (1996). *Practical bioethics for nurses*. Workshop presentation at the Bioethics Conference: A Future of Dignity. Hawaii: St. Francis Medical Center.

Moss, A.H. (1994). Narrative ethics: A patient friendly approach to 'doing ethics.' *Network of Ethics Committees Newsletter*. Morgantown, WV: Network.

Pellegrino, E.D. (1993). The metamorphosis of medical ethics. *Journal of the American Medical Association, 269,* 1158–1162.

Pellegrino, E.D., & Thomasma, D.C. (1993). *The virtues in medical practice*. New York: Oxford University Press.

Picard, A. (2000). *Critical care: Canadian nurses speak for change*. Toronto, ON: Harper Collins.

Redman, B.K. (1996). Ethical issues in the development and use of guidelines for clinical practice. *The Journal of Clinical Ethics, 7*(3), 251–256.

Rodney, P. (1988). Moral distress in critical care nursing. *Canadian Critical Care Nursing Journal, 5*(2), 9–11.

Rodney, P., Burgess, M., McPherson, G., & Brown, H. (2004). Our theoretical landscape: A brief history of health care ethics. In J.L. Storch, P. Rodney, & R. Starzomski (Eds.), *Towards a moral horizon: Nursing ethics for leadership and practice* (pp. 56–76). Don Mills, ON: Pearson Education.

Rodney, P., Pauly, B., & Burgess, M. (2004). Our theoretical landscape: Complementary approaches to health care ethics. In J.L. Storch, P. Rodney, & R. Stazomski (Eds.), *Towards a moral horizon: Nursing ethics for leadership and practice* (pp. 77–97). Don Mills, ON: Pearson Education.

Rodney, P., & Starzomski, R. (1993). Constraints on the moral agency of nurses. *Canadian Nurse, 89*(9), 23–26.

Rodney, P., & Street, A. (2004). The moral climate for nursing practice: Inquiry and action. In J.L. Storch, P. Rodney, & R. Starzomski (Eds.), *Toward a moral horizon: Nursing ethics for leadership and practice* (pp. 209–231). Don Mills, ON: Pearson Education.

Rodney, P., Varcoe, C., Storch, J.L., McPherson, G., Mahoney, K., Brown, H., et al. (2002). Navigating towards a moral horizon: A multisite qualitative study of ethical practice in nursing. *Canadian Journal of Nursing Research, 34*(3), 75–102.

Silva, M.C. (1990). *Ethical decision-making in nursing administration.* Norwalk, CT: Appleton and Lange.

Storch, J.L. (2003). Nursing: Yesterday, today, forever. [Editorial comment]. *Nursing Ethics, 10*(2), 120–121.

Storch, J.L., & Griener, G.G. (1992). Ethics committees in Canadian hospitals: Report of the 1990 pilot study. *Healthcare Management Forum, 5*(1), 19–26.

Storch, J.L., & Nield, S. (2003). Keeping codes current. *Nursing Leadership Forum, 7*(3), 103–108.

Storch, J.L., Rodney, P., Pauly, B., Brown, H., & Starzomski, R. (2002). Listening to nurses' moral voices: Building a quality health care environment. *Canadian Journal of Nursing Leadership, 15*(4), 7–16.

Storch, J.L., Rodney, P., & Starzomski, R. (2002). Ethics in health care in Canada. In B.S. Bolaria & H. Dickinson (Eds.), *Health, illness and health care in Canada* (3rd ed., pp. 409–444). Scarborough, ON: Nelson Thomson Learning.

Storch, J.L., Rodney, P., & Starzomski, R. (Eds.). (2004). *Toward a moral horizon: Nursing ethics for leadership and practice.* Don Mills, ON: Pearson Education.

Varcoe, C., & Rodney, P. (2002). Constrained agency: The social structure of nurses' work. In B.S. Bolaria & H. Dickinson (Eds.), *Health, illness and health care in Canada* (3rd ed., pp. 102–128). Scarborough, ON: Nelson Thomson Learning.

Webster, G.C., & Baylis, R.E. (2000). Moral residue. In S.B. Rubin & L. Zoloth (Eds.), *Margin of error: The ethics of mistakes in the practice of medicine* (pp. 217–230). Hagerstown, MD: University Publishing Press.

Wilkinson, J. (1987/88). Moral distress in nursing practice: Experience and effect. *Nursing Forum, 23*(1), 16–29.

Winkler, E. (1993). From Kantianism to contextualism: The rise and fall of the paradigm theory of bioethics. In E.R. Winkler & J.R. Coombs (Eds.), *Applied ethics: A reader* (pp. 343–365). Oxford, UK: Blackwell.

Yeo, M. (1993). Toward an ethic of empowerment for health promotion. *Health Promotion International, 8*(3), 225–235.

HEALTH AGENCIES AND SELF-GOVERNING PROFESSIONS: A COMPLEX RELATIONSHIP

Judith M. Hibberd

Learning Objectives

In this chapter, you will learn:

- The rights and responsibilities of professional groups in the context of health service organizations

- Similarities and differences in the way physicians and nurses are organized and represented in the decision-making processes of health service organizations

- How systems for establishing professional governance and practice standards are incorporated into the administrative structure and processes of health service organizations

- The organization of medical staff in hospitals and regional health authorities

- The evolution of contemporary professional practice models in nursing, including shared governance

- Effects of restructuring on shared governance projects and the emergence of integrated professional practice models

- Conditions that contribute to the successful implementation and maintenance of nursing professional practice models

The health care workforce comprises a broad spectrum of professional and technical workers, often referred to as knowledge workers. Many of these workers are highly specialized, having undertaken years of post-secondary education, and most, if not all, are licensed members of professional associations or colleges. Society has delegated authority and responsibility for self-governance to professional groups, allowing them to set criteria for entering and continuing in a profession, to set up methods for handling complaints and discipline, and to establish codes of ethics and standards for practice. But what happens to this authority for self-governance when the work of professionals takes place within an institution that is governed by an independent board of trustees legally accountable for all services rendered by its staff? There is potential for conflict to occur between hospital boards oriented to a business or production frame of reference and health professionals oriented to their clients and their discipline who may be unwilling to compromise on standards of clinical practice.

Although it has been argued that the employed professional should not be able to benefit from both self-governance and from collective bargaining (Beatty & Gunderson, 1979), hospital-employed professionals in Canada, such as nurses, therapists, and those in other health disciplines, continue to enjoy both forms of representation. Nurses, for example, are represented by their unions on socioeconomic issues within the workplace, and by their professional associations on a wide range of policy issues in society at large (i.e., outside the employment setting). Physicians, however, are for the most part self-employed professionals, and although licensed to practice, they are not members of employee unions. Thus, employment status is a pivotal factor in determining how health professionals fulfill their responsibilities and obligations in health agencies and how they are managed or governed.

Physicians who admit patients to hospitals are compensated on a fee-for-service basis, and their clinical practice is subject to peer review. Although there are some salaried physicians in hospitals (e.g., emergency officers and residents), physicians who wish to admit patients to a hospital and treat them on site must apply for what is known as hospital privileges. As a member of the hospital medical staff, these privileges allow physicians free access to all necessary hospital resources for treating their patients, including the services of nurses, other health disciplines, and technical staff.

In contrast, nurses are hired to fill specific employee positions, their work is subject to supervision, and they are paid a predetermined wage that is usually established through collective bargaining. It is important for nurses and managers of nursing services to understand these differences. In particular, they need to understand how the medical staff is organized, how policies and regulations governing patient care are made (many of these rules have implications for the practice of nursing), and how concerns about professional competence and quality of care are handled.

Originally, self-governance was granted as a means of regulating professionals engaged in independent practice. The issue of self-governance and professional autonomy is central to the question of how professionals are organized within health care agencies. For the purpose of this chapter, *health care agencies* refer to hospitals and regional health authorities where there is likely to be a concentration of physicians and other health care professionals as well as internal governance structures to deal with professional issues and concerns. Public health agencies, community health services, and independent health care agencies, such as nursing homes and home care, generally depend on family physicians to provide medical care to their patients and clients, and unless these agencies are an integral part of a regional health authority, they do not have an organized medical staff to the same extent as hospitals. Issues and problems that relate to professional competence and clinical standards in an independent community health agency are referred directly to the relevant licensing body under provincial legislation or are handled internally by an administrator. Thus, the focus of this chapter is on hospitals and the governance structures of medicine and nursing within those settings. Physicians and nurses comprise the two largest groups of health professionals; their work in hospitals is highly inter-dependent, but their relationships to hospitals and regional health boards differ in significant ways, as do their governance structures.

Regional health authorities with responsibility for hospitals, nursing homes, and community health agencies are operated by governing boards. The term *board* is used in this chapter to refer to all such governing bodies. The authority of the board flows from provincial legislation in the form of a hospital or health care act(s) and its regulations. Under these statutes, requirements with respect to the appointment of board members are stipulated, including their duties. Board members may be appointed provincially or locally, and in the case of Saskatchewan, some are elected. Irrespective of how membership is determined, regional health boards are made up predominantly of lay people who serve as representatives of the community. Accordingly, provincial legislation requires boards to have an organized medical staff to advise them on medical matters and to provide medical services to patients. Traditionally, by virtue of this medical organization and its advisory role to the board, physicians have enjoyed significant influence in hospitals and a number of perquisites in addition to hospital privileges.

Medical Staff Organization

All physicians and dentists appointed by the board are members of the medical staff association. Occasionally, provision is made for the inclusion of non-physician advisory scientists (Ordman, 1998). Subject to the approval of the board, members of the medical association establish bylaws and regulations to determine the following: (a) the categories of medical staff and their quali-fications (e.g., honorary, active, consulting), including the privileges afforded to each; (b) the terms of reference for the Medical Advisory Committee and its subcommittees; (c) the roles and responsibilities of chiefs of staff; (d) the policies and procedures for application and appointment to the staff; and (e) the procedures for dealing with complaints about individual physicians.

Thus, the main functions of the medical staff organization are to provide members with the framework for self-governance, to determine how the quality of patient care and the perform-ance of medical practitioners are to be monitored, and to provide a mechanism for reviewing physician applications to the staff and assigning them to appropriate categories (Lemieux-Charles, 1994). Figure 16.1 illustrates how the medical staff organization might look in a typi-cal medium-sized hospital. As noted in Chapter 8, this type of organization has been called a professional bureaucracy. It creates a matrix structure within the hospital, with two streams of authority for decision making—the board with its overall administrative power and responsibility,

Figure 16.1 Relationship of a Typical Hospital Board to its Medical Staff Organization

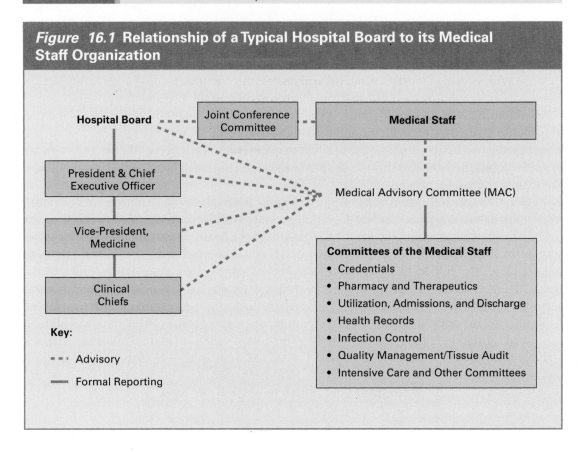

and the medical staff organization with powers derived from clinical expertise and responsibility to clients. The board is dependent on the medical staff to admit patients to the hospital.

Bylaws function as a constitution for the medical staff association. The constitution establishes the governance structures, official positions and their duties, committee structures and terms of reference, and organizational procedures. For example, leadership of the medical staff is provided through different official positions, each with a separate role and responsibilities. Five such leadership roles are described in Table 16.1. Also under these bylaws, the medical staff approve regulations that have a direct bearing on the practice of the members and, indeed, on the practice of nursing. For example, in some services, a nurse may be entitled to implement a series of standing orders for new patients without a specific order from the attending physician. The relevant medical staff committee will have authorized such procedures. The senior professional practice advisory council, under the bylaws, is known as the Medical Advisory Committee (MAC).

Table 16.1 Medical Staff Organization in a Typical Medium-Sized Hospital

Title	Definition
Chief of Staff	Appointed by the hospital board, is responsible for ensuring that the medical staff carry out their assigned functions. May or may not be chair of the medical advisory committee (MAC).
Chair/Medical Advisory Committee	Coordinates activities and chairs meetings of the MAC.
Department Head	May also be known as Chief of Service or Chief of Department. Accountable through the medical staff organization for the competence of and the quality of care given by members of the departments. Also responsible to administration for such functions as utilization review, budgeting, staff recruitment, education, and research.
President/Medical Staff	Represents and defends the interests of the medical staff as a whole and speaks on behalf of individual members.
Vice-President/Medical	May also be known as the Medical Director. As a hospital employee, is responsible for ensuring that the medical staff carry out responsibilities as outlined in the bylaws. Interprets hospital policy to the medical staff and conveys to the administration and hospital board a professional understanding of issues that concern the medical staff. Where this position exists, a chief of staff may not be required because responsibilities for the day-to-day operation of the hospital may be divided among department chiefs, chair of the MAC, and the Vice-President/Medical.

Source: Table compiled from information in various chapters of D. Gellerman (Ed.), *Medical Administration in Canadian Hospitals.* Ottawa: Canadian Medical Association, 1992.

Medical Advisory Committee

The MAC is the principal policy-making body of the organized medical staff, and, as its name implies, it makes recommendations directly to the board. Members of the MAC include the officers of the medical staff association, clinical heads or chiefs of various services, department heads, attending physicians, and the medical director or vice-president of medicine. There also may be *ex officio* members (i.e., representatives by virtue of office). For example, the administrator or chief executive officer (CEO) of the hospital and the chief nursing officer are likely to be *ex officio* members.

The MAC bears the responsibility for the professional activities of all physicians practicing in the hospital and, consequently, the quality of medical care (Blishen, 1969). In small hospitals, one or two physicians may undertake all the duties of a medical advisory committee. With regionalization, many small hospitals have been closed or merged with larger hospitals, and the organization of medical staff has become centralized. For example, rural hospitals now may have a facility medical staff committee that is part of an overall regional medical staff organization (Ordman, 1998).

The MAC has various subcommittees for carrying out its purposes (see Figure 16.1), some of which have representation from nursing and other disciplines. It is important that nurses understand the work of these committees and know who their nursing representatives are so that the nursing care implications of the decisions made by medical staff committees can be discussed and taken into account before regulations are issued. Increasingly, multidisciplinary committees (e.g., health records, infection control, and quality management) are taking over the work of medical staff committees. Two subcommittees of the MAC having considerable consequences for the practice of nursing are the pharmacy and therapeutics committee and the health records committee.

Credentials Committee

The Credentials Committee has the critical responsibility of assessing the qualifications of all applicants to the medical staff and making recommendations concerning appointments, reappointments, and the delineation of privileges for each appointee (Williams & Donnelly, 1987). The work of this committee exemplifies the process of peer review.

Nurses should be aware that there are categories of medical staff and that a physician's scope of practice varies according to her or his category. The majority of physicians appointed to the medical staff are in the active or attending category. Active members are the mainstay of the medical staff, admitting and treating patients, having access to all diagnostic resources and hospital services, and being eligible to vote and to hold office in the Medical Staff Association. There is usually provision for other categories such as honourary, consulting, and temporary medical staff. Their specific privileges are listed in the medical staff bylaws, copies of which should be made available to nurses online or in hard copy in all patient care areas.

In teaching hospitals, the majority of the physicians prescribing care for patients are residents. These physicians are completing educational or specialty programs and are supervised by the department head or active member of the medical staff affiliated with the university medical school. Residents are not members of the Medical Staff Association.

When granting privileges to a physician, the board needs to be assured that the applicant can meet the medical profession's standards of clinical performance and personal conduct. That assurance is given by virtue of a thorough review of an applicant's qualifications, experience, and reputation by the Credentials Committee, whose recommendations are ratified by the MAC before being forwarded to the board for approval. Sometimes, the MAC may wish to restrict the privileges of a member of the medical staff. Nurses who manage services such as operating rooms or case rooms must be informed of any restricted privileges of medical staff. In some hospitals, for example, a physician may not schedule or perform surgical procedures without a prior consultation with a senior member of the medical staff. If a physician attempts to exceed his or her designated privileges without appropriate supervision, the manager of the service must intervene and refer the situation to the chief of the service or the medical director, according to institutional policy and the medical staff bylaws.

Pharmacy and Therapeutics Committee

The work of the Pharmacy and Therapeutics Committee has a great impact on the administration of medications and nutritional products by nurses. For this reason, there are generally one or more nursing representatives appointed to this committee, as well as the director of pharmacy and a clinical pharmacist. This committee is responsible for developing the "policies and procedures relevant to the evaluation, selection, procurement, distribution, and therapeutic use of drugs, nutritional products and related devices" (Ordman, 1998, p. 145).

Many hospitals use a formulary, or list, of all medications that will be kept on hand in the hospital for prescription purposes. The committee may establish policies to authorize the pharmacist to substitute generic versions of brand name drugs and also may develop similar policies for controlling the utilization of the most costly drugs.

Nurses may need to refer physicians to the hospital formulary or the pharmacist if they order drugs not stocked by the hospital. The Pharmacy and Therapeutics Committee establishes regulations governing the expiry periods for narcotics and controlled medications and activities such as the administration of medications and intravenous solutions. Because nurses spend a large portion of their time administering medications and observing the effects on their patients, their expertise and practical experience is vital to the development of policies governing medication distribution and administration.

Health Records Committee

In view of the number of disciplines having access to a patient's hospital record, the original "medical records committee" is more likely to be known as the Health Records Committee or clinical records committee. Nevertheless, physicians have the responsibility for summarizing the medical treatment and progress of the patient following discharge or death. From this record, an abstract is prepared by the health records department personnel and submitted to the Canadian Institute for Health Information. The completion of medical records is considered an important aspect of medical care, and failure of a physician to complete her or his records can result in the withdrawal of hospital privileges. Nurses play an important role in safeguarding and updating the health record while the patient is in hospital, and for this reason, nurses should have a representative on the Health Records Committee. Of course, a representative from the health records department is a key member of this committee.

It should be clear from the descriptions of these committees that many of the policies and procedures governing the daily activities of health professionals, especially nurses, have their origins in one or more subcommittees of the medical staff organization. Problems arising from outdated policies and procedures or from the introduction of new products, drugs, or solutions should be communicated to the appropriate representative on these committees or to clinical leaders. Because physicians are not always reimbursed for committee work, their meetings tend to be infrequent. Serious difficulties with existing medical staff regulations should be sent in writing by managers of the unit or service to the chair of the relevant medical staff committee, with copies to the chief of service and medical director.

Medical Administration

Departmental organization of inpatients in hospitals typically is arranged according to medical specialty or subspecialty, with a chief of service or department head responsible for the administrative aspects of medical care. They are appointed to their positions by the board on the recommendation of the MAC. Theoretically, physicians are elected by their peers to the position of department head; however, in reality, physicians are sometimes persuaded by the medical director to become department heads, or they take their turn in rotation. As Lemieux-Charles (1994) explained

> Difficulty in recruiting department chiefs is not uncommon. Barriers to physician involvement can include: size of the department; physicians' concern about the impact of the role on peer relationships and referral networks; administrative requirements; and conflicts over administrative decisions directly affecting their practice (p. 132).

These difficulties and the time spent on administrative aspects of medical care are now recognized by the payment of a salary or stipend for undertaking the role of department head (Ordman, 1998).

Any serious problem that arises regarding the practice of medicine within the specialty— whether it be concerns about medical prescriptions, relations with patients, or even the unprofessional conduct of a physician that cannot be settled at the patient care level—should be referred to the department head. Thus, if nurses or their managers receive complaints or have concerns about individual physicians or any aspect of the medical care of patients, the department head must be informed. The concerns are best dealt with first on a face-to-face basis and then submitted in writing with detailed records kept to facilitate follow-up as necessary. It generally is assumed that such concerns will be addressed promptly, but in the Winnipeg case reported by Fletcher (2001), nurses' concerns were neither taken seriously by the department head, nor were they documented.

In addition to department heads, there may be an overall chief of staff as well as a medical director or vice-president of medicine.

Chief of Staff

The chief of staff is appointed by the board on the recommendation of the MAC and ultimately is responsible for ensuring that members of the Medical Staff Association fulfill their professional and clinical responsibilities. Therefore, problems associated with the competence or conduct of a member of the Medical Staff Association would be referred first to the department head and then, if necessary, to the overall chief of staff. The individual appointed as chief of staff also may be chair of the MAC and/or president of the Medical Staff Association but is not part of the hospital's administrative structure. This role should not be confused with that of the medical director (see Table 16.1).

Medical Director

The medical director, or vice-president of medicine, is an integral member of the senior management team of the region or hospital. This individual is a physician who has become an administrator and is therefore a salaried member of the hospital's senior executive team. Many have acquired administrative qualifications in addition to their medical education. As Ward (1992) remarked, medical colleagues may not readily understand this role because there is no requirement of the incumbent to represent the medical staff to the board. That responsibility falls to the chief of staff or to the chair of the MAC.

The role of the medical director involves ensuring that policies of the board concerning the medical staff are carried out. The incumbent is responsible for all medical staff affairs and is accountable to the CEO (Williams & Donnelly, 1987). The office of the medical director also may be assigned responsibility for medico-legal problems, the resolution of conflicts between administrative and medical personnel, medical student placements, and educational programming for residents.

It should be clear from this model of medical governance in Canadian hospitals that when physicians are appointed to the medical staff, they enjoy access to the full range of hospital resources and almost unfettered autonomy in practicing medicine. Collectively, physicians have been estimated to drive approximately 70% of all costs generated in hospitals, and for this reason, efforts have been made to involve them more closely in the management of resources (Lemieux-Charles, 1994). Sociologists have observed that the medical profession has achieved almost unparalleled professional power, autonomy, prestige, and income, such that other health occupations have considered their approach to self-governance as models to emulate (Hewa, 2002).

Nursing Governance

Although professional nursing associations have been granted the same privileges and responsibilities for self-governance as medicine and other health disciplines since the early 1900s, the organization and control of nursing services within health care agencies has been determined by boards and administrators. Hospitals have traditionally been influenced by the ideas of classical theorists and have operated along bureaucratic principles. They were hierarchical in structure and subdivided according to function (e.g., nursing, social work, dietary, housekeeping). The so-called "scalar principle" and the chain of command ensured a clear line of authority from top to bottom of the organization, with power and discretion concentrated at senior levels, diminishing at each level down the line. With this type of "stovepipe" arrangement, communication flowed freely up and down the line, but sometimes with difficulty along horizontal lines. Interdisciplinary coordination was inefficient and time-consuming, and rules, policies, and procedures were relied upon to govern behaviour. Such structures tended to operate in highly centralized, inflexible, and autocratic ways and generally fostered dependence and obedience. These principles were so pervasive that managers did not always realize that there were alternatives (Charns & Schaefer, 1983). The nature of bureaucracies is not conducive to feedback from employees, and so the prevalence of this type of social organization is a paradox given Western society's commitment to democratic values and ideals.

A typical nursing department organization that was prevalent in the 1950s and 1960s, that is, in the "command and control" tradition (Porter-O'Grady, 2001), appears in Figure 16.2. Directors of nursing were usually promoted on the basis of their reputations as good nurses and, therefore, had little preparation in management theory and practice. Their role was primarily to implement decisions of boards and administrators and deal with operational problems raised by the medical and nursing staffs. Many senior nurses did not control their own operational budgets, and supervisors and nurses were generally powerless as advocates for improvements in either their nursing practices or working conditions at the patient care level of the organization. As Monk (1994) noted, frustration with this type of organization increased as the pro-

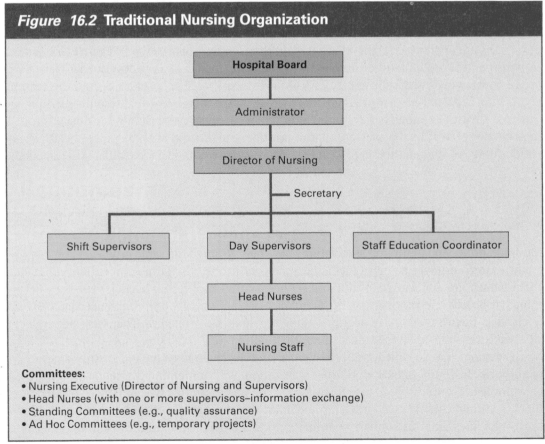

Figure 16.2 Traditional Nursing Organization

Hospital Board

Administrator

Director of Nursing

Secretary

Shift Supervisors — Day Supervisors — Staff Education Coordinator

Head Nurses

Nursing Staff

Committees:
- Nursing Executive (Director of Nursing and Supervisors)
- Head Nurses (with one or more supervisors–information exchange)
- Standing Committees (e.g., quality assurance)
- Ad Hoc Committees (e.g., temporary projects)

fessional role of nurses matured and developments in health care necessitated a paradigm shift in the way organizations were structured.

New forms of organization began to appear in the 1960s and 1970s with the recognition that productivity could be improved if the views and cooperation of employees in decision making were actively sought. Corporate sector employers began to adopt participative management practices such as quality circles, labour-management committees, autonomous work groups, and similar strategies aimed at "democratizing" the workplace. Some of these new work structures found their way into hospitals, but with varying degrees of success and sustainability. Some argued that management was the primary beneficiary of these innovations at the expense of the unionized worker (Wells, 1992). In the 1960s, Canadian nurses became active in the union movement, negotiating collective agreements and addressing their workplace concerns through these means. Employers were now obliged to deal with nurses' representatives in the workplace, to acknowledge nurses' satisfaction (or lack thereof) with the quality of care they were able to provide, and to listen to staff nurses' ideas about safe and effective patient care. Professional issues began to appear at the bargaining table, and nurses found that they had a potent means for making themselves heard (Hibberd, 1994).

In Canada, the 1990s was a decade of unprecedented reorganization in the health care field, stimulated by the rising costs of health care and the realization that the old command and control era had to be replaced with more cost-effective structures and processes. Program management gradually replaced cumbersome hierarchies, often with the loss of management positions at all levels of hospital organizations. (See Chapters 8 and 9 for more discussion of program management and the consequences of restructuring in health care agencies.)

Program management may be characterized by some or all of the following features: organizational structure is designed to address the needs of specific populations of patients or selected diagnostic categories of patients; the staff is multidisciplinary; teamwork and participatory decision making replaces top-down or unilateral practices; managers of programs are drawn from any of the health disciplines and have full responsibility for fiscal and human resources. Management of the program is sometimes shared by a physician and an administrator, often a nurse. As noted in Chapter 9, authority for professional practice issues, supervision, and development is dispersed, and individual performance appraisals may be the responsibility of someone from another discipline.

For all their shortcomings, traditional hierarchies and departmental organizations provided a sense of cohesion within the disciplines, and clear sources of authority and control over practice issues were vested in the professional leader as head of the department. This is borne out in a study of physiotherapists who moved from a departmental organization to program management. They reported feeling isolated from their colleagues with the loss of customary intraprofessional communication and collegiality. They also reported concerns about loss of control over practice, maintenance of competence, and continuing education opportunities (Miller & Soloman, 2002). Nevertheless, these changes in the structure of health agencies stimulated experimentation with new models of governance that would address the "losses" felt by health professionals in the traditional governance of their disciplines.

Professional Practice Models

The efforts of executive nurses to involve their staff in governance issues predate the restructuring trends of the 1990s by two to three decades. The seminal Magnet Hospitals Study by

McClure, Poulin, Sovie, and Wandelt (1983) revealed the importance of a professional working environment to nurses, one in which their work was valued and they were empowered by well-educated and supportive leaders. Working relationships with physicians were good, and these "magnet" hospitals had no difficulty in recruiting and retaining professional nurses. Innovative models of professional practice involving nurses in governance issues were developed with the belief that these would improve the quality of nurses' working environments and would assist in the retention of nurses. It was assumed that a more satisfied and committed nursing workforce would produce better outcomes in terms of patient care. Governance models were described in the nursing literature under a variety of labels, for example, collaborative governance, nursing or clinical practice models, shared governance, and self-managed teams to name a few.

The term *professional practice model (PPM)* generally refers to "an organizational framework designed to empower staff by supporting autonomous clinical practice with appropriate accountability" (Davis, Heath, & Reddick, 2002, p. 21). Zelauskas and Howes (1992) would add to this definition that a PPM gives nurses increased opportunities for control over nursing and the environment within which they deliver their services. Hoffart and Woods (1996) proposed five subsystems to PPMs, including professional values, professional relationships, a patient care delivery system, a management approach, and compensation and rewards. Such definitions are sufficiently broad and flexible to encompass any organizational model designed to give nurses a voice in how their discipline is governed and practiced, including shared governance. Upenieks (2000) regards PPM and shared governance as synonymous, saying

> The importance of nursing practice models (i.e., shared governance) is that these models provide an organizational framework that offers an opportunity for staff nurses to become more committed to their practice. The implementation of such models allows nurses to have an active role in decision-making, with maximal participation and accountability for the outcomes of those decisions (p. 330).

The term professional practice model should not be confused with nursing care delivery models (e.g., team nursing, primary nursing) or nursing models (e.g., nursing theories and conceptual frameworks) because these are subsystems that will be determined or reviewed once the PPM is operational. As shared governance is one of the better-known types of PPM, this model is described below.

Shared Governance

It is important to understand that it is the decision-making process that is shared between the managers and clinical staff of a discipline in a shared governance model, whether within a department, within a program, or within an entire health authority. The authorization for establishing shared governance comes from the board of the hospital or region. The board does not share its mandate to govern; rather, it delegates authority to administrators and professional leaders while retaining ultimate responsibility for all that takes place in the agency. This is why gaining and maintaining the support of the board and senior management is essential for the success of shared governance projects (Perley & Raab, 1994; Ritter-Teitel, 2002), while being mindful that all such governance models are subject to veto by the board. Shared governance does not give nurses control over operational decisions that are the prerogative of the board, and sometimes this point is not well understood by staff, especially when scarcity of resources results in major cutbacks.

In a review of some 500 articles on shared governance and PPMs, O'May and Buchan (1999) described the concept of shared governance as follows:

> The core definition [of shared governance] is a decentralized approach which gives nurses greater authority and control over their practice and work environment; engenders a sense of responsibility and accountability; and allows active participation in the decision-making process, particularly in administrative areas from which they were excluded previously (p. 281).

The decentralized approach means changes to organizational structures and processes and new expectations of nurses in relation to decision making at the patient care level, or point of service. Nurses' authority over their practice is derived from their knowledge and expertise, but in the past this knowledge has been undervalued and largely overshadowed by medical knowledge and expertise. PPMs are designed to promote professional autonomy and accountability among nursing staff, enabling them to use their expertise to define and decide what services they will provide (i.e., scope of practice) and to determine what constitutes safe and effective practice (Maas & Specht, 1994). Structures alone are not enough to make shared governance work. All participants must believe in it and commit themselves to a long process as this type of organizational change is a major cultural adaptation and cannot be achieved overnight.

The concept of empowerment of nurses is central to the notion of shared governance and provides much of the rationale for introducing it, but not all nurses will necessarily welcome the new expectations that are inherent in the concept. According to Porter-O'Grady (2001), "empowerment is an endless work effort…a dynamic, not a thing. It is a way of being and living that informs everything else that is done in the workplace" (p. 469). Adjusting to shared governance requires ongoing commitment by all participants to break out of old ways of doing things and engage in the process of adapting to new roles and relationships.

Models of Shared Governance

From their literature review, O'May and Buchan (1999, p. 283) grouped the shared governance models into four types:

Unit-based. Each unit or clinic establishes its own organization such that many models may exist throughout an individual region or hospital, and there may be no effort to coordinate them on an agency-wide basis.

Congressional. All staff belongs to a congress, and committees submit their work to an executive structure or cabinet, rather like a federal government. The medical staff organization described earlier in this chapter fits this model.

Councillor. This model consists of an overall coordinating council with subcommittees and unit-based councils. Nurses are accountable for clinical decision making.

Administrative. Both clinical and management structures exist, and a forum is used to integrate the work. An executive council may make final decisions.

Any one of these models could be adapted for institutional (hospital) or community health agency application. The councillor model pertained to around 50% of the cases reviewed by the authors, so this type is described in more detail below. It will be assumed to apply to a hospital setting. Most hospitals develop a site-specific model as it is unlikely that systems developed in other locations can be implemented without modification. Quite apart from the absence of uniformity in these models, the process of developing a site-specific model is highly instructive for everyone involved, and the participants are likely to take ownership of the model and make it work if they have been involved in its design.

The Councillor Model

An example of a councillor model appears in Figure 16.3. Like the medical model with its MAC and subcommittees, the councillor model of shared governance has a central governing council and subcouncils and thus closely resembles a medical staff organization with the exception of its relationship to the agency board.

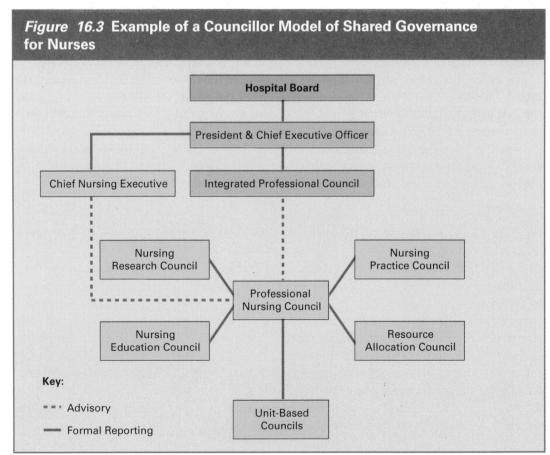

Figure 16.3 Example of a Councillor Model of Shared Governance for Nurses

Professional Nursing Council

The Professional Nursing Council is the policy-making body that oversees all other activities in the model, and although analogous to the MAC, it operates without as much scope or power. Members of the council are elected by their peers and are drawn from all nursing groups, staff nurses, managers, educators, researchers, and representatives from any affiliating faculty of nursing. If there is a chief of nursing practice or clinical leader, this person will be an *ex officio* member, with or without voting ability. The chair of this council is elected by the members and serves for a specified term (e.g., one or two years). In the absence of a senior executive nurse or professional nurse leader, the chair is considered the spokesperson for nursing in the hospital or region and represents nursing on any interdisciplinary professional council.

All other councils in the nursing organization connect with the Professional Nursing Council on a regular basis, and their recommendations for major policy changes are reviewed and either approved or ratified. The Professional Nursing Council approves the terms of reference for all subcouncils, clearly establishing the types of decisions that can be made by the subcouncils and those that must be referred to the Professional Nursing Council. Establishing and maintaining the bylaws of the model are specific responsibilities of this council, including credentialing, if any.

Clinical Practice Council

The Clinical Practice Council provides leadership for all nursing practice issues, systems, and problems. It is responsible for such areas as scope of practice, standards for evidence-based practice, care delivery models, care maps, clinical policies and procedures, and the quality of nursing care. Membership includes nurses with advanced clinical preparation as well as staff nurses with expertise in the major specialty areas. This is a key council in the organization and has a heavy workload, and projects may be reassigned on an ad hoc basis to smaller groups (e.g., the review of nursing philosophy and mission statements or the establishment of guidelines for the transfer of medical procedures). Unit-based councils work closely with members of the Clinical Practice Council, bringing practice issues or concerns to its attention.

Education Council

Areas of responsibility for the Education Council include career advancement, continuing education, orientation, mentorship, and preceptorship. The Education Council develops close liaisons with local nursing schools and faculties. This council may be responsible for administering funds for workshops, conferences, and certification courses. Membership includes nurses with teaching preparation and experience, clinical development nurses, and staff nurses.

Research Council

The main role of the Research Council is to coordinate all nursing research activities in the hospital, to promote research awareness among nurses, and to serve as a research resource. This council administers funds available for nursing research. For example, council members are responsible for reviewing all applications for funding as well as all research proposals from other disciplines requiring the involvement of nurses in the collection of data or as subjects of research. It is important to include in this council nurses who are experienced in or engaged in research. Liaison with a university school of nursing and consultation can be achieved by inviting a faculty member to serve on this council. A representative from this council also should serve on the agency-wide research committee.

Resource Management Council

The responsibility of the Resource Management Council includes all operational activities previously handled unilaterally by management personnel. Members of this council include staff nurse representatives and managers responsible for the nursing budget, staffing and scheduling, and information management. Liaison with hospital employee unions is important, and cooperation with the departments of finance, human resources, and other management support services is essential. Of all the subcommittees of the Professional Nursing Council, this council may generate the most misunderstanding as to how joint decision making works. Guidelines should be established at an early stage of implementation to promote a clear understanding of the scope of authority of the Professional Nursing Council and its subcommittees.

Unit-Based Councils

Each unit or service in the hospital or agency is entitled to form a council to address local nursing practice issues. These councils are likely to comprise small groups of nurses due to the realities of shifts, work schedules, and the day-to-day intensity of work at the patient care level. Unless supported by management personnel, these councils are difficult to sustain. Financial resources must be available so that nurses can be released from clinical activities to attend to governance work. Nurses at the unit level should be encouraged to serve on the main nursing councils to foster the information flow between the point-of-service staff and the decision makers.

Membership in all councils in this type of nursing governance model is determined by election, with the members of the individual councils electing the chairs. However, the Professional Nursing Council may reserve the right to appoint people to serve as chair if permitted to do so under the shared governance bylaws.

Planning and Implementing Shared Governance

The decision to move from a traditional nursing departmental structure to shared governance involves a profound cultural change in the beliefs, values, and customs of the participants. Full implementation may take several years to accomplish, and seeing the project through to completion can be difficult and time consuming, with unexpected roadblocks along the way. Reaching the goal of real empowerment of the nursing workforce is a continuous process, and although many shared governance structures have stood the test of time, most have not (Porter-O'Grady, 2001). With the loss of senior executive nursing administrative positions in the Canadian health care system, the momentum for sustaining new self-governing structures declined. On the other hand, medical staff organizations have tended to remain intact throughout the restructuring era due to the enduring statutory provisions in hospital and regional health authority legislation and traditional practices.

Sound planning and careful preparation of all people directly involved are key requirements for successful implementation, and the whole project needs to be informed by theories of change (see Chapters 22 and 23) and the principles of project management (see Chapter 24). Planning begins with the appointment of a Steering Committee to develop a proposal outlining the concept of shared governance; the rationale for change; the organizational structures; the time frames; the resources required, including the assistance of outside consultants; the evaluation measures; and the associated costs of the project. Senior administration must be persuaded that the project is consistent with the mission and goals of the hospital, and the proposal should be accompanied by letters of support from key people such as the chair of the MAC. This complex organizational change must have the board's approval and its continuing support throughout the project, as noted above.

Change theory suggests that potentially resistive forces need to be identified and opposition to the project addressed. If the setting is one in which the nurses' union has traditionally taken an adversarial approach to management, the introduction of a professional practice model may be perceived as a threat to the customary relationship with management. The attitude of union leaders may be that the union wants no role in governing but wants management to do its job of managing. If there is widespread support for the project by nurses caring for patients, union leaders will be expected to support their wishes. Union leaders may see the wisdom of taking part in all phases of the project in order to protect the integrity of the collective agreement. The increasing interest of American nurses in unionization has been attributed to their need to have a stronger voice, for example, in dealing with the lack of job security following radical responses to managed care in that country, and in dealing with other workforce issues (Forman, 2002). Shared governance is not incompatible with unionization—it is a complementary approach, giving nurses a voice in, as well as more control of, their professional practice.

Resistance also may come from managers whose roles change and whose positions may even disappear once the model is in place. In shared governance, the role of managers "is to facilitate, integrate, and coordinate the system and resources required for the system's maintenance and growth" (Porter-O'Grady, 1987, p. 283). In discussing the motives for introducing shared governance, Maas and Specht (1994) observed that some organizations and managers have been reluctant to relinquish power and control over decisions affecting nursing.

If the benefits of shared decision making and partnership are not accompanied with real divestment of power from traditional sources in hospitals, nurses will become frustrated and cynical and may withdraw their support for the project. Nurses may perceive that a form of pseudo-democracy is being instituted if, for example, managers monopolize the leadership roles in the various nursing councils, dominate the proceedings, and continue to make unilateral decisions. Ideally, the role of managers is to assist staff nurses to develop skills in running meetings, negotiating, dealing with conflict, and reaching consensus in decision making. The roles of managers and nurses both change in the process of implementing shared governance, and resources should be set aside for formal socialization of all nurses to their individual and collective responsibility for meeting professional and organizational goals.

Shared Governance Research

Research into the effects of shared governance on nurses and patient care underscores the challenge inherent in evaluating the outcomes of complex organizational changes. The variety in form and scope of shared governance and professional practice models makes comparative studies difficult. However, in a detailed analysis of six intervention studies, improvements in job satisfaction were reported in five of the six shared governance models. Other favourable outcomes included enhanced organizational commitment, empowerment, autonomy, and team functioning (Upenieks, 2000). The findings of this research also suggest that effective communication between managers and staff is an essential ingredient in shared governance.

Much of the literature on outcomes is based on anecdotal reports, but among the findings of studies reviewed by O'May & Buchan (1999) were improved quality of care; improved efficiency; increased sense of cohesiveness, teamwork, and collegiality; reduced turnover and absenteeism; and cost savings. These authors reported that over 90% of the studies reviewed claimed the benefits of shared governance.

Integrated Professional Practice Models

With the emergence of program management, effective interdisciplinary teamwork took on greater significance in these efficiency-driven, re-engineered organizations. New structures to facilitate collaboration, communication, and decision making among health professionals became an imperative, and integrated PPMs were introduced. Such projects are even more daunting to implement than the discipline-specific models (see Comack, Brady, & Porter-O'Grady, 1997; Perley & Raab, 1994; Davis, Heath, & Reddick, 2002; Mathews & Lankshear, 2003).

Integrated PPMs have at their core a Professional Advisory Council, directly responsible to the board, with representation from every health discipline in the agency often, however, with the exception of the medical profession (Comack et al., 1997). Porter-O'Grady, Hawkins, and Parker (1997) remarked that physicians "are accustomed to having summary authority and being the locus of control for clinical decision making" (p. 187), but it is no longer appropriate to compartmentalize the relationship of physicians to the rest of the organization. However, the provisions of hospital legislation may present a challenge to the full integration of the medical profession in multidisciplinary decision-making structures (Mathews & Lankshear, 2003).

The introduction of multidisciplinary shared governance models may threaten the continuity of an existing nursing PPM. Clearly, each profession needs its own discipline-specific system in order to retain professional autonomy and control of its unique contribution to health care. Adjustments may have to be made to nursing committee structures, but if the governance model has been well designed and built on a firm foundation of commitment from all participants, it should be able to withstand the "noise" in the hospital concerning major restructuring efforts. There is growing evidence that profession-specific structures are being regarded as an integral part of agency-wide professional governance systems (Alvarado, Boblin-Cummings, & Goddard, 2000; Mathews & Lankshear, 2003).

Leadership Implications

Nothing less than transformative leadership is required to guide the design, implementation, and maintenance of a professional practice model. In the case of integrated models, all professional leaders must be committed to collaborative teamwork, coordination, and mutual respect for each other's disciplines. They also must have a clear understanding that the project will likely be long, arduous, challenging, and often frustrating work. The continued support of an executive champion (i.e., a member of the top management team) is vital to the success of the projects.

Nurses in administrative and management positions are well placed to exercise leadership at all levels and in all phases of establishing governance models for nurses. Their customary powers for controlling and directing the workforce must be gradually relinquished as the implementation of shared governance proceeds and the need for them to become consultants, teachers, coaches, and facilitators is realized.

According to Porter-O'Grady (2001), efforts to change the patterns of leadership and behaviour of managers are critical in the early stages of initiating sustainable changes, and that failure of such projects is most likely to occur at this point. Leadership succession is another important issue that must be addressed because continuity and sustainability of the project could be placed in jeopardy (see for example, Hibberd, Storoz, & Andrews, 1992). Efforts must be made to recruit and prepare new leaders from inside and outside the organization to replace naturally occurring turnover. Projects that depend on the leadership of a single individual are vulnerable to collapse in the event of the sudden departure of that person.

Roles of nurses at the patient care level will change as nurses become increasingly involved in the process of designing the governance model and articulating the vision, mission, values, goals, principles, and decision-making processes for their nursing practice. If the stated goals for adopting a professional practice model are to increase the autonomy and accountability of nurses for their clinical practice and to involve them in organizational decision making, then nurses must be there at the planning table from the start. Nurses need to understand that senior management will retain certain administrative prerogatives even as shared governance gets underway. They also need to understand how the structures for shared governance fit into the overall structure of the hospital or health region. Staff nurses must have more than token participation in the decision-making process. Their voices need to be heard, recorded, and communicated to their colleagues through regular communication channels. To this end, resources must be found to facilitate the attendance of staff nurses at council meetings as the hectic pace at which most nurses regularly work is not conducive to temporary release from the care of patients. In other words, the budget for the project must have release time built into it. In-house educational programs will be needed to assist nurses in developing the knowledge and skills needed to be effective on the shared governance councils.

A collaborative relationship with other disciplines is a responsibility of all health professionals, but when difficulties or complaints arise at the point of service, their leaders will be required to act. Collaboration between nurses and medical staff is especially important because it affects outcomes for patients, nurses, physicians, and hospitals. In the Magnet Hospitals Study by McClure and colleagues (1983), nurse-physician relations were positive, and nurses said this was important to them in their work. The reality, however, is that clinical workplaces are full of tension and strife between these two disciplines (Ritter-Teitel, 2002). Interdisciplinary conflicts occur occasionally, but structures exist for resolving disputes in health agencies. It is effective leadership that ensures constructive resolution of conflict. Failure to address conflicts between physicians and nurses relative to patient care reinforces the perception among nurses that their professional opinions are not respected.

The lack of involvement of nurses in determining the policies and practices that affect their work has been a recurrent theme in the nursing literature for many years. This is not just a North American phenomenon. It continues to be reported as a source of dissatisfaction for nurses here and abroad (Aiken et al., 2001; Blythe, Baumann, & Giovannetti, 2001). Recognizing the value of a nursing voice at the policy level of health agencies, the Quebec government passed legislation in 1992 stipulating that all health agencies employing more than five nurses must have a nursing council answerable directly to the agency board (Monk, 1994). This gives nurses in Quebec a voice equal in prominence to their medical colleagues. Although this nursing precedent does not appear to have been emulated in other jurisdictions, councils within integrated or multi-professional practice models are being reported as having direct access to agency boards. Without the involvement of physicians, PPMs are unlikely to match the scope and power of medical staff organizations. The professional practice models being developed by nurses are positive signs that progress is being made in increasing their influence and control over the practice of nursing within their workplaces. Effective nursing leadership at all levels will be needed to sustain these developments.

Summary

- The boards of regional health authorities responsible for hospitals are required to establish medical staff associations to advise them on medical matters.
- The medical staff association operates under a set of bylaws that determines structures for self-governance, including committees with their terms of reference, credentialing procedures, peer review, and professional roles and responsibilities.
- The Medical Advisory Committee is the central governance structure of the medical staff, directly reporting to the board and meeting occasionally with the board in a joint conference forum.
- Most physicians are not employees of hospitals or health regions; they apply for privileges to practice in hospitals and most are compensated on a fee-for-service basis.
- Nurses are employees of hospital boards and have historically worked in departments that operate on bureaucratic principles. Prior to the development of professional practice models, nurses have rarely had access to senior policy-making structures, much less to opportunities to influence the decisions that affect their clinical practice.

- Widespread restructuring in the health care system during the 1990s and the emergence of program management in hospitals provided the stimulus for developing integrated professional practice models.
- Professional practice and shared governance models in nursing are designed to increase nurses' autonomy and accountability for their professional practice and to increase nurses' control over clinical decision making at the patient care level.
- The councillor model of shared governance consists of a series of nursing councils with representation from all ranks in nursing (i.e., educators, clinical specialists, staff nurses, and managers).
- The roles of managers and staff nurses change in shared governance models. Managers take on roles as coaches, facilitators, and coordinators; staff nurses take on new governance responsibilities as council members.
- Implementation of shared governance may take several years to achieve and requires careful planning and preparation of all participants as well as continuing administrative support.
- Transformative leadership is essential for successful implementation and maintenance of shared governance and professional practice models. Nurses in management and leadership positions are responsible for facilitating collaborative relations between physicians and nurses and for ensuring that the legitimate concerns of nurses regarding patient care are addressed.

Applying the Knowledge in this Chapter

Case Study

1. Dr. Michael Brandon is a family physician with admitting privileges at a regional general hospital. You are a new area manager and responsible for several surgical units including gynecology. You already have been made aware of Dr. Brandon's reputation for inappropriate behaviour with female members of staff. Today, however, you have received an incident report from a staff nurse describing a situation in which a young female inpatient alleges sexual assault by Dr. Brandon. Identify the steps you will take in responding to this report and the individuals in health agency administration and medical staff organization to whom this problem can be referred. If this incident is not satisfactorily addressed through medical staff channels, what other courses of action are available to you?

2. Mr. Krauskopf is terminally ill with lung cancer, waiting for an internal transfer to the palliative care unit. John Carmichael, one of your staff nurses caring for this patient, comes to you saying that he is in a dispute with the attending physician, Dr. Janet Tremaine, over the amount of morphine she has ordered for Mr. Krauskopf. John has indicated to this physician that, in his professional opinion, it would not be safe to administer the prescribed dose as it significantly exceeds the normal dose, as well as

the dose the patient is accustomed to receiving. The physician became angry that her order was challenged and has threatened to "take the matter further." As manager of this unit, discuss the professional and administrative resources available to you in dealing with such situations, and outline how you would handle this particular case. Under what circumstances could a physician discipline a nurse in a hospital setting?

3. You are the elected Chair of the Nursing Resources Council in a councillor model of shared governance. You are well known in the hospital as the staffing coordinator, and you have been satisfied with the way the council has been functioning. There are two other managers and three staff nurses serving on this council, which meets once per month. The staff nurses have been effectively contributing to the work of the council, but, lately, you have noticed that the attendance of the staff nurses has been variable. None of them attended the last meeting, and although all three nurses are on duty, the units where they work have not requested replacement relief for today's meeting. Assuming that this pattern continues, what could be some of the possible explanations, and how should you proceed? Keep in mind the underlying reasons for working within a shared governance framework.

Resources

ʀʋօˡʋɛ Internet Resources

The Sinclair Report:

www.pediatriccardiacinquest.mb.ca/

The full report of the Pediatric Cardiac Surgery Inquest regarding 12 deaths at the Winnipeg Health Sciences Centre in 1994, known as the Sinclair Report, is available at this Web site. Much can be learned from this case about issues of supervision and accountability within professional governance structures in a large tertiary health care complex that had adopted program management. See Fletcher (2001) for additional information.

Tim Porter-O'Grady:

www.tpogassociates.com/home.htm

Tim Porter-O'Grady is a well-known consultant and futuristic speaker and writer on health care. His extensive publications on nursing governance systems are listed on his Web site.

References

Aiken, L.H., Clarke, S.P., Sloane, D.M., Sochalski, J.A., Busse, R., Clarke, H., et al. (2001). Nurses' reports on hospital care in five countries. *Health Affairs, 20*(3), 43–53.

Alvarado, K., Boblin-Cummings, S., & Goddard, P. (2000). Experiencing nursing governance: A post merger nursing committee structure. *Canadian Journal of Nursing Administration, 13*(4), 30–35.

Beatty, D., & Gunderson, M. (1979). *The employed professional.* Working Paper # 14. Toronto, ON: Professional Organizations Committee, Ontario Ministry of the Attorney General.

Blishen, B.R. (1969). *Doctors and doctrines: The ideology of medical care in Canada.* Toronto, ON: University of Toronto Press.

Blythe, J., Baumann, A., & Giovannetti, P. (2001). Nurses' experiences of restructuring in three Ontario hospitals. *Journal of Nursing Scholarship, 33*(1), 61–68.

Charns, M.P., & Schaefer, M.J. (1983). *Health care organizations: A model for management.* Englewood Cliffs, NJ: Prentice-Hall.

Comack, M., Brady, J., & Porter-O'Grady, T. (1997). Professional practice: A framework for transition to a new culture. *Journal of Nursing Administration, 27*(12), 32–41.

Davis, B., Heath, O., & Reddick, P. (2002). A multi-disciplinary professional practice model: Supporting autonomy and accountability in program-based structure. *Canadian Journal of Nursing Leadership, 15*(4), 21–25.

Fletcher, M. (2001). The Manitoba pediatric cardiac surgery inquest report. *Canadian Nurse, 97*(2), 14–16.

Forman, H. (2002). The rising tide of healthcare labor unions in nursing. *Journal of Nursing Administration, 32,* 376–378.

Gellerman, D. (Ed.). (1992). *Medical administration in Canadian hospitals.* Ottawa: Canadian Medical Association.

Hewa, S. (2002). Physicians, the medical profession, and medical practice. In B.S. Bolaria & H.D. Dickinson (Eds.), *Health, illness and health care in Canada* (3rd ed., pp. 55–81). Scarborough, ON: Nelson Thomson Learning.

Hibberd, J.M. (1994). Professional goals and industrial strategies: An international survey. *International Nursing Review, 41,* 107–114.

Hibberd, J.M., Storoz, C.E., & Andrews, H.A. (1992). Implementing shared governance: A false start. *Nursing Clinics of North America, 27*(1), 11–22.

Hoffart, N., & Woods, C.Q. (1996). Elements of a nursing professional practice model. *Journal of Professional Nursing, 12,* 354–364.

Lemieux-Charles, L. (1994). Medical staff organization. In J.M. Hibberd & M.E. Kyle (Eds.), *Nursing management in Canada* (pp. 126–141). Toronto, ON: W.B. Saunders.

Maas, M.L., & Specht, J.P. (1994). Shared governance in nursing: What is shared, who governs, and who benefits. In J.C. McCloskey & H.K. Grace (Eds.), *Current issues in nursing* (4th ed., pp. 398–406). St. Louis, MO: The C.V. Mosby.

Mathews, S., & Lankshear, S. (2003). Describing the essential elements of a professional practice structure. *Canadian Journal of Nursing Leadership, 16*(2), 63–71.

McClure, M.L., Poulin, M.A., Sovie, M.D., & Wandelt, M.A. (1983). *Magnet hospitals: Attraction and retention of professional nurses.* Kansas City, KS: American Academy of Nursing.

Monk, M. (1994). Nursing governance. In J.M. Hibberd & M.E. Kyle (Eds.), *Nursing management in Canada* (pp. 191–211). Toronto, ON: W.B. Saunders Canada.

Miller, P.A., & Soloman, P. (2002). The influence of a move to program management on physical therapy practice. *Physical Therapy, 82,* 449–458.

O'May, F., & Buchan, J. (1999). Shared governance: A literature review. *International Journal of Nursing Studies, 36,* 281–300.

Ordman, J.A. (1998). *Medical staff organization.* [Mimeograph]. Red Deer, AB: David Thompson Health Region.

Perley, M.J., & Raab, A. (1994). Beyond shared governance: Restructuring care delivery for self-managed work teams. *Nursing Administration Quarterly, 19*(1), 12–20.

Porter-O'Grady, T. (1987). Shared governance and new organizational models. *Nursing Economics, 5*(6), 281–286.

Porter-O'Grady, T. (2001). Is shared governance still relevant? *Journal of Nursing Administration, 31*(10), 468–473.

Porter-O'Grady, T., Hawkins, M.A., & Parker, M.L. (1997). *Whole-systems shared governance: Architecture for integration.* Gaithersburg, MD: Aspen.

Ritter-Teitel, J. (2002). The impact of restructuring on professional nursing practice. *Journal of Nursing Administration, 32*(1), 31–41.

Upenieks, V. (2000). The relationship of nursing practice models and job satisfaction outcomes. *Journal of Nursing Administration, 30,* 330–335.

Ward, T. (1992). The role of the medical administrator. In D. Gellerman (Ed.), *Medical administration in Canadian hospitals* (Ch. D1). Ottawa, ON: Canadian Medical Association.

Wells, D.M. (1992). *Who gains from worker participation?* Kingston, ON: Industrial Relations Centre, Queen's University.

Williams, K.J., & Donnelly, P.R. (1987). *Medical care quality and the public trust.* Ottawa, ON: Canadian Hospital Association.

Zelauskas, B., & Howes, D.G. (1992). The effects of implementing a professional practice model. *Journal of Nursing Administration, 22*(7/8), 18–23.

Acknowledgments

The author wishes to thank Dr. Ginette Lemire Rodger, Vice-President (Professional Practice) and Chief Nursing Executive of the Ottawa Hospital, for her insights relative to professional practice models.

PROMOTING EVIDENCE-BASED PRACTICE

Carolyn J. Pepler

Learning Objectives

In this chapter, you will learn:

- The importance of scientific evidence as a basis for decision making in nursing

- That research activities include the conduct of research, the use of other researchers' findings to build practice, and the use of research techniques in daily practice

- The need for structural support, continuing education, and creativity to facilitate evidence-based practice in a health care agency

- Strategies that leaders and managers can use to promote research activities

- The costs involved in conducting and participating in research, along with the health and economic benefits of evidence-based practice

"And nothing but observation and experience will teach us ways to maintain or to bring back the state of health" (Nightingale, 1859/1980, p. 74).

Research first served as the basis for practice in the nursing care advocated by Florence Nightingale. She used detailed observation, measurement, and statistical analysis as the evidence on which to base conclusions about the nursing care during the Crimean War. Nursing knowledge and research skills have grown considerably, but what constitutes the best available evidence and its use in making decisions is not always clear.

Knowledge may be acquired in many ways: conventional wisdom is attained by thoughtful analysis of experience, and scientific knowledge is gained through research. Both constitute evidence, and in different situations, one or the other will be an appropriate basis for decision making in practice. "The key is for the decision-maker to understand the limitations of the evidence at hand, and the impact and relevance it will have on decision outcomes" (National Forum on Health, 1997, p. 6). Stetler (2001) refers to sources of knowledge in terms of *internal evidence*, based on affirmed clinical experience, consensus of local experts, or verifiable data from quality improvement or evaluation projects, and *external evidence*, based on research or consensus of national experts.

Much of the knowledge in any practice discipline is that of conventional wisdom, but, as the knowledge base expands and becomes more complex, it becomes increasingly important to build practice on scientific research. Research is a process of systematic examination of phenomena to increase knowledge of these phenomena, their characteristics, occurrence, and relation to other variables. The rigour involved in a scientific process provides for a careful examination of variables, reduces bias in data collection and analysis, and allows for critique and testing by clinicians and researchers. Clinicians are able to explain and predict outcomes of their practice and to re-examine practice as new knowledge becomes available.

The Canadian Nurses Association (1990) established three goals for nursing research: (a) to develop nurse researchers, (b) to develop nursing research, and (c) to develop a research reality. A research reality occurs when research is part of the substance of practice in all nursing fields. Decisions are based on sound research—decisions that nurses make in relation to their patients and health care, decisions that administrators make in relation to staff and policies, and decisions that educators make in relation to students and learning. The National Forum on Health (1997) defined evidence-based decision making as "the systematic application of the best available evidence to the evaluation of options and to decision-making in clinical, management and policy settings" (p. 6).

To build nursing practice on scientific evidence, four interdependent components are needed: (a) meaningful research questions that are relevant to practice, (b) sound research to answer the questions, (c) knowledgeable nurses with skills in using research findings, and (d) clinical environments open to inquiry and change. Figure 17.1 illustrates the cyclical nature of the relationship among these components.

Advantages of an evidence-based practice include improved quality of care, increased vision of the role of nursing, improved visibility of the impact of nursing care on patient outcomes, better cost-effectiveness of health care, and greater nurse satisfaction. In this chapter, nursing research activities are discussed, along with departmental strategies to promote these activities, the role of leaders and managers in developing evidence-based practice, and the costs and benefits of research.

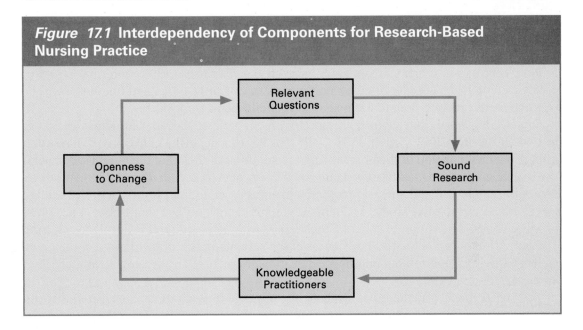

Figure 17.1 **Interdependency of Components for Research-Based Nursing Practice**

Conduct and Utilization of Nursing Research

Research activities involve both the conduct and the utilization of research. The conduct of research is the planning and implementation of a research project for the purpose of generating knowledge. The utilization of research has two major components: (a) interpretation and use of other people's research findings in practice, and (b) use of rigorous research methods in practice (Crane, 1989; Horsley, 1985; Stetler, 2001). Research utilization is an integral part of sound clinical, administrative, and educational nursing practice and is essential for quality management.

The level and type of nurse involvement in research activities require different knowledge and skills, so it is not expected that all nurses will participate in the same ways (Estabrooks, 1997). However, it is possible for all nurses to participate to some extent. For example, nurses from a 42-bed rural hospital in the United States have had an international impact on research utilization through the activities of their research committee and the production of an award-winning videotape on the topic (Horn Video Productions, 1987).

Understanding the value of research is the responsibility of all nurses. Fostering research and its utilization is the responsibility of all nursing leaders.

Models of Nursing Research Utilization

There are several models, or frameworks, for the steps needed to use research findings in nursing practice. In their project, the Conduct and Utilization of Research in Nursing (CURN), Horsley and her associates teamed researchers and clinicians who worked together to critique research reports of tested interventions that addressed relevant clinical problems (Horsley, Crane,

Crabtree, & Wood, 1983). The findings from the research were transformed into a clinical plan that could be readily understood and implemented. The teams also developed a procedure to test the intervention on a small scale. This process was used in decision making about breast-feeding information in postpartum care (Ashcroft & Kristjanson, 1994). Information about breast-feeding had been identified by staff nurses as a priority issue, and findings from the research literature were used to design an instructional booklet for nurses.

A model developed from a clinical perspective by Stetler and Marram was refined by Stetler in 1994 and again in 2001 (Stetler, 1994, 2001). The 2001 model includes five phases of research utilization: identification of the problem and preparation, validation of the findings, comparative evaluation/decision making, translation/application, and evaluation (Figure 17.2). An advantage of this model is that it allows for cognitive application of findings from descriptive studies. For example, a qualitative study of patients who refused analgesics (Schumacher et al., 2002) provided a vivid description of patients' experiences with pain and their rationale for refusing analgesia. Nurses can relate the experiences of the patients in the study to those of their own patients, thereby using a richer knowledge base in their practice. This is a cognitive application of research findings.

The Stetler model also identifies symbolic use of research findings, an application that can be extremely useful for nurse managers. This refers to the use of data from the literature or the use of scientific projects for building and supporting an argument. For instance, if a nurse manager has knowledge of the criteria for ideal computerized data management for nursing decisions (Bélanger & Grenier, 1996), the grounds for specific computer needs are stronger.

In 1991, the Registered Nurses Association of British Columbia (RNABC) launched a province-wide program to help nurses understand and use research findings in their practice. The framework it developed is similar to the Stetler model, but it also provides direction on deciding when to abandon or continue a project (RNABC, 1991). A case example of research utilization by a group of pediatric nurses interested in assessing and managing pain in children is presented in Box 17.1.

Kitson and her colleagues (Kitson, Harvey, & McCormack, 1998) in the United Kingdom developed a different type of framework that incorporated three core elements in the use of research in practice: the level and nature of evidence, the context or environment, and the process of facilitation. They examined the notion of facilitation in depth and emphasized the need for well-prepared facilitators to work with nurses in order to be successful (Harvey et al., 2002).

Research utilization may progress through several phases. For example, one group of nurses in an immunodeficiency clinic used their knowledge of social support research in a cognitive manner. The nurses knew that people with HIV have complex social support networks that influence their ability to cope with their illness. In order to use a more systematic measure of social support to track changes over time, the nurses adapted a sociogram (Maxwell, 1982) and a social support measure (Norbeck, Lindsey, & Carrieri, 1983) for their own clinical use. Clients reported that the measurement process itself helped them become more aware of their resources. The nurses completed a pilot study to test the effects of the measurement process. These nurses work in an environment that promotes research activities.

Figure 17.2 Stetler Model, Part I: Steps of Research Utilization to Facilitate EBP

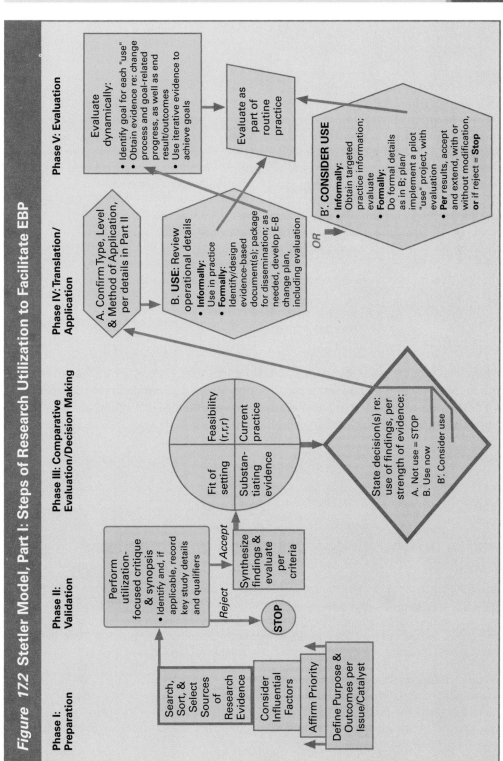

Source: From Updating the Stetler Model of Research Utilization to Facilitate Evidence-Based Practice (p. 276), by C.B. Stetler, 2001, *Nursing Outlook*, *49*(6), 272–279. Reprinted with permission.

Box 17.1

Case Example: Assessing Children's Pain

After a thorough review of the literature, nurses in a teaching hospital developed an educational program for pediatric nurses on state-of-the-art children's pain assessment and management. Program educators delivered awareness knowledge and how-to knowledge in five 30-minute classes. The classes were videotaped for nurses who were unable to attend. A pain experience history, pain observation scale, and pain flow sheet were developed that incorporated the following: the child's experience with pain, a behavioural assessment, the assessment date and time, the child's and/or parent's pain ratings, the nurse's judgment of pain intensity, and the interventions, including non-pharmacological strategies. Multiple sources of data were used to evaluate the outcomes and highlight elements of change that were important to the success of the program. Nurses reported that the assessment aids and distraction material for non-pharmacological interventions were the most useful. Six months later, nurses were using the assessment tools more often than they had during the three months immediately following the program (Howell, Foster, Hester, Vojir, & Miller, 1996).

There have been concerns for some time about the length of time between the publication of research findings and the assessment and utilization of new knowledge in practice. Box 17.2 provides a description of an emerging area of research—knowledge utilization and knowledge transfer, in which nurses are playing a significant part.

Box 17.2

Research on Knowledge Utilization and Knowledge Transfer

There is growing recognition that clinical professionals and decision makers cannot readily locate and use research findings that are appropriate and applicable to their work. Concern about the time it takes for research findings to be applied in practice has led to the emergence of new fields of funded research—knowledge utilization and knowledge transfer. Canadian nurses are at the forefront of these emerging fields of study.

Knowledge Utilization Studies in Practice (KUSP)
Dr. Carole Estabrooks is Principal Investigator of this major program of research. Its purpose is to develop knowledge and research utilization theory that can be used to increase the use of research by nurses and other allied health professionals in order to improve patient and client health outcomes.

In this program, research utilization is defined as the use of research to guide practice and is considered a special subset of evidence-based practice. It is particularly concerned with the use of research evidence (i.e., the findings of scientific studies). Both knowledge utilization and evidence-based practice are broader than research utilization, encompassing the use of other forms of evidence than just research evidence alone (Estabrooks, 1998, 1999a, 1999b). The primary objectives of the KUSP research program are to (a) improve the ability to model research utilization processes, (b) accelerate current work by nurse and other investigators, and (c) encourage new work in this field in Canada and elsewhere.

Source: Knowledge Utilization Studies Program. Retrieved May 2, 2003, from http://www.nursing.ualberta.ca/kusp/

The Centre for Knowledge Transfer

The Centre for Knowledge Transfer is a national training centre in the area of knowledge utilization and policy implementation. The centre is comprised of a consortium of universities, research institutes, and health authorities. The partnership universities are Laval, Manitoba, Saskatchewan, and Alberta. The University of Alberta houses the administrative functions of the centre. Dr. Carole Estabrooks is Academic Co-Director of the centre.

The mission of the Centre for Knowledge Transfer is to contribute to the improved transfer of knowledge for the betterment of health policy and health care services. Its mandate includes the following:

- Provide training to researchers and to students to do knowledge transfer in the health sector
- Train scholars in the field of knowledge transfer with the aim of building capacity
- Engage decision makers to maximize policy relevance of knowledge transfer training and scholarship
- Increase knowledge transfer skills among health care managers and professionals to promote evidence-based decision making

The Centre for Knowledge Transfer is funded through a multi-year award from the Canadian Health Services Research Foundation, the Canadian Institutes for Health Research, and the Alberta Heritage Foundation for Medical Research. In addition, the centre receives in-kind contributions and support from its partner universities.

Source: The Centre for Knowledge Transfer. Retrieved May 5, 2003, from http://www.ckt-ctc.ca/

Strategies to Promote Research Activities Among Nurses

A spirit of inquiry and openness to change is essential for the successful development of evidence-based practice within a department of nursing. If they are not willing to question or challenge rituals and traditions, clinical agencies will not develop practice with a sound scientific base

(Walsh & Ford, 1989). A process of building policies and procedures for research (see van Koot & Laverty, 1992) will be one of the first strategies to promote a spirit of inquiry among nurses and will encourage nurses to raise research questions. Another essential strategy for promoting best nursing practice is the creation of optimum working environments (Royle, Blythe, Ciliska, & Ing, 2000). Creating optimum working environments is an ongoing responsibility of nurse leaders.

The working environment is a major factor supporting or obstructing evidence-based practice. The four types of barriers to research utilization are related to the setting, the nurse, the research, and the presentation (Funk, Champagne, Wiese, & Tornquist, 1991a). In an American survey, Funk and her colleagues (1991b) found that eight of the ten most frequently reported barriers were related to the setting (Table 17.1).

To overcome these barriers, there must be a commitment to encourage and support nurses' questions and pursuit of knowledge. This commitment is shown in the philosophy and policies of the agency and the nursing department, in the substantive support of an infrastructure for research, and in staff development.

Research Infrastructure

The research infrastructure in clinical agencies is dependent on resources as well as philosophy and can range from a nursing research committee to a full department. Resources include an administrative structure to foster research, personnel with research training and access to literature, time, support staff, space, and equipment.

A nursing research committee is an essential component of an infrastructure that is conducive to research. The stimulation of ideas and mutual support from a group process are advantageous, and because of the many different research activities involved, the workload can be shared. A committee can review literature and disseminate findings, facilitate research utilization, provide information about research activities and resources, develop a research agenda, and review proposals for research (Vessey & Campos, 1992). Depending on the size and clinical scope of an agency, research may be best advanced by an agency-wide committee (Henderson & Brouse, 1992; Stordahl & Truitt, 2002), unit-based committees (Hoare & Earenfight, 1986), or thematic interest groups such as a pain management group (Belair, 1992).

Nurses with research training are prepared at the graduate level. They may work full time, part time, or only on consultation. Two positions that have been shown to be effective are the clinical nurse researcher, who is usually prepared at the doctoral level, and the clinical nurse specialist, who is usually prepared at the master's level. The clinical nurse researcher may conduct research, foster a research climate, provide consultation to nursing staff on research projects, advise administrators on research-based decisions, review research proposals, and coordinate a research program. The title and responsibilities vary, but the ability to develop the role and relate to staff nurses and clinical issues is crucial (Knafl, Hagle, Bevis, & Kirchhoff, 1987). The clinical nurse specialist, whose role is usually directly related to patient care, also contributes to research (Fitzgerald et al., 2003; Utz & Gleit, 1995). The clinical nurse specialist may conduct research, particularly in team projects, identify researchable clinical questions, interpret research findings for application to practice, and implement research-based innovations.

Table 17.1 Barriers to Research Utilization, Ranked and Showing Type of Barrier

Rank Order	Barrier	Type of Barrier
1	The nurse does not feel she/he has enough authority to change patient-care procedures.	Setting
2	There is insufficient time on the job to implement new ideas.	Setting
3	The nurse is unaware of the research.	Nurse
4	Physicians will not co-operate with implementation.	Setting
5	Administration will not allow implementation.	Setting
6	Other staff are not supportive of implementation.	Setting
7	The nurse feels results are not generalizable to own setting.	Setting
8	The facilities are inadequate for implementation.	Setting
9	Statistical analyses are not understandable.	Present*
10	The nurse does not have time to read research.	Setting
11	The nurse is isolated from knowledgeable colleagues with whom to discuss the research.	Nurse
12	The relevant literature is not compiled in one place.	Present
13	Implications for practice are not made clear.	Present
14	The nurse does not feel capable of evaluating the quality of the research.	Nurse
15	Research reports/articles are not readily available.	Present
16	The research has not been replicated.	Research
17	The research is not reported clearly and readably.	Present
18	The research is not relevant to the nurse's practice.	Present
19	The nurse feels the benefits of changing practice will be minimal.	Nurse
20	The nurse sees little benefit for self.	Nurse
21	The nurse is uncertain whether to believe the results of the research.	Research
22	The nurse is unwilling to change/try new ideas.	Nurse
23	The literature reports conflicting results.	Research
24	The research has methodological inadequacies.	Research
25	There is not a documented need to change practice.	Nurse
26	The nurse does not see the value of research for practice.	Nurse
27	Research reports/articles are not published fast enough.	Research
28	The conclusions drawn from the research are not justified.	Research

*Present = Presentation

Source: Adapted from Barriers to Using Research Findings in Practice: The Clinician's Perspective, by S.G. Funk, M.T. Champagne, R.A. Wiese et al., 1991b, *Applied Nursing Research*, 4(2), 92. Used with permission.

If there is no in-house staff with research training, arrangements can be made with consultants from academic settings or other agencies (Good & Schubert, 2001). Consultants with particular expertise may be sought for specific projects, or a consultant may meet with staff regularly to discuss a variety of clinical questions.

Access to literature may also depend on outside resources, and arrangements with interlibrary loan systems may be needed. Time to seek consultation or use library resources is essential in any agency with a commitment to evidence-based practice. The availability of other structural resources such as space, support staff, and equipment demonstrate leadership and organizational commitment to research (Fitch, 1992). These not only provide tangible evidence of support, they can also greatly enhance the productivity of researchers.

Demystifying Research

Research activities are often perceived by nurses as "something that somebody else does." The idea of being involved with research may be threatening for nurses without background preparation. However, staff development programs for nurses at all levels will help to demystify research. Whether nurses have had an introductory course in a baccalaureate program or not, they need to develop knowledge and skills for using research concepts in practice.

Programs in research may be offered within a health agency, or nurses may be encouraged to participate in courses outside the agency. A series of workshops for different groups of nurses may be expedient in introducing staff to ideas and strategies. It is appropriate to start with managers and senior nurses who will be leaders in an agency-wide program. A course, rather than a workshop, has the advantage of allowing nurses to use their new knowledge over time in practice between learning sessions (Pepler, 1992).

Involving the nursing staff in research activities is a powerful learning process as well (Fitch & Thompson, 1996; Parker, Gordon, & Brannon, 1992). Alliances with schools of nursing provide an opportunity for students and staff alike to raise relevant questions and gain practical experience in integrating research and practice (Good & Schubert, 2001).

Clinical Leader or Manager as Facilitator of Research Activities

A spirit of inquiry within the nursing department and the structural components of a research commitment will support nurse leaders and managers in efforts to develop research awareness in the staff. The manager at the unit level still has a key role in helping nursing staff raise questions, find answers, participate in research, conduct studies, and use findings in practice.

Raising Questions

The clinical leader or manager is the pivotal person in creating an environment open to questions. The questions may arise from any source: staff nurses, other nurse managers, senior nursing administrators, or members of other disciplines. The initial response of the front-line managers can determine the progress from the initial question—"I wonder if…" or "How come…?"—to the research activities and, finally, to improved practice. Productive responses come from managers who are at ease with not knowing. Otherwise, their initial response may be "We tried that before" or "We can't." The manager who is secure in not having an answer will be comfortable in facilitating a search for one.

To find an answer, it is essential to clarify the question. The first question raised is often either too vague or too specific. Through clarification, the nurse manager can not only show support, but also provide help to focus or expand the question that will assist in finding an answer. For instance, if the question is related to one patient, it may be useful to identify broader characteristics or commonalties across several patients to develop a meaningful question with greater relevance. If a question is vague or ambiguous, it will be helpful to clarify specific circumstances or particular variables that are of interest.

Finding Valid Answers

In any research process, the first activity is searching the literature. This takes time, but many settings now have Internet capability with direct access to online databases and literature.

Managers can facilitate the process by providing nurses the time to search online, to go to accessible libraries, and to read or bring material to the unit. Hart (2002) discusses the skills for reviewing the literature, pointing out that there are various levels and standards for integrating ideas, research, theories, and experience. Nurses can refer to resources such as the Best Practice Guidelines currently being developed by the Registered Nurses Association of Ontario or the Cochrane Collaboration—an international not-for-profit organization providing information about the effects of health care and a library of updated evidence-based health care databases. See Internet Resources at the end of this chapter for Web site information.

Electronic searching is a relatively simple process, readily learned, and invaluable for providing a comprehensive search and saving time. It also promotes browsing and stimulates curiosity. Librarians may be able to send tables of contents from relevant journals to the units so that staff can browse for articles more readily. The tables of contents from many journals are available online at no cost. It is helpful to encourage subscriptions to relevant journals for the unit. While access to a few journals is not sufficient for a comprehensive review, it is useful for keeping up-to-date in specific areas. The staff might be willing to share a subscription, costs could be negotiated with the administrator, or gifts could be directed towards a subscription.

Nurse managers can encourage staff to read research reports and think about the value and applicability of findings. It's best when reading is triggered by genuine interest in the topic, and it is most effective when a series of articles on the same topic are discussed over time. This way, the issue can be explored in depth, and the similarities and differences in research methods and findings can be examined. A review article is a good beginning because it will give an overall critique and a comprehensive reference list (see, for example, Ardery, Herr, Titler, Sorofman, & Schmitt, 2003, on pain management with elderly patients; Mercer, 2001, on umbilical cord clamping; Thomas, 2003, on stressors in mechanically ventilated patients; Wilson, 2002, on dietary restrictions for neutropenic patients).

In the clinical nursing research literature, there are three broad categories of research: (a) descriptive studies of clinical phenomena, client characteristics, or clinical problems; (b) tests of measures or instruments; and (c) experimental studies of nursing interventions. Descriptive studies increase the reader's knowledge base and can be extremely useful in working with patients and families in similar circumstances; however, they do not give directions for care. Clinicians can use the second category of research, tests of measures or instruments, to accurately measure clinical phenomena. The third category of research includes reports of interventions that, if found to be effective, can be implemented. However, nursing interventions are often complex. Whittemore and Grey (2002) have presented guidelines for integrating the four phases of clinical trials delineated by the US National Institutes of Health with elements specific to nursing interventions in order to determine their safety, efficacy, and effectiveness. These authors emphasize the differences in the purposes of pilot projects and full-scale projects and note the need to use well-recognized terminology to distinguish between these and other levels of research development. McCloskey and colleagues have discussed this issue in relation to management interventions, and nursing management interventions in particular, noting the need to specifically describe the intervention, which often takes the form of an organizational or departmental innovation (McCloskey et al., 1996).

Each research report must be critiqued to determine the potential application of the information. Nurse managers can help staff read critically by encouraging participation in courses and staff development programs and by providing opportunities for discussion with nurses who are knowledgeable about research. These may be staff nurses, managers, clinical nurse specialists, or faculty members. A number of questions about the research need to be addressed:

- Is the purpose of the study clearly explained?
- Is other relevant research reviewed adequately?
- Is the study design suitable to answer the research question?
- Is the sample population representative and adequate in terms of size?
- Are variables appropriate and clearly explained?
- Are data collection methods and measures valid and reliable?
- Are analyses appropriate and sufficiently comprehensive?
- Are findings reported clearly?
- Are findings discussed in relation to the theory and other research?
- Are conclusions and implications for practice derived from valid findings?

All these questions are important, but the last is critical. It is sometimes problematic for clinicians because the author may make a quantum leap from tentative findings to recommendations for practice. Some knowledge of research terminology, design, and methods is needed to assess the validity of such recommendations.

The clinical leader or manager needs to be supportive and creative when immediate answers are not found. In some situations, the search may be redirected. For example, there is limited research on family involvement in the care of hospitalized older adults, but two related areas from which knowledge can be gained are quite well developed: family involvement in nursing homes and family participation in the care of hospitalized children. Other times, the nurse manager may support the staff nurses in seeking help to conduct their own study in order to find an answer to their question.

Participating in Research

Answers generated through unit-based research are meaningful to informed nursing staff and are usually relevant to their practice. Nurses may help to plan a project by discussing the question, methods, and feasibility with a researcher at an early stage. Providing input to the research design increases the nurses' sense of involvement and commitment to the project.

Nurses' participation in an ongoing study could include several activities: (a) identifying potential subjects through a designated screening process, (b) asking patients if they are willing to speak to a researcher, (c) carrying out an intervention according to a protocol, (d) obtaining data (such as recording observations or collecting specimens), or (e) participating as a research subject.

Nurse managers have many responsibilities related to their unit's involvement in research conducted by nurses and other disciplines (Table 17.2). These include both facilitating participation and limiting involvement, as necessary. Both require a high level of awareness of potential projects, a clear understanding of the meaning and ramifications of involvement, and skill in facilitating approved projects. The nurse manager should be knowledgeable about all proposed research, regardless of the researcher's discipline. If nurses are likely to be involved, the manager should also review research projects in detail before they begin.

Table17.2 **Nurse Managers' Responsibilities Related to Unit Involvement in Projects Conducted by Researchers Outside Unit Nursing Staff**

- Identify opportunities for involvement
- Review proposals for feasibility, including
  - Potential for access to subjects (patients, family, staff)
  - Ongoing projects
  - Nursing skills
  - Nursing time
  - Study time frame and unit activities
- Arrange information sessions for researcher and staff
- Assure that staff on all shifts are aware of project
- Facilitate training sessions for staff, if applicable
- Collaborate with researcher regarding procedures
- Facilitate access to resources, if applicable, e.g., space, records
- Maintain regular contact with researcher for mutual updates
- Keep staff informed of study progress
- Arrange a session for researcher to report findings to staff
- Encourage staff to attend other presentations and read publications on the project

Conducting a Study

Nurses who are planning to conduct a study need the nurse manager's input and support. Research projects conducted alone are rare, so teams and consultation should be encouraged. Few staff nurses have research preparation, but many projects are manageable within normal nursing practice if the nurses can consult with others and share their workloads (Youngkins, 1991).

The nurse manager is a key person to respond to nurses' ideas for projects. It is important to be supportive but realistic about the demands of research. If the nurse manager does not have the experience or expertise, nurses can be referred to a consultant.

The details of conducting research are beyond the scope of this chapter and can be found in appropriate textbooks. Similar steps for conducting a full-scale study may be used on a small scale on one unit to test findings from previous studies. This is one stage in the process of using research findings in practice.

Using Research Findings in Practice

While every nurse can be involved in using research findings in practice, it is unrealistic to expect all nurses to lead the way. This is an important component of the manager's role, with support from administrative personnel and prepared staff, such as a clinical nurse specialist or senior staff nurse.

The first step to using research findings is a thorough critique of the research reports to determine the validity of the findings, as outlined above. The next phase, which Stetler (2001) identified as comparative evaluation/decision making, is a careful comparison between the situation reported in the research and the particular clinical situation of the reader. At this point, clinical expertise and a sound knowledge of the clinical situation are essential. Again, a series of questions is useful to consider:

- What are the similarities and differences between the problem identified in the study and the situation in the unit?
- What are the similarities and differences between the setting in the study and the setting in question?
- What are the similarities and differences between the people (patients, family members, staff) studied and those in the unit?
- How does a possible innovation fit with the philosophy and policies in the agency?
- How feasible is it to carry out the innovation on the unit?
- How feasible is it to use the same measurement techniques to assess the effectiveness of the innovation? If identical measures are not feasible, what alternatives are there?

Once a decision has been made to incorporate research findings, it must be determined whether to use the findings cognitively or to take action based on the findings (Stroud, 2002). Even cognitive application does not happen automatically. Suppose a researcher reports on the experience of specific problems or factors related to the well-being of a particular population—for instance, long-term survivors of AIDS (Barroso, 1997), psychiatric patients (Olofsson & Jacobsson, 2001), women whose family members have breast cancer (Chalmers & Thomson, 1996), postpartum mothers (Carty, Bradley, & Winslow, 1996), or children with chronic illnesses (Sartain, Clarke,

& Heyman, 2000). The nurse manager can arrange for a discussion of how the findings relate to the population in the setting and how the new knowledge might influence care.

If action is to be taken, the new information can be used as evidence of the need for change. Many groups may resist change (see Chapter 22), but with strong evidence, change agents can advocate more effectively. The research findings may prompt the nurse manager and staff to evaluate their own situation. Are they collecting enough information about patients to determine a need for change? What are the actual outcomes of current practice? What are the costs, human and financial, of current practice?

The final decision in implementing research findings is whether to use an innovation as a model for a change in practice. It is useful to plan a trial period with a comparison before and after the innovation or with a control group for whom the innovation is not used. One effective way to conduct a trial is to replicate the original study as closely as possible. Several classic sources provide clear information on this process (Haller, Reynolds, & Horsley, 1979; Horsley et al., 1983). Also, the original researcher can be consulted.

Once the new information has been in use for a period of time, an evaluation of the impact is essential. It is, therefore, important to have accurate data about the situation prior to the change. Assessment of change may be part of a regular review of nursing care or may be specific to the innovation.

Protecting Patient and Staff Rights in Relation to Research

Managers have a responsibility for protecting patient and staff rights in relation to any research. When the possibility of a research project arises, the first step is to ensure that an appropriate ethical review board has approved the project. This is essential, regardless of the researcher's discipline or institutional affiliation. A staff physician, nurse from a graduate program, university professor, or psychologist from a community agency all need approval for research projects. In teaching agencies, there is likely an established procedure, but in any agency, the manager is often the first contact researchers make. It is imperative that approval be verified. A nursing administrator or nurse researcher should sit on the review board.

It is also important that the nurse manager have an understanding of the research protocol, the purpose, the procedures, and the involvement of patients. If it is medical research or a project that does not involve nursing, the manager may still be called upon to answer questions or refer patients or family members to the researcher. The manager may be the only person who knows what other projects are in process. Patients or staff may need to be protected from "research overload." It may simply be an issue of timing. Data for one study may be collected at one time, and those for another at a different time of day or day of the week. This may not make a difference to the research, but it can make a big difference to the running of the unit. If the manager or nursing staff is involved in a screening process for research subjects, the researcher should plan this in advance with the manager. Any screening that is not built into the project can seriously jeopardize the validity of the results.

The nurse manager needs to be involved in the approval process if the study includes any nursing staff participation. Nurses need to be informed participants. They need to know why the study is being done, why specific data are being collected, what the risks and benefits are for patients, and so on. The manager may be engaged in a balancing act between encouraging and facilitating research on one hand and limiting access to patients or staff on the other.

Differentiating Between Research and Quality Management

An important distinction needs to be made between research and quality management activities. Nurse managers are responsible for the quality of care in their jurisdiction (quality management is addressed in Chapter 12). The activities of identifying problems, collecting data, testing solutions, and analyzing results may be similar, and improved nursing practice is the long-term goal of both. However, the purpose of research is to add to the knowledge base, rather than to promote a high quality of care in a specific area. Thurston and Best (1990) discuss methods for integration of the two programs to improve nursing care.

The Economics of Research

As with any other aspect of nursing, there are costs and benefits to nursing research. Knowledge of these economics in general and in relation to particular studies will help nurse managers in their research role.

Costs of Doing Research

Nurse managers need to be aware of the indirect costs of participating in research, whether nurses or researchers in other disciplines are conducting the study. Cronenwett (1987) suggested asking several questions related to the space required, changes in nursing practice, staff involvement and time, patient time, numbers of study patients at a given time, and supplies or other costs. These costs should be built into the budget of research grants.

The primary costs of nursing research involve personnel. In general, nurses do not use expensive equipment or procedures, but many clinical studies are labour intensive. Whether the study is a large funded project or a small in-house study by the nursing staff, the same time issues need to be considered. Time for planning, time for data collection, time for data analysis, and time for writing the report are essential. Pringle (1989) noted that one of the realities of research is that it is a long-term process. Benefits make the costs worthwhile, but it is also worthwhile to consider outside funding for research.

Funding Resources

Obtaining funding is a challenge in this time of restraint and limited resources available for nursing research. However, a truism also pertains. Nurses will not get funding if they do not apply. Federal and provincial government agencies fund research, as do non-governmental organizations such as the Canadian Heart Foundation or the Arthritis Society. The Canadian Nurses Foundation and some provincial nursing associations have funds for small projects. The Canadian Nurses Association regularly publishes a list of resources for research funding.

Although seeking funds adds to the overall time for a research project, having deadlines for submission can provide a major stimulus to planning. For nurses unfamiliar with the process, it is essential to get a knowledgeable consultant involved as grant applications are highly competitive.

Economic Benefits of Nursing Research

Even as health care costs soar and resources diminish, nursing research can offer economic benefits by identifying ways in which agencies can save money. The following are examples of nursing research that have resulted in substantial economic benefits.

- Fagin (1990) found that nursing programs such as long-term or hospital follow-up home care have been successful in reducing costs *"if they have served as an alternative to other types of care"* (p. 29, italics original).
- Brooten and colleagues (1986) demonstrated that an early discharge program for very-low-birth-weight infants, including counselling and home care by a hospital-based nurse specialist, yielded a net savings of US $18,560 per infant.
- Naylor and colleagues (1994) found that a clinical nurse specialist program for older cardiac patients in an acute care setting reduced the number of readmissions and total days during readmission for patients from the medical units, but not for those from the surgical units.
- Frantz, Gardner, Specht, and McIntire (2001) analyzed outcomes from a research-based pressure ulcer treatment protocol in a long-term care facility. They found that 87% of pressure sores had been healed at relatively low cost.
- An analysis of 17 studies comparing the use of a saline flush versus heparin for peripheral intravenous locks showed that saline was safe and could produce annual savings of over US $100 million in health care costs (Goode et al., 1991).
- A team in critical care encouraged all staff to identify clinical questions for which the group then performed a clinical/cost kinetics analysis to identify potential cost savings (White, Bartrug, & Bride, 1995).

Leadership Implications

Although economics is a major factor affecting choices in health care, improved patient outcomes often have long-term cost benefits that are difficult to measure. It is important for nursing researchers to consider the benefits in patient outcomes in terms of both better health and reduced health care costs, and it is important for nursing leaders to take advantage of sound research to improve care at a lower cost. Communications technology makes the most up-to-date information increasingly available at the point of service. It is the role of nurses in clinical leadership positions to promote the use and evaluation of these resources in professional practice.

Summary

- The four interdependent components that are needed for evidence-based nursing practice are (a) meaningful research questions that are relevant to practice, (b) sound research to answer the questions, (c) knowledgeable nurses with skills in using research findings, and (d) clinical environments open to inquiry and change.
- Research activities include conducting research, using other researchers' findings, and using rigorous research techniques in daily practice.
- All nurses can participate in some research activities with the help of their leaders.
- The working environment constitutes one of the major barriers to the use of research findings, and the nurse manager is the key person in creating a climate of openness and inquiry.
- Health care agencies can provide structural supports and continuing education to facilitate evidence-based practice.
- Clinical nurse leaders can help staff raise questions, find answers, participate in research, conduct studies, and use findings in practice.
- There are costs involved in conducting and participating in research, but the benefits for patients and health care costs are significant.
- Nurses in management positions have a particular responsibility to develop nursing practice in their areas that is based on sound evidence and sound economics.

Applying the Knowledge in this Chapter

Case Study

Carol Johnson and Margaret Wynan, nurses in a busy oncology day centre, are concerned about the venous irritation caused by some of the chemotherapeutic drugs. They have been trying various methods, such as hot packs and extra hydration, to prevent or relieve the irritation. They have talked to physicians, and sometimes a steroid has been given. At report one day, they ask other nurses what they have been doing, if anything, and a general discussion begins about the problems and solutions concerning various patients and their drugs.

Answer the following questions as if you were the nurse responsible for this clinic:

1. How would you assess whether this was a suitable project for research and at what level?

2. What steps would you take if you and the nursing staff thought that this topic warranted further investigation?

Resources

ⓔⓥⓞⓛⓥⓔ Internet Resources

Knowledge Utilization Studies Program (KUSP):
www.nursing.ualberta.ca/kusp/
The Centre for Knowledge Transfer:
www.ckt-ctc.ca/
The Canadian Institutes for Health Research:
http://cihr-irsc.gc.ca/index.shtml
RNAO—Best Practice Guidelines:
www.rnao.org/bestpractices/index.asp
The Cochrane Collaboration:
www.cochrane.org/index0.htm

Further Reading

Nurses looking for sound evidence upon which to base their clinical decisions can begin by searching for systematic reviews in the published literature on their topic of interest. A systematic review is limited to research drawn from pre-selected databases, using predetermined criteria for inclusion of studies in the review. The reviewer(s) assesses the scientific merit of the studies and evaluates the validity of the research findings. The Cochrane Library is a source of systematic reviews on many medical and health care subjects (see The Cochrane Collaboration Web site above). The following are examples of systematic reviews conducted by nurses.

Cummings, G., & Estabrooks, C.A. (2003). The effects of hospital restructuring on individual nurses: A systematic review. *International Journal of Sociology, 23*(8/9), 8–53.
Gillies, D., O'Riordan, E., Carr, D., O'Brien, I., Frost, J., & Gunning, R. (2003). Central venous catheter dressings: A systematic review. *Journal of Advanced Nursing, 44,* 623–632.
Peacock, S.C., & Forbes, D.A. (2003). Interventions for caregivers of persons with dementia: A systematic review. *Canadian Journal of Nursing Research, 35,* 89–107.

References

Ardery, G., Herr, K.A., Titler, M.G., Sorofman, B.A., & Schmitt, M.B. (2003). Assessing and managing acute pain in older adults: A research base to guide practice. *MEDSURG Nursing, 12*(1), 7–19.
Ashcroft, T., & Kristjanson, L.J. (1994). Research utilization in maternal-child nursing: Application of the CURN model. *Canadian Journal of Nursing Administration, 7*(5), 90–101.
Barroso, J. (1997). Restructuring my life: Becoming a long-term survivor of AIDS. *Qualitative Health Research, 7,* 57–74.
Belair, J. (1992). Pain management interest group. *Nursing Horizons, 10*(2), 12.
Belanger, G., & Grenier, R. (1996). Computerization and nursing: In search of an ideal! *Canadian Journal of Nursing Research, 28*(2), 67–84.

Brooten, D., Kumar, S., Brown, L.P., Butts, P., Finkler, S.A., Bakewell-Sachs, S., Gibbons, A., & Deliveria-Papadopoulos, M. (1986). A randomized clinical trial of early hospital discharge and home follow-up of very-low-birth-weight infants. *New England Journal of Medicine, 315,* 934–939.

Canadian Nurses Association. (1990). *Research imperative for nursing in Canada: The next five years 1990–1995.* Ottawa, ON: Author.

Carty, E.M., Bradley, C., & Winslow, W. (1996). Women's perceptions of fatigue during pregnancy and postpartum: The impact of length of hospital stay. *Clinical Nursing Research, 5*(1), 67–80.

The Centre for Knowledge Transfer. Retrieved May 5, 2003, from http://www.ckt-ctc.ca

Chalmers, K., & Thomson, K. (1996). Coming to terms with the risk of breast cancer: Perceptions of women with primary relatives with breast cancer. *Qualitative Health Research, 6,* 256–282.

Crane, J. (1989). *Factors associated with the use of research-based knowledge in nursing.* Unpublished doctoral dissertation, University of Michigan.

Cronenwett, L.R. (1987). The indirect costs of nursing research. *Journal of Nursing Administration, 17*(9), 6–8.

Estabrooks, C.A. (1997). *Research utilization in nursing: An examination of formal structure and influencing factors.* Unpublished doctoral dissertation, University of Alberta.

Estabrooks, C.A. (1998). Will evidence-based nursing practice make practice perfect? *Canadian Journal of Nursing Research, 30*(1), 15–36.

Estabrooks, C.A. (1999a). The conceptual structure of research utilization. *Research in Nursing & Health, 22*(3), 203–216.

Estabrooks, C.A. (1999b). Mapping the research utilization field in nursing. *Canadian Journal of Nursing Research, 31*(1), 53–72.

Fagin, C.M. (1990). Nursing's value proves itself. *American Journal of Nursing, 90*(10), 17–30.

Fitch, M.I. (1992). Five years in the life of a nursing research and professional development division. *Canadian Journal of Nursing Administration, 5*(1), 21–27.

Fitch, M.I., & Thompson, L. (1996). Fostering the growth of research-based oncology nursing practice. *Oncology Nursing Forum, 23,* 631–637.

Fitzgerald, M., Milberger, P., Tomlinson, P.S., Peden-Mcalpine, C., Meiers, S.J., & Sherman, S. (2003). Clinical nurse specialist participation on a collaborative research project: Barriers and benefits. *Clinical Nurse Specialist, 17*(1), 44–49.

Frantz, R.A., Gardner, S., Specht, J.K., & McIntire, G. (2001). Integration of pressure ulcer treatment protocol into practice: Clinical outcomes and care environment attributes. *Outcomes Management for Nursing Practice, 5*(3), 112–120.

Funk, S.G., Champagne, M.T., Wiese, R.A., & Tornquist, E.M. (1991a). BARRIERS: The barriers to research utilization scale. *Applied Nursing Research, 4*(1), 39–45.

Funk, S.G., Champagne, M.T., Wiese, R.A., & Tornquist, E.M. (1991b). Barriers to using findings in practice: The clinician's perspective. *Applied Nursing Research, 4*(2), 90–95.

Good, D.M., & Schubert, C.R. (2001). Faculty practice: How it enhances teaching. *Journal of Nursing Education, 40,* 389–396.

Goode, C.J., Titler, M., Rakel, B., Ones, D.S., Kleiber, C., Small, S., & Triolo, P.K. (1991). A meta-analysis of effects of heparin flush and saline flush: Quality and cost implications. *Nursing Research, 40,* 324–330.

Haller, K.B., Reynolds, M.A., & Horsley, J.A. (1979). Developing research-based innovation protocols: Process, criteria, and issues. *Research in Nursing & Health, 2,* 45–51.

Hart, C. (2002). *Doing a literature review: Releasing the social science research imagination.* Thousand Oaks, CA: SAGE Publications.

Harvey, G., Loftus-Hills, A., Rycroft-Malone, J., Titchen, A., Kitson, A., McCormack, B., & Seers, K. (2002). Getting evidence into practice: The role and function of facilitation. *Journal of Advanced Nursing, 37,* 577–588.

Henderson, A., & Brouse, J. (1992). Development of a research committee in a community hospital. *Canadian Journal of Nursing Research, 5*(2), 17–19.

Hoare, K., & Earenfight, J. (1986). Unit-based research in a service setting. *Journal of Nursing Administration, 16*(4), 35–39.

Horn Video Productions. (1987). *Using research in clinical nursing practice* [Videotape]. (Available from Horn Video Productions, 1870–360th Street, Odebolt, Iowa, USA 51458–7593).

Horsley, J.A. (1985). Using research in practice: The current context. *Western Journal of Nursing Research, 7,* 135–139.

Horsley, J.A., Crane, J., Crabtree, K., & Wood, D.J. (1983). *Using research to improve nursing practice: A guide.* New York: Grune & Stratton.

Howell, S.L., Foster, R.L., Hester, N.O., Vojir, C.P., & Miller, K.L. (1996). Evaluating a pediatric pain management research utilization program. *Canadian Journal of Nursing Research, 28*(2), 37–57.

Kitson, A., Harvey, G., & McCormack, B. (1998). Enabling the implementation of evidence based practice: A conceptual framework. *Quality in Health Care, 7,* 149–158.

Knafl, K.A., Hagle, M., Bevis, M., & Kirchhof, K. (1987). Clinical nurse researchers: Strategies for success. *Journal of Nursing Administration, 17*(10), 27–31.

Knowledge Utilization Studies Program. Retrieved May 2, 2003, from http://www.nursing.ualberta.ca/kusp/

Maxwell, M.B. (1982). The use of social networks to help cancer patients maximize support. *Cancer Nursing, 5,* 275–281.

McCloskey, J., Maas, M., Huber, D., Kasparek, A., Specht, J., Ramler, C., et al. (1996). Nursing management innovations: A need for systematic evaluation. In K. Kelly & M. Maas (Eds.), *Outcomes of effective management practice, SONA 8: Series on nursing administration* (pp. 3–19). London: Sage Publications.

Mercer, J.S. (2001). Current best evidence: A review of the literature on umbilical cord clamping. *Journal of Midwifery & Women's Health, 46,* 347-351, 402-414.

National Forum on Health. (1997). *Canada health action: Building the legacy. Synthesis reports and papers. Creating a culture of evidence-based decision-making.* Ottawa, ON: Health Canada.

Naylor, M., Brooten, D., Jones, R., Lavizzo-Mourey, R., Mezey, M., & Pauly, M. (1994). Comprehensive discharge planning for the hospitalized elderly. *Annals of Internal Medicine, 120,* 999–1006.

Nightingale, F. (1980). *Notes on nursing: What is it and what is it not.* Edinburgh, Scotland: Churchill Livingstone. (Original work published 1859 by Harrison & Sons, London).

Norbeck, J.S., Lindsey, A.M., & Carrieri, V.L. (1983). Further development of the Norbeck social support questionnaire: Normative data and validity testing. *Nursing Research, 32,* 4–9.

Olofsson, B., & Jacobsson, L. (2001). A plea for respect: Involuntarily hospitalized psychiatric patients' narratives about being subjected to coercion. *Journal of Psychiatric & Mental Health Nursing, 8,* 357–366.

Parker, M.E., Gordon, S.C., & Brannon, P.T. (1992). Involving nursing staff in research: A non-traditional approach. *Journal of Nursing Administration, 22*(4), 58–63.

Pepler, C.J. (1992). Fostering change through education. *Canadian Nurse, 88*(1), 25–27.

Pringle, D. (1989). Another twist on the double helix: Research and practice. *Canadian Journal of Nursing Research, 21,* 47–60.

Registered Nurses Association of British Columbia. (1991). *Making a difference: From ritual to research-based practice.* Vancouver, BC: Author.

Royle, J., Blythe, J., Ciliska, D., & Ing, D. (2000). The organizational environment and evidence-based nursing. *Canadian Journal of Nursing Leadership, 13*(1), 31–37.

Sartain, S.A., Clarke, C.L., & Heyman, R. (2000). Hearing the voices of children with chronic illness. *Journal of Advanced Nursing, 32,* 913–921.

Schumacher, K.L., West, C., Dodd, M., Paul, S.M., Tripathy, D., Koo, P., & Miaskowski, C. (2002). Pain management autobiographies and reluctance to use opioids for cancer pain management. *Cancer Nursing, 25,* 125–133.

Stetler, C.B. (1994). Refinement of the Stetler/Marram model for application of research findings to practice. *Nursing Outlook, 42*(1), 15–25.

Stetler, C.B. (2001). Updating the Stetler model of research utilization to facilitate evidence-based practice. *Nursing Outlook, 49*(6), 272–279.

Stordahl, N., & Truitt C.A. (2002). The nursing research committee: The James A. Haley Veterans' Hospital. *Journal of Vascular Nursing, 20,* 143–144.

Stroud, R. (2002). The withdrawal of life support in adult intensive care: An evaluative review of the literature. *Nursing in Critical Care, 7,* 176–184.

Thomas, L.A. (2003). Clinical management of stressors perceived by patients on mechanical ventilation. *AACN Clinical Issues: Advanced Practice in Acute & Critical Care, 14*(1), 73–81.

Thurston, N., & Best, M. (1990). Clinical nursing research and quality assurance: Integration for improved patient care. *Canadian Journal of Nursing Administration, 3*(2), 19–23.

Utz, S.W., & Gleit, C.J. (1995). Current developments in research-based interventions: Enhancing and advancing the CNS role. *Clinical Nurse Specialist, 9*(1), 8–11.

van Koot, B., & Laverty, P. (1992). A research foundation for policies and procedures. *Canadian Nurse, 88*(1), 39–41.

Vessey, J.A., & Campos, R.G. (1992). The role of nursing research committees. *Nursing Research, 41,* 247–249.

Walsh, M., & Ford, P. (1989). *Nursing rituals: Research and rational action.* Oxford, England: Heinemann.

White, S.K., Bartrug, B., & Bride, W. (1995). Supporting nursing innovations in a cost-conscious environment. *Critical Care Nursing Clinics of North America, 7,* 399–406.

Whittemore, R., & Grey, M. (2002). The systematic development of nursing interventions. *Journal of Nursing Scholarship, 34,* 115–120.

Wilson, B.J. (2002). Dietary recommendations for neutropenic patients. *Seminars in Oncology Nursing, 18*(1), 44–49.

Youngkins, J.M. (1991). The impact of one staff nurse's research. *American Journal of Maternal Child Nursing, 16,* 133-135, 137.

NURSING INFORMATION AND OUTCOMES

Ann E. Tourangeau

Learning Objectives

In this chapter, you will learn:

- ■ The nature and importance of nursing information and where and how it is collected and maintained

- ■ Differences between data, information, and knowledge

- ■ Why nursing processes and outcomes of care tend to be invisible in health services databases

- ■ Three categories of outcomes of interest to nursing

- ■ Responsibilities of nurse leaders related to nursing and health information, including outcomes

- ■ How and why nursing activities and outcomes can and should be made more visible in health services databases

Nursing information and outcomes are two terms that are increasingly gaining importance in nursing. In this chapter, we examine these concepts and discuss how and why they should be considered together. We explore what nursing information has been, what nursing information is currently available, whom this information is about, and why it exists. We also explore outcomes—what they are, who or what they are about, and why they are being measured.

Linking Nursing Information to Outcomes

Whether they work in clinical practice, research, education, or administrative leadership, all nurses have responsibilities and opportunities for developing and using nursing information that can be linked with outcomes (Giovannetti & O'Brien-Pallas, 1998). In fact, one important reason for developing nursing information is to be able to link that information with outcomes in order to understand the nursing determinants, or causes, of those outcomes. Once we understand what contributes to outcomes, adjustments can be made to these determinants to improve outcomes.

The role of nurse researchers is to investigate and communicate findings about the relationships between nursing (from nursing information sources) and outcomes. Nurses who provide nursing care have the most responsibilities related to nursing information. They contribute to the development of nursing information, receive and critique findings of nurse investigators, debate the meaning and usefulness of these findings, and use the findings in their nursing practice. Nurses who are educators have responsibilities for communicating the relationships between nursing information and outcomes and assisting those who provide nursing care to apply these findings to their practice. The roles of nurse leaders are (a) to communicate with other health care leaders about relationships between nursing and outcomes, (b) to secure resources that enable nurses who provide care to do so in ways that will bring about the best outcomes, and (c) to provide ongoing support and encouragement to nurses who provide care to use findings about relationships between nursing and outcomes in their practice. Because of the interrelatedness of these nursing roles, the challenge is effective communication among nurses. Nurses need to know about, understand, and support each other's primary roles so that, together, they can bring about the best outcomes.

It is now an important priority to determine and communicate the relationships between nursing (from nursing information) and outcomes. Health care systems remain under continuing pressure to account for the resources they use in bringing about the outcomes they produce. Because nursing consumes such large portions of health care resources, nursing services are easy targets for cost containment and reform activities (Aiken, Sochalski, & Anderson, 1996; Tourangeau, White, Scott, McAllister, & Giles, 1999; Tourangeau, Giovannetti, Tu, & Wood, 2002; Tourangeau, Stone, & Birnbaum, 2003). In the absence of evidence of the impact that nursing services have on outcomes, nursing services can be eroded and public access to care by registered nurses (RNs) curtailed. When evidence is available, it is possible to effectively communicate the repercussions of changes to nursing services on outcomes that are important to health care organizations and systems.

In almost every sector of health care, nurses provide the vast majority of care to patients, whether patients are individuals, families, groups, or societies and whether they are located in urban or rural geographic areas. It is, therefore, reasonable to expect that almost every important health system outcome be related to aspects of nursing care. The challenge has been and continues to be to find evidence of these relationships. To find this evidence, nurses need to develop and use information about nurses and nurses' work as well as information about patient, community, organizational, system, and societal outcomes.

Overview of Health and Nursing Information

What is meant by the term *nursing information*? It is easier to understand what information is in the context of other common terms such as *data* and *knowledge*. According to Blum (1986), *data* refers to discrete bits of information that are stored in a system or bank. Today, data are usually stored in electronic format, but there are still instances in which data are stored in paper format only. Blum described *information* as data that are interpreted, organized, and structured and described *knowledge* as information that has been synthesized so that interrelationships are formally identified.

The following example shows how data, information, and knowledge exist in a typical nursing setting. Nurse managers usually keep records about employed nursing staff. The manager may have multiple data elements for each staff member, such as professional registration or licence number, employment status, highest level of education obtained, and evidence of necessary certifications (e.g., CPR). An example of one piece of *data* is a sheet of paper recording a nurse's registration number for the current year. An organized manager keeps data about nursing staff in some sort of orderly format, such as an electronic database or a table recorded on paper. The electronic database and the paper database would likely be structured similarly, with staff names to the left of a series of rows and columns containing the data. Applying Blum's definition, this database is considered to be *information* because it is structured, organized, and easy to interpret. If the manager summarizes the information in the database and produces a report describing the percentage of staff that submitted their current registration, the number or percentage of full-time and part-time nursing staff, or the proportion of staff with a degree in nursing, then the manager has produced *knowledge* from data elements. Computers and software are used to store data elements in reservoirs or repositories of information, which can then be used to produce knowledge. The identical information could also be organized on paper and the same knowledge created from it—the process would just take a lot longer!

Management and Clinical Databases

Health system data are stored as information in every jurisdiction across North America. There are different kinds of databases in health care that are often categorized by the type of information in the database. Management databases are generally used to record information about topics like organizational activity statistics, finances and accounting, human resources (including payroll), and inventory or resource management control. Generally, these databases are not specific to patients or care recipients, but are used to collect and organize data related to the operation of organizational departments. Management databases are developed to account for and control resource use, produce accountability reports, automate or standardize repetitive activities, and assist in decision making.

On the other hand, clinical databases generally contain specific information about people who receive health care. They may include personal information about the individual (e.g., age and gender), the services and procedures received, results of diagnostic tests, outcomes associated with care, and even some information about providers of care. In the past, clinical databases have focused on medical components of care, but efforts are currently underway to expand the perspective to include the structures, processes, and outcomes of care that health care consumers receive from a broader health care team, including nurses. Generally, clinical databases contain patient-specific information such as medical diagnoses, processes of care (e.g., surgical procedures), outcomes associated with the health care encounter, and so on.

Management databases can exist within an organization for internal use only or can be used to build larger databases developed across health care organizations at the system level. For example, most hospitals have administrative databases used to organize financial expenditures and income. However, provincial departments of health have also established databases that summarize financial expenditures and income for hospitals in their jurisdictions. Data are exported from individual health care organizations to build system-level databases. Some provinces call this the Management Information System. In Ontario, the Ministry of Health and Long-Term Care has established the Ontario Hospital Reporting System that contains, among other information, summaries of Ontario hospital expenditures and incomes.

Clinical databases can also exist exclusively within an organization or can be exported to build a system-level clinical database. For example, most Canadian hospitals collect important clinical data about each discharged patient by coding and abstracting each patient chart according to national guidelines. These data are collected in health records databases and used to develop both information and knowledge about the patients served by that hospital. These data are also routinely exported by hospitals to a national organization called the Canadian Institute for Health Information (CIHI). The CIHI organizes and edits these patient-level data before sending them back to hospitals and to each respective provincial department of health. Thus, provincial health departments receive standardized and credible information about each patient discharged from a hospital within their province, and they are able to use this aggregated information for a variety of purposes.

Canadian Institute for Health Information (CIHI) Databases

For many decades, health care information has been amassed in jurisdictions across Canada at both the health care organization and the system level. However, there were few standards for what data should be collected and how that data should be collected and stored. During the 1990s, great advances were made in Canada to begin to address these issues. Perhaps the most important initiative was the creation of the CIHI in 1994 to foster the development of reliable, meaningful, and believable health care information.

The CIHI is a not-for-profit national agency mandated by Canada's health ministers to coordinate the development and maintenance of a comprehensive and integrated approach to health information for Canada (CIHI, 2003a). The role of the CIHI is to provide and coordinate provision of accurate, meaningful, and timely health information required to develop health policy, effectively manage Canadian health care systems, and generate public awareness about factors affecting good health. CIHI is far more than a health data and information reservoir. Though a vast array of health data are collected, edited, and managed in CIHI databases, the CIHI also plays a key national role in producing health care knowledge through analysis of its health information databases. For example, the CIHI uses information in its databases to produce a yearly national report, *Health Care in Canada* (see CIHI, 2002, 2003b).

The CIHI (2003a) has a number of core functions, including the following:
- Identifying health information needs and priorities
- Conducting analyses and leading or participating in special health care research initiatives
- Funding and facilitating population health research, conducting policy analyses, and developing policy options
- Supporting the development of national health care indicators
- Coordinating and promoting development and maintenance of national health information standards
- Developing and managing health databases and registries
- Providing appropriate access to health data
- Publishing reports and disseminating health information.

Information of importance to nursing may be about nurses, patients, or health care systems; it might also reflect structures, processes, or outcomes for nurses, patients, or health care systems. The CIHI has the largest national health database holdings, which are categorized into three groups: (a) health services databases, (b) health professionals databases, and (c) health expenditure databases. Health services databases contain information about health services provided to individual patients. Health professionals databases track information about the professionals working in the health care system, and health expenditure databases provide summary information on health expenditures in Canada. Some of the important health databases held by the CIHI are briefly described in the tables throughout the chapter. The following sections describe a key database from each of the three categories and provide examples of how the databases have been used to develop nursing knowledge.

A Health Services Database: The Discharge Abstract Database

The Discharge Abstract Database (DAD) is one example of a large health services database held by the CIHI. Table 18.1 briefly describes some others. Health records departments extract information from patient charts using coding guidelines to create abstracts of the charts for approximately 75% of all patients discharged from Canadian acute care, chronic, and rehabilitation hospitals. Hospitals in Quebec and some parts of Manitoba do not contribute to the DAD (Richards, Brown, & Homan, 2001). The abstracts are then submitted to the CIHI and entered into the DAD.

Table 18.1 Select Health Services Databases of the Canadian Institute for Health Information (CIHI)

Database	Key Elements	Source	Availability
Discharge Abstract Database (DAD)	Contains demographic, clinical, and administrative data for patients discharged from acute care (including day surgery), chronic, and rehabilitation hospitals across Canada (except Quebec and some Manitoba facilities)	Hospital data submitted directly to the CIHI from abstracted charts of discharged patients (about 4.3 million records annually)	1979–1980 to current fiscal year
National Ambulatory Care Reporting System (NACRS)	Contains demographic, clinical, administrative, and financial data for hospital- and community-based ambulatory care, including emergency department care (to date, data are primarily from Ontario)	Client/patient data submitted to the CIHI at time of service	2001–2002 to current fiscal year
Continuing Care Reporting System (CCRS)	Contains data on demographics, cognitive, behavioural, and physical functioning, medication use, nutritional status, and special treatments and procedures for patients in designated continuing care beds across Canada	Patient assessment data collected by nurses and other health care providers using the Resident Assessment Instrument (RAI) Minimum Data Set (MDS 2.0)®	2002–2003 (first year available) to current fiscal year

Source: © (2001–2003) Canadian Institute for Health Information (CIHI). The contents of Table 18.1 is adapted from page 7 of the "Discharge Abstract Database (DAD)"; page 8 of the "National Ambulatory Care Reporting System (NACRS)"; and page 9 of the "Continuing Care Research Database (CCRD)" as published by CIHI. Used with permission.

The DAD is a patient-specific database containing information about patients discharged from hospitals during each fiscal year, April 1 through March 31. For each discharged patient, the DAD lists personal information (e.g., birth date, age, address, health card number, pre-admission medical diagnosis, comorbidities), administrative information (e.g., hospital identifier number, admission date and time, discharge date and time), and medical information (e.g., initial reasons for admission; medical diagnoses; medical care received, including surgical and diagnostic procedures; medical complications; identifiers for the physician(s) most responsible for diagnoses and procedures).

The DAD also contains information related to some patient outcomes. For example, there is a data field that identifies the status of each discharged patient as being either dead or alive. Thus, patient mortality and survival can be identified with this database. Because admission and discharge dates are listed for each patient, the length of each patient stay can be calculated. Other outcomes, such as readmission to hospital, can be calculated or derived from data in the DAD. The CIHI not only collects these data from each hospital, but also edits them for accuracy and plausibility before sending the edited data back to the hospital and on to provincial and territorial departments of health for their use.

Nurses' Contribution to the DAD

Though most information abstracted from patient charts for the DAD is extracted from medical care documentation, nurses contribute to DAD data by documenting patient care and other patient activities. For example, admission and discharge times are recorded in the DAD and are usually verified by admitting department records and nursing documentation.

The DAD has frequently been used in research examining medical processes and outcomes of care, but it has been used less often in studies examining nursing care processes and their determination of important patient and organizational outcomes. An example of the use of the DAD in nursing research is a study of the determinants of 30-day mortality for hospitalized patients (Tourangeau et al., 2002). The authors of this study used a variety of data sources, including the DAD, to examine the effects that nursing structures and processes of care have on patient mortality in Ontario hospitals. DAD data were used to develop risk-adjusted mortality rates for acute care medical patients who were discharged from Ontario hospitals during the 1998 and 1999 fiscal years.

What is noticeably absent from the DAD is information about nursing processes of care and the many patient outcomes that are believed to be particularly sensitive to nursing care. A nursing-sensitive outcome is defined as a patient state, behaviour, or perception that is responsive to nursing intervention (Irvine, Sidani, & McGillis Hall, 1998; Maas, Johnson, & Moorhead, 1996). For example, there are no data in the DAD that identify the nursing interventions delivered or what categories of nursing personnel delivered those interventions to patients. Important nursing information such as symptom management interventions and discharge teaching given to patients is also missing from the DAD. Correspondingly, patient outcomes believed to be particularly sensitive to nursing care, such as pain symptoms, functional status, and ability to manage one's own care, are also absent from the DAD.

Nursing Minimum Data Sets

Much effort has been made over the past 15 years to improve this lack of patient information important to nursing. Since the 1960s, there have been calls for the development of a nursing minimum data set consisting of a "minimum set of information with uniform definitions and categories concerning the specific dimension of professional nursing, which meets the information needs of multiple data users in the health care system" (Werley, 1988, p. 7).

Several of the areas deemed as essential components of this nursing minimum data set for each hospitalized patient include nursing intensity use (O'Brien-Pallas & Giovannetti, 1993), nursing interventions received (Giovannetti, Smith, & Broad, 1999; McCloskey & Bulechek, 1993), and the outcomes of nursing care (Giovannetti et al., 1999; Marek & Lang, 1993). A more detailed description of nursing minimum data sets can be found elsewhere (see Mallette, 2003).

Much work has been completed over the past decade to develop classification schemes that use a common language and have common definitions to identify typical patient problems and nursing interventions that address these problems (Bowles & Naylor, 1996; Henry, Holzemer, Randell, Hsieh, & Miller, 1997) and related nursing-sensitive patient outcomes (Maas et al., 1996; Micek et al., 1996; Nielsen & Mortensen, 1997, 1998). Though, in principle, agreement has been reached with agencies such as the CIHI about the importance of nursing minimum data sets across Canadian health care sectors, there is still limited movement toward routine collection of such patient and nurse-specific data elements in health care databases (Tourangeau, 2001). The result of such a lack of information perpetuates the invisibility of nursing care in the delivery

Table 18.2 Select Health Professionals Databases of the Canadian Institute for Health Information (CIHI)

Database	Key Elements	Source	Availability
Registered Nurses Database (RNDB)	Contains demographic, employment, and education data for each registered nurse licensed in a Canadian province or territory (data edited to remove duplications for nurses licensed in more than one jurisdiction)	Nurses complete yearly mandatory licensure form and submit to provincial/territorial licensing body; Licensing body submits data annually to the CIHI	Annually since 1980
Licensed Practical Nurses Database (LPNDB)	Contains demographic, employment, and education data for each practical nurse licensed in a Canadian province or territory (data edited to remove duplications for practical nurses licensed in more than one jurisdiction)	Licensed practical nurses complete yearly mandatory licensure form and submit to provincial/territorial licensing body; Licensing body submits data annually to the CIHI	Annually since 2002
National Physician Database (NPDB)	Contains sociodemographic, payment, and service utilization data for fee-for-service physicians	Data submitted to the CIHI from provincial/territorial medical health care insurance plans	Available from 1972–1973 until 1990–1991 fiscal year as Medical Care Database and annually since then as NPDB

Source: © (2001–2003) Canadian Institute for Health Information (CIHI). The contents of Table 18.2 is adapted from page 14 of the "Registered Nurses Database (RNDB)"; page 14 of the "Licensed Practical Nurses Database (LPNDB)"; and page 15 of the "Registered Psychiatric Nurses Database (RPND)" as published by CIHI. Used with permission.

and outcomes of health care (Giovannetti & O'Brien-Pallas, 1998; Giovannetti et al., 1999; Tourangeau, 2001). This lack of information also impedes development of knowledge about the contribution that nursing care makes to patient and organizational outcomes.

A Health Professionals Database: The Registered Nurses Database

The Registered Nurses Database (RNDB) is an example of a health professionals database held by the CIHI. Table 18.2 lists some other examples. To facilitate nursing human resource planning and policy development, the CIHI prepares timely reports about the supply and distribution of RNs in Canada (CIHI, 2003a). The CIHI develops the RNDB yearly by collecting nurse-specific data from each of the 13 provincial and territorial nursing associations responsible for registered nurse licensure in Canada. Data collected include demographic information (e.g., nurse age and gender), employment information, and nurse education. Nurses contribute to the development of this national database when they complete and submit their licensure forms to their provincial/territorial licensing body. To protect the privacy of nurses, some data elements are not released to the public, and reports contain aggregated data that preserves the anonymity of nurses.

The *Supply and Distribution of Registered Nurses in Canada, 2001 Report* (CIHI, 2001) describes trends in the supply of RNs between 1997 and 2001 in all provinces and territories. The report also describes gender and age trends as well as education and employment trends of RNs across Canada. This CIHI report provides governments and professional nursing organizations with useful knowledge that can be used to build health policy and related strategies.

A Health Expenditure Database: The Canadian Management Information System Database

One of the health expenditure databases held by the CIHI is The Canadian Management Information System Database (CMDB). Table 18.3 lists some others. The CMDB contains financial and statistical information on hospitals and regional health authorities across Canada (CIHI, 2003a). This is one of the oldest databases in Canadian health care and was established in 1932 by Statistics Canada under the name *Annual Return of Health Care Facilities –Hospitals*. It was known by that name until 1994.

The CMDB contains information about financial expenditures and statistical information on personnel and patient activity in hospitals. For example, the total number of paid nursing hours over the fiscal year in each hospital's functional centre is recorded in this database (a *functional centre* is a grouping of like hospital departments such as medicine units or surgical units). Expenditures by hospital functional centres are also listed in this database by various categories of expenses (e.g., staffing, medical-surgical supplies). Activity statistics such as the number of patient days in each hospital's functional centre, the average daily census, or the number of beds staffed and in operation are also held in this database.

Nurses contribute directly to this database when they report admissions and discharges to their hospital units and when they complete midnight census reports, either electronically or through paper reports. Information from this database is frequently used to develop nursing knowledge and to assist in managerial decision making at hospital, health region, and system levels. It is in this database that Canadian hospitals provide evidence of reconciliation of their

Table 18.3 Select Health Expenditure Databases of the Canadian Institute for Health Information (CIHI)

Database	Key Elements	Source	Availability
Canadian Management Information System Database (CMDB)	Contains financial and statistical information on hospitals and regional health authorities across Canada, at functional level of organization	In provinces/territories where a central database of management information system (MIS) data is maintained, data are transferred directly from the Ministry of Health for that jurisdiction; Otherwise, individual facilities or regional health authorities are surveyed for this information	Available from 1932 to 1933 and 1993 to 1994 under the name *Annual Return of Health Care Facilities-Hospitals*. Available as CMDB annually since 1994–1995
National Health Expenditure Database (NHEX)	Contains data for over 40 spending categories from five sources of finance (federal and provincial/territorial/municipal governments, workers' compensation boards, social security funds, and the private sector)	Data manually extracted from public documents, public government accounts and other financial reports, private insurance companies, and AC Nielsen Canada	Annually since 1960
Organization for Economic Cooperation and Development (OECD) Health Database (Canadian segment)	Contains information on health care spending, health care services, and health status among member countries of the OECD. Consists of 10 parts: health status, health care resources, health care utilization, expenditure on health, financing and remuneration, social protections, pharmaceutical market, non-medical determinants of health, demographic references, and economic references	Canadian data primarily originates from the CIHI and Statistics Canada databases	Annually since 1960

Source: © (2001–2003) Canadian Institute for Health Information (CIHI). The contents of Table 18.3 is adapted from page 16 of the "Canadian MIS Database (CMDB)"; page 16 of the "National Health Expenditure Database (NHEX)"; and page 17 of the "Organisation for Economic Co-operation and Development (OECD) Health Database" as published by CIHI. Used with permission.

expenditures and the outputs or products arising from these expenditures. Hospitals demonstrate accountability for resources consumed when they report to this database.

Because the CMDB contains vital information about nurse staffing in hospitals, data elements from this database have been used frequently in nursing research. For example, Tourangeau and colleagues (2002) used a subset of the CMDB, the *Ontario Hospital Reporting System for 1998-1999,* in their study of the determinants of 30-day mortality for hospitalized patients. Indicators of three of the hypothesized predictors of mortality were developed for Ontario hospitals using the Ontario subset of the CMDB: nurse staffing dose, nursing skill mix, and the proportion of hours worked by full-time registered nurses.

Other Sources of Nursing Information

Other important health information is collected outside of the CIHI, and some of this information may be important for nursing. For example, most provincial and territorial jurisdictions maintain vital statistics information on residents, which usually includes birth and death information. Provincial and territorial jurisdictions also maintain databases related to medication benefits provided to residents. An example of this is the Ontario Drug Benefits Database that records claims for prescriptions received under the Ontario Drug Benefit Program. This database contains information such as the age of the medication recipient, the medication dispensed, estimated days' supply of the medication, supplier information, cost, and so on. Provinces and territories also maintain data on fees paid directly from their health insurance plans. For example, in Ontario, the Ontario Ministry of Health and Long-Term Care maintains a database of all claims made by physicians, groups, and laboratories to the *Ontario Health Insurance Plan.*

Other sources of nursing information may exist in databases created explicitly for research purposes. For example, two nationally funded studies are currently underway to examine the nursing-related determinants of mortality and unplanned readmission for medical and surgical patients in acute care hospitals in Ontario. As part of this study, approximately 13,000 Ontario RNs and registered practical nurses (RPNs) are being surveyed to collect information about themselves, their work environments, their responses to work environments (e.g., burnout), their level of job satisfaction, and some important processes of care that cannot be found in current health system databases. A rich database of Ontario nurse and nursing information will be available to develop nursing knowledge. These data will be linked with other databases to investigate the determinants of patient mortality and unplanned readmission to hospital outcomes.

Outcomes of Interest to Nursing

A discussion of outcomes should start with clarification of what is meant by the term. The meaning of *outcomes* depends, in part, on to what or whom the outcome refers. For example, health-related outcomes might relate to any of the following: (a) patients who receive care, (b) organizations in which care is delivered, (c) groups of people (e.g., communities, regions) who receive care, (d) providers of care (e.g., nurses, physicians), or even (e) systems of health care. In this section, nursing care outcomes, health organization or system outcomes, and patient care outcomes are discussed. *The Canadian Oxford Dictionary* defines outcome as a result or a visible effect (Barber, 1998). In nursing practice, *patient outcomes* refer to the end results of care (Hegyvary, 1991; Jennings & Staggers, 1998) and include those measurable changes in patients' health status that reflect the response to a nursing (or other) intervention (Sidani & Braden, 1998). Here, *nurse outcomes* refer to the results or visible effects that being employed as a nurse has on nurses.

Nurse Outcomes

Nurse outcomes such as job satisfaction, burnout, violence or abuse, and intention to remain in one's job are of interest to nurses and the nursing profession, but they also interest other health system stakeholders, including health care administrators and other providers of health care (Aiken, Clarke, Sloane, Sochalski, & Silber, 2002; Clarke, Rockett, Sloane, & Aiken, 2002; Duncan, Estabrooks, & Reimer, 2000; Hesketh et al., 2003; Ingersoll, Olsan, Drew-Cates, DeVinney, & Davies, 2002; Lake, 1998; Langemo, Anderson, & Volden, 2002; Rafferty, Ball, & Aiken, 2001). There are multiple reasons for this interest in nurse outcomes.

First, there is increasing recognition of the importance of nurses and nursing care in the health of all communities. The outbreak of sudden acute respiratory syndrome (SARS) in 2003 heightened awareness of the importance of nurses and nursing care to the health of the population.

Second, there is some evidence that nurse outcomes are related to patient outcomes. Nurses' job satisfaction has been shown to influence patients' satisfaction with their care (Atkins, Marshall, & Javalgi, 1996; Kaldenberg & Regrut, 1999). Therefore, if an organization wants to improve patient satisfaction, it also needs to develop strategies aimed at improving the job satisfaction of nurses.

Third, nurse outcomes are related to organizational outcomes, such as employee retention. Nurse burnout and job dissatisfaction have been shown to be precursors of nurse turnover (Goodman & Boss, 1999; Lake, 1998). With the current and impending shortage of RNs in the Canadian health care system, health care employers and governments responsible for health care need to be concerned about nurse turnover and committed to implementing strategies to retain qualified RNs in their places of work. Health care organizations will continue to be in competition with each other to attract and retain competent and motivated nurses. Those organizations that facilitate desirable nurse outcomes will be better able to recruit and retain such nurses. Unfortunately, nurse outcome data are not routinely collected and stored in databases; therefore, available nurse outcome information is generally collected as part of specific research studies.

Organization and System Outcomes

Health care organizations and even health care systems are concerned with a variety of patient, employee, and financial status outcomes. Health care organizations and systems are also held accountable for the results of their efforts in producing the health-related outcomes desired by communities and societies. Traditionally, health care organizations and systems have focused on outcomes such as average length of patient stay, hospital-acquired infection rates, employee satisfaction, employee (including nurse) retention and turnover, overall patient satisfaction, mortality, and financial outcomes such as cost per patient stay. Health care organizations often summarize or "roll up" individual care recipient and employee outcomes to identify organization level outcomes. For example, though patient survival or death is an individual patient outcome, hospitals calculate death rates for all discharged patients or for various subgroups of patients receiving care in their organizations.

Patient Outcomes

It has become increasingly important that providers of health care, including nurses, gather evidence accounting for the resources used to deliver health care and the outcomes attained by this resource use. Nurses are becoming more interested in examining patient outcomes as part of their accountability obligations (Pringle & Doran, 2003). Examining patient outcomes with the inputs of health care, such as nursing care, is an important component in accountability activities. However, one of the challenges is to determine which patient outcomes should be considered as important to nursing. A growing number of nurse scholars are addressing this challenge. The range of answers varies depending on the patients or recipients of care being considered. Sidani and Braden (1998) identified four categories of outcomes that are of interest to nurse researchers:

- Clinical end points such as mortality and survival
- Functional status, encompassing physical, mental, and social functioning
- Perceptual outcomes related to well-being, life satisfaction, and satisfaction with care received
- Financial outcomes related to use of resources.

A group of Canadian nurse scientists have developed an outcome framework within their Nursing Role Effectiveness Model (Irvine, Sidani, & McGillis Hall, 1998). Groups of outcomes of interest for nursing were identified as functional status, self-care, symptom control, safety/adverse occurrences, and patent satisfaction.

Perhaps the most developed nursing sensitive outcome classification scheme has been developed by a group of scholars at the University of Iowa College of Nursing and is referred to as the *Nursing Outcome Classification (NOC)* (Johnson, Maas, & Moorhead, 2000). The NOC system consists of 260 outcome labels, each with definitions, measures, and indicators. Within the NOC, nursing-sensitive outcomes have been identified for individual patients, families, and communities. The 260 outcomes are grouped into seven domains: functional health, physiological health, psychological health, health knowledge and behaviour, perceived health, family health, and community health. It is important to note that financial outcomes are not included in the NOC as they reflect outcomes of importance to organizations rather than to recipients of care. Currently, nurses use the NOC in many health care organizations as a framework to document the results of patient care activities.

One of the most significant challenges related to understanding patient outcomes and their nurse-related causes or determinants is the lack of databases that routinely collect such nursing-sensitive outcome data. Pringle and Doran (2003) suggest that the next major breakthrough in outcomes investigation will be the establishment of databases that contain nursing-sensitive outcomes collected for all patients who receive nursing care. In fact, in 2002, Dr. Doran undertook leadership of a major project funded by the Ontario Ministry of Health and Long-Term Care to investigate the feasibility of instituting data collection of nursing-sensitive outcomes in all Ontario health care sectors, including acute care, long-term care, complex continuing care, and home care. The foundation of this project is built on the Nursing Role Effectiveness Model previously developed (Irvine et al., 1998). The results will guide the establishment of a permanent source of data that documents nursing-sensitive outcomes of care provided to recipients of nursing care within Ontario.

Because data reflecting the structures of nursing care (e.g., the amount, dose, or skill mix of nurse staffing) have been more accessible in health care databases by researchers, there is a growing body of literature about the effects of nurse staffing on patient outcomes. Examples of the patient outcomes studied include, among many others, medication errors, patient falls, cardiopulmonary arrests, pressure ulcers, pneumonia, urinary tract and other infections, intravenous complications (see Blegen, Goode, & Reed, 1998; Blegen & Vaughn, 1998; Heinemann, Lengacher, VanCott, Mabe, & Swymer, 1996; Krapohl & Larson, 1996; Lichtig, Knauf, & Milholland, 1999; Tourangeau et al., 1999; Wan & Shukla, 1987), patient satisfaction with nursing care (Aiken, Sloane, Lake, Sochalski, & Weber, 1999; Bostrom & Zimmerman, 1993; Heinemann et al., 1996), length of patient stay (Bryan et al., 1998; Czaplinski & Diers, 1998), and patient mortality (Aiken et al., 2002; Needleman, Buerhaus, Mattke, Stewart, & Zelevinsky, 2002; Tourangeau et al., 2002).

Leadership Implications

Current and future nurse leaders have a number of responsibilities related to developing and using nursing and health information. Perhaps one of the biggest challenges is to synthesize the research evidence that links the structures (e.g., nurse staffing and nurse characteristics) and processes (e.g., interventions) of nursing care with the outcomes of care at the patient and organizational levels. However, this alone is insufficient. Nurse leaders must communicate these links to nurses, other health care providers, health system administrators, and those who develop and establish health policy. At no time has this been more important as health care systems and their organizations struggle to contain costs while improving the quality and outcomes of health care services.

The body of knowledge that accounts for the impact of the structures and processes of nursing care on patient and organizational outcomes is rapidly expanding. Nurse leaders must use the information and knowledge created from the data to make decisions about best uses of scarce and expensive nursing resources in order to bring about the best possible patient and organizational outcomes. When there is lack of knowledge, or insufficient assimilation and dissemination of knowledge, health policy decisions may be made without objective consideration of the positive and negative impacts on patient and organizational outcomes.

However, developing and disseminating this knowledge has challenges and costs. The work and outcomes of nurses and nursing care must be made visible. Nurses, other health care providers, administrators, and those who establish policy must understand and appreciate the need to document nursing care plans, activities, and outcomes. Over the past decade, many health care organizations have sought solutions that allow for more allocation of nursing time to direct patient care. It is sometimes suggested that charting nursing care and patient care outcomes be done "by exception." The information structure and documentation contained in nursing assessments and care plans are often lost because these records are not retained. These common practices contribute to and perpetuate the difficulty in studying and improving nursing care and nursing-sensitive patient outcomes; therefore, all health system leaders need to advocate for improved documentation of nursing care in health records. Nursing leaders and expert clinical nurses need to participate actively in decisions about nursing information that should be permanently and continually recorded in health services databases.

Nurse leaders should also become familiar with current sources of health and nursing information within their organizations and health care systems so that they are better prepared to encourage and assist nurses in their accurate and timely data contributions to this information. When leaders are well informed about the various sources of health and nursing information, they can ask relevant questions and find answers in order to develop practical knowledge from these sources of information. For example, when planning and developing a new program led by a nurse practitioner to manage acute stroke patients during hospitalization and rehabilitation, the nurse leader would ask the health records department for a report about the number of such patients discharged over the past year, their average age, their average length of hospital stay, their survival or death rate, their frequency of discharge to particular locations, and so on. Nurse leaders can also access health information from other sources (e.g., the CIHI and provincial/territorial nurse licensing organizations) to assist in planning and making decisions.

Summary

- All nurses, regardless of their focus in clinical practice, research, education, or administration, have roles in developing and using nursing information, including patient outcomes.
- It has never been more important for nurses to develop and communicate knowledge of relationships between nursing and patient outcomes that is uncovered in nursing information.
- Data are discrete bits of information. When data are stored in an organized manner, they are referred to as information. Information that has been analyzed and synthesized becomes knowledge.
- The Canadian Institute for Health Information (CIHI), a national not-for-profit organization, has the largest holding of health-related databases in Canada. It primarily holds three categories of databases: health services, health professionals, and health expenditure. The CIHI not only collects and edits these data, but also analyzes and synthesizes them to produce health-related knowledge that is disseminated in its reports.
- Nursing information, particularly about nursing processes and outcomes of care, is not very visible in most health services databases. There is more information available in health professionals and expenditure databases about the supply of nurses, patterns of nurse staffing in health care organizations, and nurse characteristics.

- Outcomes may reflect end results for nurses, patients/recipients of care, organizations, and even systems of health care.
- One of the most highly developed patient outcome classification schemes is the Nursing Outcome Classification (NOC) developed by scholars at the University of Iowa College of Nursing.
- Nurse leaders have responsibilities related to developing, using, and communicating nursing information, including evidence of relationships between the structures and processes of nursing care and patient and organizational outcomes.

Applying the Knowledge in this Chapter

Exercise

1. Interview one nurse leader and one non-nurse leader within a health care organization. Ask them to share their perspectives about the value of nursing and patient outcome information. Ask these leaders whether they use this information and, if so, how they use this information. Compare responses from both leaders.

2. Log on to the Canadian Institute for Health Information Web site (www.cihi.ca). Search for current health care related reports. Review at least two reports to determine what health information was used to develop these reports. Search for information or knowledge about, and of interest to, nursing.

Resources

evolve Internet Resources

Canadian Institute for Health Information (CIHI):
  www.cihi.ca

University of Iowa College of Nursing:
  Nursing Intervention Classification (NIC)
  www.nursing.uiowa.edu/centers/cncce/nic/nicoverview.htm

  Nursing Outcome Classification (NOC)
  www.nursing.uiowa.edu/centers/cncce/noc/

International Council of Nurses (ICN):
  International Classification for Nursing Practice
  www.icn.ch/icnpupdate.htm

Canadian Nurses Association (CNA):
  National Nursing Informatics Project
  www.cna-nurses.ca/pages/resources/nni/nnicausn.htm

Further Reading

Doran, D.M. (Ed.). (2003). *Nursing-sensitive outcomes: State of the science*. Boston: Jones and Bartlett.

Canadian Institute for Health Information. (2002). *Privacy and confidentiality of health information at CIHI: Principles and policies for protection of personal health information and policies for institution-identifiable information*. Ottawa, ON: Author.

Canadian Institute for Health Information. (2003). *Canadian Institute for Health Information: Products and services catalogue*. Ottawa, ON: CIHI.

Harbeson, G. (2003). Meeting information challenges. In Springhouse Publishing (Ed.), *Five keys to successful nursing management* (pp. 456–488). Philadelphia: Lippincott Williams & Wilkins.

Kennedy, M.H. (2003). Supporting administrative decision making. In S.P. Englebardt & R. Nelson (Eds.), *Health care informatics* (pp. 81–113). St. Louis, MO: Mosby.

Morris, M. (2003). Managing the data. In Springhouse Publishing (Ed.), *Five keys to successful nursing management* (pp. 432–455). Philadelphia: Lippincott Williams & Wilkins.

Papers from the Nursing Minimum Data Set Conference: October 27-29, 1992. (1993). Ottawa, ON: Canadian Nurses Association.

Thede, L.Q. (2002). Understanding databases. In S.P. Englebardt & R. Nelson (Eds.), *Health care informatics* (pp. 55–80), St. Louis, MO: Mosby.

References

Aiken, L.H., Clarke, S.P., Sloane, D.M., Sochalski, J., & Silber, J.H. (2002). Hospital nurse staffing and patient mortality, nurse burnout, and job satisfaction. *Journal of the American Medical Association, 288*(16), 1987–1993.

Aiken, L.H., Sloane, D.M., Lake, E.T., Sochalski, J., & Weber, A.L. (1999). Organization and outcomes of inpatient AIDS care. *Medical Care, 37,* 760–772.

Aiken, L.H., Sochalski, J., & Anderson, G. (1996). Downsizing the hospital nursing workforce. *Health Affairs, 15*(4), 88–92.

Atkins, P.M., Marshall, B.S., & Javalgi, R.G. (1996). Happy employees lead to loyal patients. *Journal of Health Care Marketing, 16*(4), 15–23.

Barber, K. (Ed.). (1998). *The Canadian Oxford dictionary.* Toronto, ON: Oxford University Press.

Blegen, M.A., Goode, C.J., & Reed, L. (1998). Nurse staffing and patient outcomes. *Nursing Research, 47*(1), 43–50.

Blegen, M.A., & Vaughn, T. (1998). A multisite study of nurse staffing and patient occurrences. *Nursing Economics, 16,* 196–203.

Blum, B.I. (1986). *Clinical information systems.* New York: Springer-Verlag.

Bostrom, J., & Zimmerman, J. (1993). Restructuring nursing for a competitive health care environment. *Nursing Economics, 11*(1), 35-41, 54.

Bowles, K.H., & Naylor, M.D. (1996). Nursing intervention classification systems. *Image: Journal of Nursing Scholarship, 28,* 303–308.

Bryan, Y.E., Hitchings, K.S., Fuss, M.A., Fox, M.A., Kinneman, M.T., & Young, M.J. (1998). Measuring and evaluating hospital restructuring efforts: Eighteen month follow-up and extension to critical care. *Journal of Nursing Administration, 28*(9), 21–27.

Canadian Institute for Health Information. (2001). *Supply and distribution of registered nurses in Canada, 2001 report.* Ottawa, ON: Author.

Canadian Institute for Health Information. (2002). *Health care in Canada 2002.* Ottawa, ON: CIHI.

Canadian Institute for Health Information. (2003a). *Products and services catalogue.* Ottawa, ON: CIHI.

Canadian Institute for Health Information. (2003b). *Health care in Canada 2003.* Ottawa, ON: CIHI.

Clarke, S.P., Rockett, J.L., Sloane, D.M., & Aiken, L.H. (2002). Organizational climate, staffing, and safety equipment as predictors of needlestick injuries and near misses in hospital nurses. *American Journal of Infection Control, 30,* 207–216.

Czaplinski, C., & Diers, D. (1998). The effect of staff nursing on length of stay and mortality. *Medical Care, 36,* 1626–1638.

Duncan, S., Estabrooks, C.A., & Reimer, M. (2000). Violence against nurses. *Alberta Registered Nurse, 56*(2), 13–14.

Giovannetti, P., & O'Brien-Pallas, L. (1998). From nursing data to information to evidence: Are we prepared? *Canadian Journal of Nursing Research, 30*(1), 3–7.

Giovannetti, P., Smith, D.L., & Broad, E. (1999). Structuring and managing health information. In J.M. Hibberd & D.L. Smith (Eds.), *Nursing management in Canada* (2nd ed., pp. 297–318). Toronto, ON: Saunders.

Goodman, E.A., & Boss, R.W. (1999). Burnout dimensions and voluntary and involuntary turnover in a health care setting. *Journal of Health and Human Services Administration, 21,* 462–471.

Hegyvary, S.T. (1991). Issues in outcome research. *Journal of Nursing Quality Assurance, 5*(2), 1–6.

Heinemann, D., Lengacher, C.A., VanCott, M.L., Mabe, P., & Swymer, S. (1996). Partners in patient care: Measuring the effects on patient satisfaction and other quality indicators. *Nursing Economics, 14,* 276–285.

Henry, S. B., Holzemer, W.L., Randell, C., Hsieh, S., & Miller, T.J. (1997). Comparison of nursing interventions classification and current procedural terminology codes for categorizing nursing activities. *Image: Journal of Nursing Scholarship, 29,* 133–138.

Hesketh, K.L., Duncan, S.M., Estabrooks, C.A., Reimer, M.A., Giovannetti, P., Hyndman, K., & Acorn, S. (2003). Workplace violence in Alberta and British Columbia hospitals. *Health Policy, 63,* 311–321.

Ingersoll, G.L., Olsan, T., Drew-Cates, J., DeVinney, B., & Davies, J. (2002). Nurses' job satisfaction, organizational commitment, and career intent. *Journal of Nursing Administration, 32,* 250–263.

Irvine, D., Sidani, S., & McGillis Hall, L. (1998). Linking outcomes to nurses' role in health care. *Nursing Economics, 16*(2), 58-64, 87.

Jennings, B.M., & Staggers, N. (1998). The language of outcomes. *Advances in Nursing Science, 20*(4), 72–80.

Johnson, M., Maas, M.L., & Moorhead, S. (2000). *Nursing outcomes classification (NOC)* (2nd ed.). St. Louis, MO: Mosby.

Kaldenberg, D.O., & Regrut, B.A. (1999). Do satisfied patients depend on satisfied employees? Or, do satisfied employees depend on satisfied patients? *The Satisfaction Report Newsletter, 3,* 1–4.

Krapohl, G.L., & Larson, E. (1996). The impact of unlicensed assistive personnel on nursing care delivery. *Nursing Economics, 14,* 99-110, 122.

Lake, E.T. (1998). Advances in understanding and predicting nurse turnover. *Research in Sociology and Health Care, 15,* 147–171.

Langemo, D.K., Anderson, J., & Volden, C.M. (2002). Nursing quality outcome indicators: The North Dakota study. *Journal of Nursing Administration, 32*(2), 98–105.

Lichtig, L.K., Knauf, R.A., & Milholland, D.K. (1999). Some impacts of nursing on acute care hospital outcomes. *Journal of Nursing Administration, 29*(2), 25–33.

Maas, M.L., Johnson, M., & Moorhead S. (1996). Classifying nursing-sensitive patient outcomes. *Image: Journal of Nursing Scholarship, 28,* 295–301.

Mallette, C. (2003). Nursing minimum data sets. In D.M. Doran (Ed.), *Nursing-sensitive outcomes: State of the science* (pp. 319–353). Sudbury, MA: Jones and Bartlett.

Marek, K.D., & Lang, N.M. (1993). Nursing sensitive outcomes. In Canadian Nurses Association (Ed.), *Papers from the nursing minimum data set conference* (pp. 100–120). Ottawa, ON: The Canadian Nurses Association.

McCloskey, J.C., & Bulechek, G.M. (1993). Nursing intervention schemes. In Canadian Nurses Association (Ed.), *Papers from the nursing minimum data set conference* (pp. 77–91). Ottawa, ON: The Canadian Nurses Association.

Micek, W.T., Berry, L., Gilski, D., Kallenbach, A., Link, D., & Scharer, K. (1996). Patient outcomes: The link between nursing diagnoses and interventions. *Journal of Nursing Administration, 26*(11), 29–35.

Needleman, J., Buerhaus, P., Mattke, S., Stewart, M., & Zelevinsky, K. (2002). Nurse-staffing levels and the quality of care in hospitals. *The New England Journal of Medicine, 346*(22), 1715–1722.

Nielsen, G.H., & Mortensen, R.A. (1997). The architecture of ICNP: Time for outcomes—Part I. *International Nursing Review, 44,* 182-188, 176.

Nielsen, G.H., & Mortensen, R.A. (1998). The architecture of ICNP: Time for outcomes—Part II. *International Nursing Review, 45,* 27–31.

O'Brien-Pallas, L.L., & Giovannetti, P. (1993). Nursing intensity. In Canadian Nurses Association (Ed.), *Papers from the nursing minimum data set conference* (pp. 68–76). Ottawa, ON: The Canadian Nurses Association.

Pringle, D., & Doran, D. (2003). Patient outcomes as an accountability. In D. M. Doran (Ed.), *Nursing-sensitive outcomes: State of the science* (pp. 1–25). Sudbury, MA: Jones and Bartlett.

Rafferty, A.M., Ball, J., & Aiken, L.H. (2001). Are teamwork and professional autonomy compatible, and do they result in improved hospital care? *Quality in Health Care, 10*(Suppl), ii32–ii37.

Richards, J., Brown, A., & Homan, C. (2001). The data quality study of the Canadian discharge abstract database. *Proceedings of Statistics Canada Symposium 2001: Achieving data quality in a statistical agency.* Ottawa, ON: Canadian Institute for Health Information.

Sidani, S., & Braden, C.J. (1998). *Evaluating nursing interventions: A theory driven approach.* Thousand Oaks, CA: Sage.

Tourangeau, A.E. (2001). *The effects of nursing-related hospital factors on 30-day medical mortality.* Unpublished doctoral dissertation, University of Alberta, Edmonton, Alberta, Canada.

Tourangeau, A.E., Giovannetti, P., Tu, J.V., & Wood, M. (2002). Nursing-related determinants of 30-day mortality for hopitalized patients. *Canadian Journal of Nursing Research, 33*(4), 71–88.

Tourangeau, A.E., Stone, P.W., & Birnbaum, D. (2003). Hidden in plain view: The importance of professional nursing care. *Clinical Governance: An International Journal, 8,* 158–163.

Tourangeau, A.E., White, P., Scott, J., McAllister, M., & Giles, L. (1999). Evaluation of a partnership model of care delivery involving registered nurses and unlicensed assistive personnel. *Canadian Journal of Nursing Leadership, 12*(2), 4–20.

Wan, T.T., & Shukla, R.K. (1987). Contextual and organizational correlates of the quality of hospital nursing care. *Quality Review Bulletin, 13*(2), 61–64.

Werley, H.H. (1988). Introduction to the nursing minimum data set and its development. In H.H. Werley & N.M. Lang (Eds.), *Identification of the nursing minimum data set* (pp. 1–15). New York: Springer.

NURSING ADMINISTRATION RESEARCH

Heather K. Spence Laschinger

Learning Objectives

In this chapter, you will learn:

- The purpose and domain of nursing administration research
- The process of building evidence-based knowledge for nursing administration and leadership practice
- Current priorities in nursing administration research
- Uses and importance of theory in nursing administration research
- About Canadian nursing administration research
- About nursing involvement in health services research in Canada

Nursing administrators require a body of knowledge upon which to base their practice in today's rapidly changing health care organizations. The recent emphasis on evidenced-based practice in the clinical setting is equally important for nursing administration settings. In 2002, the Canadian Nurses Association (CNA), in a position statement on evidenced-based decision making and nursing practice, stated that "evidence-based decision-making is an important element of quality care in all domains of practice," including nursing administration (CNA, 2002, p. 1). Nursing administration or nursing systems research is the mechanism by which this evidence base for nursing administrative practice is produced. Until recently, however, there have been few systematic programs of nursing administration research targeted at building a cumulative body of knowledge in which to ground nursing administration practice. This chapter describes the purpose of nursing administration research and its evolution from a scattered collection of unrelated studies to the development of a more focused programmatic approach aimed at providing evidence for administrative decisions and policy making in today's ever-changing health care settings.

Purpose of Nursing Administration Research

In 1986, the American Organization of Nurse Executives (AONE) defined nursing administration research as the scientific inquiry of factors that influence the effective and efficient delivery of high quality nursing services. This involves investigating relationships among the structures, processes, and outcomes of nursing service delivery with an eye to discovering mechanisms for improving both patient care and nurse outcomes that can be translated into policies that affect the workplace.

With the broadening focus of nurse administrator roles over the past decade, this definition has expanded to include the wider perspective of health services research in general. This is logical given nursing's central role in the delivery of health services in all health care settings. Nurse administrators are responsible for large groups of nurses and ancillary workers and are accountable for managing large budgets to ensure the provision of high quality patient care at a reasonable cost. Health services research is concerned with cost, use, access, and quality issues and is inherently multidisciplinary in nature. Nursing researchers have only recently begun to get involved in health services research. However, there is a movement in the nursing research community to build capacity in this area (Bowman & Gardner, 2001).

The Domain of Nursing Administration Research

Research in nursing administration can be grouped into various topic areas, such as (a) nursing productivity, (b) nursing care quality, (c) work environment quality, (d) patient outcomes, and (e) studies examining interactions among these factors. *Nursing productivity* studies address issues relating to nursing care requirements and the resource allocation processes and costs associated with meeting these requirements. Evaluations of *nursing care quality* include assessments of the impact of nursing interventions on patient outcomes and patient satisfaction with nursing care. Studies of *nursing work environments* deal with factors that affect nurses' ability to accomplish their work in meaningful ways and that promote job satisfaction and organizational commitment. *Patient outcome* studies have become more prevalent over the past decade as part of an effort to encourage nursing to document its contribution to the health care process. Finally, studies that incorporate a variety of these factors into a multi-dimensional analysis are becoming the norm in current nursing administration research. Nurse researchers' entry into health services research has resulted in greater use of both primary data collection methods and analysis of administrative data to examine complex questions relating to nursing service delivery.

Building Evidenced-Based Knowledge for Nursing Administration Practice

Lynn and Layman (1996) have characterized much of nursing administration research as "fire-stomping or problem solving research" (p. 9), suggesting that rather than developing a body of accumulative knowledge on a substantive topic, researchers have typically responded to trendy topics of the day, jumping from topic to topic over time and never building knowledge that can guide future nursing administration practice. They advocate the development of research programs that address topics of concern to the discipline, topics that are studied systematically from a variety of perspectives by a group of researchers, thereby generating critical dialogue about the nature of the phenomenon and leading to new ideas.

Several approaches have been taken to creating an agenda for useful research in nursing administration. A consensus of several reviews in the late 1980s and the early 1990s was that nursing administration research tended to have an internal focus on nursing roles, although there was a trend in the 1990s of expanding the focus to include characteristics of the organizations in which these roles were enacted (Hermansdorfer, Henry, Moody, & Smyth, 1990; Ingersoll, Hoffart, & Schultz, 1990; McDaniel, 1990).

In a series of articles, Lynn and colleagues reviewed attempts to characterize areas of concern to nursing administration (Lynn & Layman, 1996; Lynn, Layman, & Englebardt, 1998; Lynn, Layman, & Richard, 1999). A variety of priority-setting initiatives have been conducted to identify priorities for nursing administration research, particularly in the United States. However, Lynn and Layman (1996) could find little evidence that published research reflected the contents of these priority lists when they tried to categorize over 133 published reports according to these priorities. Using a Delphi process, Lynn and colleagues (1998) generated a list of 44 nursing administration research priorities, categorized into four substantive conceptual domains: (a) outcomes (patient, organizational, practice), (b) financial concerns (costs of care and impact of financial constraint), (c) provider configuration/role issues, and (d) informatics. In a follow-up study, both researchers and the literature were surveyed to ascertain how ongoing research and published literature reflected these categories of priorities. The researchers who were surveyed identified activity in most of the 44 priority areas, but several important priorities were not listed: (a) nursing's contribution to hospital costs, (b) the impact of staffing levels on patient outcomes, and (c) optimizing health care system redesign to ensure patient care quality. Researchers emphasized outcome evaluations, database development, informatics, and evaluation of organizational change to a greater extent than staffing and work environment issues. The literature reflected similar foci. However, there were few literature citations relating to factors influencing nurses' decision making, such as the practice environment, work team, and information technology. The authors of this follow-up study noted that, contrary to the belief that funding for nursing administration research was not available, most of this research was funded and published in a timely manner. The authors emphasized the importance of building multidisciplinary research teams to address these priorities and the need to create a systematic body of knowledge that can inform approaches to solving problems concerning the discipline in the future (Lynn et al., 1999).

Current Priorities in Nursing Administration Research

Nursing administration research priorities at the turn of the 21st century reflect the dramatic changes that have occurred in health care systems in the 1990s and the demographic factors that exacerbate problems associated with these changes. These priorities reflect the dynamic interplay between social factors in the external environment and intellectual efforts to find a solution to these problems (Ingersoll et al., 1990). With hospitals downsizing in the face of financial constraints, fewer nurses are available to care for patients who are much sicker than patient populations prior to restructuring. This situation led to concerns about patient care quality and patient safety. At the same time, the aging of the nursing workforce and the decline in new recruits to the profession have resulted in a nursing shortage crisis, making recruitment and retention a major priority. These themes are reflected in the four priorities put forward by the AONE in 2003: (a) work environment and workforce, (b) patient care advocacy, (c) technology, and (d) patient safety (Ritter-Teitel, 2003).

Theory Development and Testing in Nursing Administration Research

Until recently, much of nursing administration research has been atheoretical. Researchers focused on describing phenomena of interest, for instance, job satisfaction. When relationships among variables were examined, they were usually based on implicit hunches rather than explicit theory. Few studies reported in the literature had explicit theoretical frameworks that guided the research questions under investigation. Although many studies examined the same variables or concepts, the lack of an explicit theoretical framework for these variables resulted in different modes of operationalization, making comparisons across studies difficult. Moreover, the lack of specified relationships among variables, based on sound reasoning within a logical nomological network of concepts, made it difficult for researchers to replicate results and build coherent explanations of phenomena. Thus, the process of building theory for nursing administration was hampered by a lack of articulation of logical relationships among concepts to explain nursing administration phenomena of interest, and by a lack of cumulative empirical results that could form the basis for theoretical explanations of these phenomena. This, in turn, denied nurse administrators a source of empirically supported and theory-driven interventions.

The Iowa Model

However, there have been attempts to develop conceptual models of the nursing administration domain. Researchers at the University of Iowa School of Nursing proposed a conceptual model of nursing administration intended to serve as a framework for building theory for nursing administration practice (Johnson, Gardner, Kelly, Maas, & McCloskey, 1991). The model delineates important variables of concern to nursing administration practice and suggests relationships among these variables. The authors suggest that this model provides a guide to action/decision making for nursing administrators and for framing research questions to explain nursing administration phenomena. They argue that the model provides a useful way of developing evidence-based knowledge for nursing administration practice, addressing the lack of a systematized body of knowledge in the science of nursing administration (Malasanos & Dougherty, 1989).

The Iowa Model posits two major clusters of variables that interact to influence nursing administration practice: systems and outcomes. Each of these consists of three levels of concern: patient aggregates, organization, and health administration system. Within each level, the model identifies concepts important to nursing administration. The authors suggest that relationships exist among the elements of the model and among the levels within each of the systems and outcomes variable clusters. For instance, systems factors, such as structure, process, controls, and resources, have an influence on outcomes factors, such as quality, costs, and systems performance. As an open system model, the impact of the external environment on these variables is an important aspect of the model.

While the Iowa model is potentially useful as a structure for organizing a comprehensive body of knowledge for nursing administration, it is probably too broad and ill-defined to provide specific knowledge in definitive areas that can be used to guide nursing administration practice. What are needed are more mid-range theories that can be tested in programs of research over time to evolve a substantive body of evidence that can be used for nursing administration decision making. This approach has been adopted by a variety of nursing administration researchers with some success.

Mid-Range Theories and Programs of Research

Several nursing administration scholars have selected a specific area of concern to nursing administration practice and have either developed their own theoretical explanations of the phenomena or have tested established theories from the nursing or organizational literature. For instance, in her program of research, Alexander studies nursing work environments from a contingency theory perspective (Alexander & Bauerschmidt, 1987; Alexander & Kroposki, 2001). Laschinger and colleagues have tested Kanter's (1993) theory of structural power in organizations in a series of studies of nursing work environments (Laschinger, 1996; Laschinger, Finegan, Shamian, & Wilk, 2001). McDaniel (1990) has examined nursing leadership from the perspective of Bass' (1998) transformational leadership theory, and McNeese-Smith (1995, 1999) has tested Kouzes and Posner's (1995) leadership theory in nursing settings.

The advantage of using well-established theories to test propositions about nursing administration phenomena of interest is that these theories are usually well thought out, with clearly articulated descriptions of constructs and relationships among these constructs. There is usually empirical support for the proposed relationships within the theory that is obtained from studies within systematic programs of research. When hypotheses derived from these theories are empirically supported across multiple studies, strategies suggested by the theory can be justifiably employed as theory-driven solutions to organizational problems.

Many organizational solutions advocated by management consultants have never been empirically tested. Adoption of these untested models can be a risky and costly decision for organizations; therefore, it is also important to test theories developed in other disciplines for their applicability to nursing and health care settings. While there may be empirical support for the theory in a business setting, it is possible that the proposed relationships will not hold in health care settings. There are many examples of inappropriate applications of industrial models to health care settings that may have been avoided by prior testing. Researchers in nursing administration can make a major contribution to theory-driven, evidence-based nursing administration practice by establishing programs of research designed to test promising theoretical explanations of nursing administration phenomena.

Other nursing researchers have developed their own conceptual models as frameworks for studying nursing administration problems. These models have served as the framework for programs of research to build a body of knowledge about specific aspects of nursing administration practice. The Iowa Model of nursing administration described earlier is one such example.

Magnet Hospitals Model

Another model that has received considerable attention in the literature over the past decade is the "magnet hospitals" model, originally developed by researchers sponsored by the American Nurses Association in an effort to describe hospitals that were able to attract and retain nurses even in times of fiscal restraint (McClure, Poulin, Sovie, & Wandelt, 1983). Kramer and her colleagues conducted further research with this model (Kramer, 1990; Kramer & Hafner, 1989; Kramer & Schmalenberg, 1988).

Since 1994, Aiken and her colleagues at University of Pennsylvania have used the magnet hospitals model to describe aspects of nursing work environments that result in positive nurse and patient outcomes. The results of several studies have shown that magnet hospitals characteristically have higher levels of autonomy, control over the practice environment, and good nurse-physician relationships. Aiken, Sochalski, and Lake (1997) argue that this model is an important attempt to open the "black box" of health services research by examining the intermediate processes that influence how structural conditions affect provider and patient outcomes. The results of this research have shown that magnet hospitals have lower patient mortality rates and lower nurse burnout levels than non-magnet hospitals (Aiken, Smith, & Lake, 1994). The model provides direction for administrators interested in creating positive work environments that attract and retain nurses and ensure positive patient outcomes.

Canadian Nursing Administration Research

In Canada, nurse researchers in the Nursing Effectiveness and Utilization Research Unit (NEURU) at the University of Toronto and McMaster University have made major contributions to the development of a systematic knowledge base for nursing administration. O'Brien-Pallas (1994) has built a program of research around her Client Care Delivery Model. The model evolved from a focus on nursing workload measurement in the 1980s to a more comprehensive model of the multivariate nature of patient care delivery systems. O'Brien-Pallas and her colleagues have conducted a series of studies designed to establish empirical links between constructs in the model (Irvine et al., 2000; O'Brien-Pallas, Doran, et al., 2001a, 2001b).

More recently, the NEURU has focused more intensively on human resource planning in response to the impending nursing shortage in Canada. This work is guided by a theoretical model of health human resources planning developed by NEURU scholars (Birch, O'Brien-Pallas, Alksnis, Murphy, & Thomson, 2003; O'Brien-Pallas & Baumann, 2000; O'Brien-Pallas, Baumann, et al., 2001), and there are currently several studies underway to test this model (Holgate et al., 2001; Murphy et al., 2000).

The Nursing Role Effectiveness Model (NREM) developed by Irvine, Sidani, and McGillis Hall (1998) is an example of a nursing theoretical model intended to explain how nurses' execution of their roles impacts patient outcomes. This theoretical model addresses the critical need to empirically demonstrate the effect of nursing interventions on patient outcomes. Nurses' role enactment is conceptualized as the mediating process through which workplace structures affect patient outcomes. This model has been tested in actual nursing settings, resulting in empirical support for propositions derived from the model. Sidani and Irvine (1999) used the NREM to develop a conceptual framework to guide their evaluation of the acute care nurse practitioner role. Others evaluated the model in a tertiary care hospital and found that it provided a well-defined conceptual framework to guide the evaluation of outcomes of nursing care (Doran, Sidani, Keatings, & Doidge, 2002). The NREM has also been used to link nurse staffing levels to patient outcomes with significant results (McGillis Hall et al., 2003). McGillis Hall and Doran (2003) examined the linkages between nurse staffing and care delivery models in relation to patient care quality. Finally, the model was also used to evaluate the feasibility of collecting nurse-sensitive outcomes in different health care sectors (Doran et al., 2004).

At the University of Western Ontario, the Workplace Empowerment Research Program, led by Dr. Heather Laschinger, has conducted numerous studies over the past decade that have contributed a substantial body of knowledge supporting the usefulness of Kanter's organizational empowerment theory as a model for creating healthy work environments in nursing settings (Laschinger, 1996). Over 40 studies, by both faculty and graduate students, designed to systematically test Kanter's theory within a variety of nursing populations have produced evidence to support the claim that when work environments provide employees access to information, resources, support, and opportunities to learn and grow, they are more motivated and committed to the organization, more satisfied with their job, and more effective at work.

The results of this body of work have consistently linked nurses' perceptions of empowerment to numerous organizational outcomes that are important to nurse retention and recruitment, such as job satisfaction (Laschinger, Finegan, & Shamian, 2001; Manojlovich, & Laschinger, 2002), organizational commitment (Laschinger et al., 2001; Laschinger, Finegan, Shamian, & Casier, 2000; McDermott, Laschinger, & Shamian, 1996), and autonomy or control over practice (Laschinger, Almost, & Tuer-Hodes, 2003; Laschinger & Havens, 1996; Sabiston & Laschinger, 1995). Publications of this body of knowledge have stimulated numerous replication studies in nursing and health care populations in other parts of the world and in non-health care settings. The cumulative results of this research provide strong evidence for the value of creating working conditions that incorporate the empowerment structures described in Kanter's theory in the effort to create satisfying healthy work environments for nurses.

Other researchers across Canada have conducted research relevant to nursing administration practice. These researchers have used various theoretical frameworks to study a variety of nursing administration phenomena, such as Hackman and Oldham's Work Redesign Model (1975), Karasek's Demand-Control Model (1979), and Siegrist's Effort-Reward Imbalance Theory (1996). At the University of Alberta, Professor Donna Lynn Smith has developed a conceptual model to advance research and develop research capacity to examine continuity of care as a health services and nursing outcome, and Dr. Greta Cummings has initiated a program of research focused on nursing leadership variables and impact.

These programs of research are situated in graduate programs in nursing administration and provide graduate students with opportunities to contribute to the development of systematic knowledge for nursing administration. Graduate student involvement in ongoing investigations of phenomena of interest to nursing administration allows them to contribute to a growing body of evidence for theories pertinent to nursing administration practice. Students work with faculty to develop studies that test these theories in an area of interest to them. They are encouraged to build on previous work and to critically challenge tenets of these theories in dialogue with peers and faculty researchers. A positive outcome of this process is that students learn how systematic knowledge is built through research, building on previous work and seeing where their own work fits within the larger body of knowledge generated by others in the research program. Another advantage is that students become aware of how results of this research can be used to implement theory-driven, evidence-based strategies in their own workplaces upon beginning or returning to work. Thus, students' knowledge of the theory-practice-research cycle is reinforced.

Current Priorities in Nursing Administration Research

Building a body of knowledge for nursing administration is dependent on the existence of a cadre of researchers and scholars who work together to develop this knowledge. The logical home for these scholars is the university setting, in graduate programs in nursing administration and/or health services delivery.

Until the late 1960s and 1970s, most graduate programs in nursing offered a major in nursing administration. However, in the 1960s, there was a move in the discipline to emphasize the preparation of nurses with advanced clinical practice expertise. This change was brought on by the recognition that nursing lacked a strong substantive base for clinical practice, and thus, there was a perceived need to focus on the development of a clinical nursing knowledge base. Unfortunately, this change in emphasis was accompanied by the closure or dramatic reduction of programs of nursing administration in both the US and Canada. A consequence of this change in focus was a decline in both the number of nursing systems researchers and the number of graduate students entering the field of nursing administration. This change in emphasis coincided with a reduction in available funding for nursing systems research. With fewer researchers conducting studies to address important problems in nursing administration, the knowledge base for nursing services delivery was weakened. Furthermore, the cadre of nursing systems researchers was severely curtailed as there were fewer graduates from graduate programs of nursing administration. Thus, the field was deprived of fresh ideas that could be used to understand the complexities of the demands inherent in the dramatically changed health care systems of the 1980s and 1990s.

Nursing Involvement in Health Services Research

In response to dramatic changes in health care delivery systems that resulted from massive restructuring initiatives in the 1990s, the need for nursing systems research has become apparent. In light of the prominent role played by nursing in the production of high quality care in health care settings, many recognized the importance of having nursing input and/or leadership in studies of health services delivery. Early health services research had focused on costs and regional variations in hospital utilization patterns with little involvement of nurse researchers. However, when cost and quality of health care delivery, and more recently, patient safety, became a prime focus of health services research, the importance of nurse researchers' involvement in study teams became obvious. Lack of nursing involvement in health services research often meant that key variables were omitted from investigations of health services delivery models, often limiting the credibility of the results for policy development. However, to optimize their contribution, nurse researchers needed to develop their knowledge of health services research skills and techniques. Graduate programs in nursing administration have slowly begun to reappear and have added course work in quality management, costing, and program evaluation. Funding bodies have begun to support health services and systems research; for example, centres funded by the federal government, such as the Canadian Health Services Research Foundation (CHSRF) Training Centres, have been established across the country to build capacity in health services research methods. Fellowships are available to support nurse researcher's involvement in these programs. (See Internet Resources at the end of the chapter for more information.)

Leadership Implications

These efforts are encouraging signs for the development of a sound body of knowledge to guide nursing administrative practice. Nursing leadership roles have dramatically changed as a result of health care restructuring, and nurse leaders now carry widely expanded roles that require knowledge of system-wide structures and processes and the skills to manage the problems that arise in these complex systems. To optimize their ability to accomplish their work goals, they must be able to draw upon a solid body of up-to-date, research-based evidence. Programs of nursing administration research are the foundation for creating a systematic body of evidence in which to ground nursing administration practice in today's chaotic health care environments.

Summary

- The purpose of nursing administration research is to investigate relationships among the structures, processes, and outcomes of nursing service delivery with an eye to discovering mechanisms for improving both patient care and nurse outcomes that can be translated into policies that affect the workplace.
- The domain of nursing administration research encompasses the areas of nursing productivity, nursing care quality, work environment quality, patient outcomes, and the interaction among these areas.
- Current priorities in nursing services research are considered to be in the following four areas: nurses' work environment and workforce, patient care advocacy, technology, and patient safety.
- Ongoing issues include theory development and testing in nursing administration research, building and strengthening the cadre of current and future nursing systems researchers, and supporting the involvement of nurses in interdisciplinary health services research.

Applying the Knowledge in this Chapter

Exercise

1. Review the topic areas in The Domain of Nursing Administration Research discussed on page 482. Write a research question for each topic area.

2. Select an article from a journal that publishes research on nursing leadership and administration. Answer these questions about the article:
   a) Is the study part of a program of research?
   b) What is the theoretical perspective of the research?
   c) Is the organizational context of the research described?
   d) How does the study relate to previous research?
   e) What are the variables? Do they fit with the theoretical framework?
   f) What methodological approach is used?
   g) Is there an intervention in the study? If so, what is it?
   h) Do the results support hypotheses derived from the theoretical framework?
   i) Do the results add to an existing body of knowledge on the topic? Do they expand understanding of the topic under study?
   j) Are the results of the study transferable or generalizable? Why or why not?
   k) What were the strengths of the study? How could the study have been improved?
   l) Were there any innovative aspects of the study?

Resources

𝑒𝑣𝑜𝑙𝑣𝑒 Internet Resources

Canadian Health Services Research Foundation (CHSRF):

www.chsrf.ca/

The CHSRF funds management and policy research in health services and nursing, supports the synthesis and dissemination of research results, and supports the use of research results by managers and policy makers in the health system.

Canadian Institute of Health Research (CIHR):

www.cihr-irsc.gc.ca/index.shtml

The CIHR is a federal agency for health research. Its objective is to excel, according to internationally accepted standards of scientific excellence, in the creation of new knowledge and its translation into improved health for Canadians, more effective health services and products, and a strengthened health care system.

Canadian Policy Research Networks Inc. (CPRN):

www.cprn.org

CPRN's mission is to create knowledge and lead public debate on social and economic issues important to the well-being of Canadians. Its research is organized under four networks—Family, Work, Health, and Public Involvement.

CHSRF/CIHR Regional Training Centres:

www.chsrf.ca/cadre/regional_training_centres_e.php

These centres are designed to increase the number of well-qualified applied health services and nursing researchers. Emphasis is placed on the creation of opportunities to share issues and ideas through placements with decision-making organizations. These placements also ensure that awareness and understanding of decision makers' concerns are included in the training experience. There are four Regional Training Centres (Western, Ontario, Atlantic, and FERASI in Quebec) and one National Centre for Knowledge Transfer.

CHSRF National Chair in Nursing Health Human Resources:

www.hhr.utoronto.ca/

Dr. Linda O'Brien-Pallas is the National Chair in Nursing Health Human Resources.

Institute of Medicine (IOM):

www.iom.edu/

The IOM provides science-based advice about issues of medicine and public health. It was chartered in 1970 as a component of the National Academy of Sciences. The IOM provides a vital service by working outside the framework of government to ensure scientifically informed analysis and independent guidance.

McMaster University Site:

www.fhs.mcmaster.ca/nru/

The NEURU is a collaborative project of the University of Toronto, Faculty of Nursing and McMaster University, School of Nursing. The Unit consists of Co-Principal Investigators, Dr. Linda O'Brien-Pallas at the Toronto site and Dr. Andrea Baumann at McMaster site, along with 46 co-investigators and more than 50 researchers. The NRU has been recognized internationally, nationally, and provincially for its comprehensive team approach to problem identification and resolution.

Nursing Effectiveness Utilization and Outcomes Research Unit (NEURU):

University of Toronto Site :

www.nursing.utoronto.ca/research/units/nru.aspx

Office of Nursing Policy (ONP):

www.hc-sc.gc.ca/onp-bpsi/

Health Canada's ONP was established by the Minister of Health in 1999 to provide evidence-based nursing perspectives on a wide range of policy issues and contribute to health policy and program development. The creation of ONP signaled that nursing and nurses' perspectives would be influential in shaping the future of health care in Canada because optimal nursing care means improved health care and healthier Canadians.

The Change Foundation:

    www.changefoundation.com/

    The Change Foundation brings together researchers, health care providers, health care managers, and policy makers in Ontario and around the world to understand the impact of change on the health of consumers and the delivery of health care services. Together with its stakeholders, the Foundation is researching, creating, innovating, and networking at the forefront of trends and change in health and health care delivery.

Further Reading

Journals Publishing Nursing Administration/Nursing Services Research

Canadian Journal of Nursing Leadership
Journal of Nursing Administration
Journal of Nursing Care Quality
Nursing Administration Quarterly
Nursing Economics

Health Services Research Journals

Health Care Management Review
Health Services Research
Medical Care

References

Aiken, L.H., Smith, H.L. & Lake, E.T. (1994). Lower medicare mortality among a set of hospitals known for good nursing care. *Medical Care, 32,* 771–787.

Aiken, L.H., Sochalski, J., & Lake, E.T. (1997). Studying outcomes of organizational change in health services. *Medical Care, 35*(11), NS6–NS18.

Alexander, J.W., & Bauerschmidt, A.D. (1987). Implications for nursing administration of the relationship of technology and structure to quality of care. *Nursing Administration Quarterly, 11*(4), 1–10.

Alexander, J.W., & Kroposki, M. (2001). Using a management perspective to define and measure changes in nursing technology. *Journal of Advanced Nursing, 35,* 776–783

Bass, B.M. (1998). *Transformational leadership: Industrial, military, and educational impact.* Mahwah, NJ: Lawrence Erlbaum Associates.

Birch, S., O'Brien-Pallas, L.L., Alksnis, C., Murphy, G.T., & Thomson, D. (2003). Beyond demographic change in human resources planning: An extended framework and application to nursing. *Journal of Health Services Research and Policy, 8,* 225–229.

Bowman, C.C., & Gardner, D. (2001). Building health services research capacity in nursing: Views from members of nursing's leadership. *Nursing Outlook, 49,* 187–192.

Canadian Nurses Association. (2002). *CNA position statement: Evidence-based decision-making and nursing practice.* Ottawa, ON: CNA.

Doran, D., Harrison, M., Laschinger, H.K.S., Hirdes, J., Rukholm, E., Sidani, S., et al. (2004). *An evaluation of the feasibility of instituting data collection of nursing sensitive outcomes in acute care, long-term care, complex continuing care and home care.* Toronto, ON: Ministry of Health and Long Term Care.

Doran, D., Sidani, S., Keatings, M., & Doidge, D. (2002). An empirical test of the Nursing Role Effectiveness Model. *Journal of Advanced Nursing, 38*(1), 29–39.

Hackman, J.R., & Oldham, G.R. (1975). Development of the Job Diagnostic Survey. *Journal of Applied Psychology, 60,* 159–170.

Hermansdorfer, P., Henry, B., Moody, L., & Smyth, K. (1990). Analysis of nursing administration research, 1976–1986. *Western Journal of Nursing Research, 12,* 546–557.

Holgate, V., Jeans, M.E., Marshall, S., McPherson, D., Osted, A., & Sholzberg-Gray, S. (2001). *Building the future: An integrated strategy for nursing human resources in Canada.* Funded by Human Resources Development Canada. Retrieved March 3, 2004, from http://www.buildingthefuture.ca/

Ingersoll, G.L., Hoffart, N., & Schultz, A.W. (1990). Health services research in nursing: Current status and future directions. *Nursing Economics, 8,* 229–238.

Irvine, D., O'Brien-Pallas, L.L., Murray, M., Cockerill, R., Sidani, S., Laurie-Shaw, B., & Lochhaas-Gerlach, J. (2000). The reliability and validity of two health status measures for evaluating outcomes of home care nursing. *Research in Nursing & Health, 23*(1), 43–54.

Irvine, D., Sidani, S., & McGillis Hall, L. (1998). Linking outcomes to nurses' roles in health care. *Nursing Economics, 16,* 58–64, 87.

Johnson, M., Gardner, D., Kelly, K., Maas, M., & McCloskey, J.C. (1991). The Iowa Model: A proposed model for nursing administration. *Nursing Economics, 9,* 255–262.

Kanter, R.M. 1993. *Mean and women of the corporation* (2nd ed.). New York: Basic Books.

Karasek, R.A. (1979). Job demands, job decision latitude and mental strain: Implications for job redesign. *Administrative Science Quarterly, 24,* 285–306.

Kouzes, J.M., & Posner, B.Z. (1995). *The leadership challenge: How to get extraordinary things done in organizations.* San Francisco, CA: Jossey-Bass.

Kramer, M. (1990). The magnet hospitals: Excellence revisited. *Journal of Nursing Administration, 20*(9), 35–44.

Kramer, M., & Hafner, L.P. (1989). Shared values: Impact on staff nurse job satisfaction and perceived productivity. *Nursing Research, 38,* 172–177.

Kramer, M., & Schmalenberg, C. (1988). Magnet hospitals. Part 1. Institutions of excellence. *Journal of Nursing Administration, 18*(1), 13–24.

Laschinger, H.K.S. (1996). A theoretical approach to studying work empowerment in nursing: A review of studies testing Kanter's theory of structural power in organizations. *Nursing Administration Quarterly, 20*(2), 25–41.

Laschinger, H.K.S., Almost, J., & Tuer-Hodes, D. (2003). Workplace empowerment and magnet hospital characteristics: Making the link. *Journal of Nursing Administration, 33*(7/8), 410–422.

Laschinger, H.K.S., Finegan, J., & Shamian, J. (2001). The impact of workplace empowerment and organizational trust on staff nurses' work satisfaction and organizational commitment. *Health Care Management Review, 26*(3), 7–23.

Laschinger, H.K.S., Finegan, J., Shamian, J., & Casier, S. (2000). Organizational trust and empowerment in restructured health care settings: Effects on staff nurse commitment. *Journal of Nursing Administration, 30,* 413–425.

Laschinger, H.K.S., Finegan, J., Shamian, J., & Wilk, P. (2001). Impact of structural and psychological empowerment on job strain in nursing work settings: Expanding Kanter's Model. *Journal of Nursing Administration, 31,* 260–272.

Laschinger, H.K.S., & Havens, D. (1996). Staff nurse work empowerment and perceived control over nursing practice. Conditions for work effectiveness. *Journal of Nursing Administration, 26*(9), 27–35.

Lynn, M.R., & Layman, E.L. (1996). Research priorities. The nature of nursing administration research: Knowledge building or fire stomping? *Journal of Nursing Administration, 26*(5), 9–14.

Lynn, M.R., Layman, E.L., & Englebardt, S.P. (1998). Research priorities. Nursing administration research priorities a national Delphi study. *Journal of Nursing Administration, 28*(5), 7–11.

Lynn, M.R., Layman, E.L., & Richard, S. (1999). Research priorities. The final chapter in the nursing administration research priorities sage: The state of the state. *Journal of Nursing Administration, 29*(5), 5-9, 20.

Malasanos, L., & Dougherty, M. (1989). Foreword. In B. Henry, C. Arndt, M. DiVincenti, & A. Marriner-Tomey (Eds.), *Dimensions of nursing administration* (pp. xiii–xiv). Boston, MA: Blackwell Scientific Publications.

Manojlovich, M., & Laschinger, H.K.S. (2002). The relationship of empowerment and selected personality characteristics to nursing job satisfaction. *Journal of Nursing Administration, 32*, 586–595.

McClure, M.M., Poulin, M.A., Sovie, M.D., & Wandelt, M.A. (1983). *Magnet hospitals: Attraction and retention of professional nurses*. Kansas City, MS: American Nurses Association.

McDaniel, C. (1990). Nursing administration research as a paradigm reflection. *Nursing and Health Care, 11*, 191–193.

McDermott, K., Laschinger, H.K.S., & Shamian, J. (1996). Work empowerment and organizational commitment. *Nursing Management, 27*(5), 44–48.

McGillis Hall, L., & Doran, D. (2003). Nurse staffing, care delivery model and patient care quality. *Journal of Nursing Care Quality, 19*(1), 27–33.

McGillis Hall, L., Doran, D., Baker, R. Pink, G., Sidani, S., O'Brien-Pallas, L., & Donner, G. (2003). Nurse staffing models as predictors of patient outcomes. *Medical Care, 41*, 1096–1109.

McNeese-Smith, D.K. (1995). Job satisfaction, productivity and organizational commitment: The result of leadership. *Journal of Nursing Administration, 25*(9), 17–26.

McNeese-Smith, D.K. (1999). The relationship between managerial motivation, leadership, nurse outcomes and patient satisfaction. *Journal of Organizational Behavior, 20*, 243–259.

Murphy, G.T., O'Brien-Pallas, L.L., Alksnis, C., Birch, S., Darlington, G., Kephart, G., et al. (2000). *Health human resource planning: An examination of relationships among the use of nurses and population health in the province of Ontario*. Project RC1-0618-06. Funded by Canadian Health Services Research Foundation.

O'Brien-Pallas, L. (1994). *Skill-mix in nursing*. Paper presented at the Annual Meeting of Ontario Chief Nursing Executives, Toronto, Ontario, Canada.

O'Brien-Pallas, L., & Baumann, A. (2000). Toward evidence-based policy decisions: a case study of nursing health human resources in Ontario, Canada *Nursing Inquiry, 7*, 248–257.

O'Brien-Pallas, L., Baumann, A., Donner, G., Murphy, G.T., Lochhaas-Gerlach, J., & Luba, M. (2001). Forecasting models for human resources in health care. *Journal of Advanced Nursing, 33*(1), 120–129.

O'Brien-Pallas, L., Doran, D.I., Murray, M., Cockerill, R., Sidani, S., Laurie-Shaw, B., & Lochhaas-Gerlach, J. (2001a). Evaluation of a client care delivery model, part 1: Variability in nursing utilization in community home nursing. *Nursing Economics, 19*, 267–276.

O'Brien-Pallas, L., Doran, D.I., Murray, M., Cockerill, R., Sidani, S., Laurie-Shaw, B., & Lochhaas-Gerlach, J. (2001b). Evaluation of a client care delivery model, part 2: Variability in nursing utilization in community home nursing. *Nursing Economics, 20*(1), 13–36.

Ritter-Teitel, J. (2003). Nursing administrative research: the underpinning of decisive leadership. *Journal of Nursing Administration, 33*, 257–259.

Sabiston, J.A., & Laschinger, H.K.S. (1995). Staff nurse work empowerment and perceived autonomy: Testing Kanter's theory of structural power in organizations. *Journal of Nursing Administration, 25*(9), 42–50.

Sidani, S., & Irvine, D. (1999). A conceptual framework for evaluating the nurse practitioner role in acute care settings. *Journal of Advanced Nursing, 30*(1), 58–66.

Siegrist, J. (1996). Adverse health effects of high effort–low reward conditions at work. *Journal of Occupational Health Psychology, 1*, 27–43.

LEADERSHIP CHALLENGES AND DIRECTIONS

Ginette Lemire Rodger

Learning Objectives

In this chapter, you will learn:

- The evolution of the concept of leadership

- Characteristics of the nursing workplace in the 21st century

- Common characteristics of effective contemporary leaders

- The changing nature of formal nursing leadership in health care agencies

- How leadership skills may be exercised at the clinical level within health care agencies

- The challenges that nurse managers will face in developing new forms of leadership

Leadership has become the major theme of nursing conferences and organizational redesign in health care and therefore of key relevance for the management of nursing services. The theme of leadership has replaced the theme of political action, which was the priority of the late 1990s and early 2000s, as the most pressing issue requiring concerted action by the nursing profession. As the health care system is in a constant re-engineering mode, trying to meet the challenges of finite resources, political choices, and the transition to a new era, leadership has become a central concept for nurse managers. Leadership is critical for shaping this emerging era into one that pursues the ultimate goal of health for all people.

In discussing the topic of leadership challenges and directions, this chapter starts with a short review of the evolution of the concept of leadership, followed by a description of the social and organizational changes created by the transition from the industrial age to the information age. Next, the focus is on new forms of leadership at the individual, organizational, and global levels. The last section of the chapter highlights the challenges faced by nurse managers and the nursing profession in moving in the desired directions toward the future.

Evolution of the Concept of Leadership

"Leadership is one of the world's most sought-after and valued skills. It sets certain individuals apart, signaling to the world that they have the 'edge' over others" (Leatt & Porter, 2003, p. 15). What is leadership and what makes a successful leader? These questions have been studied throughout the ages. At a time when society as a whole is undergoing transition to the information age, or new era, the concept of leadership is under intense scrutiny because leadership is central to the creation of the new reality. The literature on this topic and its many definitions is abundant.

In this chapter, leadership means the process of influencing and persuading a group in its activities and efforts toward goal setting and goal achievement (Bass & Stogdill, 1990; Stogdill, 1950). Other definitions are a variation on the same theme. For example, Drucker (1996), who has studied this phenomenon for 50 years, describes leaders as guided by the goal or mission, influencing the process and relationships with the followers in a joint venture. Most definitions of leadership include three elements, namely, influence, group, and goal. "First, leadership is viewed as a process of influence whereby the leader has an impact on others by inducing them to behave in a certain way [i.e., to achieve some task or goal]. Second, that influence process is conceptualised as taking place in a group context. Group members are invariably taken to be the leader's subordinates and hence the person for whom the leader has some responsibility" (Bryman, 1996, p. 276).

Bryman (1996) reviewed the scholarly work of social scientists and psychologists and concluded that these fields of study lacked an agreed upon conceptual framework and that leadership research and theory have been trivial and contradictory. Although the concept of leadership is difficult to define, Bryman identified four stages in its development: the trait approach, the style approach, the contingency approach, and the new leadership approach. A more detailed explanation of the evolution of the concept of leadership can be found in Chapter 14.

New Era in Health Care

At the 1994 United Nations Conference entitled "The World's Transformation: Conflict or Harmony?", Dr. Keith A. Bezanson, Canadian Director General of the International Development Research Council, concluded that the transformation we are experiencing is so profound that no one can foresee the journey or the outcomes. However, those nations, groups, and individuals able to create and access knowledge and technology are having an increasing influence over the destiny of the world (Bezanson, 1994).

This unsettling reality is part of the transition to a new era—the information age. Champy (1995) writes that we are the last generation of the industrial age and the first generation of the information age or, as Toffler (1980) called it, the third wave. Words such as cyberspace, genetic hardware, and trade patterns are reflections of this new era. Other words in our vocabulary have now taken on new meanings. For example, the word "chaos," which was understood as a total lack of organization and confusion, now means randomness of systems constrained by a type of order that is non-linear (Hamilton, West, Cherri, Mackey, & Fisher, 1994). Similarly, the word system, which used to mean a machine of some sort, now has a more complex definition such as "an assembly or combination of parts that form a complex unitary whole" (*Webster's*, 1989). The word paradox, defined as "a seemingly absurd or self-contradictory statement which, when investigated or explained, may prove to be well-founded or true" (Barber, 1998), is now part of the reality in the new era. For example, the request for services that are customized, high quality, low cost, and immediately available seems to be contradictory, but organizations and groups are meeting goals that seemed impossible just a few years ago. These words are part and parcel of everyday life now, and new sciences are being created that come from the convergence of empirical evidence in all fields of study. One such new area of study is complexity science.

Complexity Science

Complexity science is defined as "a description of phenomena demonstrated in systems characterized by non-linear, interactive components, emergent phenomena, continuous and discontinuous change, and unpredictable outcomes. Complexity is usually understood in contrast to simple, linear and equilibrium-based system[s]" (Zimmerman, Lindberg, & Plsek, 1998, p. 263).

What does all this have to do with nursing leadership? A lot, actually, because it has a direct effect on the type of leader the new era demands. Since the information era is grounded in knowledge and technology, leaders must understand the world around them and also be well prepared in their discipline.

In March 2003, four organizations convened an international summit at the University of Minnesota where 150 scholars, scientists, educators, and practitioners from fields as diverse as cognitive psychology, computer sciences, genetics, critical care, and business management discussed the application of complexity science to health care and thought up new ways to care for patients and to lead organizations and the health care system as a whole.

At the summit, Holland (2003) elaborated on the concept of complex adaptive systems and described complexity science as the science of the 21st century, distinct from Newtonian reductionism that has guided scientific thinking for over three centuries. Holland elaborated on how "complexity science can guide our understanding of the health care system, a multi-layered system largely driven by rapidly changing technology and information. In health care…practitioners…make up a continuously evolving system because of their innovative, diverse, and progressive adaptations. Knowing the building blocks of the organization…and its core processes, is critical" (Holland, 2003, p. 2). Holland describes many other possible interfaces of the building blocks of the health care system and the corresponding questions and plans needed to manage effectively and efficiently in this environment. How does such complexity in health care translate into the organization of work?

Organization of Work in the Information Age

Rapidly changing technology and its impact on organizations have been described by Toffler (1980) in his book *The Third Wave* as a profound social shift, a social upheaval created by the replacement of the industrial age by high technology, network relationships, and the information age.

The description of the organization of work in the third wave (Toffler & Toffler, 1995) is very important for nurse managers because it will drive the new era of leadership required in nursing. The nature of organizations has changed. There are often multiple units of operation that are quasi-autonomous with a tendency toward integration; there are very few control points and little standardization, but there is flexibility, fluidity, and movement; and the units are part of multiple networks of partners and alliances in multiple sites. This reality is already evident in many health care environments. The units are more autonomous and so are the programs; the nurses have more affinity to the profession than to the organization (Mintzberg, 1997), and many have multiple employers. Committees, work groups, and teams of multiple professionals meet for a limited period of time to redesign services, improve processes, innovate, allocate resources, and study the effectiveness of interventions. These groups disband and regroup for other projects, issues, or reviews. Models and strict procedures are being deconstructed, and systems and processes are being re-engineered so that they are more adapted to the uniqueness of each service. The work is done at multiple sites within merged organizations, regionally, provincially, nationally, or internationally.

If these characteristics of the information age are not yet visible in your organization, it is only a matter of time before they become overt because they are part of a social transformation. One change that has been implemented in every province except Quebec (which, in 2003, did introduce some organizational changes in this direction) is program management.

Program Management

Program management is a form of organizational design that comes from the business world and is adopted from the concept of product line management (Harber & Eni, 1989). It is a design where the individuals and resources are aligned by program rather than by discipline. The program designation may vary from medical specialties to generic foci such as women's health or long-term care. (See Chapter 8 for more on program management.)

Many goals are pursued by this form of design, including the following: (a) a more flexible organization with shared responsibility and decision-making power and fiscal responsibility closer to the point of service delivery (Harber & Eni, 1989); (b) improved accountability and effectiveness; (c) better managed costs (Monaghan, Alton, & Allen, 1992); and (d) more client-centred care with improved outcomes (Verrier, 1993).

Baker (1993) has reviewed the advantages and disadvantages of program management in health care and noted that the focus of the program is more generic and multidisciplinary, the authority and responsibility have shifted from the leaders of the health disciplines to the program managers, and the information system, including costing and budgeting, is transferred to the program. Further, in order to have greater responsiveness to patient care needs, quality assessment and improvement are focused on the outcomes of the program. This new design raises several issues for professionals, including the loss of professional identity, lower visibility of professional standards, interdisciplinary assessment and review with little focus on specific disciplinary standards or assessment, and a new emphasis on managerial structure, values, and career advancement.

The shift to program management in the 1990s and the corresponding emphasis on the bottom line have had important positive impacts for health care as documented by Baker, for example, the streamlining of costs, more multidisciplinary participation with a patient focus, and the new drive toward quality improvement and clinical pathways, to name a few. But it also brought with it major negative impacts on outcomes for patients (Aiken et al., 2001; Tourangeau, Giovannetti, Tu, & Wood, 2002), nurses, and organizations. Many of these effects have been documented in the unanimous report of the Canadian Nursing Advisory Committee (2002), which represented all levels of government, regions of the country, employers and unions, educators and researchers, associations, and nurses from all areas of practice.

As mentioned in Chapter 14, leadership positions in nursing are needed to support and guide the development of professional practice in health agencies, and this is also true for other health professionals. Many nurse leaders are experiencing difficulty in leading the transformation of services within a reformed health care system because they are progressively becoming generic executives who are less visible to their profession. Fagin (1996) calls the phenomenon in the United States a crisis of national discipline leadership in health care. She wrote, "Our institutions can boast of superb leaders in nursing (and medicine) responding to current political and managerial challenges. However, there seems to be an absence of the visionary, transforming nursing (and medical) leaders who not only respond to their institutional challenges but also speak for their professions and for the public they serve"(p. 30). So what kind of leadership is called for in light of the new era in health care?

New Nursing Leadership

According to Vance (1977), the movement, growth, and value of a profession are inextricably tied to its leadership. In the transition to a new paradigm, the discipline of nursing with its knowledge and professional practice requires transformational leadership. This is the kind of leadership that thrives on change and innovation and empowers by exercising "power 'with' not power 'to' others" (Barker, 1990, p. 39). Leaders in clinical nursing, management, education, and research must lead within nursing and alongside or parallel to other stakeholders in the new reality or risk becoming lost and out of touch with their professional roots. The road is not easy and the map not very precise, but how this is done will most likely determine the ability of the nursing profession to contribute to the new paradigm into the next century.

The Effective Contemporary Leader

There are four key attributes required of individual leaders in nursing, and these are vision, knowledge, confidence, and visibility.

Vision

One definition of vision is "the ability to dream [and] translate those dreams into a reality" (Deveraux, 1989, p. 3). Another is that vision is an image of a possible and desirable future that is realistic, attainable, credible, and attractive (Barker, 1990). Visions that have proven to be successful in transforming organizations have several common characteristics:

- They reflect the core purpose of the organization.
- They are feasible, yet challenging.
- They have significance that transcends the organization and impacts society as a whole.
- They appeal to the moral values, emotions, and imagination of the people in the profession and the organization.

Because the goal of health system leadership is to get people to invest their talents, knowledge, and skills in health services with a view to the ultimate success of the system, having a vision is vital. These ideas are illustrated in a simple model suggested by Barker (1990):

$$\text{Vision} \longrightarrow \text{Energized Action for Change} \longrightarrow \text{Success and Excellence}$$

Vision is essential because it generates the energy necessary to produce action and the results of that action, that in turn, lead to success. Although the model may seem simple, nurse leaders enrolled in an international nursing leadership training program found vision to be the most difficult skill to master (Deveraux, 1989). Even though they felt they had good ideas, few were accustomed to creating detailed plans and crafting strategies to achieve those ideas. Evidently, moving from the idea (i.e., the vision) to the feasibility of implementing the idea was the difficult part.

Even if the power of the mind alone is not sufficient to make a vision a reality, it is, nevertheless, the key element. For example, Bennis and Nanus (1985) suggest that, in envisioning, the leader must have the following:

- Foresight—a sense of the possible future of the organization
- A world view—an awareness of the impact of new trends in society and health care
- Hindsight—an appreciation for cultural and traditional roots
- Depth of sight—an ability to survey internal and external environments
- Peripheral vision—an awareness of competitors and stakeholders

* Revision—a willingness to revisit the vision with changes

Thus, while visions are important assets en route to the new era, intelligence, imagination, and knowledge are essential resources, and it is the effective use of these resources that creates a vision.

Knowledge

The knowledge base for effective leadership has been the subject of much scrutiny and the basis of an educational agenda that attempts to contend with contemporary megatrends. Paul (1989), for example, identified the megatrends for which leaders of the information age must be educated, and we need to be mindful of these megatrends if nursing leadership is to guide the profession through this era. In educational programming, there is a shift from

* strategy to structure;
* centralization to decentralization;
* functions to systems;
* hierarchy to horizontal networking;
* hands to brains;
* individuals to teams;
* "soft" culture to "hard" culture (i.e., outcomes); and
* *laissez-faire* to social accountability.

Awareness of these changes is essential knowledge for all leaders in the contemporary transition. Nursing leaders must concern themselves with how these trends will fashion our clinical, educational, and research agendas as well as our management structure into an integrated whole for the nursing profession.

Confidence

Leaders must have confidence if they are to be successful in implementing reform. Using Stuart's (1986) strategic contingency model, it is possible to identify three important variables that nurse leaders must keep in mind when bringing about reform. The first is *centrality*. Traditionally, it has been the role and responsibility of nurses to coordinate the services around the delivery of nursing care and to integrate their work with all other disciplines. Nursing has therefore enjoyed a central role in the delivery of institutional patient care.

The second variable is *substitutability*. This means that if the nursing profession is viewed only as the co-coordinator of care done by others, it will be a great disservice because other workers could then be easily substituted for nurses. We have to be mindful of the precise contribution of nurses to health care delivery. We know through clinical research, for example, that certain nursing interventions for neonatal infants have a direct impact on the infants' future illness patterns and growth and development. We also know that particular types of nurse-client interaction with cancer patients have physiological and psychological impacts, helping to reduce patients' stress and conserve their energy. Moreover, we know that, through interdisciplinary collaboration in diabetes education, complications in diabetics can be reduced by as much as 80%. When impacts or outcomes such as these can be attributed to nursing interventions, it becomes clear that knowledge-based nursing interventions are not substitutable. Knowledge of the contributions of nursing is what confident nursing leadership can articulate as the health system undergoes reform.

Finally, the third variable is *uncertainty*. Nursing needs confident leaders who have self-esteem and are able to live with insecurity. Confident and knowledgeable leaders can articulate issues and speak out for health services and the contributions that nurses make within the system. Such leaders are able to think critically, consider the options before them, as well as the possibilities, and still confront those options that differ from the management vision. For example, if public participation is part of the management model, but the public is only consulted and does not participate, nursing leaders will raise this issue in debate and obtain modification to the management model. Leaders are not paralyzed; they do not despair in times of insecurity and do not shrink from the constant challenges that lie ahead.

The confident leader, then, is armed with a vision of nursing and health services as a clear agenda. This energizes and mobilizes staff in pursuing their goals and dealing with change. The confident leader works with a team of colleagues to pursue common goals. Functioning under an umbrella of confidence makes the road of daily crises easier to travel and allows the leader to address and overcome vested interests, resistance to change, and quick-fix solutions.

Visibility

The fourth characteristic needed by leaders is visibility. Remaining visible is particularly challenging for nursing leaders as so many of the redesigning efforts in health services have introduced organizational models that replace existing professional models with management ones. The present wave of organizational changes has characteristically eliminated nursing positions at the policy and senior management levels of health care agencies. Some administrators, however, want to have nurses as incumbents in newly created positions because of their nursing knowledge and skills in organizing the delivery of patient care, without regard for the knowledge required for other aspects of the position. As a result, nursing becomes both invisible and disposable. Moreover, there is little consistency across regional health authorities.

In one Alberta regional health authority (RHA), for example, there are seven senior managers, six of whom are nurses. In the RHA next door, there is not one nurse among the seven senior management positions. This sort of inconsistency is occurring in the US and is of concern to nursing leaders there. Fagin (1996) noted the following at an invitational conference on executive leadership in major teaching hospitals and academic health centres:

> In examining some written descriptions of these models, one notes that discipline-specific requirements exist only for physicians. Surely nurses exist and participate in some of the leadership roles, but [their] credentials do not appear. This dangerous situation appears to be part of a growing trend and has implications for the profession and for the public. For the profession, by deliberately leaving out the credential of the nursing license, nursing's power, ethic, roles, and future are made as invisible as the most stereotypic view of nursing we all decry. For the public, the potential absence of professional nurses could lead to lower quality of care and in some cases to life-threatening events (p. 32).

Since the end of the 1990s, some positions of vice-president or chief of nursing responsible for nursing professional practice have been reintroduced. Where these positions do not exist, vice-president positions responsible for other programs often carry the title of nursing as well. It is very difficult to have sufficient time to combine program responsibility with the massive redesign of the nursing professional practice environment that is needed following the deconstruction of the 1990s. In any case, this re-emergence of nursing positions is recognition of the profession and is the result of the leadership of nurses who are making nursing more visible.

Nursing Leadership in all Domains

The most significant and challenging new direction for nursing leadership is to develop leadership in all domains of the profession, namely, clinical practice, education, management, and research. To date, nursing leadership has been exercised mostly by managers, educators, and researchers. Clinical nurses are providing excellent care to their patients and clients, but they have not been part of the critical decision making regarding their practice or patient care policies. So, the biggest challenge facing nursing is in the clinical domain.

The new matrix structures, such as program management, and the prevalence of semi-autonomous teams in clinical areas have, as explained in Chapter 8, dissipated the authority and points of control formerly available to administrative nurses in traditional pyramidal hierarchies. All nurses who are members of semi-autonomous and interdisciplinary teams must be willing to assume leadership roles; otherwise, nursing will be absent from the deliberations and decisions regarding patient care. The familiar, top-down hierarchical structure (Figure 20.1), in which the vice-president, chief, director, and manager provided a chain of command for the team, is being replaced by multiple teams of individual professionals who work in a temporary matrix that is fluid and changes with circumstances (Figure 20.2).

The network requires that all professionals exercise their leadership in their areas of expertise and that they not defer to a few colleagues in positions of authority. Clinical nurses should be able to make decisions about their clinical practice based on their expertise. Nurse educators should exercise their leadership in areas of learning, teaching, and career development. Similarly, nurse researchers should be able to make decisions concerning the discovery, dissemination, and integration of new nursing knowledge. And, finally, for nurse managers, their leadership should be in the areas of resources, processes, infrastructure, and goal attainment in the discipline. It is the interdependence of these areas of expertise and leadership that is needed to provide an integrated and global nursing approach in the information age.

The practice of nursing crosses multiple domains, so it will be possible for one professional nurse to exercise expertise in several domains. For example, the academic may also be practicing with a specific population in the community while teaching and managing a team of researchers. The advanced practice nurse may also have a case load, carry out research, teach, and manage a team of clinical nurses. This interdependence is experienced within multidisciplinary teams and corporate teams; therefore, networks are complex webs of interactions for meeting the goals that have been set.

Figure 20.1 Nursing Hierarchy from the Industrial Age

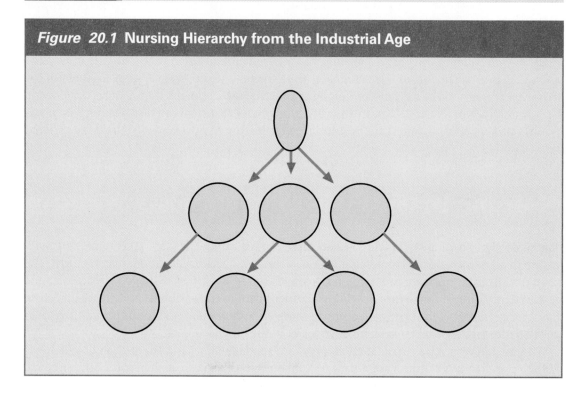

Shared Governance

Is the development of leadership in all domains of practice a restatement of the concept of shared governance? Porter-O'Grady (2001) raises the question of whether shared governance is still relevant. He notes that the concept of shared governance has been advocated for the last two decades as a strategy to empower nurses and provide a framework for organizing nursing work. "No matter how much nursing leaders identify the value and role of the nurse in critical decision-making, health policy or leadership in healthcare, not much has changed for...most practicing nurses.... It seems surreal at best to hear the same complaints and problems voiced today that I heard voiced 30 years ago.... One is led to wonder what set of circumstances keeps the oppressive conditions of nursing practice constant as the rest of the world changes almost in every way" (p. 468).

The four critical principles of shared governance (partnership, accountability, equity, and ownership) are as relevant today, but obviously nursing has not embraced the concept (see Chapter 16 for further discussion of shared governance). Why not? Maurer (1995) states that empowerment is based on the recognition of power already present, and it does not need a

Figure 20.2 **Nursing Matrix from the New Era**

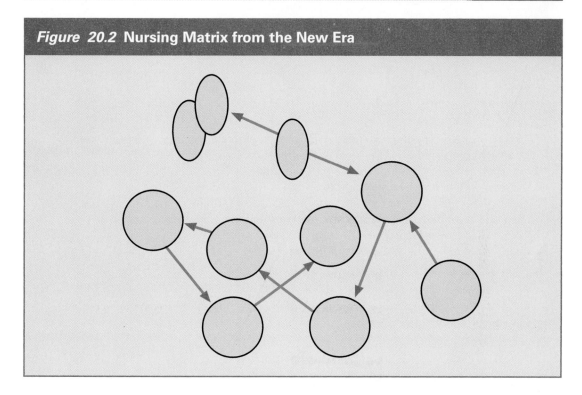

transfer of locus of control, but recognition of the location of legitimate decisions. In the last two decades, neither locus of control nor structural changes have been made to ensure that clinical nurses can legitimately make decisions about their practice. For example, the policies, procedures, and protocols that guide clinical practice are usually developed by educators and managers with very little input from clinicians. Yet, clinical nurses are the experts, and if they do not have legitimate areas of decision making, they will not be able to exercise their leadership nor will they wish to. This is often why the unit councils or unit nursing clinical practice committees in shared governance have found it difficult to survive.

The principles of shared governance are still valid today, but like any vision, unless there is a strategic plan and action taken to realize the vision, it is unlikely to make a difference. In summary, to ensure nursing leadership in all domains, changes must take place in the locus of control and in decision structures in order to carve a legitimate role for clinical nurses, and strategic plans must be implemented to ensure that organizational behaviour changes as well. Box 20.1 provides examples of how organizational change can support clinical leadership and decision making.

Box 20.1

Clinical Leadership

The following are three real-life examples of organizational support for clinical leadership and decision making.

1. The Ottawa Hospital has created a corporate nursing clinical practice committee (CNCPC) composed of one clinical nurse representative from each of the 120 units/services within the hospital's six organizations. The committee meets four hours a month and is lead by an elected executive of clinical nurses. The committee is responsible for the corporate nursing clinical agenda. Some of their successes include the implementation of a new standardized medication administration schedule, nursing assessment documentation, a program to reduce violence, better equipment, and a health passport for patients.

2. New Brunswick Health Region Two has created a clinical forum similar to that of the Ottawa Hospital above called G57, the grouping of 57 units with a similar agenda.

3. In 2002, the Regina Qu'Appelle Health Region implemented a clinical practice nursing council for the region.

Global Nursing Leadership

The other new direction for nursing leadership is in the area of global nursing leadership. Globalization is created by the movement of information, material, and people across borders, and this calls for leaders with a global perspective. Major worldwide trends point to increased global interdependency and interrelatedness. This translates to a growing need to overcome barriers that separate cultures as well as the need to develop new leadership that is culturally fluent and aware of cross-cultural opportunities and problems (Smith & Lischin, 1987). According to Maznevski and DiStefano (2000), "global leaders must develop a strong portfolio of technical, interpersonal and conceptual skills appropriate for managing the most complex of all possible situations" (p. 195). They suggest that an effective strategy for developing global leaders is to work with global teams. Individuals, however, must have in-depth knowledge of their own area of specialty, and this must be coupled with knowledge of other functions. Global leaders also must develop strong skills in three areas: learning and adapting, managing relationships, and managing ambiguity.

Nursing is fortunate to have had very effective global leaders through the work of the International Council of Nurses (ICN) and the Canadian Nurses Association (CNA) International Affairs Department. The need for global leadership is now reaching our individual workplaces where multi-site and multi-country projects are underway. These projects are likely to increase exponentially in the next decade. Global nursing leadership is not the affair of the few anymore but of all nurses at all levels—locally, provincially, nationally, and internationally.

The Challenge Ahead

Developing a new model of nursing leadership depends, in great part, on the leadership of nurses in management roles. In order to guide the transition, innovation will be needed to redesign strategies and structures that will help reduce co-dependency, provide knowledge and skills to all nurses, and let go of areas of power while guiding the growth and the attainment of goals. Some of the challenges in developing this new model of nursing leadership include the following:

- Reconceptualization of nursing leadership to ensure that the notion of leadership is not equated only with management
- Reorganization of the work environment to value all forms of leadership (i.e., creation of climate, structure, and processes)
- Moving toward a professional leadership model in all domains, at all levels, and in an interdependence mode
- Helping nurse managers and educators facilitate the transition as they change their own roles
- Preparing a generation of nurses who are able to exercise their leadership knowledge and skill (including the art of persuasion)
- Working on teams (processes and dynamics), not only in teams
- Innovation, innovation, innovation…. We should no longer hear the expression "it has never been done before."

Leadership Implications

It is the current nurse leaders who will have to guide the transformation of the nursing profession. When we are in the centre of a tornado, however, it is difficult to see the big picture, so we need to be guided by "radar." This radar for nurses in leadership positions consists of (a) management and leadership knowledge and skills to adapt to the information age, (b) professional values and accountability for excellence in nursing practice, and (c) the ability to work in networks that include nurse leaders in all domains and at all levels.

The shift in our views on leadership is one of the greatest professional challenges because it confronts some of our fundamental beliefs. For example, leadership has been understood to mean leaders and followers, but we need to develop leadership in everyone if we are to exercise influence throughout the web of networks. The shift confronts the nature of the nursing infrastructure to which nurses have been socialized in order to redistribute power. It demands that we become the instrument of our own destiny in order to share control over professional decisions. For the profession, the new iteration of nursing leadership will ensure that nursing thrives in the new era of health care and that nurses will increase their ability to serve the Canadian public even better. This chapter is a call for nursing leadership.

In conclusion, the last word will be from Dr. Mo Im Kim, past president of the ICN: "There is nothing around us to reverse the direction of development and change …thus we are posed with the question of being the master of these changes or their servant" (as cited in White, 2003, p. 98).

Summary

- Leadership is defined as the process of influencing a group in its efforts toward goal setting and goal achievement. The movement, growth, and value of a profession are inextricably tied to its leadership.
- Since the 1940s, four stages in the development of the concept of leadership have been identified in the scholarly work of social scientists, namely trait, style, contingency, and new leadership approaches.
- A new era in health care is the result of a social upheaval created by the replacement of the industrial age with the information age.
- The organization of work in the information age is in multiple units of operation that are quasi-autonomous and tending toward integration. There are few points of control and little standardization in these units, but there is flexibility, fluidity, and movement. These units are part of multiple networks of partners and alliances and operate in multiple sites.
- Characteristics of the information age are more or less visible in our workplace and constitute a social transformation. One visible change is the advent of program management.
- New forms of leadership—in all domains of practice and at all levels—are required for nursing to be effective in the new era.
- Effective contemporary nurse leaders possess four primary attributes. These leaders are visionary, knowledgeable, confident, and visible.
- New leadership is needed in all domains of practice so that nurses make decisions regarding their own areas of expertise.
- Creation of an environment in which clinical nurses make decisions regarding their areas of expertise demands a change in the locus of control, in decision structures, and in strategic plans to ensure behavioural changes.
- Preparation of global nursing leaders is required not only for international work, but for work at all levels because globalization is reaching local levels.
- Challenges for first-line nurse managers include guiding the transition to the new era, redesigning strategies and structures to help reduce co-dependency, providing knowledge and skills to all nurses, and letting go of areas of power while guiding the growth and professional development of nurses and the attainment of nursing goals.
- Whether nurses are passive or active in the redesign of the new era of nursing leadership, they co-create the reality they will live.

Applying the Knowledge in this Chapter

Case Study

A clinical manager would like to create opportunities for clinical nurses on her unit to be involved in clinical decision making and, eventually, to exercise leadership in their domain. The unit is a medical unit with approximately 60 full-time and part-time registered nurses and licensed practical nurses. A few years ago, a unit clinic practice committee existed but, due to lack of interest, it folded.

At a recent staff meeting, the clinical manager brought forward the idea of creating a unit clinical practice committee or a unit council, but no one volunteered or showed any interest. From this response, it was clear to the clinical manager what the problems were and that it was her job to fix them. Nurses had no time for committee work due to their workload.

At the request of the Chief of Nursing, the clinical manager named a nurse representative from the unit to attend the corporate nursing clinical practice committee, which is responsible for setting the clinical agenda for the organization. The nurse who attended the corporate committee meeting was overwhelmed with the corporate role clinical nurses played, the number of issues they dealt with, and their accomplishments. She did not realize that several changes in the hospital were the result of the clinical nurses' work, for example, the new medication administration schedule, the new nursing assessment documentation, and the health passport for patients to facilitate their transfer to the community. She came back to her unit wanting to share the information and to help create a unit committee, but when she talked to a few of her colleagues, she could not find anyone interested. The clinical manager and the nurse representative met to develop a plan to promote clinical leadership on the unit.

Using the ideas presented in this chapter, identify the underlying problems in this case study. Develop a strategy that both the clinical manager and clinical nurses might implement in order to create a new forum for clinical decision making. What elements of participation, partnership, education, communication, locus of control, and so on will the plan have to address? What are the clinical issues that could be on the agenda of the committee?

Resources

evolve Internet Resources

Canadian Nurses Association (CNA):
   Position Statement
   www.cna-nurses.ca/_frames/policies/policiesmainframe.htm
   This 2002 position statement, *Nursing Leadership*, identifies the beliefs of the profession on the issues of leadership and the quality professional practice environment.

International Council of Nurses (ICN):
 Position Statement
 www.icn.ch/psmanagement00.htm
 The ICN's Position Statement for the year 2000, entitled *Management of Nursing and Healthcare Services,* can be found on this site.

Further Reading

Canadian Nurses Association. (2003). *Succession planning for nursing leadership*. Ottawa, ON: Canadian Nurses Association.
 The Board of Directors of the CNA has approved a background document to facilitate the development of strategies to support leadership development in nursing organizations or associations. The "acceleration pool" system and the six steps to successful succession planning are described.

Ferguson-Paré, M., Mitchell, G., Perkin, K., & Stevensen, L. (2002). *Academy of Canadian Executive Nurses – Background paper on leadership*. Toronto, ON: Academy of Canadian Executive Nurses (ACEN).
 In this paper, the ACEN describes the need for nursing leadership and the turbulent Canadian environment within which nursing leadership is exercised. They identify the six behaviours that support autonomous professional practice and the role of executive nurses.

References

Aiken, L., Clarke, S.P., Sloane, D.M., Sochalski, J.A., Busse, R., Clarke, H., et al. (2001). Nurses report on hospital care in five countries. *Health Affairs, 20*(3), 43–53.

Baker, G.R. (1993). The implications of program management for professional and managerial roles. *Physiotherapy Canada, 45*(4), 221–224.

Barber, C. (Ed.). (1998). *The Canadian Oxford dictionary*. Toronto, ON: Oxford University Press.

Barker, A.M. (1990). *Transformational nursing leadership*. Baltimore: Williams & Wilkins.

Bass, B.M., & Stogdill, R.M. (1990). *Bass and Stogdill's handbook of leadership: Theory, research, and managerial applications* (3rd ed.). New York: Free Press.

Bennis, W.G., & Nanus, B. (1985). *Leaders: The strategies for taking charge*. New York: Harper & Row.

Bezanson, K.A. (1994). From megatrends to sustainability: The challenge for international development organizations. *UNPD roundtable on global change: Social conflict or harmony?* Ottawa, ON: International Development Research Council.

Bryman, A. (1996). Leadership in organizations. In S.R. Clegg, C. Hardy, & W.R. Nord (Eds.), *Handbook of organizational studies* (pp. 276–292). Newbury Park, CA: Sage Publications.

Canadian Nursing Advisory Committee. (2002). *Our health, our future, creating a quality workplace for Canadian nurses*. Ottawa, ON: Advisory Committee on Human Health Resources, Health Canada.

Champy, J. (1995). *Reengineering management*. New York: Harper Business.

Deveraux, M.O. (1989). *Leadership development: Key to effectiveness at the policy level*. Paper presented at the Conference on Nursing Leadership: Using Research for Policy Making in Primary Health Care. Yonsei University, Seoul, Korea.

Drucker, P.F. (1996). Foreword: Not enough generals were killed. In F. Hesselbein, M. Goldsmith, & R. Beckhard (Eds.), *The leader of the future: New visions, strategies, and practices for the next era* (pp. xi–xv). San Francisco: Jossey-Bass.

Fagin, C.M. (1996). Executive leadership: Improving nursing practice, education, and research. *Journal of Nursing Administration, 26*(3), 30–37.

Hamilton, P., West, B., Cherri, M., Mackey, J., & Fisher, P. (1994). Preliminary evidence of non-linear dynamics in births to adolescents in Texas, 1964 to 1990. *Theoretic and Applied Chaos in Nursing, 1*(1), 15–22.

Harber, B.W., & Eni, G.O. (1989). Issues for consideration in the establishment of a program management structure. *Forum, 2*(3), 6–14.

Holland, J. (2003). *Applying complexity science to health and healthcare.* Minneapolis, MN: Center for the Study of Health Care Management, University of Minnesota.

Leatt, P., & Porter, J. (2003). Where are the health care leaders? The need for investment in leadership development. *Healthcare Papers, 4*(1), 14–31.

Maurer, G. (1995). True empowerment: From shared governance to self-managed work teams. *Journal of Shared Governance, 1*(1), 25–30.

Maznevski, M.L., & DiStefano, J.J. (2000). Global leaders are team players: Developing global leaders through membership on global teams. *Human Resources Management, 39*(2/3), 195–208.

Mintzberg, H. (1997). No formulas or management model allowed. *Forum, 10*, 8–9.

Monaghan, B.J., Alton, L., & Allen, D. (1992). Transition to program management. *Leadership,* (Sept/Oct), 33–37.

Paul, J.P. (1989). The consequences of megatrends on business education. *European Management Journal, 7*(3), 284–285.

Porter-O'Grady, T. (2001). Is shared governance still relevant? *Journal of Nursing Administration, 31*(10), 468–473.

Stogdill, R.M. (1950). Leadership, membership and organization. *Psychological Bulletin, 47,* 1–14.

Smith, R.C., & Lischin, S. (1987). *Intercultural relations and the development of global measurement.* Columbus, OH: Bureau of Business Research, Ohio State University.

Stuart, G.W. (1986). An organizational strategy for empowering nursing. *Nursing Economics, 4*(2), 69–73.

Toffler, A. (1980). *The third wave.* New York: William Morrow.

Toffler, A., & Toffler, H. (1995). Getting set for the coming millennium. *The Futurist, 29*(5), 13–14.

Tourangeau, A.E., Giovannetti, P., Tu, J.V., & Wood, M. (2002). Nursing related determinants of 30-day mortality for hospitalised patients. *Canadian Journal of Nursing Research, 33*(4), 71–88.

Vance, C.N. (1977). *Group profile of contemporary influentials in American nursing.* Unpublished doctoral dissertation, Teachers College, Columbia University, New York.

Verrier, M.C. (1993). Program management: A professional opportunity. *Physiotherapy Canada, 45*(4), 225.

Webster's encyclopedic unabridged dictionary of the English language. (1989). New York: Portland House.

Zimmerman, B., Lindberg, C., & Plsek, P. (1998). *Edgeware: Lessons from complexity science for health care leaders.* Irving, TX: VHA Inc.

SECTION

V

LEADERSHIP AND MANAGEMENT SKILLS

The authors of the chapters in Section V have drawn substantially from their experiences in senior leadership roles in the health system, government, and private industry. Most have also taught in the fields of nursing and administration, and many have provided consultation services or conducted management research. This section focuses on some of the major functions of management and the knowledge and skills required of leaders and managers. All the topics contribute either directly or indirectly to the quality of working environments; therefore, all nurses need to have knowledge of this material whether or not they are, or aspire to be, managers.

Effective teamwork is now a necessity in all organizational environments. In Chapter 21, *Leadership for Teamwork and Collaboration*, the authors discuss the skills and responsibilities of leaders who must ensure that groups are appropriately structured so they can remain productive with all participants focused on achieving the objectives. This is important for all RNs who, at one time or another, will find themselves working with or leading groups.

Change is a pervasive phenomenon in the health care system. Chapter 22, *Leading and Managing Change*, concerns the responsibility of managers to plan, implement, and evaluate change in constructive ways without disrupting or frustrating workers. A basic understanding of theories of change is of value to all nurses because, throughout their careers, they will constantly need to participate in change processes. A case example is used to illustrate the application of various theories of change when introducing a new model of nursing care delivery.

Chapter 23, *Intraorganizational Politics*, will help readers to understand the sources of power in organizations and how nurses can capitalize on their knowledge of power dynamics in order to achieve needed changes for improving nursing care.

In Chapter 24, the concepts and skills of *Project Management* are introduced. These can be immediately applied to work being conducted by students, clinical nurses, and nurse managers. The project management approach is now widely used in complex organizations as a framework for assuring successful and timely implementation of planned change. The approach is illustrated by a case example involving a change in the staff mix in a long-term facility.

Developing Human Resources in Health Agencies is the focus of Chapter 25. Competence in this area directly affects the day-to-day work life of all employees in health agencies and has an immediate bearing on the morale and productivity of the workforce. It is important that all nurses have a general knowledge of the processes, practices, and systems to which they will be exposed as potential employees. This chapter provides a basic overview of the employer's responsibilities in relation to hiring, developing, and supervising the workforce.

Chapter 26, *Human Resource Allocation: Staffing and Scheduling*, provides a detailed explanation of how work schedules are designed and how staffing decisions are made. Staffing affects patients, employees, and managers, and appropriate work schedules are essential for achieving safe patient care and promoting the quality of work life of employees. These decisions involve the allocation of both human and financial resources and are a means through which values, priorities, and standards of care are operationalized.

Day-to-day conflicts that emerge in practice are discussed in Chapter 27, *Conflict Resolution and Negotiation*. The principles and tactics for managing conflict and negotiating agreements between parties are applicable in the workplace and beyond. It is expected that most readers will know the basic concepts and skills required to recognize and deal with conflict. However, it is the responsibility of leaders to select appropriate strategies for resolving conflicts that threaten to disrupt the workplace and to ensure that the outcomes are constructive. Principled bargaining is an effective method for resolving interpersonal and inter-group conflicts.

Chapter 28, *Working with Unions*, contains a model of the legal framework that governs relations between employers and unions, including structures and processes for settling disputes (i.e., strikes, lockouts, and grievances) between the parties. In Canada, almost all nurse employees, with the exception of senior managers, are members of unions, and their terms and conditions of employment are contained in collective agreements. The knowledge in this chapter is vital to undergraduates, RNs, leaders, and managers, who may play different roles within these processes at various stages in their careers.

Everyone working in the health system is subject to budget constraints. *Business Planning and Budget Preparation*, Chapter 29, is not exclusively a management function as budgets must be prepared for research proposals, projects, and even educational travel. Most publicly funded health care programs are required to have a written business plan with clear goals and objectives before funding is considered. Knowledge of business plans and the budget process allows all nurses to understand the importance of efficiently managing scarce resources and to contribute to the budget process.

Influential Writing, Chapter 30, is an important instrument of change and is frequently underrated as a professional and managerial skill. Good writing skills are required of all health workers, and they are essential for effective leadership practice. Written documentation is required in clinical practice as well as in the reporting of issues requiring the attention of senior decision makers. The author provides accepted norms and practical guidelines to assist in the composition of reports, memoranda, and other documents required for formal communication.

All participants in applied research are motivated to identify the policy implications of their work, and readers who are pursuing graduate studies may wish to consider conducting policy research. Chapter 31, *Policy Analysis: From Issues to Action*, introduces the reader to several models of policy and decision making and to the terminology associated with these processes. The role and skill set of the policy analyst is presented with an emphasis on the conceptual and writing skills required to carry out this professional role successfully. This chapter will be of particular interest to nurses working in government departments or in positions in health agencies where the specialized professional skills of policy analysis are applied.

LEADERSHIP FOR TEAMWORK AND COLLABORATION

Donna Lynn Smith, Shirley Meyer, and Dorothy M. Wylie

Learning Objectives

In this chapter, you will learn:

- The importance of teamwork in health organizations
- Similarities and differences between workgroups and teams
- Basic concepts about group structure, process, and development that provide a background for understanding workgroups, teams, and collaboration
- Roles and behaviours of members and leaders in effective teams
- Characteristics of and challenges facing health care teams
- How organizational context and leadership affect the performance of teams
- The growing importance of collaboration as a leadership behaviour and an organizational norm
- Types of collaboration and the conditions for effective collaboration

The importance of effective teamwork and collaboration is now recognized in most professional fields and work settings. In health care, as knowledge expands and service is provided in increasingly complex environments, a single individual or discipline is rarely able to provide the range of clinical services that a patient or group of similar patients might need. Managers and leaders in health settings must be able to effectively work together across disciplinary and departmental boundaries, and often across boundaries between care settings and organizations. As explained in Chapter 7, there are many stakeholder groups that provide services for or have an interest in how services are provided. Failure of collaboration among stakeholders, including government departments and various levels of government, creates costly inefficiencies and mistakes that can have far-reaching public consequences. Therefore, all stakeholders have an interest in understanding how teams work and how obstacles to effective teamwork and collaboration may be overcome.

Leaders and managers at all levels and in all professional fields must now be skilled as team members. More importantly, they must be able to help others develop the skills of teamwork and collaboration. The standards of the Canadian Council on Health Services Accreditation (CCHSA) reflect this view (CCHSA, 2002). In the past, health care organizations were assessed on how well each department or profession met the standards developed in their own discipline. The current approach is one in which accreditors interview teams of professionals who care for particular client groups, thereby assessing the performance of the workgroup or team and not individual disciplines or departments. Leaders of health care agencies have become aware of the importance of effective teamwork and their responsibilities for achieving it (Beverley, Dobson, Atkinson, & Caldwell, 1997; Young, Ang, & Findlay, 1997).

Collaboration is now widely seen as a favoured approach to providing patient care, leading organizations, educating future health professionals, and conducting health care research, and it is particularly relevant to work that is dynamic and unpredictable (Sullivan, 1998). A review of the literature and analysis of the concept of collaboration led Sullivan (1998) to the following definition:

> Collaboration is defined as a dynamic, transforming process of creating a power-sharing partnership for pervasive application in health care practice, education, research, and organizational settings for the purposeful attention to needs and problems in order to achieve likely successful outcomes (p. 6).

The critical attributes of successful collaborative practice were identified by Bailey and Armer (1998) and include cooperation, assertiveness, responsibility, communication, autonomy, and co-ordination. Equality and complimentary expertise are key to successful collaboration at all levels.

Why Is Teamwork so Important?

All organizations, and the subunits within them, must coordinate their activities, and this is a particular need for knowledge-intensive enterprises (Elmore, 2000). Teamwork has always been necessary in the delivery of health services where work is complex and interdependent, involving the application of expert knowledge and specialized techniques under changing clinical, organizational, and environmental circumstances; however, the need for teamwork and collaboration has intensified in the health care environment as part of a larger social transformation from individual work to teamwork (LaFasto & Larsen, 2001).

Coordination between individual professionals and within and among organizational units is achieved through mutual adjustment processes that involve interpersonal interaction between individuals and groups to bridge the formal and informal structures in the organization. As explained in Chapter 8, the need for mutual adjustment processes increases with the complexity of work being performed. Therefore, in the delivery of clinical health services, it is almost always necessary for individuals and groups to be able to work effectively together to achieve common objectives for the care of the patient or client. Activities and processes within and between the departments or subunits of health agencies also need to be coordinated. Some horizontal coordination is achieved through policies and procedures and through the activities of centralized departments such as finance and human resources. However, most coordination occurs through the work of groups and teams. Structures for horizontal coordination take many forms, including temporary or permanent workgroups, teams, committees, networks, task forces, and project teams. These coordinating mechanisms vary in the formality of their structure and in their permanence, but to succeed, all require the application of skills of leadership and collaboration.

An underlying premise of this chapter is that the skills of teamwork and collaboration can be learned and improved through reflective practice. Since the late 1960s in Canada, educational programs for registered nurses (RNs) have incorporated specific learning objectives and experiences to develop the knowledge and skills for effective workgroup and team participation. Nurses also learn the skills needed to collaborate with patients, families, and communities when planning and providing care. This learning provides a strong foundation for the leadership and development of teams and collaboration at other levels.

The chapter continues with a brief review of group dynamics and structure, functions, and norms. Roles of group members and models of group development are highlighted. This knowledge provides a basis for understanding similarities and differences between workgroups and teams. The role of the leader of workgroups and teams is then discussed with emphasis on how group and team performance can be improved. Finally, goals and approaches to collaboration are discussed with a focus on the decision-making and behavioural roles of health care leaders.

Group Dynamics and Structure

Much of the basic knowledge of how small groups function was developed between the 1950s and 1970s as social psychologists observed small group interaction, often under controlled circumstances. Group dynamics was defined by Luft (1970) as the "study of individuals interacting in small groups" (p. 1). An understanding of basic concepts about the way small groups work is the starting point for effective group and team leadership and participation. A group consists of two or more people who come together, or who are brought together, to achieve a purpose through communication and interaction. Individuals usually belong to several groups, whether in the home, workplace, classroom, or as members of associations or clubs. Many groups are formed for the purpose of accomplishing a task, but people often voluntarily join groups to meet their own needs for affiliation, self-esteem, or recognition. Groups may be needed to accomplish organizational goals in the workplace, but they can also meet the personal needs of group members.

A group is a social system with its own boundaries, structure, and culture. The structure and culture of a group can become so firmly established that it can be extremely difficult to change the ways the group has developed for doing business (Dimock, 1987). Group membership tends to become inclusive for the members and exclusive for those who are not members. Non-members may be viewed as outsiders or may see themselves that way. In fact, it may be easier to start a new group than to get an existing group to change behaviours. Many changes in organizational structure and processes are introduced because it is assumed or asserted that groups of people cannot, or will not, change the way they work.

The size of a group can be a significant factor in its effectiveness. Group interaction tends to decrease as the number of people in a group increases (Zander, 1986). As a result, people who belong to large groups are often less satisfied with membership in the group because there are fewer opportunities for participation and interaction. In large groups with limited interaction, a group member may feel anonymous, which can result in a lack of cooperation or commitment.

Not all individuals contribute equally to the groups in which they participate. Slavin (1992) pointed out that achievement can be difficult to assess because group products are the result of pooled, rather than individual, learning and accomplishment. Individual responsibility can be diffused because the group, rather than its individual members, is held accountable for the product or outcome. The term *free-rider effect* was introduced to describe the situation in which a group member reduces individual effort by taking advantage of the efforts of others (Kerr & Bruun, 1981, 1983). Alternatively, some group members may reduce their individual efforts if they perceive that others in the group are "free riding" by contributing less than they are able or less than other members of the group. This has been termed the *sucker effect* (Kerr & Bruun, 1983). These behaviours fall within a broader category of behaviour that has been described as *social loafing* (Slavin, 1992; Latane, 1986). This term refers to a reduction of effort and performance when a group shares a single goal but individual contributions toward it cannot be readily monitored. Social loafing has been observed in small groups but is more likely to occur in larger groups where an individual may feel lost in the crowd.

Group Functions and Norms

Tasks, interaction, and self-orientation are the three basic functions that affect the group process (Boshear & Albrecht, 1977).

- *Task behaviours* achieve the goals of the group and can be called the work of the group. They include gathering facts, developing goals, sharing information, clarifying issues, problem solving, or reaching consensus in decision making.

- *Interaction activities* are the processes that determine how the group performs. They include communicating, expressing feelings, attempting to resolve disagreements, and establishing the norms of behaviour for the group.

- *Self-oriented behaviours* are behaviours that the group members use to meet their individual needs. These may not always be useful for achieving group goals or positive interaction. For example, members may dwell on personal concerns and issues, waste time, dominate the discussion, have side conversations with others, not listen, or continually interrupt.

The functions of task, interaction, and self-orientation can be carried out directly or indirectly. Direct activities are open, and group members share the reasons for their behaviour with the group. Open communication, including the sharing of personal needs and wishes by group members, can sometimes lead to resolution of interpersonal issues. Sometimes, however, undisclosed intentions or motivations of group members may be reflected in hidden agendas.

Individuals who are attempting to pursue a hidden agenda within a group may do so by undermining projects, making secret agreements with other members, promoting personal needs above others, and suppressing or avoiding interpersonal issues. Hidden agendas may arise around the group task, group leadership, or individual members. Groups may work well at the surface level when the hidden agenda is resting or has been settled, but at times of crises, unresolved hidden agendas may give rise to an increase in indirect activities within the group. All groups have surface agendas and hidden agendas and work on both at the same time (Bradford, 1978).

Groups often establish norms of behaviour early in their development. Norms are the expectations of the group about how their members will behave in the achievement of the task. Norms may be formalized into written statements of procedure or may be informal and unexpressed. Regardless of their format, norms can strongly influence an individual's behaviour in a group. When groups demand strict adherence to group norms, there is a high degree of conformity and cohesiveness. In some situations, this is positive; in others, it may not be constructive and can lead to "groupthink." This term was coined by Janis (1983) and is defined as an extreme occurrence in which poor group decisions result from a limited exploration of alternative solutions to problems. The groupthink phenomenon was discussed in Chapter 13 as it applies to organizational leadership.

Models of Group Development

Many different models of group development have been described (Bales, 1950; Bion, 1961; Jones, 1991; Lacoursiere, 1974; Schutz, 1958; Tuckman, 1965; Tuckman & Jensen, 1977). Although the terminology differs, each model portrays the tasks and interpersonal behaviours within a group as it moves through various stages. All groups do not necessarily progress through a predictable or "normal" development process. Sometimes groups become bogged down in the early stages of development and cannot achieve the stage of interdependence where roles and functions are shared among group members.

In one five-stage model of group development (Tuckman, 1965; Tuckman & Jensen, 1977), the first stage, *forming,* is described as a time of orientation when members seek guidance from the leader and direction on rules and functions. During this phase, they also determine their commitment to the group. The second stage, *storming,* is characterized by competition and conflict, with resistance to other members' roles and ideas. Members experience discomfort in this stage; some become passive and others, vocal and hostile. During the third stage, *norming,* a sense of cohesion starts to develop. Team members buy into the group as trust and open communication emerge. There can be a sense of energy and creativity during this phase. When the group reaches the fourth stage, *performing,* it operates interdependently and its goals and roles are clear yet flexible. Members are more confident, morale is good, and productivity related to the task is high. At the fifth stage, *adjourning,* the task has been completed and the relationships that have developed may be given up. A similar model described by Lacoursiere (1974, 1980) categorized the developmental stages as orientation, dissatisfaction, production, and termination.

Figure 21.1 illustrates how groups move through the task and interpersonal dimensions in a four-stage model (Pheiffer, 1991). In stage one, as they are becoming oriented to the task, group

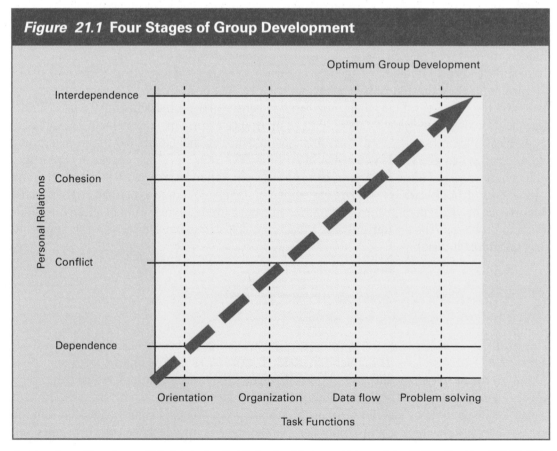

Figure 21.1 Four Stages of Group Development

Source: From *Theories and Models in Applied Behavioral Science,* Volume 2 (p. 100), edited by J.W. Pfeiffer, 1991, San Diego, CA: Pfeiffer & Company. Reprinted with permission.

members are dependent on the leader for guidance and direction. At stage two, members begin to organize their own approaches to the task, and conflict may develop among members as differing ideas, methods, and behaviours begin to surface. In stage three, as some level of trust begins to emerge and members get to know each other better, there is movement toward group cohesion. Information begins to flow as members share perceptions, feelings, and ideas at the task level as well as the personal level. In stage four, interdependence is evident as members begin to feel more comfortable working together, can openly share and communicate, and can work toward a higher level of problem solving.

Regardless of the model chosen to illustrate group development, specific elements must be in place for groups to be effective. The goals of the group need to be clear and will need to be clarified occasionally to keep the group on track. The necessary group roles and functions must be carried out to maintain the life of the group, and every group member has a responsibility to see that functions are fulfilled. Open, two-way communication is essential and should provide opportunities for members to express perceptions, feelings, and ideas. Positive norms need to be established to create a climate of trust and to allow for participation by each member of the group. There should be opportunities for group leadership to be shared among the members and for leadership to alternate according to the skill requirements, the functions to be fulfilled, and the abilities of the group members.

Workgroups and Teams: Similarities and Differences

Most organizations are composed of numerous workgroups, but these will not inevitably become teams. It is not always necessary for a workgroup to develop into a team; however, most teams will first function as effective working groups.

The differences between workgroups and teams were demonstrated in research conducted by Katzenbach and Smith (1993). Workgroups are characterized by the following: a strong clearly focused leader; a purpose that fits with the broader organizational mission; individual members who are accountable for individual work products or outcomes; delegated work; decision making; and efficient meetings. These authors stated that "the best working groups come together to share information, perspectives, and insights; to make decisions that help each person to do his or her job better; and to reinforce individual performance standards. But the focus is always on individual accountability" (p. 112).

Larson and LaFasto (1989) defined teams as consisting of two or more people with specific performance objectives or goals to be achieved. Collaboration within the team is required to coordinate the activities of members and to attain the objectives or goals. The team has a specific purpose and produces work products or outcomes that are the result of collective efforts. The performance of the team is assessed based on these collective accomplishments. The focus on group goals and the satisfaction of achieving them creates a direction, momentum, cohesion, and commitment that go beyond that seen in workgroups.

As explained in Chapters 8 and 9, organizational structure, horizontal coordinating mechanisms, role descriptions, and the arrangements for allocating and coordinating work responsibilities are factors that affect the composition and productivity of workgroups at all levels of the organization. Most workgroups are led by individuals who are acting in their positions of formal authority within the organization. For example, the chief executive officer leads the team of executive-level leaders, usually vice-presidents and directors, who report directly to her or him. Other groups are led by middle managers, first-line managers, or by individuals who have been delegated specific leadership responsibilities, such as team leaders, shift supervisors, or nurses assigned shift-by-shift "in-charge" responsibilities. Appropriate leadership is necessary for workgroups to function cohesively and to accomplish their work. Many organizations provide in-service programs designed to improve the skills of managers in group, team, and project leadership.

Workgroups and teams also differ in their composition. The membership of a workgroup is often determined by environmental and administrative factors such as past recruitment decisions and shift schedules. Membership in many workgroups automatically includes all personnel in a unit or program. In contrast, teams require the right mix of technical and functional expertise, interpersonal skills, and problem-solving and decision-making abilities; therefore, members are selected for their skills and skill potential. A critical factor for team success is support for team efforts from higher levels of management. This enables the team to focus on collective goal achievement and to develop a form of discipline that includes commitment and clear rules of behaviour. A majority of the high performance teams that were studied by Katzenbach and Smith (1993) had no more than 10 members. Their composition is stable when compared to that of many workgroups. Members of teams frequently have fun together and develop a synergistic energy. Teams are not necessarily better than workgroups in every situation, which is fortunate because highly effective teams are relatively rare; however, when such teams do emerge, they are a valuable organizational resource.

Within the organizational context, senior management provides teams with a mandate and a "performance challenge." When the goal is clear and stable and team members have equal power, highly developed relationship skills, and complementary knowledge, teams can often act independently and flexibly in establishing their own specific goals and work plans in response to demands or opportunities presented to them. To be effective, teams must have relatively stable membership, and members must have complimentary knowledge and equal power. This, in turn, facilitates shared leadership and mutual accountability for team outcomes.

Roles of Group Members

The effectiveness of workgroups and teams depends upon the roles, skills, and behaviours of members. Fourteen roles that group members carry out to achieve the functions of the group were described by Dimock (1985). These roles are summarized in Box 21.1. The task roles and the group building and maintenance roles contain 11 functions, all of which are essential to development of the group. The self-orientation role is carried out through three individual functions. Group roles can be assessed by observing the group and keeping a record of the roles each member plays.

Box 21.1

Roles of Group Members

Task Functions
1. Defining problems. Defining the group problem and overall purpose of the group.
2. Seeking information. Clarifying a suggestion or requesting factual information about the group problem or methods to be used.
3. Giving information. Clarifying a suggestion or offering facts or general information about the group problem or methods to be used.
4. Seeking opinions. Asking for the opinions of others relevant to discussion.
5. Giving opinions. Stating beliefs or opinions relevant to discussion.
6. Testing feasibility. Questioning reality, checking practicality of suggested solutions.

Group-Building and Maintenance Functions
1. Coordinating. Clarifying a recent statement and relating it to another statement in such a way as to bring them together. Reviewing proposed alternatives.
2. Mediating/harmonizing. Interceding in disputes or disagreements and attempting to reconcile them. Highlighting similarities in views.
3. Orienting/facilitating. Keeping the group on track, pointing out deviations from agreed upon procedures or from direction of the group discussion. Helping the group progress along, proposing other procedures to make the group more effective.
4. Supporting/encouraging. Expressing approval of others' suggestions, praising others' ideas, being warm and responsive to others' ideas.
5. Following. Going along with the movement of the group, accepting ideas of others, expressing agreement.

Individual Functions
1. Blocking. Interfering with the progress of the group by arguing, resisting, or disagreeing beyond reason, or by coming back to same "dead" issue later.
2. Out of field. Withdrawing from discussion, daydreaming, doing something else, whispering to others, leaving the room, etc.
3. Digressing. Getting off topic, leading discussion in some personally oriented direction, or making a brief statement into a long nebulous speech.

Source: From *How to Observe Your Group* (2nd ed.), by H.G. Dimock, 1985, Guelph, ON: University of Guelph. Copyright 1985 by University of Guelph. Reprinted with permission.

Not all individuals are effective members of groups or teams. Researchers conducted a study to identify specific qualities and behaviours of effective team members by asking 15,000 members of teams in organizations to assess fellow teammates. They developed the *Connect Model*™, a one-page checklist that enables team members to complete a self-assessment of their contributions to collaboration within the team on the dimensions of experience, problem solving, openness and supportiveness, personal initiative, and positive or negative style (LaFasto & Larsen, 2001).

The ability of team members to develop and maintain constructive relationships within the team is also critical to team effectiveness. Based on their studies of 15,000 team members' assessments of each other and data gathered on 35,000 work relationships in organizations, LaFasto and Larsen (2001) concluded that the following behaviours and conditions are necessary for effective relationships within teams:

- Commitment to the work of the team
- Contributing to a feeling of safety by showing respect for others' points of view
- Narrowing discussions to one issue at a time so discussion can move forward in a non-threatening way
- Neutralizing defensiveness
- Explaining one's own position and echoing what others have said to facilitate understanding
- The willingness of each team member to change one behaviour to help the group move forward
- Tracking progress by monitoring agreed-upon indicators

Improving the Performance of Workgroups and Teams

The performance of workgroups and teams can be improved through the efforts of individuals within the group, but it also requires support from the organizational culture and the management practices of organizational leaders.

Shared leadership often characterizes effective teamwork. Blanchard (1991) has emphasized that a group's overall levels of productivity and morale are shaped by specific behaviours that can be performed by any member of the group. The two key behaviours are giving direction and giving support. Direction is given by creating structure through the use of tools like agendas and role and task descriptions; by controlling teamwork through the use of scheduling and time management tools; and by supervising, including identifying areas of activity where the group needs assistance in order to reach its goals. Support is given by praising constructive contributions, listening to various points of view, and facilitating participation so that all members of the group develop an appreciation for each other's contributions and experience a growing sense of commitment to one another and to the goals of the unit, program, or organization.

Training can be a key factor in improving the performance of workgroups and teams. Anderson (1993) cited a number of authorities, including Edward Deming, founder of the quality improvement paradigm that gained prominence in the 1980s. Deming advocated that training in team processes and process improvement should be supplemented by developing skills in communication, chairing, participating, resolving conflict, and problem solving. These skills benefit both the organization and the individual. However, the most important factor in the successful performance of workgroups and teams is leadership and management practices.

Leadership Competence

Leaders often lack insight into the ways their behaviour and priorities affect organizational performance and the performance of teams. The extensive research conducted by LaFasto and Larsen (2001) reveals the importance of effective team leadership at all organizational levels and emphasizes the following leadership behaviours:

- **Focus on the goal:** "Time and time again, we hear team members complain about the 'mission of the month' or the 'vision du jour.' They are referring to team leaders who make changes in the goal with almost no explanation and almost no reference to the past. Such cavalier and amnesiac behavior erodes faith in the leader, the goal, and ultimately the team itself" (LaFasto & Larsen, 2001, p. 100).

- **Ensure a collaborative climate:** This involves making communication safe, but it also involves demanding a collaborative approach, intentionally rewarding collaborative behaviour, and guiding the team's problem-solving efforts.

- **Build confidence:** This is accomplished by helping teams achieve results. It requires that information be shared with team members and that individuals within the team, and the team as a whole, be assigned and trusted with the responsibility to carry out tasks. Micromanagement of the team disempowers team members.

- **Demonstrate sufficient technical know-how:** Team leaders must understand the content or body of knowledge directly related to achievement of the goal, and this can include expert professional knowledge. Knowledge of the organization, its culture, and its external environment may also be necessary. LaFasto and Larsen (2001) state that there is a strong connection between the leader's technical knowledge and the team's goal achievement because "an intimate knowledge of how something works increases the chance of the leader helping the team address the more subtle technical issues that must be addressed to accomplish an objective" (p. 133).

- **Set priorities:** In organizational teamwork, LaFasto and Larsen (2001) advocate that "leaders must scrape away the inessentials and concentrate on a handful of critical initiatives that will advance the team toward its goal" (p. 136).

- **Manage performance:** Team leaders have a responsibility to make performance expectations clear and to give constructive feedback to resolve performance issues. If this is not done, relationships and productivity within the team will deteriorate and there will be no incentive for individuals to strive for above-average performance.

Management Practices

Management practices have the greatest influence on shaping an organizational environment that supports teamwork and collaboration (LaFasto & Larsen, 2001). The responsibilities of senior leaders for the culture of the organization were discussed in Chapters 8 and 13. More specifically, LaFasto and Larsen concluded from their extensive studies that the following three management practices were critical to enabling teams to perform effectively:

1. **Setting a clear direction and a focus on priorities:** When goals and priorities are constantly changing, the time and energy of employees is wasted, and leaders cause confusion and disarray. However, when "management directives and requests are selective and aligned with the overarching objective," they are "more likely to be trusted as making sense rather than one more dartboard attempt at the right strategy" (p. 165).

2. **Balancing resources and demands:** The control of organizational priorities and resources is the prerogative of managers in positions of formal authority. "Temporary imbalances in demands and resources are inevitable but a sustained imbalance is debilitating" (p. 167). Managers must either "scale back" demands or increase resources to enable teams to function. One member of a hospital surgical team who contributed to the research on teams is quoted as saying, "When demands are real, resources shouldn't be imaginary" (p. 168). By listening more carefully to their teams, executives may be able to learn how priorities can be adjusted in order to enable teams to do their best possible work with available resources.

3. **Establishing clear operating principles:** LaFasto and Larsen emphasize the importance of accountability as an operating principle necessary for effective performance of teams, stating: "Any management practice that leaves out accountability is useless, and lack of accountability—for some or for all—causes slippage and impedes teamwork and collaboration" (p. 169). Values of collaboration must be exemplified in leadership behaviour. Organizational politics are "antithetical to collaboration" and should not be allowed to divert valuable time and effort. Organizational structures and processes must support teamwork, and "when structure works well, it adds clarity, stability, and discipline to the coordination of effort" (p. 175). Processes can sometimes overcome constraints caused by structure if they bring the right people together to make decisions and keep interrelated tasks and people appropriately connected with one another.

Challenges of Teamwork in Health Care

Workgroups and teams in health care settings must address and overcome certain challenges that are specific to their environment. These challenges affect both intradisciplinary and interdisciplinary workgroups and teams.

Intradisciplinary teams, composed of members of the same profession, have been common in health organizations for many years. Physicians who work together in a practice or specialty area frequently do so as a team, and in teaching hospitals, such teams often include medical students in various stages of their training. In the early 1950s, the concept of team nursing began to be promoted in order to provide care more efficiently and effectively to groups of patients during severe nursing shortages. Team building within nursing organizations has been advocated as a means of sharing leadership and optimizing accountability (Jacobsen-Webb, 1985).

An interdisciplinary team was defined as "a functioning unit, composed of individuals with varied and specialized training, who coordinate their activities to provide services to a client or group of clients" (Ducanis & Golin, 1979, p. 3). The first intentional efforts to establish health care teams were in community and mental health, child development, and rehabilitation centres. Today, interdisciplinary teams exist in both community and hospital settings, and many include nurses, physicians, social workers, rehabilitation therapists, recreation therapists, respiratory therapists, dieticians, pastoral-care professionals, and volunteers. Although the concept of interdisciplinary teams has been in place for many years, studies to examine the effectiveness and outcomes of the team approach are relatively recent and few.

Although there is broad agreement that teamwork is necessary in health care settings, a number of problems associated with interdisciplinary teamwork in health care have been identified in the literature (see Anderson, 1993; Baggs, Ryan, Phelps, Richeson, & Johnson, 1992; Baggs & Schmitt, 1997; Briggs, 1991; Chavigny, 1988; Deber & Leatt, 1986; Ducanis & Golin, 1979; Fagin, 1992; Fried & Leatt, 1986; Fried, Leatt, Deber, & Wilson, 1988; Temkin-Greener, 1983). These problems include lack of clarity of roles, confusion over accountability, leadership issues, lack of clearly defined mutual goals, poor communication skills, inadequate problem-solving skills, inadequate decision-making methods, infringement of the disciplinary boundaries, and lack of conflict management skills. The group development models provide some insights into how these problems can prevent teams from functioning effectively. Many of these weaknesses in team function arise from lack of group process skills and poor team management in health care situations.

Ducanis and Golin (1979) used a team system model to explore the various and complex dimensions of health care team interaction (Figure 21.2). The health team is conceptualized as an open system incorporating a feedback loop. This feedback loop provides information that will influence and change goals and activities. Three components affect the goals, activities, and outcomes of a team. These are the professional team members, the client and family, and the organizational context.

Professional Team Members

The professionals who come together to make up an interdisciplinary team have each been educated and socialized into the professional norms and standards of their own discipline. Historically, in health care, rigid boundaries have existed around professional disciplines. Stereotypes, distorted perceptions of the roles of other professionals, overlapping of roles, status issues, and varying points of view all contribute to interprofessional conflict and can lead to a poorly functioning team. Structural issues, such as the imbalance of power between physicians and other health professionals, also affect the performance of professional teams and were discussed in Chapter 8.

Figure 21.2 The Team System Model

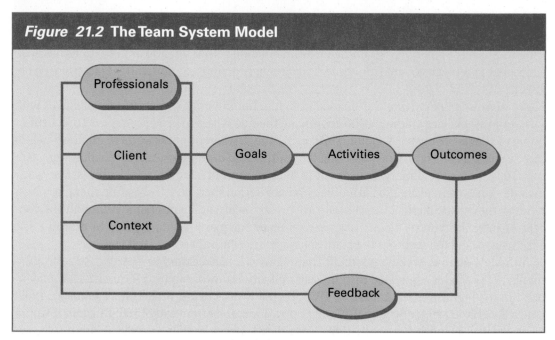

Source: From *The Interdisciplinary Health Care Team: A Handbook*, by A.J. Ducanis and A.K. Golin, 1979, Germantown, MD: Aspen Systems.

Traditional stereotypes colour interactions between professionals and can be illustrated by the "doctor-nurse game" described by Stein in 1967 (Stein, Watts, & Howell, 1990; Copnell et al., 2004). The relationships between physicians and nurses have traditionally appeared to be those of superiors and subordinates. Open disagreement between the two players was to be avoided at all costs. In communication and consultation, the nurse assumed a passive manner and made recommendations in a way that made them appear to have been initiated by the physician rather than the nurse. Nurses working in contemporary health organizations are better educated and more assertive than their earlier counterparts; they seek greater autonomy and expect to have more equal relationships with physicians. The former hierarchical arrangements are beginning to crumble and dissolve, but at a rather slow pace (Ornstein, 1990; Stein et al., 1990). Shortages of primary care providers, consumer demand for holistic care, and the demonstrated cost-effectiveness of advanced nursing practice roles have fuelled the development of collaborative practice between individual professionals and in national, state, and provincial demonstration projects (Sullivan, 1998; Reay, Golden-Biddle, & Germann, 2003a, 2003b). Effective teamwork and collaboration characterize some of the many innovations now seen as key to the sustainability of the health system (Rachlis, 2004; Long, 2001).

Other barriers that contribute to tension between nurses and physicians include the inability of nurses to describe their roles and scope of practice, differences in education levels, sex-role stereotyping and gender differences, social differences, and a tendency among nurses to accord status to "hands-on" activities rather than intellectual activities (Fagin, 1992). These barriers are not unique to nurse-physician relationships. The same types of issues are played out between and among the other professional groups that make up interdisciplinary teams. In a study of multi-disciplinary renal teams across Canada and in Michigan, Deber and Leatt (1986) contrasted descriptions by health care team members of their ideal roles in decision making with their perceptions of their actual roles. The teams consisted of nephrologists, physicians, surgeons, nurses, social workers, dieticians, and technicians. The findings showed that the nephrologists took leadership roles on the teams and assumed the major responsibility and accountability for clinical decision making. Team members from other disciplines deferred to physicians. Nevertheless, the members maintained the ideal of a collaborative multidisciplinary renal team with equal representation and equal decision-making powers.

Status differences among the professions often fuel issues that relate to leadership of the team. Physicians have traditionally assumed, or have been placed in, team leadership roles, but they have often lacked the interpersonal skills needed to develop team cohesion or the values needed to share leadership with other team members when appropriate. As independent practitioners who are also in private business, many have been reluctant to devote time to team conferences or other collaborative activities that are not directly remunerated through fee-for-service. Alternative payment mechanisms for physicians have been widely advocated, and when implemented, may enable physicians to fulfill their potential for non-hierarchical teamwork and collaboration. This would benefit individual patients and the community and make teamwork more rewarding for all professional participants.

Where there are differences between perceptions of the ideal role and the actual role, role conflict and role ambiguity can occur. Role deprivation occurs when the person who occupies a role cannot behave as he or she thinks appropriate. Nurses have expressed feelings of role deprivation in numerous job satisfaction surveys—burnout, frustration, and high turnover have been some of the results. Lack of role clarity among the group members contributes to dysfunction in health care teams.

Specific training for collaborative health teamwork has become a priority (Casto & Julia, 1994; Lowry, Burns, Smith, & Jacobson, 2000). Beginning in 1995, at the University of Alberta, an interdisciplinary course has been offered to undergraduate students from the disciplines of pharmacy, rehabilitation medicine, nursing, medicine, dentistry, and physical education. This course has been designed to promote an appreciation for the contributions of each health discipline and to help students develop skills in collaborative problem solving. A self-directed team of faculty from all participating disciplines leads the course, assisted by tutors from health agencies in the community. This course is now compulsory for students in all health science faculties and related clinical experiences, and advanced courses have also been developed.

Clients and Families in the Health Team

Traditionally, the client has not been seen as part of the interdisciplinary team, but as consumers become more knowledgeable, they have made it clear that they wish to be actively involved in decisions affecting their own health. Today, clients and their families or significant others (often called informal caregivers) are being acknowledged and included as members of the health care team. One psychologist has described how family and friends can supplement the work of professionals in the creation of a team that works with both the "outer environment" of the patient or client as well as that person's "mindfulness" and use of self: "I've seen teams of helpers bring the principles of basic attendance into assisting childbirth, elder-care, and attending the injured, ill and dying. Sometimes these teams have been only loosely knit together; other times they have been well organized and have had team leaders" (Wegela, 1996, p. 198). The evolution of a team like this is described in detail in Callwood's account (1986) of how a group of acquaintances in Toronto, Ontario were drawn together through their concern for an older friend who was dying. Although most had not previously known each other, they became a team to achieve the common purpose of providing palliative care for their friend in her home until she died.

Recent changes in the structure of the health care system have resulted in the need for informal caregivers (a majority of whom are women) to provide many health services to family members in their homes. These structural changes have increased both the level of responsibility and the costs that are borne by families. For example, when intravenous medications were administered in hospital, professionals were responsible for the administration and the equipment, and medications were provided to patients at no charge. Many intravenous medications are now administered at home by family members, and in some provinces, the costs of these medications are now an expense for the patient and family. As these and other direct costs are transferred to individuals and families, it is not surprising that families and informal caregivers now expect to be included in the planning, decision making, and evaluation of the health care they receive and often help to provide.

In the past, when clients and families were occasionally included in care conferences, the purpose was to obtain their cooperation or compliance for a plan that had already been developed by the professional team. Understandably, the experience of "being conferenced" was often intimidating. Clients and their significant others are no longer content with this passive role. Teams of health professionals must become more proactive in developing the values and skills required to include the patient and informal caregivers as equal partners in planning care. This need is also being recognized at the level of the health care system. In many sectors of the health care system today, public advocates have been appointed to represent patients or clients who feel that their needs and interests are not appropriately recognized by health professionals and health care organizations.

Although efforts are being made to increase patient involvement in health care teams, it is worth noting that Spitzer and Roberts (1980) raised several questions about whether people are better off being cared for by teams at all. They asked: Do teams further depersonalize medical care? Do patients prefer health teams? Do they have a choice? Ducanis and Golin (1979) pointed out that the relationship between client and individual professional becomes diluted in the team approach. There is an impact on both the client and the professional. Clients may experience less structure and support with the group approach and feel the loss of the one-to-one relationship. The individual professional may feel a loss of autonomy when decisions made in a one-to-one discussion with the client are subject to team review. There is also the possibility that the client may receive conflicting information from various team members. Some clients and families may feel intimidated by the size and professional composition of the group and, therefore, not see the process as helpful or supportive to them. Few studies of client satisfaction with interdisciplinary teams have been carried out, and studies are needed to provide a basis for continuous improvement by health teams.

The introduction of increased numbers of multi-skilled workers into health care teams and the substitution of other providers for RNs is another issue that directly affects health care consumers. Citizens consistently express higher levels of trust in RNs than in any other professional group (Picard, 2000), yet the composition of workgroups providing health services in hospitals, continuing care, and home care programs increasingly relies upon other workers. The rhetoric accompanying the introduction of patient-focused or patient-centred care models to replace nursing care delivery models in the 1990s de-emphasizes the importance of clinical and leadership expertise of RNs and, instead, presents the notion of "mutual accountability" as a desirable outcome (Schweikhart & Smith-Daniels, 1996). Professional expertise may be diluted in some interdisciplinary teams when educational preparation is unequal and responsibilities overlap (as between RNs and multi-skilled workers). The term *collaboration* is not appropriate to describe such teams since collaboration is a relationship characterized by equal power and complementary expertise.

Self-directed teams have been advocated by management consultants and some health services executives as a way of improving service to patients (Hassen & Lindenburger, 1993), but patient's opinions on this matter are not generally known. However, patients and citizens regularly complain that they do not know who is "in charge" of their care.

Members of the community now expect to be treated as partners in their interactions with the health care system and health professionals. Some client support groups have been successful in making changes to the health care system, and advocacy by such groups can be expected to increase as the population ages and more out-of-pocket expenses are associated with health services. In notorious instances, such as the "tainted blood scandals" in several Western countries and the deaths of children at the Winnipeg Health Sciences Centre (Sinclair, 2001) and the Bristol Infirmary (Bristol Royal Infirmary Enquiry, 2001), patients were deceived and treated disrespectfully. Public tolerance for such behaviour by health professionals and leaders has been exhausted, and increased transparency and accountability are now required to meet consumer expectations. This issue is discussed in greater depth in Chapter 13. Teams that share knowledge, values, and leadership among professionals and with clients can be mechanisms for constructive change in the health care system.

The Organizational Context of Teamwork

An organization is a social system and therefore has a unique culture and climate. Teamwork and collaboration require organizational support to develop and be successful (Wellins, Byham, & Dixon, 1994; Zenger, Musselwhite, Hurson, & Perrin, 1994).

In traditional organizations, work was determined and planned by managers. Managers were the custodians of information and made most organizational decisions, which were then communicated to workers. Employees, for the most part, had narrowly defined roles or skill sets, and training opportunities, when available, were usually focused on upgrading technical skills. When support staff or specialized skills were needed, staff specialists were usually imported from outside the working group to fulfill the needs. Rewards were based on individual performance, and there were hazards associated with risk taking.

In team-centred organizations, by contrast, managers and team members jointly define goals and tasks. Where positions and roles need broader knowledge, training in interpersonal and administrative skill areas is provided to supplement technical knowledge. Cross-training, in which workers learn skills and roles additional to those associated with their own positions, was once viewed as inefficient but is now widely advocated. Support staff and skills as well as leadership skills are now often incorporated into teams rather than being provided from a central source. To improve the climate for teamwork and collaboration, health organizations must review their philosophies, reward systems, supervisory practices, and organizational support systems to ensure that they support and encourage teamwork.

In the 1980s and early 1990s, there were attempts to decentralize decision making and empower workgroups and teams responsible for patient care through the introduction of quality improvement programs. However, many such initiatives were introduced in parallel with organizational downsizing and restructuring that included the introduction of program management. These management decisions were touted as an approach that would create improved coordination and more egalitarian teamwork among the professionals and departments who served particular patient groups (Hassen & Lindenburger, 1993). As explained in Chapters 8 and 9, some functional departments, including nursing, were broken down, although other disciplinary and professional structures remained in place, reinforcing the structural differences in power already present in health organizations and teams. Multi-skilled workers were introduced, accountability in work teams was diffused, and self-directed teams were advocated as the way of the future. It was assumed and claimed that these changes would improve teamwork, clinical outcomes, and patient satisfaction while reducing costs, but this has not yet been conclusively demonstrated. However, there is now a consensus that the organizational instability created by these changes is a root cause of adverse occurrences in hospitals (National Steering Committee on Patient Safety, 2002). Evidence from studies such as those carried out by LaFasto and Larsen (2001) suggests that the idea of self-directed clinical teams in hospitals may be misplaced unless team members have the complimentary levels of expertise, power, and interpersonal and relationship skills that are required for successful collaboration. If leaders of clinical teams do not possess the necessary skills for team leadership, these teams cannot perform in a timely and effective manner. Health outcomes such as death and complication rates, and organizational outcomes such as the ability to attract and retain registered nurses, have been linked to dysfunctional relationships in clinical teams. The results of attempting to introduce quality improvement initiatives, which depend on active teamwork, at the same time as massive downsizing have been described as "disastrous" (Rondeau & Wagar, 2004).

In organizational forms such as program management, there is a need for increased communication, coordination, and collaboration. Senior leaders in the organization are responsible for creating a culture and modelling behaviours that assure such collaboration. Leaders at all levels of the organization must be proficient as members or leaders of teams that may form and re-form frequently. Within regionalized health care systems, the need to implement, manage, and coordinate regional systems has led to more centralized organizational structures and management approaches. In larger and centrally administered organizations, it can be more difficult to provide meaningful leadership to workgroups and teams at the level of care units and worksites.

Hackman (1990) pointed out that groups cannot flourish when members have multiple tasks to perform, when staff assignments continually shift or group membership changes, and when organizational rewards are based on the individual rather than the team. Under these conditions, issues of quality of service arise, and tension develops concerning how to work effectively and efficiently within limited time constraints.

Health care teams associated with teaching hospitals face particular challenges because these settings often include learners who rotate in and out of teams. These learners may not yet have acquired group skills, and the development of their clinical expertise may also be in the early stages. However, they may be more likely than some permanent members of the group to see issues and situations from a client's perspective, and it is incumbent upon the leaders and permanent members of the team to find ways of including and maximizing the contributions of students.

Another context-related problem faced by interdisciplinary health teams in recent years has been the impact of personnel changes that are the result of layoffs and "bumping," particularly of nurses, but also of some other professionals. In many health organizations, the number of permanent full-time and part-time positions decreased, and the number of casual or call-in workers increased through restructuring in order for the organization to reduce costs associated with employee benefits. Ironically, this happened at a time when the importance of teamwork was being presented to professionals as the reason for organizational re-design and restructuring activities. Evidence of the importance of stability and effective relationships in high-performance teams suggests that eliminating permanent positions to save benefits costs in the short term is a false economy. When the membership of workgroups and teams is constantly changing, the cohesiveness, group competence, and commitment that are necessary for high team productivity cannot be achieved.

Leading and Developing Workgroups and Teams

Managers at all levels in health organizations must assume greater responsibility for effective leadership of workgroups and teams, and nurse managers have multiple roles in this regard. First and foremost, they lead working groups of staff, in particular, nursing units or programs. At this level, workgroups are responsible for many outcomes, including meeting the health needs of clients and ensuring client and family satisfaction with the care being provided. Staff satisfaction often results when working groups and teams accomplish this work effectively. In addition, the nurse manager and the unit or program staff may participate in one or more interdisciplinary teams or serve on various inter- and intradisciplinary committees, task forces, or project teams of the kind described in Chapter 24. The manager may take a leadership role in some cases, a membership role in others. As explained in Chapter 24, the skills of successful teamwork and team leadership are critical to the success of projects (see Glaser, 2004; Loo, 2003; Nordqvist, Hovmark, & Zika-Viktorsson, 2004; Thamhain, 2004; Turner, 2004; Vaaland, 2004). Reay and colleagues (2003a, 2003b) have pointed out that successful introduction of new roles, such as that of nurse practitioner, depends on managerial activities and effectiveness and not merely on the knowledge and abilities of individual nurse practitioners. Varney (1989) believed that managers must not only know what constitutes effective teamwork, they must also develop the abilities to observe, diagnose, and problem solve to promote effectiveness. Managers need to know the abilities and readiness of team members to take on the responsibility of the tasks they have been assigned, and they must be able to adjust their leadership style to fit the situation. As groups become empowered and self-managed, managers need to know when to step aside and support the group in other ways.

Studies have shown that leadership styles can range from an autocratic, authoritarian style to a democratic, more participative style. The situational leadership model (Hersey & Blanchard, 1982) is discussed in Chapter 14. It is a particularly useful model for group or team leaders because it suggests ways of varying leadership style to match the abilities and motivations of group members. Within the situational leadership framework, leadership style is described as the behaviour pattern of an individual, as perceived by others, when that person is attempting to influence a group.

A leader's own perception of his or her behaviour (self-perception) may be very different from that of the group members. Leadership style is determined by the combination of two factors: task behaviours and relationship behaviours. Task behaviours are behaviours by which the leader organizes the group and establishes the channels of communication and the ways of getting the task done. Relationship behaviours are behaviours that facilitate relationships between the leader and the group members, open up communication, and provide socioemotional support. The effectiveness of the leadership style is determined by the appropriateness of that style to the environment in which it is being used.

Both the readiness level of individuals and the readiness level of the group as a whole can be considered in this model. Groups that come together frequently and interact to achieve tasks can reach a high level of readiness in their group behaviour. The leader may then choose to deal with the group as a whole with an approach that matches its readiness level. However, the leader also understands that there are differing levels of readiness among the individuals who make up the group and therefore uses a variety of styles when interacting with individual members. Building on this notion, Dimock (1987) suggests that the group members and the situation determine the appropriate leadership style. He advises group leaders to start groups off with a structured and directive approach. At the same time, the leader should assess the abilities of the group members and then slowly move along the continuum to a more facilitative coaching style according to member readiness.

In contemporary organizations, leaders at all levels must have the skills and willingness to provide leadership to groups and teams. A specific performance challenge that is clear and compelling to all team members can be as important as the team leader in determining a team's performance (Katzenbach & Smith, 1993). This speaks to the need for leaders to engage workers in goal setting, decision making, and developing new initiatives. Workgroups or teams are sometimes brought together precisely because the diverse perspectives and skills of their members are needed to accomplish a task or carry out a project. When participants possess high levels of skill, readiness, and a shared commitment to the task at hand, there is often a natural sharing of task leadership among group members, as well as consideration and support. Under these conditions, a self-directed team may naturally evolve.

Some organizations provide specific in-service training to employees to assist them in developing skills of group leadership and followership. Farley and Stoner (1989) presented a useful model that can assist leaders in evaluating their team building efforts by suggesting "ideal outcomes" that characterize various stages of the team building process.

Collaboration

Collaboration is a complex concept that involves shared power as well as shared goals and commitments (Henneman, Lee, & Cohen, 1995). In recent years, extensive nursing literature on collaboration has focused on the need for collaborative skills in emerging advanced practice roles (Sullivan, 1998). Many benefits of clinical collaboration have been discussed, and it has been demonstrated that patient outcomes are improved when nurses and physicians collaborate to provide care.

The values and skills of collaboration can also be applied to relationships with clients and their significant others and to interdepartmental relationships. Nursing and health care leaders can create structures and an organizational culture that will foster and accelerate these types of collaboration. However, they must also be concerned with other forms of collaboration that go beyond the relationships between clinical professionals, disciplines, and organizational departments to the relationships between health sectors and organizations.

Intersectoral Collaboration

The various settings in which health care has been delivered, and their governing or organizational structures, are commonly referred to as *sectors* of the health system. Examples of these sectors are acute care, long-term or continuing care, community health, home care, rehabilitation, and mental health. These sectors have sometimes been referred to as "silos" or "stovepipes," and one focus of health system restructuring has been to alter the traditional arrangements between the sectors in order to align policies and create incentives and structures to accelerate the pace and effectiveness of collaboration between them. To achieve intersectoral collaboration, care providers and leaders from more than one sector work together to plan for services for a particular population across the continuum of care. For example, to plan for a comprehensive and integrated array of services for older people, representatives from the sectors listed above would work with each other and also with providers of services that are outside the health care system, such as housing, transportation, and income support.

Efforts to improve intersectoral collaboration have been actively underway in most provinces since the early 1990s. In the province of Saskatchewan, specific structural changes were made by the provincial government to integrate ambulance services and mental health services (which remain separate sectors in some provinces) with other health services. Other government-level incentives have encouraged voluntary organizations (e.g., church-owned hospitals and long-term care centres) to collaborate with the boards of health regions. The Saskatoon Health Region has developed and sustained a unique structure in which the responsibilities of regional vice-presidents and senior managers cut across sectoral boundaries for particular client populations. Intersectoral collaboration is particularly important for the care of people with chronic illnesses, who use many services that are not provided by hospitals and physicians.

Interorganizational Collaboration

Interorganizational collaboration is collaboration between independent organizations or corporations. Organizations may undertake collaborations for the purposes of planning, policy making, political action, or knowledge development. There is usually the expectation of mutual benefit, and one benefit of collaboration between organizations is the sharing of risks and costs. Interorganizational collaboration is illustrated by the common efforts of several professional associations to advocate for seat belt legislation or by the efforts of health regions to achieve economies of scale through bulk purchasing. Citizens and consumer advocacy organizations sometimes collaborate with one another to influence the policy-making process. Although health regions, government, and professional associations often attempt to gain the support of consumer organizations on particular issues, citizen participation through interorganizational collaboration with health boards is still relatively rare. Organizations may choose to collaborate with one another on specific issues, or they may formalize collaborative practices and goals through formal partnership agreements or contracts. In some instances of intersectoral collaboration, interorganizational collaboration is necessary to facilitate or achieve the collaboration (van Eyk & Baum, 2002).

Collaboration Between Researchers and Decision Makers

Collaboration between researchers and decision makers has been actively encouraged in recent years by agencies that fund health services research. The need to accelerate the application of knowledge to policy and management decisions has been identified in a broadly based consultation with stakeholders in the health care system. Certain kinds of research funding are now contingent upon the ability of the research team to develop and sustain partnerships with executive-level decision makers who are responsible for policy decision making or with program-level decision makers who implement and manage programs and services. As discussed in Chapter 17, such partnerships are proving to be an effective mechanism for knowledge transfer. Three types of collaboration between researchers and decision makers have been described (Ross, Lavis, Rodriguez, Woodside, & Denis, 2003). Decision makers may collaborate with researchers as formal supporters, responsive audiences, or integral partners. By creating opportunities for staff members to become involved in research and by becoming involved as research partners themselves, leaders are making a long-term investment for their organizations and for the health care system.

Collaboration is the way of the future, and skills of collaboration are now synonymous with leadership. References that describe various types of collaboration have been included at the end of this chapter in the Further Reading section.

Leadership Implications

The study of groups has a long history, but knowledge specific to designing and maintaining effective workgroups in organizations has not been consolidated and systematically applied (Goodman & Associates, 1986). It is now recognized as important to study the processes and outcomes of teamwork and collaboration, but unfortunately, available evidence from such studies is not always applied in organizational decision making. More knowledge about the functioning and outcomes of various types of health care teams is needed. The growing body of knowledge on collaboration emphasizes the importance of equal power and complementary expertise in collaborative relationships (Sullivan, 1998). The importance of organizational values, culture, and leadership to the outcomes of clinical teamwork has been acknowledged in recent studies (Cummings, 2003; Cummings & Estabrooks, 2003; Rondeau & Wagar, 2004).

Whatever the focus or goal of workgroups, teams, and organizations, three dimensions of group effectiveness are important (Hackman, 1990). These are productivity, the process of the work, and the personal well-being of the members. In terms of productivity, the results of the group's work need to conform to a standard of quality, quantity, and timeliness for the client; in other words, clients must be satisfied with the results. The process of doing the work should contribute to achieving the purpose of the group. Ideally, relationships are established whereby members enjoy the work and feel they have had developmental opportunities that contribute to their well-being. Because groups, teams, and organizations are social systems, they will behave at various levels within a climate of incentives. Leaders who hope to improve the quality and quantity of teamwork and collaboration must find ways to create conditions that enhance and reward the behaviours and values of the group.

When environmental conditions are uncertain and the pace of change is rapid, it is challenging for leaders to be able to create the conditions in which risk taking is encouraged and rewarded. However, these conditions are usually required for optimal productivity by groups, teams, and collaborating partners. Trust occurs in an organizational culture that is characterized by honesty and integrity, openness and willingness to share and receive information, consistency of responses and behaviour, and respect, including treating each other with fairness and dignity (Larson & LaFasto, 1989). Recent research suggests that another critical factor in the development and maintenance of trust in a group over time is the experience of working together to achieve real results (Katzenbach & Smith, 1993). Other research has highlighted the key role of organizational leaders and team leaders in assuring that teamwork and collaboration are effective, pointing out that "teams without formal leadership are consistently poor at managing their own performance...[and] when such teams come off track they are much less likely to be self-corrective" (LaFasto & Larsen, 2001, p. 149). These findings point to the need for leaders to be careful in the way they structure teams and set goals; the need to develop organizational capacity for teamwork, collaboration, and team leadership; and most importantly, the need for conservation of the human and organizational capital represented by existing or developing teams.

Summary

- Health care organizations now recognize the necessity for members and leaders in all health disciplines to be able to work effectively together in the interests of the client.
- The characteristics of professional roles, accompanied by traditional hierarchical relationships among professions, can produce conflict and dysfunction in workgroups and teams in health care settings. This can interfere with meeting client needs and achieving organizational goals. Health care managers must learn ways to address these obstacles to enable groups to function more effectively.
- Groups and teams develop a shared history and life of their own, as demonstrated in the various models of group development. Knowledge about stages of group development and awareness of strategies to shape the course of group development are vital strengths for health care leaders, today and in the future.
- Group or team members can assume various roles, and the best approach to leading a group is one that takes into account the maturity, abilities, and motivation of group members.
- The skills involved in assuming, sharing, and delegating leadership within groups or teams are of critical importance. These skills will become increasingly indispensable as the complexities of client care and organizational life dictate the need for groups and teams to form, perform, and disband quickly and effectively according to needs and circumstances.
- Workgroups and teams in health care organizations face some unique and complex challenges. Gaps, duplication, and a lack of coordination in providing service are some consequences of delaying or failing to overcome these challenges. Mistakes or unnecessary costs may also be consequences.
- Progressive health organizations are now developing management approaches, training programs, and organizational and leadership supports to facilitate effective teamwork and collaboration.
- The ability to contribute to groups and teams as a participating member is now an essential professional skill that can be improved upon throughout one's career.
- The values and skills of collaboration are now needed by leaders at all levels and in all sectors of the health care system.
- Collaboration works best when collaborators have equal power and complimentary expertise.
- Self-directed or leaderless teams have been shown to be poor at managing their own performance or correcting performance problems.
- Effective team leadership and management practices are needed if teams are to achieve results. When team members have the necessary knowledge and skills, participatory and empowering leadership strategies contribute to effective team performance.

Applying the Knowledge in this Chapter

Exercise

Think of a group or team that you have worked with or are now working with, and answer the following questions with that group or team in mind:

1. What is the purpose of the group/team?

2. Why or how was it formed?

3. Does the group have a leader?

4. How was the leader chosen?

5. Refer to Box 21.1, Roles of Group Members. Describe how the task functions, building and maintenance functions, and individual functions are handled by the group.

6. Is the group you have described a workgroup or a team? Use examples to support your answer.

7. Describe an example of collaboration from your own experience. Was the collaboration clinical, intersectoral, interorganizational, or between researchers and decision makers? Why was collaboration necessary, and what were the outcomes?

Resources

Further Reading

Chaleff, I. (1995). *The courageous follower: Standing up to and for our leaders*. San Francisco: Berrett-Koehler.
The author of this book is a consultant to leading industries and governments. He points out that a follower is not necessarily a subordinate, but shares with the leader a common responsibility for the organization's purpose and stakeholders. The practical and values-based approach outlined in this book challenges individuals to assume responsibility for sharing leadership, supporting leaders, and where necessary, challenging leaders.

Douglass, M., & Douglass, N. (1992). *Time management for teams*. New York: Amacom.
This publication of the American Management Association reflects the new organizational reality in which teams assume responsibility for their own leadership and productivity. It includes practical suggestions and worksheets to assist groups in managing their time, as well as sections on making meetings productive, managing "the boss," and teaming up with support staff.

Katzenbach, J.R., & Smith, D.K. (1993). *The wisdom of teams: Creating the high-performance organization*. New York: Harper Business.
The authors have conducted research with large numbers of teams in business, volunteer, and public organizations. They describe the differences between teams and workgroups and discuss factors involved in improving the performance of teams. An abridged version of the original book (without bibliographical references and index), published in 1994, contains a question-and-answer guide that contrasts the commonly assumed answers to questions about teams with the research findings of the authors.

Zenger, J.H., Musselwhite, E., Hurson, K., & Perrin, C. (1994). *Leading teams: Mastering the new role*. New York: Irwin Professional Publishing.
The authors of this book have had varied careers in business education as corporate executives and leaders of teams. They link the need for high-level team performance to the widely acknowledged need for organizations to move from being internally driven to customer driven, to move from a focus on process to a focus on function, and to move from a management-centred approach to greater employee involvement. Practical approaches for developing teams are presented. The final section of the book is a series of profiles in team leadership that are excerpts from research interviews. These provide insight into the thinking and skills of effective team leaders.

References

Anderson, L.K. (1993). Teams: Group process, success, and barriers. *Journal of Nursing Administration, 23*(9), 15–19.

Baggs, J.G., Ryan, S.A., Phelps, C.E., Richeson, J.F., & Johnson, J. (1992). The association between interdisciplinary collaboration and patient outcomes. *Heart & Lung, 21*(1), 18–24.

Baggs, J.G., & Schmitt, M.H. (1997). Nurses' and resident physicians' perceptions of the process of collaboration in an MICU. *Research in Nursing and Health, 20*(1), 71–80.

Bailey, J., & Armer, J.M. (1998). Registered nurse-physician collaborative practice: Success stories. In T. J. Sullivan (Ed.), *Collaboration: A health care imperative* (pp. 225–249). New York: McGraw-Hill.

Bales, R.F. (1950). *Interaction process analysis: A method for the study of small groups*. Reading, MA: Addison-Wesley.

Beverley, L., Dobson, D., Atkinson, M., & Caldwell, L. (1997). Development and evaluation of interdisciplinary team standards of patient care. *Healthcare Management Forum, 10*(4), 35–39.

Bion, R.W. (1961). *Experiences in groups*. New York: Basic Books.

Blanchard, K. (1991). Get your group to perform like a team. *Inside Guide, 12,* 13, 16.

Boshear, W.C., & Albrecht, K.G. (1977). *Understanding people: Models and concepts*. San Diego, CA: University Associates.

Bradford, L.P. (1978). *Group development* (2nd ed.). San Diego, CA: University Associates.

Briggs, M.H. (1991). Team development: Decision-making for early intervention. Infant-toddler intervention. *The Transdisciplinary Journal, 1*(1), 1–9.

Bristol Royal Infirmary Enquiry. (2001, July). *The report of the public inquiry into children's heart surgery at the Bristol Royal Infirmary 1984–1995: Learning from Bristol*. London: Stationery Office.

Callwood, J. (1986). *Twelve weeks in spring*. Toronto, ON: Key Porter.

Canadian Council on Health Services Accreditation. (2002). *AIM: Achieving improved measurement: Accreditation program*. Ottawa, ON: Author.

Casto, R.M. & Julia, M.C. (1994). *Interprofessional care and collaborative practice*. Pacific Grove, CA: Brooks/Cole Publishing Co.

Chavigny, K.H. (1988). Coalition building between medicine and nursing. *Nursing Economics, 6*(4), 179–184.

Copnell, B., Johnston, L., Harrison, D., Wilson, A., Robson, A., Mulcahy, C., et al. (2004). Clinical nursing related to specific groups: Doctors' and nurses' perceptions of interdisciplinary collaboration in the NICU, and the impact of a neonatal nurse practitioner model of practice. *Journal of Clinical Nursing, 13*(1), 105–113.

Cummings, G. (2003). *The effects of hospital restructuring on nurses: How emotionally intelligent leadership mitigates these effects*. Unpublished doctoral dissertation, University of Alberta, Edmonton, Alberta, Canada.

Cummings, G. & Estabrooks, C.A. (2003). The effects of hospital restructuring that included layoffs on individual nurses who remained employed: A systematic review of impact. *International Journal of Sociology and Social Policy, 23*(8/9), 8–53.

Deber, R., & Leatt, P. (1986). The multidisciplinary renal team: Who makes the decisions? *Health Matrix, 4*(3), 3–9.

Dimock, H.G. (1985). *How to observe your group* (2nd ed.). Guelph, ON: University of Guelph.

Dimock, H.G. (1987). *Groups: Leadership and group development* (Rev. ed.). San Diego, CA: University Associates.

Ducanis, A.J., & Golin, A.K. (1979). *The interdisciplinary health care team: A handbook*. Germantown, MD: Aspen Systems.

Elmore, R.F. (2000). Building a new structure for school leadership. Washington, DC: Albert Shanker Institute. Retrieved December 4, 2003, from http://www.shankerinstitute.org/Downloads/building.pdf

Fagin, C.M. (1992). Collaboration between nurses & physicians: No longer a choice. *Nursing & Health Care, 13*(7), 354–363.

Farley, M.J., & Stoner, M.H. (1989). The nurse executive and interdisciplinary team-building. *Nursing Administration, 13*(2), 24–30.

Fried, B.J., & Leatt, P. (1986). Role perceptions among occupational groups in an ambulatory care setting. *Human Relations, 39*(12), 1155–1173.

Fried, B.J., Leatt, P., Deber, R., & Wilson, E. (1988). Multidisciplinary teams in health care: Lessons from oncology and renal teams. *Healthcare Management Forum, 1*(4), 28–34.

Glaser, J. (2004). Back to basics: Managing IT projects. *Healthcare Financial Management, 58*(7), 34–38.

Goodman, P.S. & Associates. (1986). *Designing effective workgroups*. San Francisco: Jossey-Bass.

Hackman, J.R. (1990). *Groups that work (and those that don't): Creating conditions for effective teamwork*. San Francisco: Jossey-Bass.

Hassen, P., & Lindenburger, S. (1993). *Rx for hospitals: New hope for Medicare in the nineties*. Toronto, ON: Stoddart Publishing.

Henneman, E.A., Lee, J.L., & Cohen, J.I. (1995). Collaboration: A concept analysis. *Journal of Advanced Nursing, 21*(1), 103–109.

Hersey, P., & Blanchard, K. (1982). *Management of organizational behaviour: Utilizing human resources* (4th ed.). Englewood Cliffs, NJ: Prentice-Hall.

Jacobsen-Webb, M.L. (1985). Team building: Key to executive success. *Journal of Nursing Administration, 15*(2), 16–21.

Janis, I.L. (1983). *Groupthink* (2nd ed.). Boston: Houghton Mifflin.

Jones, J.E. (1991). A model of group development. In J.W. Pfeiffer & A.C. Ballew (Eds.). *Theories and models in applied behavioral science. Vol. 2*. San Diego, CA: Pfeiffer and Company. (Original article published in 1974.)

Katzenbach, J.H., & Smith, D.K. (1993). The discipline of teams. *Harvard Business Review, 71*(2), 111–120.

Kerr, N.L., & Bruun, S.E. (1981). Ringelmann revisited: Alternative explanations for the social loafing effect. *Personality and Social Psychology Bulletin, 7*, 224–231.

Kerr, N.L., & Bruun, S.E. (1983). Dispensability of member effort and group motivation losses: Free-rider effects. *Journal of Personality and Social Psychology, 44*(1), 78–94.

Lacoursiere, R.B. (1974). A group method to facilitate learning during the stages of psychiatric affiliation. *International Journal of Group Psychotherapy, 24*, 342–351.

Lacoursiere, R.B. (1980). *The life cycle of groups: Group development stage theory*. New York: Human Science Press.

LaFasto, F., & Larsen, C.E (2001). *When teams work best: 6,000 team members and leaders tell what it takes to succeed*. Thousand Oaks, CA: Sage Publications.

Larsen, C.E., & LaFasto, F. (1989). *Teamwork: What must go right/what can go wrong*. Newbury Park, CA: Sage.

Latane, B. (1986). Responsibility and effort in organizations. In P.S. Goodman & Associates (Eds.), *Designing effective workgroups* (pp. 277–304). San Francisco: Jossey-Bass.

Long, K.A. (2001). A reality-oriented approach to interdisciplinary work. *Journal of Professional Nursing, 17*(6), 278–282.

Loo, R. (2003). Project management: A core competency for professional nurses and nurse managers. *Journal for Nurses in Staff Development, 19*(4), 187–193.

Lowry, L., Burns, C.M., Smith, A., & Jacobson, H. (2000). Compete or complement? An interdisciplinary approach to training health professionals. *Nursing and Health Care Perspectives 21*(2), 76–80.

Luft, J. (1970). *Group processes: An introduction to group dynamics* (2nd ed.). Palo Alto, CA: Mayfield.

National Steering Committee on Patient Safety. (2002). *Building a safer system: A national integrated strategy for improving patient safety in Canadian health care*. Ottawa, ON: Author.

Nordqvist, S., Hovmark, S., & Zika-Viktorsson, A. (2004). Perceived time pressure and social processes in project teams. *International Journal of Project Management, 22*(6), 463–468.

Ornstein, H.J. (1990). Collaborative practice between Ontario nurses and physicians: Is it possible? *Canadian Journal of Nursing Administration, 3*(4), 10–14.

Pheiffer, J.W. (Ed.). (1991). *Theories and models in applied behavioral science, Vol. 2.* San Diego, CA: Pheiffer & Company.

Picard, A. (2000). *Critical care: Canadian nurses speak for change*. Toronto, ON: Harper Collins.

Rachlis, M. (2004). *Prescription for excellence: How innovation is saving Canada's health care system*. Toronto, ON: Harper Collins.

Reay, T., Golden-Biddle, K., & Germann, K. (2003a). *How nurse practitioners and middle managers are acting to create work role changes*. Best Papers Proceedings of the Academy of Management in Seattle, Washington.

Reay, T., Golden-Biddle, K., & Germann, K. (2003b). Challenges and leadership strategies for managers of nurse practitioners. *Journal of Nursing Management, 11*(6), 396–403.

Rondeau, K.V., & Wagar, T.H. (2004). Implementing CQI while reducing the work force: How does it influence hospital performance? *Healthcare Management Forum, 17*(2), 22–29.

Ross, S., Lavis, J., Rodriguez, C., Woodside, J., & Denis, J.L. (2003). Partnership experiences: Involving decision-makers in the research process. *Journal of Health Services Research and Policy, 8*(Suppl 2), 26–34.

Schutz, W. (1958). *Firo: A three dimensional theory of interpersonal behavior*. New York: Holt, Rinehart and Winston.

Schweikhart, S.B., & Smith-Daniels, V. (1996). Reengineering the work of caregivers: Role redefinition, team structures, and organizational redesign. *Hospital & Health Services Administration, 41*(1), 19–35.

Sinclair, C.M. (2001, May). *The report of the Manitoba pediatric cardiac surgery inquest: An inquiry into twelve deaths at the Winnipeg Health Sciences Centre in 1994*. Winnipeg, MB: Provincial Court of Manitoba.

Slavin, R.E. (1992). When and why does cooperative learning increase achievement: Theoretical and empirical perspectives. In R. Hertz-Lazarowitz & R. Miller (Eds.), *Interaction in cooperative groups* (pp. 145–173). New York, NY: Cambridge University Press.

Spitzer, W.O., & Roberts, R.F. (1980). Twelve questions about teams in health services. *Journal of Community Health, 6*(1), 1–5.

Stein, L.I., Watts, D.T., & Howell, T. (1990). The doctor-nurse game revisited. *The New England Journal of Medicine, 322*(8), 546–549.

Sullivan, T.J. (1998). *Collaboration: A health care imperative*. New York: McGraw-Hill.

Temkin-Greener, H. (1983). Interprofessional perspectives on teamwork in health care: A case study. *Milbank Memorial Fund Quarterly, 61*(4), 641–658.

Thamhain, H.J. (2004). 15 rules for consulting in support of a client project. *Consulting to Management, 15*(2), 42–46.

Tuckman, B.W. (1965). Developmental sequence in small groups. *Psychological Bulletin, 63*(6), 384–399.

Tuckman, B.W., & Jensen, M.A. (1977). Stages of small group development revisited. *Group & Organization Studies, 2*(4), 419–427.

Turner, J.R. (2004). Five necessary conditions for project success. *International Journal of Project Management, 22*(5), 349–350.

Vaaland, T.I. (2004). Improving project collaboration: Start with the conflicts. *International Journal of Project Management, 22*(6), 447–454.

van Eyk, H., & Baum, F. (2002). Learning about interagency collaboration: Trialling collaborative projects between hospitals and community health services. *Health and Social Care in the Community, 10*(4), 262–269.

Varney, G.H. (1989). *Building productive teams*. San Francisco: Jossey-Bass.

Wegela, K.K. (1996). *How to be a help instead of a nuisance*. Boston: Shambhala Publications.

Wellins, R., Byham, W., & Dixon, G. (1994). *Inside teams: How 20 world-class organizations are winning through teamwork*. San Francisco: Jossey-Bass.

Young, J.M., Ang, R., & Findlay, T. (1997). Interdisciplinary professional practice leadership within a program model: BC's rehab experience. *Healthcare Management Forum, 10*(4), 48–50.

Zander, A. (1986). *Making groups effective*. San Francisco: Jossey-Bass.

Zenger, J., Musselwhite, E., Hurson, K, & Perrin, C. (1994). *Leading teams: Mastering the new role*. New York: Irwin Professional Publishing.

LEADING AND MANAGING CHANGE

Judith Skelton-Green

Learning Objectives

In this chapter, you will learn:

- Changes affecting the health care system

- Basic types of change, and different models of change management

- The difference between change and transition and the interdependence of these concepts

- Processes that a nurse leader may use in responding to, and championing, change

- Tools and strategies that can be used to implement change

- How to create a change-ready culture in your nursing unit

Changes in the health care system, and in the world at large, place unprecedented pressure on health service organizations and have particular impact on the ways in which these organizations are led and managed. Vaill (1989) used the image of "permanent whitewater" to describe the environment of chaotic change prevalent in most organizations. This image is intended to capture the speed, unpredictability, novelty, complexity, and excitement of the world in which business exists today. Those involved in the health care system often feel as if they are caught in whitewater situations and are paddling upstream. Today, and for the future, nurse leaders require an ability to deal with change positively. They are challenged to embrace change in a way that will allow them to position themselves and their organizations effectively for the future.

Nurse leaders who wish to promote and facilitate change need (a) knowledge about change and change management, (b) the ability to differentiate between change and transition, (c) a positive attitude toward change, and (d) a set of tools and strategies that they can apply to the specific changes they encounter.

Changes Affecting the Health Care System

Like all businesses in North America, the Canadian health care system is experiencing a period of significant and widespread change. Some of the changes are spontaneous; others have been planned. Still others are seriously needed but have not yet begun. In the past few years, there have been a number of landmark reports documenting the current state of our health care system and making recommendations for its future (see Commission d'étude, 2001; Commission on Medicare, 2001; Commission on the Future, 2002; Premier's Advisory Council, 2001; Standing Senate Committee, 2002). In these reports, there is remarkable consistency both in the descriptions of the present challenges and in the desired characteristics of the future. The signing of the *2003 First Ministers' Accord on Health Care Renewal* (Health Canada, 2003), known as the Health Accord, signaled significant agreement on the kinds of changes that we will see in the next decade.

Funding

In the 1990s, the federal government dramatically reduced the amount of money it was transferring to the provinces for health care. Provincial governments, struggling with their own debt and deficit problems, in turn decreased health care funding in most if not all sectors. In some provinces, funding responsibility was further devolved to municipalities by creating funding "envelopes" held and managed by boards located in smaller geographic regions. Since 2000, the federal government has been increasing its contribution to health care. The 2003 Health Accord confirms that this trend will continue in the near future (Health Canada, 2003). Any time there is a significant adjustment in funding, whether it is a decrease or an increase, there will be dramatic changes in the system as it struggles to make the best possible decisions on what services to provide and how to provide them within the current budget.

Service Delivery

Restructuring of Canadian health care services has been initiated at a variety of levels to achieve a number of basic objectives, most of which can be summarized as attempts to increase the efficiency or effectiveness of health care interventions. Examples of changes in service delivery include the following:

- Hospital closures and amalgamations and reductions in inpatient hospital beds
- Increases in non-invasive and outpatient surgery
- Increases in the number and kinds of services offered to patients through ambulatory care clinics and home care
- Increases in the number of services targeted to older adults
- Development of primary care teams of physicians, nurse practitioners, and other professionals to replace traditional solo-practice family physicians
- Increases in the number and range of services offered by the private sector, particularly in the area of alternative therapies
- Establishment of regional health authorities, whose mandate is to coordinate and integrate multiple aspects of care delivery, from acute care in hospitals to community care and mental health services

Health Promotion and Wellness

The benefits of health promotion and wellness are slowly becoming driving forces for system restructuring. A plethora of literature outlines the benefits, both tangible and intangible, of health promotion and illness prevention. Appropriate patient screening, education, and monitoring are key components to avoiding unnecessary illness, hospitalization, and disability. Additionally, improved access to health information and health education permits improved care management and early identification of at-risk individuals in the community.

Home Care

Technological advances in communication and monitoring equipment now permit effective home management of patients previously requiring hospitalization. At the same time, the public is expressing a distinct preference for receiving certain kinds of care at home, particularly chronic and palliative care. Increasingly, health care leaders are searching for ways to shift the focus of care from inpatient care to outpatient management. However, as care at home increases, it brings with it new challenges, such as the obligation to attend to the respite and financial needs of family caregivers. With increasing home care services, we also see increasing requirements to demonstrate accountability for the use of resources.

Aboriginal Health

There are serious disparities between Aboriginal and non-Aboriginal Canadians, both in health status and in ability to access health care services. The reasons for these differences are complex, some of them historical, some structural and/or jurisdictional, and some social. As a result, the answers to addressing the disparities do not come easily. Work has begun, however, and suggestions for the kinds of changes needed have been outlined in numerous reports, the most recent of which is the Romanow Report (Commission on the Future, 2002).

Health Human Resources

We have seen dramatic shifts from a period of oversupply of nurses and physicians in the early 1990s to a situation where the supply of nurses, physicians, and other professionals is expected to be critically short. This shift is due to a variety of factors, including aging of the provider population, workload and working conditions, and the availability of a wider range of career opportunities for young people. Furthermore, health care leaders have become increasingly aware that the future viability of the health care system in Canada requires more and better attention to its human resources. Specifically, it is clear that changes must be made in order to strengthen national health human resources planning, to improve recruitment and retention of needed health providers, and to address the concerns of these providers about the quality of their work life.

Health Information Technology and Telecommunications

Virtually all the studies of health reform in Canada have emphasized the crucial link between health care reform and the effective use of information technology. Indeed, many believe that needed system reforms will only be achieved through the effective application of new information and telecommunications technologies, including the introduction of an electronic patient record. As a result, many provinces are currently working toward developing core health information network infrastructures around which a wide variety of services and patient-based applications can be developed and delivered. At the same time, many (if not most) individual health care organizations are implementing automated systems in a variety of areas, from patient care management to finance.

Beyond these provincial initiatives, it is widely recognized that we need a nationwide information network that can transcend traditional organizational, program, and geographic boundaries to integrate health-related information that meets the needs of a wide range of users, including health providers, researchers, policy makers, and the general public. Support for a national health information infrastructure was also highlighted in the 2003 Health Accord. Major system-wide changes such as this inevitably have an impact on the administration of health agencies, giving rise to organizational changes within these agencies. People in leadership and management positions are responsible for dealing with new and ongoing changes, often simultaneously, as well as dealing with different types of change.

Types of Change

Change may take three forms: developmental, spontaneous, or carefully planned. Leaders and managers need to know how to respond to all types of change.

Developmental Change

Developmental change occurs as an organization grows and becomes more complex. Organizations grow and develop according to their needs, often in highly predictable ways. Imagine, for example, that a small clinic opens in a rural community and is staffed for eight hours a day by a full-time registered nurse (RN) and a full-time receptionist. A physician is available two days a week. Staff communication is simple, usually one to one, and problems are generally discussed over lunch and solved in a collaborative manner. Staff members are enthusiastic about the potential role of the clinic in community health promotion, and their efforts in this regard prove highly successful. Over time, several members are added to the staff to provide support for a variety of new services. Staff communication patterns become more complex and often break down, "turf protection" begins, the receptionist feels overworked and angry at being "everybody's servant," and clients remark that the place is "less user friendly." These unwanted changes are the result of the evolution to a larger and, therefore, more complex organization. Change was necessary to meet the predefined objectives of the clinic and could not have been avoided; nonetheless, the manager could, and should, have anticipated some of the changes and planned to minimize their negative outcomes.

Spontaneous Change

Spontaneous change often is called a "reaction" and may be compared to the invasion of a human organism by a cold virus. Such an invasion may cause major disruption to the health of one person but be only a minor inconvenience to another depending on the overall condition, both physical and psychological, of the host. Unexpected invasions of health care organizations take various forms. They may be events with short-term repercussions, such as an air crash near a small regional hospital, a wildcat strike that virtually closes acute care beds in a region, or an unusually heavy snow storm in a widespread rural community served by visiting nurses. They may also be events with longer term repercussions: a recent example is the dramatic impact of Severe Acute Respiratory Syndrome (SARS) on the policies and practices of health care agencies; another example is the prolonged effect of fiscal restraint on the health system.

An organization can neither fully anticipate nor avoid spontaneous change and therefore has little or no time to plan its response. Nonetheless, leaders and managers can reduce the reactive impact through general planning and the use of mechanisms such as disaster plans and assorted communication strategies. Successful responses to spontaneous change require flexibility, cohesiveness, and a level of trust within the organization.

Planned Change

In planned change, a desired future result is achieved by deliberately determining deficiencies within the current state, deciding on one or more possible improvements, and enacting a plan to implement them and achieve the change. Individuals use planned change when they read to gain new knowledge, take courses to develop their management skills, or decide to improve their health through exercise and better eating habits.

Organizations are constantly involved in planned change. Changes may be
- department specific, such as a nursing unit changing its care delivery model;
- organization-wide, such as deciding to expand the services of a visiting nurses association;
- cross-institutional, such as a number of health care organizations deciding to merge their operations to form an integrated delivery system; or
- system-wide, such as the introduction of a large number of new nursing home beds into a region or community.

Leaders and managers can prepare for the potential results of developmental or spontaneous change, but they cannot actually plan for these changes in a systematically controlled manner, as they can with planned change. Success in bringing about planned change is a major part of the nurse manager's role.

Models of Change Management

The study of change is longstanding. Over the past 50 years, innumerable views and models of change and change management have emerged. This section describes four models of change management; some are long-standing and some are more recent, but all are useful to nurse managers today. They are referred to by the names of the authors who first described and tested them.

The case study presented in Box 22.1 will be used to illustrate how the four models of change management might be applied to bring about change.

Lewin's Theory of Change

Classical change theory has its origins in the work of Kurt Lewin (1951), who described change in terms of *field* and *force*. When applying Lewin's theory of change to an organization, the organization is considered an open system (see Chapters 8 and 10), and the change occurs in three phases: (a) the unfreezing phase, (b) the moving phase, and (c) the refreezing phase.

Box 22.1

Case Study: A Nursing Care Delivery System

As nurse manager of a patient care unit, Sandra Charleston is concerned about several problems that she believes are related. The satisfaction ratings that the unit has been receiving from patient questionnaires are mediocre, and patients have complained that no one is taking responsibility for coordinating and managing their plan of care. Staff members are complaining about workload, yet they are not using one another's skills and abilities to their best advantage. Sandra believes it is time to introduce a new model of care—one that will simultaneously improve the quality and coordination of care, enhance accountability, and enable all her nurses to work to their full scope of practice.

In the unfreezing phase, organizational members identify the desired change or problem. In the case presented in Box 22.1, what needs to be "unfrozen" is the way in which care is currently being delivered and the attitudes of some of the staff toward that care. As part of the unfreezing phase, information must be gathered. Lewin recommended conducting a force-field analysis to gather preliminary data regarding the problem or desired change and to gain information about the driving and restraining forces. Figure 22.1 shows a sample force-field analysis for the case study. In this example, the nurse manager is considering a change to the care delivery system in her unit and is therefore the change agent in this situation.

Following the force-field analysis, the change agent shares initial information with the target group (i.e., the nursing staff) so that a joint diagnosis of the change issue can be made. Together, they develop a joint action plan to achieve the desired change. The focus of the action plan is to increase the forces facilitating change and/or decrease those inhibiting change.

If Sandra applied Lewin's theory of change to her situation, she would tell her staff about the patient complaints and the information from the patient satisfaction surveys. She also would research the literature on different care delivery systems, and she would gather information directly from patient testimonials and site visits. Sandra would share this information with her staff, and together they would develop a plan for change. Staff members with experience in alternative systems (especially the staff level or team leader) would need to be fully engaged in

Figure 22.1 **Force-Field Analysis of Change in Nursing Care Delivery System**

Target System
the nursing staff

Driving Forces

✔ Some staff are frustrated with the current system
✔ There is administrative support for the change
✔ Satisfaction surveys and complaints show that patients are not happy with the results of the current system
✔ Some staff have worked with and liked other care delivery systems
✔ There is a staff nurse leader who is keen to "try something different"; she is admired and respected by the others

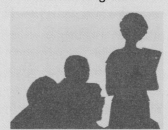

Goal
To implement a new care delivery system

Restraining Forces

✘ Staff are comfortable with the way they have always done things
✘ Some RNs may be threatened by practical nurses taking on roles and functions that only RNs previously provided
✘ Some physicians and other health professionals may be threatened by nurses taking on an expanded role in case management
✘ Some nurses (both RNs and practical nurses) do not have the knowledge and skill to take on an expanded scope of practice

selecting the new system for the unit and planning how to move forward. Fears, concerns, and knowledge and skill deficits must be addressed in the plan.

In the moving phase, actions identified within the action plan are carried out. Change begins as the system moves from its present state to its envisioned future state. In the refreezing phase, the goal is to integrate and stabilize the change and withdraw the change agent from the system.

Rogers and Shoemaker's Theory of Change

Rogers and Shoemaker (1971) also proposed a three-phase model of change. Their model focuses on the goal of change and the communication of that goal to all concerned. The three phases are (a) invention of the change, (b) diffusion or communication of information regarding the change, and (c) consequence of the change, which is either an adoption or rejection of the change. The Rogers and Shoemaker model is based on the assumption that people are rational and will adopt change if it is logically justified and they can see some possible gain in making the change. The focus of the approach is to provide the knowledge necessary for making a rational choice.

If applying this model to her situation, Sandra would need to identify or "invent" one or more models of care that would be better than the current model. She would then consider how to communicate key information to her staff and the other professionals about what her proposed change is and how it can be implemented. She would also anticipate and address any factors that might lead to rejection of the new model, while taking advantage of any factors that could enhance the chances of success.

Rogers and Shoemaker also labelled types of individuals according to how they respond to change:
- *Innovators* actively seek and look forward to change.
- *Early adopters* help make change possible.
- The *early majority* provides a support system for the change.
- The *late majority* provides peer pressure to support the change.
- *Laggards* strive to keep doing things the way they have been done before.
- *Rejectors* work actively against the change.

Sandra, therefore, would attempt to identify how members of her staff and significant others would likely respond to the proposed change. She would carefully consider how she could take advantage of those individuals who might assist and limit the influence of those who might resist or sabotage the proposed change.

Kanter's Innovational Theory of Change

In *The Change Masters*, Kanter (1983) described a model of change designed to guide executives in promoting innovation and entrepreneurship within their organizations. She argued that innovation and change could be fostered, promoted, and initiated at all levels within an organization. In her research, Kanter found that innovation flourishes in organizations possessing a culture of pride, which encourages teamwork, consensus building, communication, and fosters a sense of personal value. In contrast, organizations that inhibit innovation tend to advocate a top-down approach characterized by multiple formal structures. Kanter concluded that change initiated in this top-down manner reinforces a culture of inferiority, which leads to members feeling complacent, anxious, and distrustful.

In her change model, Kanter (1983) described three sequential "waves of activity" that characterize innovation leading to change: (a) problem definition, (b) coalition building, and (c) mobilization. During the problem definition wave, information is gathered in order to shape a feasible focused project for action. The coalition-building wave involves communication and collaboration within the organization to garner support and resources for the project. During the mobilization wave, resources are invested to bring the innovation from idea to reality.

Inherent in Kanter's conceptualization of innovation is the concept of empowerment. She argued that leaders who wish to promote innovation should do so using a collaborative and participative approach that involves team building, seeking input, persuading (rather than ordering), being sensitive to the interests and priorities of others, and sharing rewards and recognition.

Applying Kanter's model to her situation, Sandra would continue to collect the information she needs to "define the problem." She already has information from patients and families regarding their dissatisfaction with the way in which care is currently delivered, and she has a good understanding of the knowledge and skill levels of her staff. She could collect more information by investigating other care models. In order to build a coalition, she would have to ensure that she had the support of her supervisor (the nurse administrator). After careful consideration, she might have serious concerns about how some of the nursing staff, physicians, and other health care professionals will respond to a proposed change. At this point, Sandra's greatest efforts would be spent engaging the skeptics and opponents in the process of choosing and planning for a better future so that when the plan is mobilized, it will have a good chance of success. One strategy that Sandra might consider is to establish a multidisciplinary task force empowered to address the problem and place the front-line staff leader in the role of chair. Sandra would then move into the background, acting as coach, enabler, and supporter to the task force through the staff nurse leader.

Bridges' Transitional Theory of Change

In the literature on change, several authors emphasize the importance of attending to the human side of change in organizations. The most comprehensive work in this area is that of William Bridges, a leading expert on organizational transition.

Bridges (1991), and together with Mitchell (2000), differentiated between organizational change and transition. Change, he argued, is about what will be altered; transition is about how the change will *feel* for those who are required to make it. He suggested that change can be planned and managed using a more or less rational model. Transition, in contrast, is a three-part psychosocial process that extends over a long period of time and requires different skills and strategies. Bridges described three phases in the transition experience. The first is the ending phase, which involves letting go of the old situation and the old identity that went with it. The second is the neutral zone, which exists between the old familiar reality and a new reality that is yet very unclear. The third is the new beginning phase, when people actually face the new way of doing things.

The ending phase is a time of loss. During this phase, people have to let go of the way things always were; in the process, they also let go of how they previously functioned and what they believe made them successful. Bridges asserted that people who have particular difficulty letting go are those whose identity is tied to relationships, status, role, or feelings of belonging. When people experience a loss, their coping behaviours often include denial, anger, bargaining, and despair (Bridges, 1991; Kübler-Ross, 1969). Change at work may result in feelings of loss. Bridges believed that the only way to deal with employees' behaviours associated with feelings of loss is to allow employees to express themselves openly within the organization. Support and open communication on the part of the manager are essential during this phase.

According to Bridges, it is not clear where the ending phase of transition stops and the second phase, the neutral zone, begins. As its name suggests, the neutral zone is an in-between time when people recognize that the old way of being is no longer an option yet are unclear about where they are headed. It is a time filled with great uncertainty and confusion, and it consumes a lot of emotional energy. People describe being in the neutral zone as feeling that everything is falling apart. These feelings can be so powerful that there is a real risk that a person may leave the organization. Because the neutral zone is uncomfortable, people try to get out of it. Some will try to rush ahead into the future but perhaps without a clear idea of where they are going or how they will get there. Others will try to back-pedal and retreat into the past. The difficult aspect of the neutral zone is that it cannot be avoided or rushed. In planning for change, the change leader must allow time and provide support for this phase because it is in the neutral zone that the best creativity and energy of transition occur. Bridges suggested that people could be assisted through the neutral zone by being given the opportunity to redefine themselves and their future.

Just as transition begins with an ending, it ends with a new beginning. In the new beginning phase, it is clear what is expected of people in the future state and what needs to be done to get there. However, some individuals may not be confident about their ability to behave in the desired new fashion. This feeling is very disconcerting because it calls their sense of competence and value into question. Their inclination will be to hold back, waiting to see how others are going to behave. This may be particularly difficult in an organization that has a history of punishing mistakes. A great deal of support is needed to help these individuals through this stage.

In Sandra's case, the process of moving to a different model of care means that she will be asking the staff to give up familiar routines, disrupt comfortable work habits, and develop new modes of communication; in effect, she will be asking them to exchange the familiar past for an uncertain future. Sandra should anticipate all of the characteristics of transition. She should be prepared for the emotional reactions and give careful thought to how she will engage and support her staff during the transition.

Tools and Strategies for Leading and Managing Change

Successful nurse managers recognize that change can be more of an opportunity than a threat. They create working environments in which nurses are ready to take risks and be active participants in change, and they make use of the many tools and strategies for implementing change, some of which are discussed in this section.

Diagnosing Change

Sometimes when anticipating a change, nurse managers may not know where to focus their energies. Dannemiller and Jacobs (1992) proposed the following formula for change planning:

$$D \times V \times F > R$$

where,

  D is discomfort (or dissatisfaction with the status quo)
  V is vision (of the preferred future)
  F is first steps (the clarity of the plan for how to move forward)
  R is resistance.

What this means is that the product of discomfort, vision, and first steps must be greater than the resistance or else the change will fail. In attributing values to the four variables in this formula, it is necessary to use the same scale (i.e., a percentage, expressed as a decimal). For example, if you think you are 80% clear on the vision of what the change will accomplish, you would give V a score of 0.8.

Consider the case study and decide how Sandra might apply the formula to her situation. Sandra may estimate that some staff members, physicians, and a few other professionals may significantly resist her proposed change. This resistance will be offset to some extent by staff who have worked in other models and by one nurse in particular who is keen to try a different approach. Sandra decides that the R (resistance) quotient is currently 60%, so R gets a value of 0.6. Not many staff are dissatisfied with the current system, so Sandra gives D a value of 0.4. Her vision of the preferred model is developing but is not yet clear, so she assigns V a value of 0.5. Finally, the concrete steps that must be undertaken to move forward have not yet been defined, so she assigns F a value of 0.3. After plugging these values into the model, Sandra readily sees that

$$D\,(0.4) \times V\,(0.5) \times F\,(0.3) = 0.06$$

This value is not nearly great enough to overcome the anticipated resistance of 0.6. Sandra knows she must attend to all three factors on the left side of this equation in order to succeed.

Suppose that in approaching the challenge, Sandra shares the patient satisfaction and complaint information with all of the members of the interdisciplinary team, they are all are shocked, and many are motivated to address the situation. Suppose Sandra establishes a multidisciplinary task force that identifies a model it believes will be an improvement and also identifies many issues that will have to be considered when implementing the change. At this point, the values in the change formula might begin to look more like this: $D = 0.8$, $V = 0.9$, $F = 0.5$, and $R = 0.4$. The product of the first three factors has increased to 0.36, which is much closer to the resistance. Now, the key to success will lie in increasing the F quotient (i.e., developing a clear plan for implementing the change) and decreasing the resistance.

Leading Change

Bridges and Mitchell (2000) suggested that there are seven essential steps for leading a group through a time of transition. It is interesting how well these steps align with the change formula described above. The first step is for the leader to "learn to describe the change and why it must happen, and do so succinctly—in one minute or less". The description of what the change will look like strengthens the *V* (vision) quotient, and the description of why it is needed helps strengthen the *D* quotient (i.e., staff members' dissatisfaction with the current state).

Next, the leader must "be sure that the details of the change are planned carefully and that someone is responsible for each detail, that timelines for all the changes are established; and that a communications plan explaining the changes is in place". This step addresses the *F* quotient (first steps).

Third, the leader must "understand (with the assistance of others closer to the change) just who is going to have to let go of what".

Fourth, armed with that knowledge, the leader must "make sure that steps are taken to help people respectfully let go of the past". Understanding the losses and supporting people as they accept change will help decrease the *R* (resistance) quotient. It should be noted that some individuals, particularly powerful highly placed individuals within the organization, might not support the change. In that case, it may be necessary to adjust the vision or first steps to make the change a better fit with the priorities of these individuals.

The last three steps that Bridges and Mitchell proposed build upon the first four outlined above. They emphasize that it is important for the leader to "help people through the neutral zone with communication (rather than simple information) that emphasizes connections with and concern for the followers". Along the way, the leader must be prepared to "create temporary solutions to the temporary problems and the high levels of uncertainty". In the Case Study (Box 22.1), for example, Sandra could make interim changes in assignments or help staff members who are unlikely to adjust find work in other units where they will be more comfortable. Finally, the leader must "help people to launch the new beginning by articulating the new attitudes and behaviors needed to make the change work—and then modeling, providing practice in, and rewarding those behaviors and attitudes".

Effective Questioning—A Powerful Change Tool

It has been suggested that the most powerful tool a manager can use to promote change is the Effective Question, or EQ (Oakley & Krug, 1991). Effective questions are those that empower people, release their positive energy, and get them thinking and acting proactively rather than reactively. Table 22.1 contrasts ineffective questions with effective questions.

Creating an Environment that Is Change Ready

Successful nurse leaders recognize and show others that change can be an opportunity rather than a threat. They create a trusting environment for risk taking in which nurses are ready to be active participants in change. Kriegel and Brandt (1996) stated that managers who wish to minimize resistance to change must deliberately cultivate a fundamental attitude of change readiness in themselves and their staff members. Change readiness, they say, is an attitude that is open and receptive to new ideas; excited rather than anxious about change; challenged, not threatened, by transitions; and committed to change as an ongoing process. They emphasized

Table 22.1 Ineffective versus Effective Questions as a Tool for Change

Ineffective Questions	Effective Questions
✘ What is wrong with this situation?	✓ What is already working? (Here? Other places?)
✘ Why does this always happen to us?	✓ What makes it work?
✘ Who's to blame for this? How can we avoid being blamed for this?	✓ What is the objective of this change?
✘ How is this going to hurt me/us?	✓ What are the benefits of achieving this objective?
✘ What do we have to do to fix the problem?	✓ What can we do to move closer to our objective?

Source: Adapted from *Enlightened Leadership: Getting to the Heart of Change* (pp. 137–166), by E. Oakley and D. Krug, 1991, New York: Simon & Schuster Adult Publishing Group. Copyright 1991 by Key to Renewal, Inc. Adapted with permission.

that individuals and teams demonstrate change readiness when they "anticipate and initiate change; challenge the status quo; create instead of react to change; and lead rather than follow" (Kriegel & Brandt, 1996, pp. 8–9). The authors suggested a number of strategies for managers to use in coaching themselves and their staff to be change ready:

- *Rounding up "sacred cows":* Challenging traditional beliefs, assumptions, and practices in order to identify and discard those that are no longer useful
- *Developing a change-ready environment:* Changing the focus of the management style from controlling to coaching, and building a work environment that is characterized by trust and caring (a trusting environment is one built on honesty, integrity, and reliability; caring involves treating individuals with respect and empathy and acknowledging their efforts and contributions)
- *Turning resistance into readiness:* Recognizing and overcoming the four major forms of resistance to change: fear, powerlessness, inertia, and absence of self-interest (or inability to see how the change would benefit them)
- *Motivating people to change:* Using urgency, inspiration, ownership, and rewards and recognition to get people excited about change and willing to initiate it
- *Continuously developing traits of change readiness:* Developing traits such as resourcefulness, optimism, adventurousness, drive, adaptability, confidence, and a tolerance for ambiguity

The Power of a Positive Attitude

People frequently resist change when others impose it upon them. They also usually resist change because they assume it will be disruptive, time-consuming, result in conflict, or will create a new state that is less desirable than the present one. Such attitudes can seriously handicap an organization's efforts to move forward. Sometimes, it is the nurse manager who struggles with maintaining a positive attitude toward change. Morgan (1988) summarized the fundamental shifts in attitude that managers must make in order to embrace, rather than resist, change:

- They must adopt a proactive, positive, and optimistic view of the future by anticipating emerging problems, reframing them as opportunities, and planning ahead for them.
- They must view their organizations "from the outside in" by identifying strengths and weaknesses from the perspective of their customers and developing competencies to address the deficits.
- They must constantly stimulate new initiatives and explore new directions by promoting, celebrating, and rewarding creativity, learning, and innovation of individuals and groups within the organization.
- They must identify and forge new partnerships with diverse stakeholders (both internal and external) in order to mobilize meaningful action on shared problems.
- They must develop and demonstrate a much greater sense of social responsibility than they have in the past.

Leadership Implications

Nurses today are functioning in complex corporations and in whitewater environments that are placing ever-increasing demands for change upon them: demands from multiple constituencies, from the outside environment, from changing values (of society and its workers), and from increasingly complex tasks. Some of these changes can be anticipated; others cannot. Among the most important skills for nurse leaders in these rapidly changing environments are the abilities to anticipate the demands, to engage in planned change in order to stay ahead of the pressures, and to prepare and support staff to cope with the changes. In the words of Kanter (1983), if they are to be successful, nurse leaders need to become change masters:

Change masters are—literally—the right people in the right place at the right time. The right people are the ones with the ideas that move beyond the organization's established practices, ideas they can form into visions. The right places are the integrative environments that support innovation, encourage the building of coalitions and teams to support and implement visions. The right times are those moments in the flow of organizational history when it is possible to reconstruct reality on the basis of accumulated innovations to shape a more productive and successful future (p. 306).

Summary

To behave proactively, rather than reactively, in a changing environment, nurse leaders and managers must be able do the following:

- Recognize that there are different types of change—developmental, spontaneous, and planned—and that different approaches are required for each
- Become familiar with common models and terminology of change so that comfort with change is increased and the best model is selected for a given situation
- Understand the difference between change and transition (the human reaction to change) and attend carefully to both
- Develop and cultivate in others a positive attitude toward change
- Recognize that planned change is a complex process that, in order to succeed, requires an organized approach and attention to numerous risk factors
- Identify and use strategies and tools not only to advance a particular change effort, but also to create an environment that is consistently open and ready for change

Applying the Knowledge in this Chapter

Exercise

Eileen Chang has been attending planning meetings to discuss the planned merging of the regional health authority's two orthopedic services. Eileen is the first-level manager responsible for the orthopedic unit on the site where both services will be brought together. Plans for the merger have been approved by the board, which means that, in addition to her own unit, Eileen will be responsible for a new pre-admission clinic for the combined orthopedic services. The clinic will be set up in renovated space adjacent to her unit. Her unit and the clinic will be managed as a single administrative unit. She is excited about this change and believes that it will offer some challenging opportunities for her staff.

In responding to the following questions, state your assumptions in advance; for example, you may want to assume that nurses have a collective agreement and that the new clinic will not be operational for another six months.

1. Select a model of change management discussed in this chapter, and apply the ideas in the model to the change implementation process. For example, if you choose Lewin's model, describe what Eileen will do to begin the unfreezing phase.

2. What are some of the possible responses Eileen may get from her staff? How should these responses be handled?

3. What are some of the staffing and scheduling issues that may be of concern to Eileen's staff (refer to Chapter 26)?

4. Describe the leadership skills that Eileen will need to effectively achieve this planned change.

Resources

evolve Internet Resources

Change Management Resource Library:

www.change-management.org/

University of Alberta School of Business. A Multidisciplinary Study of Organizational Change in Canadian Health Care:

www.healthorgchange.com/

Further Reading

Drucker, P.F. (Writer), & Senge, P.M. (Writer). (2001). *Leading in a time of change: What it will take to lead tomorrow* [Videotape]. (Available from John Wiley & Sons Canada, Ltd., 22 Worcester Road, Etobicoke, Ontario, M9W 1L1).

The Drucker Foundation presents a conversation between Peter Drucker and Peter Senge—visionary leaders who have long been involved in setting the agenda for organizational leadership and change. In this package, which includes a video and companion workbook, these men share their wisdom on how leaders can prepare themselves and their organizations for change.

Kotter, J. (1996). *Leading change.* Boston: Harvard University Press.

Kotter's books are of particular interest to those who are faced with the challenge of implementing large-scale change. This book describes an eight-stage process for creating major change.

Kotter, J.P., & Cohen, D.S. (2002). *The heart of change: Real-life stories of how people change their organizations.* Boston: Harvard Business School Press.

Kotter's books are of particular interest to those who are faced with the challenge of implementing large-scale change. This book delves deep into the subject of change to get to the heart of how change actually happens. Through real-life stories of front-line people in different kinds of organizations, the authors address the fundamental problem of how to go beyond getting your message across to fundamentally changing people's behaviour.

Kouzes, J.M., & Posner, B.Z. (1999). *The leadership challenge planner: An action guide to achieving your personal best.* San Francisco: Jossey-Bass Pfeiffer.

The "leadership planner" is a step-by-step workbook that guides readers through a real-life change initiative of their own choosing.

Kouzes, J.M., & Posner, B.Z. (2003, Spring). Challenge is the opportunity for greatness. [Electronic version]. *Leader to Leader, 28,* 16–23.

In this article, Kouzes and Posner make the case that when times are stable and secure, no one is severely tested and thus no significant change occurs. They say, "Only challenge produces the opportunity for greatness," and go on to provide guidance for leaders and managers on how to lead in the chaos and uncertainty of present times.

Meyerson, D.E. (2001). *Tempered radicals: How people use difference to inspire change at work.* Boston: Harvard Business School Press.

This book describes the critical role of "tempered radicals"—rank and file employees who are "different" and who use this difference to inspire change at work every day. It shows how these individuals have learned to navigate successfully between "fitting in and selling out" and how they are able to successfully advance their own careers without compromising their values. It describes how they rely on conviction, patience, and courage and how they use a variety of strategies to inspire change. Finally, it describes how, through their actions, they help their organizations to learn and adapt.

Weisbord, M.R. (1976). Why organizational development hasn't worked (so far) in medical centers. *Healthcare Management Review, 1*(2), 17–28.

Hospitals have historically been resistant to broad system change. In this classic article, Marvin Weisbord—an internationally recognized organizational development guru—provides fascinating insight into why this is by examining how the task, identity, and governance systems of hospitals differ from those of other businesses.

Wheatley, M. (2001). *Turning to one another: Simple conversations to restore hope to the future.* San Francisco: Berrett-Koehler.

In this book, Meg Wheatley suggests that we can learn much about each other by resurrecting the simple art of true conversation, by simply talking to one another about things that matter. Out of these conversations, Wheatley argues, comes an incredible force for change in the world.

References

Bridges, W. (1991). *Managing transitions: Making the most of change.* Reading, MA: Addison-Wesley.

Bridges, W., & Mitchell, S. (2000, Spring). Leading transition: A new model for change. [Electronic version]. *Leader to Leader, 16,* 30–36. Retreived January 2005, from http://www.pfdf.org/leaderbooks/L2L/spring2000/bridges.html

Commission d'étude sur les services de santé et les services sociaux. (2001). *Emerging solutions: Report and recommendations.* Chair: M. Clair. Quebec City, QC: Ministry of Health and Social Services.

Commission on Medicare. (2001). *Caring for medicare: Sustaining a quality system.* Commissioner: K. Fyke. Regina, SK: Government of Saskatchewan.

Commission on the Future of Health Care in Canada. (2002, November). *Building on values: The future of healthcare in Canada – Final report.* Commissioner: R. Romanow. Ottawa, ON: Parliament of Canada.

Dannemiller, K.D., & Jacobs, R.W. (1992). Changing the way organizations change: A revolution of common sense. *Journal of Applied Behavioral Science, 28*(4), 480–498.

Health Canada. (2003). *2003 First minister's accord on health care renewal.* Retrieved March 31, 2004, from http://www.hc-sc.gc.ca/english/hca2003/accord.html

Kanter, R.M. (1983). *The change masters: Innovation and entrepreneurship in the American corporation.* New York: Touchstone.

Kriegel, R., & Brandt, D. (1996). *Sacred cows make the best burgers: Paradigm-busting strategies for developing change-ready people and organizations.* New York: Warner Books.

Kübler-Ross, E. (1969). *On death and dying.* New York: MacMillan.

Lewin, K. (1951). *Field theory in social science.* New York: Harper & Row.

Morgan, G. (1988). *Riding the waves of change: Developing managerial competencies for a turbulent world.* San Francisco: Jossey-Bass.

Oakley, E., & Krug, D. (1991). *Enlightened leadership: Getting to the heart of change.* New York: Simon & Schuster.

Premier's Advisory Council on Health. (2001). *A framework for reform. Report of the Premier's Advisory Council on Health.* Chair: D. Mazankowski. Edmonton, AB: Government of Alberta.

Rogers, E., & Shoemaker, S. (1971). *Communication of innovations.* Glencoe, NY: Free Press.

Standing Senate Committee on Social Affairs, Science and Technology. (2002). *The health of Canadians – The federal role. Final report on the state of the health care system in Canada.* Volume 6, Recommendations for reform. Chair: The Honorable M. J. L. Kirby. Ottawa, ON: Parliament of Canada.

Vaill, P.B. (1989). *Managing as a performing art: New ideas for a world of chaotic change.* San Francisco: Jossey-Bass.

23

INTRAORGANIZATIONAL POLITICS

Ginette Lemire Rodger

Learning Objectives

In this chapter, you will learn:

- The role of politics within organizations and its impact on the process of change

- Definitions of concepts such as politics, power, and political action

- A five-step political process framework that helps nurses and their leaders prepare strategies to accomplish their goals

- Commonly recognized sources of power available to nurses in health care agencies

- The importance of temporary alliances and coalitions among subgroups in organizations (e.g., administrators, physicians, nurses, and other health professionals)

- Challenges facing nurses in front-line leadership and management positions

Intraorganizational politics is an important concept for nurses to understand because it plays a significant role in every aspect of their professional lives. Important questions in health care are often political issues, such as which health goals are pursued, who receives what type of care and when, which health care programs are maintained or deleted, which resources are allocated to these programs, and which organizational models will be implemented and by whom. Intraorganizational politics is directly related to the ultimate goal of nursing—the health of the consumer.

This chapter begins with an explanation of why nurses need to develop political knowledge and skills. Key terms that are central to organizational politics are defined, and the five steps in a political process framework are discussed. The chapter concludes with a discussion of the challenges front-line nurses and managers must overcome when they use the political process. In view of the loss of many senior and middle level managers following the widespread restructuring activities in the health care system during the 1990s, nurses can no longer assume that the use of power and politics is the prerogative of senior management and agency boards. Inasmuch as the majority of nurses work in health care organizations, the information in this chapter is relevant for all nurses whether they are engaged in clinical practice, first-level and middle management, clinical leadership, or senior administration. Accordingly, when the term nurse or nurses is used in this chapter, it is intended to be inclusive of individuals in all nursing positions, no matter at what level of the organization.

The Need for Political Awareness

Canadian nurses must possess political knowledge and skills in order to respond to the unprecedented changes as the health care system is overhauled and the role and value of nursing are re-examined and modified. The rate and intensity of change in the health care system exemplifies Erik Erikson's theory of change (1963). Over 40 years ago, Erikson predicted that the rate of change in the world would continually accelerate and that people and institutions would face multiple simultaneous changes. He believed that the limits of human and institutional adaptability were not known. Today, change is still accelerating and intensifying.

Kurt Lewin (1951), a well-known theorist of change, would call the period of change that the Canadian health care system is experiencing "the moving stage." Change, according to his theory, has three stages: *the unfreezing stage*, a cognitive phase in which the individual is exposed to the idea of the need for change; *the moving stage*, a cognitive redefinition in which the change is planned and initiated; and *the refreezing stage*, in which the change is integrated and stabilized (Lewin, 1951). During the unfreezing and moving phases, the next direction is initiated and movement begins. This is usually a time of insecurity, repositioning, and challenges; it is a time with no clear answers. However, it is also a time of opportunity. During this period, effective politics can make a great difference in setting the course of action for a project, a department, or an organization.

As Starke and Rempel (1988) observed, "Because politics is so common, managers in all kinds of organizations must understand what it is and why it occurs. They must also learn to cope with its manifestations if they wish to be successful in their careers" (p. 12). Nurses must be knowledgeable about politics and related concepts, such as power, influence, and the political process. Theoretical knowledge is important, but not sufficient. Managers must develop abilities and skills in using these concepts if they are to influence decisions to support nursing goals. It is one thing to know about politics, and another thing to be political.

Definitions

The term *intraorganizational* in this chapter refers to an organization within a health care agency. *Politics*, as used in this chapter, can be defined broadly as "the capacity to influence." More specifically, Laswell (1936) defined politics as "the study of influence and the influential" (p. 13). He said that, to comprehend politics, one must look not only at who draws power, but also at the relationship that person has with those affected by the actions. The same notion of politics is apparent in the work of Stevens (1980b), in which she described politics as "a process by which one influences the decisions of others and exerts control over situations and events" (p. 208). Pfeffer (1981) defined *organizational politics* as the behaviours of individuals as they attempt "to acquire, develop, and use power and other resources to obtain their preferred outcomes in a situation where there is uncertainty…about choices" (p. 7). Like politics, *power* is also defined in terms of influencing and controlling. Shiflett and McFarland (1978) defined power as "one person's degree of influence over others, to the extent that obedience or conformity are assumed to follow" (p. 19).

It is also important to define the actions that we associate with the concepts of politics and power. *Political action* and *political process* can be defined as a systematic series of actions directed toward influencing others into conformity with a pursued goal. It is interesting to note that the definitions of politics, power, influence, and political process have similar roots. The mechanism central to politics and power is the process of planned change. The terms *planned change* and *political process* are used interchangeably in this chapter.

Political Process Framework

For more than a decade, the political process framework described in Box 23.1 has been used to show nurses how to successfully bring about organizational and social change. This framework highlights some elements of intraorganizational politics, and it can serve as a guide for front-line managers who want to use a political process to bring about change. The same five-step process is followed whether a manager wants to bring about a change, guide a change in a different direction, or prevent a change that could be detrimental to client care. A more detailed analysis of the five steps of the process follows.

Box 23.1

Political Process Framework

1. Establish goal and objectives
2. Assess positive and negative factors
    *   Social values and trends
    *   Key individuals or groups
    *   Sources of power
    *   Resources
    *   Timing
3. Plan the strategy
4. Implement the strategy
5. Evaluate and readjust the strategy

Step 1: Establish Goal and Objectives

Since change is multifaceted and constant, the setting of a definite goal and objectives is an important step in the political process. There is a need to set priorities among the competing issues. Which issues must be dealt with and in what way? Some issues play a pivotal role in an organization because they control other secondary or dependent issues; therefore, dealing with essential issues will, in fact, influence the resolution of other issues.

The political process is most effectively exercised when the purpose is clear. The process of clarifying objectives can take time and involve a lot of thought, consultation, and research, depending on the scope of the issue being addressed. You may begin with a general idea of the desirable results—the goal—but you also need to refine the objectives, including what needs to be done, when, and where. The changes made by nurses to the *Canada Health Act* in 1984 provide a well-known example. When refining the objectives, nurses had to be as precise as possible in suggesting exactly what words in the legislation would be removed, what words would be added, and when the changes would be proposed at which seating of the House of Commons Committee.

Similarly, before initiating change on a unit, service, or department, nurse managers must clarify the goals and objectives of the change. Effectively completing this first step achieves the following outcomes: (a) a clear goal, (b) a specific set of objectives, (c) a definite target (i.e., identifying the person or group who has the authority to bring about the desired goal and who needs to be persuaded), (d) a specific message that conveys the value of the endeavour and that can be used to persuade, and (e) the formation of a core strategy group consisting of people who are interested in attaining the goal.

Stevens (1980a) stressed that unity among those desiring the change is a prerequisite for effectiveness in such endeavours; therefore, ensuring that the entire group agrees upon the goal and objectives is an essential component of this first step. Stevens urged nurses working toward change to debate their policies (goal and objectives) internally, make decisions, and then present a united front to the public or the organization they are trying to influence.

Two important goals for nurse managers to consider are (a) the allocation of health care resources and (b) the leadership position of nursing in the health care system. These two issues are pivotal in the current climate of health care reform, and managers are currently pursuing specific objectives to address them.

Health Care Resources

Allocation of scarce resources is often the most vital issue in an organization, and this is reflected in the organization's political struggles, or "power plays." Del Bueno (1986) noted that, in times of economic scarcity, "political activity increases as individuals compete for those declining resources. A power holder must not only have control of valued resources, but must be willing to use them to influence others. When power is hoarded it atrophies and blocks achievement" (pp. 125–126).

In an ideal world, nursing care would be as highly valued as other types of care, and allocation of resources would be a non-issue because objective data about the effects of such care would guide allocation. However, this is not the way health care resources are allocated in the real world. In fact, the people who control the resources influence the delivery of client care and determine who receives what care. For example, the way a hospital allocates its material resources, such as supplies and equipment, usually reflects the power and influence of physicians (Mason & McCarthy, 1985).

There is ample research evidence that nurses can efficiently and cost-effectively deliver many health care services for which they are not now responsible, both in hospitals and the community (Bissinger, Allred, Arford, & Bellig, 1997; Canadian Nurses Association, 1993; Lasater, 1996; Shamian, 1997; Weeks, 2002). However, despite the need for cost reductions in health care, there have been major roadblocks to the introduction of these changes because stakeholders who control the resources favour the medical and hospital models rather than primary health care, public health, and nursing models.

Nursing has responsibility for an important part of the health care resources and should use this fact as part of a political process. The ability to influence decisions and gain support for the efficient use of health care resources will be enhanced by developing political alliances within multidisciplinary teams. This will be discussed later in the chapter.

Leadership Position of Nursing

The other pivotal issue to consider when establishing goals and objectives is the leadership role nurses must play in a time of transition. Prescott (1993) said that registered nurses "are one of the hospital's most important resources for achieving and maintaining a competitive advantage because they contribute in important ways both to cost savings and to delivering high-quality care" (p. 192). Prescott documented nursing utility and assets by means of outcomes research, such as the impact of nurses on hospital mortality rates, lengths of stay, costs, and morbidity outcomes. She concluded that nursing is an important component of hospital survival in a reformed health care system.

Several organizational models introduced in the present wave of organizational change eliminate nursing positions at policy and senior management levels. Some administrators have hired nurses as incumbents for the new management positions at this level because these managers recognize the need for nurses' knowledge and skills. In most instances, however, the job description does not refer to the nursing knowledge that is needed, and the nursing component consequently becomes invisible and disposable. Would any other industry wipe out its senior production managers or put them in advisory positions to the production line? Of course not!

In light of this disconcerting state of affairs, the Canadian Nurses Association (CNA) (2002) takes the position that, in order to support quality professional environments, there must be a chief executive nurse to provide visionary leadership for the discipline, with sufficient authority and resources to ensure nursing standards are met. As well, the CNA has identified 16 principles as a framework for supporting quality, efficient, and effective nursing services, including among other points, middle managers who are registered nurses and nurses involved in strategic planning and decision making at the board and executive levels.

Allocation of resources and leadership positions are two examples of goals to be attained through intraorganizational politics. Once the goal is set and the objectives clarified, the second important step of the process is assessing the positive and negative factors that will help or hinder the achievement of the goal.

Step 2: Assess Positive and Negative Factors

The political process, or the exercise of power, requires that consideration be given to what will help achieve the objectives and what will impede progress. These elements are what Lewin (1951) called "driving forces" and "resisting forces." Each has to be assessed if a nurse manager wishes to develop an effective strategy for change. Driving forces must be used and maximized, and resisting forces must be minimized. When negative factors are encountered—whether related to values or trends in the environment or to key players, resources, or timing—there are ways to deal with them appropriately and thereby increase chances of success. These options include avoiding, minimizing, or confronting. To marshal these options, thus maximizing the positive forces and dealing with the negative forces, nurse managers need to recognize prevailing values and trends within the organization.

Values and Trends

Nurses need to know and recognize prevailing social values, trends, and beliefs. If reaching a goal means going against these factors, it will be difficult, if not impossible, to accomplish it. Predominant values and trends in an organization are often referred to as the "organizational culture." Schein (1985) defined organizational culture as "a pattern of basic assumptions—invented, discovered, or developed by a given group as it learns to cope with its problems of external adaptation and internal integration—that has worked well enough to be considered valid and, therefore, to be taught to new members as the correct way to perceive, think, and feel in relation to those problems" (p. 9). Each organization has its own culture, but within a large organization, subcultures also develop within specialized groups, departments, or units (Sovie, 1993). As Drucker (1992) noted, culture does not change, behaviour does. Therefore, if a nurse wishes to influence decisions, it is vital in intraorganizational politics to analyze the climate, values, and trends of the work environment.

An example of the effect of trends is the case of an agency that attempted to regroup all long-term care patients into one area; that attempt failed because, in the organizational culture at the time, it had been considered unacceptable to mix different types of care. The change was successful five years later, however, because values and trends had changed. It was then considered desirable to have the full continuum of care in one agency as an efficient way of utilizing beds and containing costs.

How can a nurse assess organizational culture? Fleeger (1993) identified two types of clues: (a) explicit clues, which include formal contracts, written mission statements, policies and procedures, organizational charts, and job descriptions; and (b) implicit clues, which include the informal unwritten rules and expectations (e.g., regarding dress, communications, and behaviours). Both explicit and implicit clues must be used as indicators of values and trends in the organization.

Key Players

When planning or coping with change, nurses must identify which individuals or groups will affect and be affected by the planned change and evaluate who might support or oppose the goal. These people are key players in the change process because they can influence the target individual or groups identified in the first step of the process and can affect your ability to persuade the target of the value of the goal. It is necessary to assess the key players' strengths and identify their particular goals. It may not be possible to identify all the forces for and against the change, but nurses should make an effort to gather as much useful information as possible to plan the nursing strategy.

Key players who support the goal can be considered a resource for the project, and key players who oppose the goal are likely to create conflict. Unfortunately, many nurses are not skillful at dealing with conflict. The choices are fairly limited when dealing with negative key players: they can be deliberately avoided; their impact can be minimized by identifying the specific area they oppose and trying to convince them either to support the goal or, at least, to be neutral; or they can be confronted by developing arguments that demonstrate why the proposed goal is better.

Del Bueno (1986) discussed these interfaces among individuals at different levels, from different departments, or with different values. She stated that considerable managerial skill and tactics are necessary to resolve such conflicts and offered suggestions that have a high probability of success. Her suggestions include the following: build your team; choose your second-in-command carefully; establish alliances with superiors as well as with peers; maintain a flexible position and maneuverability; and project an image of status, power, and material success.

Sources of Power

What kinds of power will the key individuals or groups use to support or oppose the set goal? Does a group have different types of power than an individual? What are some effective strategies to ensure that nurses in management positions have the capacity to influence each situation? What are the key variables that affect attainment of power?

There are various ways of describing types of individual power. French and Raven (1959) identify five sources of power:

- *Legitimate power*: Authority vested in a role or position that is accepted and recognized by others in the organization, such as a front-line manager position
- *Reward power:* Power based on a person's use of positive sanctions such as money, positive evaluation, or other forms of gain
- *Coercive power:* Power based on the use of negative sanctions such as threats or punishment
- *Expert power:* Power based on valid knowledge or information in a given domain, such as nursing knowledge and skills
- *Referent power:* Power based on positive personal appeal to which others respond; often identified as charisma

Davidhizar (1993) also identified charisma as a source of power or political strength, and she recognized that charismatic power was an emerging paradigm for managers at the time. The same is true today for modern managers. Wieland and Ullrich (1976) discussed two derivative forms of power, usually not mentioned in the nursing literature: (a) associative power, derived from associating with others who are perceived as powerful, and (b) lower participant power, in which those lower in the hierarchy hold power over their managers. Fergusson (1985) also described a form of associative power but referred to it as "power through interdependence."

Similar types of power can be attributed to a group or an organization. In assessing the power of a group, however, the relative or potential influence should be considered by looking at a combination of factors. Versteeg (1979) identified five factors that need to be considered:

1. *Size.* In terms of political power, the number of members in a group in relation to the percentage they represent of the total group is an important factor. For example, if a group represents 50% of the nurses in a specialty or a unit and another group represents 90% of the nurses in their unit, the latter group has a higher size factor.

2. *Information base.* This includes the information possessed by the membership, especially what it knows about the goal and relevant professional and social issues.

3. *Expertise.* This refers to the knowledge base or special expertise the group offers. It is similar in nature to the expert power of individuals.

4. *Physical resources.* Time and money enable a group to exercise power.

5. *Personal attributes.* Similar to the referent power or charismatic power of individuals, personal attributes refer to the personal appeal of the group collectively and of its spokespersons.

What are some tactics that nurses can use with these types of power? The power of an individual is relative to that of others in influencing the behaviour of others or, in the context of this discussion, in influencing decisions. For example, in a hospital or a community health centre, nurse managers have legitimate power because of their position. As well, individual nurse managers may have various degrees of the other forms of power, such as expertise and charisma.

It is useful for a nurse manager to determine the sources of power for key participants in the objectives and to use these to maximum benefit. The nurse manager needs to weigh the relative importance of positional power over expert power. Using the source of power of key individuals and groups to plan the strategy is known as a "power strategy." A power strategy means that individuals with similar sources of power will be on both sides of the argument. If physicians use their expertise in medicine to influence the debate about a nursing issue in a specialty area, and if nurses with expertise in that area engage in this debate, the nurses' influence would be greater. If the nurses did not have expertise in the specialty area but had legitimate power for that area, they would have considerably less influence. This scenario would not be a power strategy because the sources of power would be different and, therefore, would not carry the same weight in the debate.

Several tactics can be used to acquire and maintain the derivative forms of power—associative power and lower participant power. For associative power, some of the tactics recommended in the literature include forming coalitions, negotiating or making trade-offs, lobbying, being present on key committees, and getting involved in social activities. In other words, the person planning a change needs to be at the right place, at the right time, with the right people.

As an example, forming a coalition (a temporary alliance between individuals or groups with a common goal) can be effective in influencing others into conformity. Caplow (1969) studied traditional coalitions in organizations and distribution of power among organizational triads. Sills (1976) later discussed Caplow's theory in terms of relative power among the three parts of the triad, in particular, the relationships in a hospital management triad formed by administrator, physician, and nurse.

Even though the size and complexity of hospitals and the position titles have changed in recent years, the basic mechanisms of the organizational triads are still valid today. Figure 23.1, which is adapted from the work of Caplow, shows the relationship between a hospital administrator (A), the medical director (B), and the senior nurse manager (C). In the triad, one must keep in mind that the positions are imbedded in the status order of the organization, which is

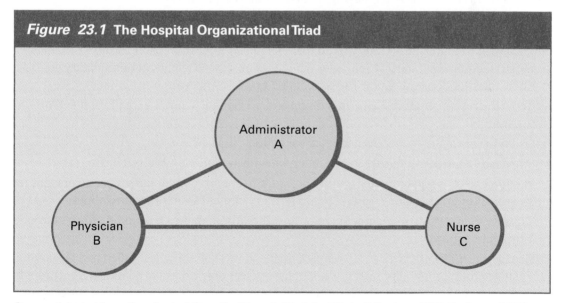

Figure 23.1 **The Hospital Organizational Triad**

Source: Adapted from *Two Against One: Coalitions in Triads* (p. 55), by T. Caplow, 1969, Englewood Cliffs, NJ: Prentice-Hall. Reprinted with permission.

represented by the size of the circles. In fact, the power distribution is largely determined by the actual behaviour of the incumbent. Furthermore, socialization of roles in adult life is often the result of primary and secondary socialization.

Applying Caplow's theoretical discussions, one sees that hospital administrators often share with physicians their primary socialization as men and their secondary socialization as being university-educated. Physicians and nurses share their secondary socialization in the "laying on of hands" and in being educated in closed, caste-like professions with specific codes, entrance requirements, and rituals. So, in health care, a coalition between A and B is considered a "conservative coalition" because it respects the primary and secondary socialization. A coalition between A and C is considered an "improper coalition" because it negates the primary and secondary socialization. A coalition between B and C is considered a "revolutionary coalition," a winning coalition that has the potential to dominate the more powerful member of the organizational triad. This theory can be applied to a debate over the need for bed closures. For example, a conservative coalition would be one in which the administrator, in coalition with physicians, decides how many beds to close and presents the recommendation to the board or the executive committee; such a recommendation would be accepted. An improper coalition exists when the administrator, in coalition with nurses, presents a bed-closure plan despite opposition from physicians; such a recommendation also would likely be accepted. However, if an administrator recommended bed closures, but nurses and physicians in a revolutionary coalition opposed that recommendation, the administrator, the board, or the executive committee would be hard-pressed to accept the recommendation.

Sills concluded that the system is kept in balance through rapid intermittent coalitions between administrators and physicians or administrators and nurses, which, in fact, prevent revolutionary coalitions from taking place. An understanding of these patterns can help nurses analyze ways in which decision making is carried out in organizations.

On a regular basis, nurses discuss and negotiate issues with other nurses and physicians, but they are not as skillful at influencing interdisciplinary politics or team processes. A political alliance with the multidisciplinary team members is an important asset for nurse managers today. Devereux and Dirschel (1985) offer guidelines on how to apply interdisciplinary politics:

- Know the situation (e.g., know the patient and problem the team must handle).
- Know the resources available from nursing and, in general, from the institution and/or community.
- Listen to colleagues' concerns and plans for action.
- Emphasize mutuality of goals shared among members of the multidisciplinary team.
- Reinforce what is legal practice of nursing; work to ensure that all nurses are competent in their areas of practice and be alert to casual encroachment from other disciplines.
- Expand nursing goals to include those of the other disciplines to help build alliances for future interactions.

Managers can also use tactics of lower participant power. For example, Shiflett and McFarland (1978) noted that a nurse administrator might have power over a hospital administrator through "1. control of resources upon which the administrator is dependent; 2. control of the access of others to that person; 3. control of techniques, procedures or knowledge vital to the administrator; and 4. personality attributes such as charm, likeableness, or charisma recognized by the administrator as desirable in subordinates" (p. 20). The authors (Shiflett and McFarland, 1978) also noted that staff members could use this same type of power with the front-line manager. One should also remember that derivative forms of power are more uncertain than other forms and that some forms of power are considered more legitimate than others, depending on the circumstances.

What are the key variables affecting the attainment of power? Instead of focusing on individual or group sources of power, Hickson and colleagues concentrated on horizontal power, or relationships between groups and subunits within an organization (Hickson, Hinings, Lee, Schneck, & Pennings, 1971). Stuart (1986) also highlighted the importance of interdisciplinary alliances within an organization and referred to this as the strategic-contingencies model. "Such an approach views intraorganizational conflict and negotiation as ongoing processes with the balance of power to effect change distributed dynamically among the various subunits. The division of labor among these subunits is then the source of intraorganizational power, and each subunit's tasks, functioning, and links with the activities of other subunits are crucial power variables" (p. 69).

In Stuart's (1986) model, three variables govern a subunit's power within the organization (nursing being a subunit, and a department being a subunit): (a) centrality, the degree of the subunit's interdependence with other subunits; (b) substitutability, the possibility of replacement by others; and (c) coping with uncertainty, the ability to handle, through a variety of mechanisms, inevitable but unpredictable occurrences. In light of these variables, Stuart recommended four principles for improving the quality of nursing care and maintaining power:

* Increase connections with other subunits and maintain the centrality;
* Become irreplaceable;
* Demonstrate nursing assets; for example, focus on the research showing the impact of nurse staffing on patients and nurses (e.g., Aiken, Clarke, Sloane, Sochalski, & Silber, 2002);
* Participate in high-level decision making about goals, resources, and activities desirable for the organization.

Physical Resources and Timing

In addition to assessing trends and values, key players, and sources of power, nurse managers also must consider resources such as time, money, and the willingness of individuals to support the project. What kinds of people and what mix of each different element will be needed? Will the project require the assistance of consultants or staff with special skills? Often, the value of the time and energy of the people committed to the goal is underestimated; belief and dedication to a cause is a resource of great value. Any deficiencies in resources can be compensated for when the strategy is planned; for example, increasing the number of volunteers can offset the shortcoming created by a limited amount of time. If special skills are needed, hiring or enlisting the help of an expert (even a student in that specialty) may be an option.

The timing of an issue is another critical factor. Timing is often so critical that it may be necessary to wait to implement a plan until conditions are more favourable. On the other hand, it may be necessary to be ready to move forward when opportunities present themselves.

Favourable and unfavourable times should be identified early in the process and a range of possible deadlines set for accomplishing the goal.

Step 3: Plan the Strategy

The two first steps (establishing the goal and assessing positive and negative forces) require the most time and are the most important. Once these are completed, the next step is to plan the strategy. The strategy is the framework within which necessary activities are carried out. It involves an action plan or a defined approach to reaching the goal.

Robbins (1986) noted that, whereas passion and belief provide the fuel for achieving power, intelligence and logical strategies (i.e., a sound plan) provide the road maps by which success is eventually achieved. Once the goal and objectives are clear and positive and negative factors that will influence change are assessed, it is time to use that knowledge to develop a strategy. A viable strategy may be devised by first developing strategies for each individual or group that has been targeted in the first step. At this point, all pieces of the puzzle must be brought together. The choice of activities used in an overall plan should be congruent with the assessment of the positive and negative factors identified in the second step of the process.

Steps 4 and 5: Implement and Evaluate the Strategy

Once the plan is complete, implementation begins. The effectiveness of the tactics selected and the strategy as a whole must be evaluated on an ongoing basis. Some activities or tactics may not be effective and should be replaced by others.

There is always a need to monitor the political process and adapt the strategies in the light of progress and changing conditions. Successful approaches can be duplicated and shared with other groups involved in the political process, and unsuccessful approaches can be modified.

Challenges for the Manager

Understanding intraorganizational politics and using the political process are challenging endeavours. Most studies on the topic identify nurses, in general, and nursing administrators, in particular, as ill-prepared and apathetic political spectators (Byers, 1990; Cronkhite, 1991; Small, 1989). In light of the serious consequences of this state of affairs in a time of reform, the situation creates important challenges for nurse leaders and managers.

The first challenge comes from a bias that can be traced back to the Western philosophical view that men are rational thinkers and thus responsible for affairs of the state, whereas women are emotional thinkers and therefore responsible for affairs of the family and for the support of men (Lloyd, 1984). Professions that are predominantly female, such as nursing, are affected by these stereotypes. Although much progress has been made, these ingrained cultural views explain why such topics as politics and power begin to appear in the nursing literature only in the late 1970s and why many nurses are still uncomfortable with these concepts today. The second challenge is to provide positive role models for other nurses by using the political process, encouraging educational programs, and rewarding political participation and behaviour among colleagues. The third is to provide a climate that encourages nurses to promote unity and to consolidate their political power by applying the four principles for attaining power: increasing connections, becoming irreplaceable, demonstrating nursing assets, and participating in high-level decision making (Stuart, 1986).

Leadership Implications

Knowledge and skills related to intraorganizational politics are essential for effective nurse leaders and managers of the 21st century. Nurses must learn about the effectiveness of political action in health care through courses, literature, mentoring, and projects that garner political expertise and positions of power or influence. The effectiveness of intraorganizational politics is not conditional upon the professions or educational backgrounds of the players, but it is conditional upon a clear goal, a systematic process, and determination. Nursing professionals can be part of the solution in restructuring health care, but their involvement depends on the political abilities and knowledge of intraorganizational politicsof their leaders. These leaders are instrumental in facilitating the acquisition of knowledge and abilities for nurses in all domains of practice: clinical, educational, research, and management.

An effective strategy to achieve goals can be planned and implemented through the judicious choice of priorities and the use of a political process drawing on multiple sources of power. These ingredients, plus the determination of nurses in senior positions, will ensure success in influencing decisions that support the goals of nursing.

Summary

- The Canadian health care system is experiencing the "moving state," as described in Lewin's theory of change (1951). During this time, effective politics can make a great difference in setting the course of a project, department, or organization.
- The political process framework has five steps: (a) establish goal and objectives; (b) assess positive and negative factors related to trends and values, key individuals or groups, and sources of power, resources, and timing; (c) plan a strategy; (d) implement the strategy; and (e) evaluate and readjust the strategy.
- Two pivotal issues for nurse managers are the allocation of health care resources and the leadership position of nurses.
- Commonly recognized sources of power include legitimate, reward, coercive, expert, and referent power. Two derivative forms are associative power and lower participant power.
- Associative power coalitions are formed among the organizational triad (i.e., administrator, physician, and nurse) in health care.

- Nurses must become proficient in the application of essential variables (centrality, substitutability, and coping with uncertainty) that affect attainment of power.
- Factors that affect the relative or potential influence of a group in an organization include size, information base, expertise, physical resources, and personal attributes.
- Challenges for nurses include the bias in society regarding women and politics, the need for positive nurse role models, and the creation of a climate that encourages attaining power in an organization.
- Knowledge and skills in intraorganizational politics are essential to be effective in nursing leadership and management.

Applying the Knowledge in this Chapter

Case Study

A corporate committee of clinical nurses in a large hospital decided to standardize the way nursing clinical practice was organized. Several models were in existence across the units (e.g., primary nursing, team nursing, total patient care, case management). A workgroup was created to tackle the issue, composed of clinical nurses working with different models (majority of the group), clinical managers, nurse educators, patient representatives, advanced practice nurses, and a university representative. From their work and multiple internal and external consultations over a period of almost a year, a new model was developed. The model was reached by consensus among the members of the workgroup, and it was developed from the best of all models in existence and in the literature. The model was designed to promote full scope of practice, autonomy, and accountability for all nurses. It provided a safety net for novice nurses by assigning a clinical expert on each shift.

Senior management, clinical directors, the Medical Advisory Committee, and the Professional Advisory Committee all agreed that this new model would help improve patient care and outcomes, and implementation began. The implementation included information sessions with nurses and other health professionals, including physicians, a steering workgroup consisting of nurses and other health professionals, as well as unit subgroups with nurses and other health professionals.

The implementation of the model implied that, on some units, the team leader position would disappear, and each nurse would interface directly with physicians and other health professionals for the care of their patients. On other units, the team leader role would be retained because of the size of the unit, but the role would become more administrative rather than clinical in order to avoid erosion of clinical nurses' autonomy. Some physicians and other professionals feared that the new model would affect their practice. They were worried that they would have to communicate with more than one nurse for the patients on a unit, they would be called often for unimportant reasons, and that novice nurses would not be able to interface with them adequately. Some of the team leaders encouraged the physicians to use their influence to prevent the model from being implemented on their unit. Physicians, other health professionals, and some nurses mounted petitions, wrote letters to the Chief Executive Officer and Vice-President of Medical Affairs, and held departmental meetings on this topic. One physician threatened to leave the hospital if the model was implemented.

Using the ideas presented in this chapter, identify the underlying problems in this case study. Analyze the sources of power utilized to influence the implementation, and consider what you would do to plan a power strategy. What resources are required to overcome the problem? Are there any potential alliances to be made? Plan appropriate change strategies for ensuring the implementation of the nursing model.

Resources

evolve Internet Resources

Canadian Medical Association (CMA):
www.cma.ca/
Canadian Nurses Association (CNA):
www.cna-nurses.ca/
The CNA's 2002 position statement on nursing leadership can be found on this site.

Further Reading

Canadian Medical Association & Canadian Nurses Association. (2004). *The taming of the queue: Toward a cure for health care wait times.* Ottawa, ON: Authors.
This paper is the result of the formation of a "revolutionary" coalition of two national professional associations who joined forces to write a discussion paper that would inform the public policy process on an issue of mutual concern. The Liberal Party of Canada had identified waiting times for access to health services as a major issue in the 2004 Canadian general election. This paper is available on the association Web sites listed above.

References

Aiken, L.H., Clarke, S.P., Sloane, D.M., Sochalski, J., & Silber, J.H. (2002). Hospital nurse staffing and patient mortality, nurse burnout, and job satisfaction. *Journal of the American Medical Association, 288*(16), 1987–1993.

Bissinger, R.L., Allred, C.A., Arford, P.H., & Bellig, L.L. (1997). A cost-effectiveness analysis of neonatal nurse practitioners. *Nursing Economics, 15,* 92–99.

Byers, S.R. (1990). *Relationship among staff nurses' beliefs, nursing practice and unit ethos.* Unpublished doctoral dissertation, Ohio State University, Columbus. (From CIHNAL 1983-1993, Abstract No. 142524).

Canadian Nurses Association. (2002). *Nursing leadership: Position statement.* Ottawa, ON: Author.

Canadian Nurses Association. (1993). *New directions in health care: Cost effective nursing alternatives.* Ottawa, ON: Author.

Caplow, T. (1969). *Two against one: Coalitions in triads.* Englewood Cliffs, NJ: Prentice Hall.

Cronkhite, L.M. (1991). *The role of the hospital nurse administrator in a changing health care environment: A study of values and conflicts.* Unpublished doctoral dissertation, University of Wisconsin, Milwaukee. (From CIHNAL 1983-1993, Abstract No. 161175).

Davidhizar, R. (1993). Leading with charisma. *Journal of Advanced Nursing, 18*(4), 675–679.

Del Bueno, D.J. (1986). Power and politics in organizations. *Nursing Outlook, 34*(3), 124–128.

Devereux, P.M., & Dirschel, K.M. (1985). Interdisciplinary politics. In D.J. Mason & S.W. Talbot (Eds.), *Political action handbook for nurses* (pp. 240–250). Menlo Park, CA: Addison-Wesley.

Drucker, P. (1992). *Managing for the future: The 1990s and beyond.* New York: Truman Tally Books/Dutton.

Erikson, E.H. (1963). *The challenge of youth.* Garden City, NY: Doubleday.

Fergusson, V.D. (1985). Two perspectives on power. In D.J. Mason & S.W. Talbot (Eds.), *Political action handbook for nurses* (pp. 88–93). Menlo Park, CA: Addison-Wesley.

Fleeger, M.E. (1993). Assessing organizational culture: A planning strategy. *Nursing Management, 24*(2), 39–41.

French, J.R.P., & Raven, B. (1959). The bases of social power. In D. Cartwright (Ed.), *Studies in social power* (pp. 150–167). Ann Arbor, MI: University Press.

Hickson, D., Hinings, C., Lee, C., Schneck, R., & Pennings, J. (1971). A strategic contingencies' theory of organizational power. *Administrative Science Quarterly, 16*(2), 216–229.

Lasater, M. (1996). The effect of a nurse-managed CHF clinic on patient readmission and length of stay. *Home Healthcare Nurse, 14,* 351–356.

Laswell, H.D. (1936). *Politics: Who gets what, when, how.* New York: The World Publishing.

Lewin, K. (1951). *The nature of field theory.* New York: Macmillan.

Lloyd, G. (1984). *The man of reason.* London: Methuen.

Mason, D.J., & McCarthy, A.M. (1985). The politics of patient care. In D.J. Mason & S.W. Talbot (Eds.), *Political action handbook for nurses* (pp. 38–52). Menlo Park, CA: Addison-Wesley.

Pfeffer, J. (1981). *Power in organization.* Boston: Pitman.

Prescott, P. (1993). Nursing: An important component of hospital survival under a reformed health-care system. *Nursing Economics, 11*(4), 192–199.

Robbins, A. (1986). *Unlimited power.* New York: Simon & Schuster.

Schein, E. (1985). *Organizational culture and leadership: A dynamic view.* San Francisco: Jossey-Bass.

Shamian, J. (1997). How nursing contributes towards quality and cost-effective health care. *International Nursing Review, 44*(3), 79-84, 90.

Shiflett, N., & McFarland, D.E. (1978). Power and the nursing administrator. *Journal of Nursing Administration, 7*(3), 19–23.

Sills, G.M. (1976). Nursing, medicine, and hospital administrator. *American Journal of Nursing, 76*(9), 1432–1434.

Small, E.B. (1989). *Factors associated with political participation.* Unpublished doctoral dissertation, North Carolina State University, Chapel Hill. (From CIHNAL 1983-1993, Abstract No. 119031).

Sovie, M.D. (1993). Hospital culture–Why create one? *Nursing Economics, 11*(2), 69–75.

Starke, A., & Rempel, E. (1988). Organizational politics and nursing administration. *Canadian Journal of Nursing Administration, 1*(4), 11–14.

Stevens, B.J. (1980a). Development and use of power in nursing. In *Assuring a goal-directed future for nursing* (Publication 52-1814). New York: National League for Nursing.

Stevens, B.J. (1980b). Power and politics for the nurse executive. *Nursing and Health Care, 1*(4), 208–210.

Stuart, G.W. (1986). An organizational strategy for empowering nursing. *Nursing Economics, 4*(2), 69–73.

Versteeg, D.F. (1979). The political process: Or the power and glory. *Nursing Dimensions, 7*(2), 20–27.

Weeks, M.B. (2002). Determining the cost-effectiveness of the registered nurse first assistant: The research link. *Canadian Operating Room Nursing Journal, 20*(4), 16–21.

Wieland, G.F., & Ullrich, R.A. (1976). *Organizations: Behavior, design, and change.* Homewood, IL: Richard D. Irwin.

PROJECT MANAGEMENT

Donna Lynn Smith and Michelle Salesse

Learning Objectives

In this chapter, you will learn:

- How the project management approach is used to structure the implementation of planned change

- The characteristics of a project and the features that distinguish projects from routine organizational operations

- How and why projects are initiated

- Some of the structural elements of projects and why these are important to the success of a project

- The roles of a project sponsor, project manager, and project team

- The importance of planning, scheduling, and evaluation as they pertain to project development and management

- Key elements of a project work plan

- How to recognize situations or examples in which the project management approach might be applicable

- Features of the culture of projects

Organizations in the health care system are being challenged to maintain and improve upon the services they offer while responding to the pressures created by emerging scientific developments and technologies, financial restraint, and changes in clients' expectations and social values. It is clear that change in the health care system will continue to be an everyday occurrence. Managers at all organizational levels often want to spend more time on planning and innovation, but find it difficult to do so because of the relentless pressures of their everyday work. Some aspects of this dilemma can be dealt with by using time management strategies, but new initiatives cannot be effectively accomplished without dedicated time and human resources. Organizations must find ways to maintain and continuously improve upon their routine operations through incremental change, but paradoxically, they must also find ways to make strategic and innovative responses to rapidly changing external circumstances. Projects are temporary management structures established to energize and speed up the process of diffusing innovations through an organization or to accelerate the pace of change. As a model, project management provides a structured approach for implementing planned change in complex contexts.

Organizations create structure to facilitate the coordination of activities and to control the actions of their members (Bishop, 1999). Matrix structures and project management technologies were initially developed in the 1950s and 1960s in the aerospace, defense, and construction industries (Glasser, 1963). They began to appear in business and public sector organizations in the 1970s, and since that time they have contributed to what Kerzner (1984) has described as an "organizational revolution." He explained that "commonly used organizational structures proved inadequate in responding to an ever changing environment," (p. 307) and that the complexities faced by organizations forced them to consider and implement structures that could facilitate more timely responses to external pressures. The project management approach has also been advocated as a way for nursing executives to achieve professional and corporate goals (Hermann, Alexander, & Kiely, 1992; Loo, 2003).

In this chapter, the characteristics of a project are described, including a brief explanation of what a project is, why and how it is initiated, and the role of the stakeholders. The structural elements of projects, including sponsorship and reporting mechanisms, committees, project managers, project team members, objectives, and work plans, are discussed, and the importance of planning, scheduling, and monitoring activities in projects is emphasized. The role of a project manager is described, and the chapter concludes with a discussion of the culture of projects.

What Is a Project?

A project is a temporary structure created for a specific period of time to accomplish a specific task that has a defined end product or service. Projects vary in size, scope, and design; however, a common feature of most projects is that they cut across the departmental, functional, or programmatic lines of an organization to bring together groups of people or activities to formalize plans and schedules for achieving specific outcomes. By establishing formal projects and allocating resources to facilitate project work, organizations can overcome resistance to change or an unacceptably slow pace of change within line departments and functional areas. Projects are often created to accelerate changes considered strategically necessary for organizational adaptation and survival or to coordinate complex organization-wide initiatives that occur infrequently.

The central processes of organizations involve recurring activities or patterns of activities that adapt incrementally over time. Changes in the external environment, such as public expectations or the funding policies or incentives of government agencies, may create the need to introduce or develop new technologies, products, services, or programs; to reposition an organization or program so that it can become more effective; to develop new competencies; or to plan and bring into operation new systems, structures, and processes. When this happens, a concentrated effort is needed to achieve specific and predetermined results (sometimes called *deliverables*) within a defined period of time and a specified budget. These conditions define a project and differentiate it from the more routine activities of an organization. Projects and project management are a means of managing, monitoring, and achieving planned change. Project management has been defined as a set of management disciplines and practices that, if executed well, increase the likelihood that a project will deliver the desired results (Glaser, 2004).

How Are Projects Initiated?

The impetus for a project can come from leaders or stakeholders. Projects may be initiated to address the priorities of provincial health departments or governing boards. Executive management may initiate a project to achieve particular organizational changes (e.g., the implementation of a new information system) or organization-wide compliance with new policies or practices. Sometimes, internal stakeholders identify issues and propose policy and program innovations that gain the support of other organizational stakeholders and an executive champion who can help to secure support and resources to initiate a project. Stakeholders outside the organization may also raise issues that become policy priorities and result in the initiation of projects.

The Role of Stakeholders in Initiating Projects

Stakeholders are individuals or groups with an interest in a particular issue or objective: their influence may initiate projects, and they are often involved in project steering or advisory committees where they influence the structure, allocation of resources, and schedules. The involvement of stakeholder groups in initiating and monitoring a project is often a critical factor in achieving project goals and diffusing the knowledge and experience developed in a project throughout the organization.

Projects are often initiated at the executive level of the organization in order to make changes in structure or processes in a climate of increased demand and shrinking resources; for example, an organization-wide, total quality management program may be launched, pharmacy or other clinical services may be decentralized, or a work redesign initiative or injury prevention program may be undertaken. New buildings, systems, programs, and research projects are usually planned and implemented by means of a project management structure. New information systems are developed, acquired, and implemented by means of formal projects.

Sometimes, projects originate at the grassroots of the organization when a group of staff within a program or work unit brings forward a project idea. For example, the nurses within an extended care unit might advocate for the implementation of a self-medication program for residents of the unit. With the support of their leader, they could form a committee and develop plans for implementing the program. Their leader would assist them in communicating the objectives and potential benefits of the program to the senior level of the organization. The unit leader could also help to facilitate the work of the group through staff scheduling, financing planning and learning time for the committee, or by obtaining commitments for such necessities as renovations, supplies, and expert consultation. If the innovative idea becomes a project, the goals and plans of the committee are supported and formalized, and human or financial resources are allocated to it so that the goals can realistically be accomplished within the time specified.

Projects may also be initiated in response to community pressure. As client groups become more effective in coordinating their activities and communicating their needs, they may put pressure on health organizations to become more responsive to clients who have not previously been a high priority. For example, advocacy organizations for victims of sexual assault and domestic violence may urge police departments, hospital emergency services, and health professionals to initiate educational programs and develop customized approaches that address the needs of these people in a more focused and coordinated manner. One well-known example of a major project resulting from citizen and client advocacy is the innovative Northeast Community Health Centre in Edmonton, Alberta. The impetus for this centre came from a citizens group that originally advocated for hospital and emergency services in the northeast part of the city.

Structural Elements of Projects

Each project is different, and there is no one way to manage projects. Pilot projects and experiments may be hampered by excessive formal oversight, whereas large, multi-year, multi-million dollar undertakings cannot be accomplished without elaborate structures, management, communications, decision making, and reporting. Glaser (2004) notes that all projects benefit from having a well-defined approach in the areas of roles, committees, charters, plans, and status reporting.

The structural elements of projects include a sponsorship and reporting mechanism, a committee structure for planning and monitoring the project, a project manager, and a project team. Other structural elements are the objectives (i.e., the goals) and the work plan for the project. The work plan identifies the expected outcomes or deliverables, the activities required to complete them, and the completion dates for all activities and deliverables. Often, a monitoring or evaluation process is set up in parallel with a project, and this is sometimes completed with the assistance of experts and stakeholders who are outside of the organization so that impartial audits and assessments of project management and results can be obtained. In large and costly projects that take place over a period of several years, such parallel monitoring mechanisms are often critical to a successful outcome. In complex projects, the structural elements are sometimes summarized in a project chart (Glaser, 2004).

Sponsorship and Reporting Mechanism

A project must often be marketed throughout the organization, particularly if resources such as staff time, expert consultation, or special funding are needed to initiate and complete it. The project must go beyond the idea stage to become a formally approved organizational priority and investment. Organizational endorsement is important, even if the amount of money required to initiate and manage the project is minimal, because the project will consume time and intellectual capital and may therefore be a distraction from other corporate objectives. Senior management support is critical for the success of projects; for a project to gain this support, it must be closely aligned with the needs and objectives of the organization.

The term *executive champion* is sometimes used to describe the role of a person at the executive level of an organization who can assist the project in the following ways: communicate and interpret the goals and benefits of a project to the executive team, assign or obtain needed resources, enlist and sustain the support of other departments or stakeholder groups, remove barriers, provide recognition, and assist in disseminating and adopting the new knowledge developed through the project. Some projects begin as the executive champion's own ideas, but others originate elsewhere in the organization, perhaps from front-line leaders or work teams. In the latter case, for a project to succeed, someone at a more senior level of the organization must be persuaded to become an advocate for the project on behalf of the unit or workgroup, as in the example of the self-medication program described earlier.

Obtaining the interest and support of an executive champion is usually essential for the success of a project that begins at the grassroots level of the organization. Although projects that are congruent with corporate vision and overall management strategy are most likely to attract corporate support, some organizations purposely accommodate a few low-key and inexpensive grassroots projects as a way of fostering innovation and creativity. The term *skunk works* is sometimes used to describe unofficial projects of this nature (Kanter, 1989), and they have also been referred to as "havens for safe learning" (Galbraith, 1982). Such projects can enhance the adaptive capacities of an organization by allowing new ideas and emergent leadership to flourish.

Committees and Sponsors

To be successful, most projects require a broader base of support than can be provided by an individual project leader or even a single executive champion. When a project has influence or impact across more than one organizational unit, there is a need for support from other parts of the organization. In fact, projects were among the first of the various forms of matrix structures that are now common in complex organizations (Meredith & Mantel, 2000; PMBOK, 2000). A project (i.e., the project manager and team) is usually linked to the rest of the organization through a designated individual or business sponsor who holds overall accountability for the project. A project that affects a very large part of the organization may have the chief executive officer (CEO) as the business sponsor.

A steering or sponsoring committee is needed to market a project and then support its initiation, planning, and eventual implementation. An existing committee can be a project sponsor if its members include stakeholders in the project. There may be a number of business owners for a project—these are line managers of departments or functions affected by the project. If an existing committee does not already bring the business owners together, or if the project is of sufficient importance to the organization, a committee structure may be established with the goal of providing specific support and direction to the project. Occasionally, such a committee becomes the project sponsor, and the project manager will report to it for purposes of the project, rather than to his or her usual supervisor.

Whatever the nature of the supporting committee structure, it is important that terms of reference be established to guide committee members, the project manager, and the project team. This is particularly important when special committees are established to advise or oversee projects. The formal terms of reference should include clear statements about the committee's decision-making mandates and procedures, where or to whom it reports, and the role of its chair. The terms *steering committee* and *advisory committee* are sometimes used interchangeably, but these two types of committees have different roles. A steering committee is made up of individuals who have formal decision-making responsibilities within the organization; an advisory committee is made of individuals who offer their perspectives but do not have the authority to actually make decisions about the project. An advisory committee is a means of including and informing project stakeholders and can sometimes prevent stakeholders who are not supportive of the project mandate from obstructing the progress of a project. However, token stakeholder representation wastes time and other resources and can produce cynicism and ill will if it appears that the concerns and recommendations of advisory groups are not take seriously.

The sponsor of a project is the individual and/or group in the organizational structure that is responsible for the project and has the authority or ability to validate, clarify, or if necessary, alter its mandate. The reporting structure for a project should clearly spell out the authority and responsibility of the project sponsor, whether an individual or committee. In the case of committees, existing or specially developed terms of reference should be available to all those concerned with the project. The sponsor may be identified by the executive and may sometimes be a member of the executive team. Occasionally, a person who has no interest in, or knowledge of, a particular project is appointed as a sponsor. This is an undesirable situation that can discourage project team members and the project manager, and it is potentially a waste of organizational resources. The skills of a project manager, combined with cohesion and productivity of the project team, can sometimes overcome the inherent difficulties of such a situation, but it is preferable that the sponsor and executive champion of a project believe in its value, concur with its objectives, understand the difficulties it is likely to face, and feel a commitment to supporting the project manager and team.

The Project Manager

In general, the role of a project manager is to:

- lead and coordinate the activities of a project;
- recruit or develop and coach the project team;
- keep the project moving forward by identifying and resolving issues and problems;
- manage the multiple communications processes and relationships required to keep the project moving forward;

- manage the project budget and other resources; and
- ensure that project goals are achieved within the agreed upon time frame and resources.

If projects are relatively simple and grow from the grassroots of the organization, the role of project manager may be added to the regular responsibilities of a staff member with interests, knowledge, and leadership abilities relevant to the project. This approach has the advantage of building support for the project from within the operating units of the organization, but it can sometimes result in overload for the individual who is trying to maintain all regular responsibilities in addition to managing the project. Occasionally, a project manager is seconded from regular responsibilities to lead a project on a part-time or full-time basis. For complex projects, a full- or part-time project manager may be seconded or even recruited to the role.

However a project manager is chosen, it is critical that the role and reporting channel for this individual be clearly defined. This is sometimes more easily said than done because the project manager must (a) obtain or communicate information important to the success of the project in a timely fashion, (b) develop support for project activities, (c) get agreement or commitment on scheduling issues that affect other departments, and (d) maintain the necessary level of staffing support for the project. To do this, the project manager usually needs access to a variety of people and resources in different departments and at different levels of the organization. Project managers may be assigned to report to the same vice-president as do their departmental supervisors. Occasionally, a project manager will report directly to the CEO or a board committee. Although such arrangements can be inherently stressful, they are necessary. A project can rarely remain on schedule and succeed if the project manager is confined to communication through a traditional bureaucratic hierarchy.

Good project managers have strong planning and operational management skills. They must have the necessary background and experience, technical expertise, leadership ability, and interpersonal competence. Skills in communication, consultation, persuasion, and negotiation assume greater prominence in project management when the staff assigned or seconded to the project continue to report to, and be assessed by, the managers of their home departments. The project manager gains authority from the project mandate and the degree of high-level organizational support that exists for the project. Developing commitment to the goals and demands of the project within the project team and across the organization as a whole is often a complex process that depends upon the integrity, credibility, and interpersonal and political skills of the project manager. Project managers must understand the issues and skills involved in developing shared commitment, behavioural norms, and high productivity among members of workgroups and teams. In addition, project managers must be able to lead the team in structuring its goals and tasks, developing a work plan, framing issues, and resolving conflicts within the project team or between the team and other parts of the organization.

There are a variety of project management methods available to assist project managers in structuring project activities. Box 24.1 presents a list of steps that will serve as a useful guide to project managers. It was prepared by Nancy Rowan, a graduate of the nursing program at McMaster University, who has managed many projects within organizations and now works as a management consultant.

Box 24.1

Steps in the Project Management Process

Step 1. Project Initiation
- Analyzing the market
- Defining the scope
- Identifying the constraints
- Developing the conceptual framework
- Confirming the mandate
- Developing/negotiating the terms of reference
- Defining the organizational structure

Step 2. Planning the Project Work
- Establishing a shared vision
- Recruiting and training personnel for the project
- Preparing a budget (financial integrity)
- Designing systems to assure a quality product (technical integrity)
- Establishing a communication and/or marketing plan
- Establishing an evaluation plan
- Identifying the competition
- Identifying pockets of resistance
- Identifying potential areas of conflict
- Identifying milestones
- Writing measurable objectives
- Identifying decision points and reporting intervals
- Identifying decision-making processes and criteria
- Establishing a detailed work plan

Step 3. Executing the Project Work
- Performing project activities
- Anticipating and managing operational problems
- Ongoing environmental scanning
- Adjusting priorities and schedules
- Tracking actual work
- Tracking and controlling costs
- Negotiating changes/commitments
- Managing conflict
- Reporting to stakeholders
- Monitoring performance
- Communicating with both internal and external audiences (formal and informal)
- Marketing the product

Step 4. Concluding the Project
- Evaluating outcomes
- Developing a final report
- Publishing results
- Terminating the project or re-establishing it in a new context
- Finalizing contracts or agreements
- Acknowledging participants
- Acknowledging stakeholders/funders
- Planning for the continuance of the initiative (if indicated)

Source: Nancy Rowan, BScN, MHSA. Used with permission.

Project managers are responsible for managing and allocating project resources and, sometimes, are responsible for obtaining resources at the outset of the project or throughout its life. They also manage the many relationships necessary to implement the project, including those involving other facets of the organization and external stakeholders. If important relationships are neglected, the result can be major difficulties, delays, and costs for the project. Consulting firms that manage large projects now recognize this by assigning the responsibility for "relationship management" in a project to a very senior individual. SMART Project Management, developed by Hartman (2000), is an example of one project management method.

The Project Team
The project team is made up of the project manager and the individuals who have been recruited, seconded, or assigned to the project team or to other roles critical to the project. The time, skills, and effort of project staff are a major project and organizational resource. In some instances, a project manager is appointed and then has an opportunity to choose the individuals to be recruited or seconded to the project team. More often, people are assigned to the team because of their professional knowledge and skills, their previous experience in similar projects, or because they have uncommitted time. Occasionally, departmental managers decide to solve problems in a local workgroup by loaning or transferring people who are "troublemakers" to a project. These people can sometimes be an asset to a project if they have high levels of initiative and good interpersonal skills. Knowledge directly pertinent to a project is an asset and is required by a critical mass of project team members; however, most projects can manage to absorb one or more individuals with generic skills as long as they are willing to learn from others and have reasonably high interpersonal competence.

A mix of technical and conceptual skills is required in most projects. Selection of the project team depends upon a number of factors, including the nature of the technical work to be done, the level and type of expertise required at each phase of the project, reporting relationships, and the availability of staff in the organization. Teams are brought together to implement projects precisely because the combined knowledge and skill of a group usually surpasses that of individuals. A skilled project manager recognizes the need to share leadership within the project team

591

so that the full potential of the team can be realized. Creation, modification, and implementation of the project work plan and schedule are among the many group problem-solving tasks faced by project teams.

The team must communicate and agree about who is doing what. It also must become expert at identifying the issues that affect the project in order to resolve them within the team or to be able to communicate them and seek support for their resolution in various departments and at various levels of the organization. In addition to work done individually by team members with particular knowledge and skills, the identification and resolution of issues is a central activity throughout the life of a project. Project teams are more likely to overcome obstacles and achieve their goals when team members commit to completing the project goals, share responsibility and power, and demonstrate initiative, creativity, flexibility, and perseverance.

Developing shared knowledge, behavioural norms, group history, and *esprit de corps* is also critical to the successful management and implementation of projects. The literature indicates that the development process for projects is very knowledge intensive but that is also generates knowledge at a rapid rate (Hartman, 2000; Kanter, 1989; Scholtes, Joiner, & Streibel, 1996). Projects frequently engender secondary innovations; therefore, the cumulative expertise of a high-performance project team is an irreplaceable corporate resource and should be nurtured and protected as such.

In Box 24.2, a case study is presented that describes how a project originated and was managed in a regional multi-site continuing care organization. In this situation, a middle manager

Box 24.2

Case Study: A Middle Manager becomes a Project Manager

Carewest is a multi-site, publicly funded continuing care organization. In 2002, it operated nine sites throughout the Calgary Health Region, including 182 rehabilitation and recovery beds, 40 designated assisted living beds, 958 continuing care beds, and a variety of community outreach services. Services were being expanded to include regional rehabilitation and recovery programs. Regulatory changes in the provincial context had increased the scope of practice for licensed practical nurses (LPNs). Within this context, a decision was made at the executive level of the organization to introduce the LPN role within the organization. This decision dictated the need to redesign the roles of registered nurses (RNs) and other nursing personnel.

In this work redesign project, the key activity was to redesign the role of the RN and then to implement the new roles of RNs and LPNs. The work of unlicensed health care attendants would remain the same, and LPNs would be introduced to the care setting with a role description that enabled them to fully enact their recently expanded scope of practice. It was critically important to achieve "buy in" from all affected staff to assure that the RNs and LPNs did not duplicate each other's work and that health care attendants understood from whom to take direction.

Important background work on role design was completed before the new roles were implemented. A series of charts were prepared by a senior nursing leader in the organization to illustrate the alignment of roles and responsibilities for all members of the care team. These charts confirmed the leadership responsibilities of RNs and provided consistent guidance to all staff about the goals and substance of the change being made.

The project was initiated within the Carewest George Boyack Care Centre, a 221-bed continuing care facility located in northeastern Calgary. Carewest has a relatively flat organizational structure. The executive director is responsible for management of the organization, and the site and service leaders, who report directly to the executive director, are responsible for the administration of client services of one to three sites each and for the business-enabling operations of the organization. Together, these leaders form the organization's Senior Executive Committee. Program leaders, who report to the site leaders, are responsible for program and facilities operations while providing clinical expertise for front-line staff within specific programs and facilities.

The senior management team was interested in the development of a prototypical implementation plan that could be pilot tested in one centre and then adapted for the others. A newly recruited program leader in the organization, with responsibility for the overall operational management of the Capable Seniors Program (a program for physically frail but cognitively intact older adults) at the Carewest George Boyack Care Centre, was asked to be the project manager for this implementation project. As a program leader, she had the administrative authority to initiate and implement the project within her own program.

The new program leader assumed the role of project manager in addition to her operational responsibilities. Management support for the project was secured via a communication memorandum that detailed the mandate for the change. A "management sponsor" was identified in each department, and this leader communicated the project and its mandate within her or his own department. The project manager worked closely with each department manager to negotiate and confirm the availability of staff members who had been assigned to work on the project, to follow up and monitor those resources committed, and to take action if a mishap occurred.

The Steering Committee for this project, called the LPN Implementation Working Group, consisted of all site leaders, the service leader of human resources, and the service development leader. It was a high-level planning group assembled to discuss the general impact of implementation of LPNs into long-term care and to plan for such implementation across the organization. The project manager continued to report weekly to the site leader of her own care centre. At the mid-point of the project, she attended a meeting of the Steering Committee (LPN Implementation Working Group) to report on the project.

Before calling upon the departments and people whose resources or time had been committed to the project, the project manager made a courtesy telephone call or informal in-person visit to remind the various department managers of corporate level commitment to the project, to review the project timelines, and to negotiate and confirm the availability of staff members who had been assigned to work on the project.

A project management approach was used to conduct the work required to implement the change of incorporating the role of the LPNs within the multidisciplinary care team structure of Carewest. The framework for the project management process that incorporated relationship building as the foundation was used to guide the process (Table 24.1).

The original project was considered finished when the new LPN roles took effect. Subsequently, the initial project was used as a prototype for implementation in other centres.

Source: Adapted from *Workforce Redesign in a Multisite Continuing Care Organization: Implementing a Planned Change,* by M. Salesse, 2002, unpublished report of Nursing 900 Project presented to complete requirements for the MN degree, Faculty of Nursing, University of Alberta, Edmonton, Alberta.

in the organization was asked to manage the project in addition to her day-to-day responsibilities for managing a program. Implementation of the project in this manager's program was seen as a pilot project or prototype for implementing the change in other units and programs within the organization.

Project Objectives and Work Plan

A project is unlikely to succeed without clearly formulated objectives that are agreed upon by all stakeholders. It is sometimes necessary to revise project objectives, and recognizing when and why this may be necessary is a key skill of the project manager. Whether objectives remain the same or are modified during the life of a project, they must be effectively communicated to stakeholders throughout the organization. The project objectives provide a high-level framework within which other project parameters (e.g., the budget and timelines) are determined. The objectives should specify the project outcomes or deliverables and provide guidance for evaluating project outcomes and effectiveness.

In its simplest form, a project work plan is a list of activities that specifies the dates each activity will begin and finish and identifies the individual or group that has primary responsibility for ensuring the activity is completed properly and on time. This type of work plan may be all that is necessary for an uncomplicated project. A Gantt chart is commonly used to summarize activities, accountabilities, and timelines in simple projects (Hartman, 2000; Meredith & Mantel, 2000; PMBOK, 2000). The example shown in Figure 24.1 illustrates the work plan for a generic project.

Large projects that involve many stakeholders, require large resource commitments, and take place over extended periods of time need to use more elaborate project planning, scheduling, and monitoring technologies. Two limitations of the Gantt chart are that it does not show the interdependencies between activities and it does not distinguish between primary and supplementary activities. These limitations are overcome by using complex network diagrams (Meredith & Mantel, 2000; PMBOK, 2000) such as that shown in Figure 24.2.

Figure 24.1 Gantt Chart for a Generic Project

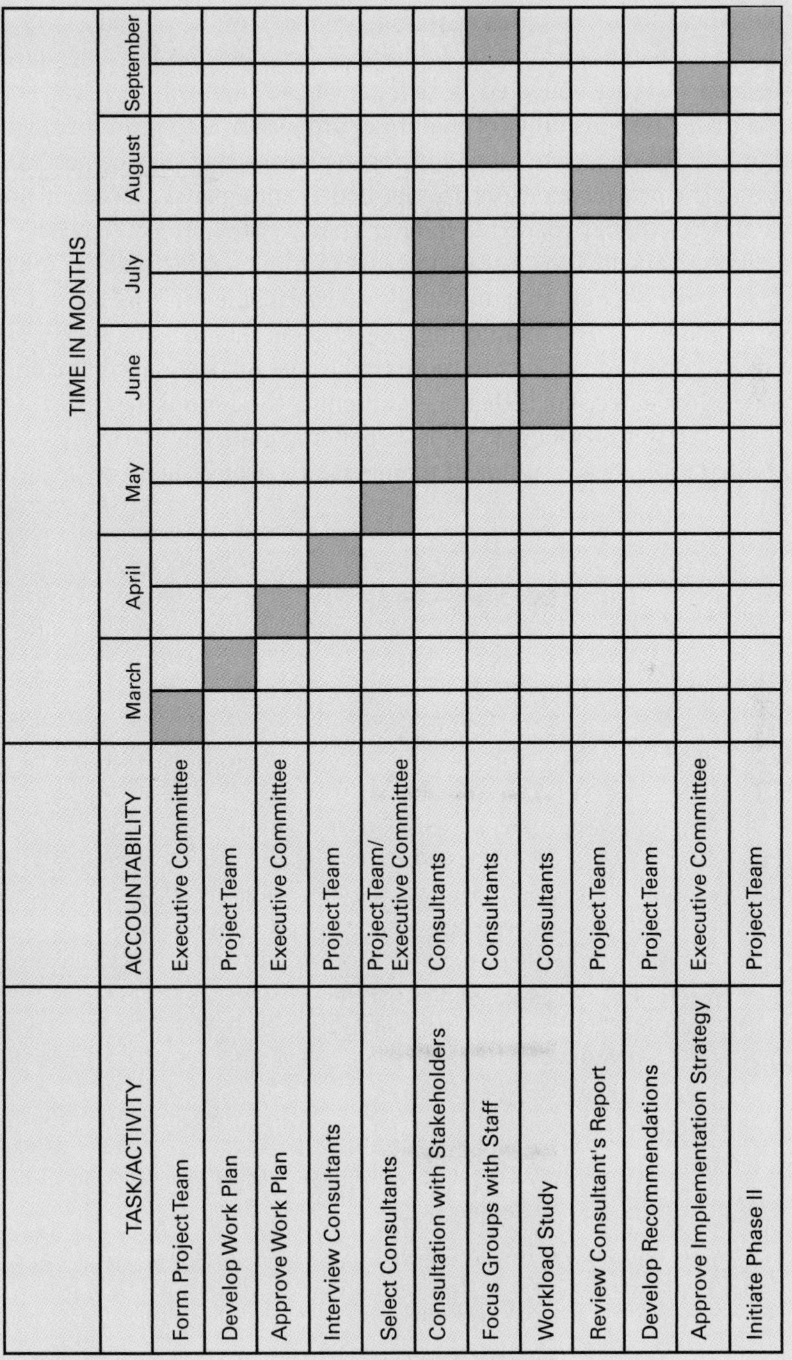

TIME IN MONTHS

TASK/ACTIVITY	ACCOUNTABILITY	March	April	May	June	July	August	September
Form Project Team	Executive Committee	■						
Develop Work Plan	Project Team	■						
Approve Work Plan	Executive Committee		■					
Interview Consultants	Project Team		■					
Select Consultants	Project Team/Executive Committee			■				
Consultation with Stakeholders	Consultants			■	■	■		
Focus Groups with Staff	Consultants			■	■			■
Workload Study	Consultants				■	■		
Review Consultant's Report	Project Team						■	
Develop Recommendations	Project Team						■	
Approve Implementation Strategy	Executive Committee							■
Initiate Phase II	Project Team							■

In Figure 24.2, there are nine major activities (A1 through A9), several of which are comprised of sub-activities (S1, S2, etc.). In this diagram, activities A1 through A3, including the sub-activities of each, will be taking place at more or less the same time in order to complete A4 on schedule. These three activities must be completed on time, and a delay in any one of them can result in a delay in starting A4. In large and complex projects, person-hours or days and their associated costs are budgeted to each activity and sub-activity. Even small delays can be costly, and a major responsibility of the project manager is to monitor the completion of activities and to lead the development of contingency plans that may be necessary if unavoidable delays occur. The project sponsors are notified of anticipated delays and any unexpected costs that may arise. Activities occurring in later phases of the project may have to be speeded up or done in different and less costly ways in order to compensate for delays in the early stages of the project. An array of computer software is now available to assist project teams in planning, scheduling, budgeting, and monitoring projects, and skill in using such tools will increasingly be seen as an important adjunct to more traditional managerial competencies.

An even more complicated skill is that of maintaining the commitment and morale of a project group so that it can stay on schedule while responding positively and quickly to the inevitable obstacles that most projects encounter. If members of a project team continue to have other

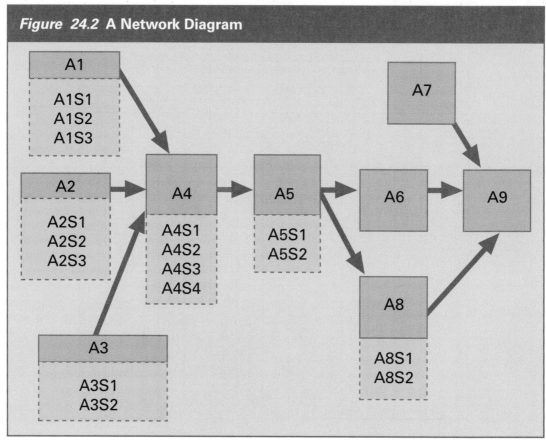

Figure 24.2 A Network Diagram

responsibilities within the organization, or if there is not clear and continuous direction and support from the project sponsors, this can be particularly difficult.

In the Case Study described in Box 24.2, the leadership and project management skills of a middle manager were recognized when she was asked to manage the project for the organization. This example highlights the way a project is structured and illustrates the type of matrix-reporting relationships that are common when projects are developed using the human resources already available within the organization.

The Culture of Projects

Noted management researcher and consultant Rosabeth Moss Kanter has discussed a number of differences between "mainstreams" (the operational departments and functions of an organization) and "newstreams" (the channels and mechanisms set up to change the organization). She noted that the operating logic of a newstream often conflicts with that of the mainstream. "Mainstreams and newstreams differ in performance criteria, predictability, and the need to shed the burden of the past" (Kanter, 1989, p. 202). She pointed out that in creative projects, regardless of type, people share the following experiences:

- the need to move quickly when opportunity or inspiration strikes;
- missed deadlines and encounters with the unexpected;
- the constant need to justify the project, especially as new or more attractive options come up;
- extreme emotional swings, frustrations, and moments of despair alternating with clear highs;
- difficulty keeping up with what everyone on the project is doing and thinking;
- being completely absorbed in the project.

These and other factors combine to produce a unique culture in each project as well as a project-oriented culture that characterizes some organizations. The framework for the project management process shown in Table 24.1 illustrates the interrelationships and the importance of organizational and project culture.

The very advantages attributed to project-oriented cultures can also hinder their progress. Project-oriented cultures can provide flexibility and balanced decision making, but they are also complex and have potential for conflict. Disadvantages arise from the confusion that may result from the shared and overlapping responsibilities, the potential for power struggles, and the stress placed on individuals. Recognizing the characteristics of newstream culture and the people who work within it is important, both to those who are a part of it and to those who work in parallel or management roles. Project managers must be aware of shifts of power and be able to focus on issues rather than people when they are forced to take sides. The use of information, decision support systems, and extensive staff training can help to develop attitudes and behaviours consistent with the more collegial nature of project-oriented cultures, making it easier to deal with operational problems that may arise.

Table 24.1 **Framework for Project Management Process**

Pre-Planning	Planning	Action
• Environmental analysis • Creating a shared vision and common direction • Developing guiding principles for implementation process • Identifying resource requirements	Crafting an implementation plan: • Assigning responsibility • Sequencing and scheduling deliverables • Scheduling resources • Protecting the plan	Strategies for change: • Developing supportive coalitions • Dealing effectively with staff resistance • Communicating throughout the change process • Creating a sense of urgency • Involving staff in creating their own future **Monitoring Strategy** Creating symbols of change throughout the work environment: • Separating from the past • Communicating the vision and goal • Modelling the vision and goal

Success and Failure of Projects

Using a project management approach can enhance the likelihood of success for change initiatives and the implementation of innovations. However, not all projects are successful. For example, Glaser (2004) reports that the failure rate of information technology projects is surprisingly high, with an estimated one-third of these projects being cancelled before completion, and only 10% achieving their original plan. Failure of some projects is due to a lack of appropriate and well-understood structure and organizational support for the project, or a failure to properly align the project with the existing structures, relationships, and culture of the organization (Thamhain, 2004). Imposing excessive time pressure on the project team or too much supervision of the project manager may result in demoralization of the project team and prevent flexible responses to uncertainties that arise (Nordqvist, Hovmark, & Zika-Viktorsson, 2004; Turner, 2004). Turner (2004) identified the following conditions necessary for project success:

1. Success criteria for the project should be agreed upon with the stakeholders before the start of the project and repeatedly at configuration review points throughout the project.

2. A collaborative working relationship should be maintained between the project owner and the project manager, with both viewing the project as a partnership.

3. The project manager should be empowered, with the owner giving guidance as to how he or she thinks the project should be best achieved, but allowing the project manager flexibility to deal with unforeseen circumstances.

4. The owner should take an interest in the performance of the project and should receive regular written and face-to-face progress and status reports.

Leadership Implications

Projects and their culture are now an integral feature of the life and work of health agencies, programs, regions, and government ministries, and project management has been described as an emerging profession with its own vocabulary and an emerging body of generally accepted knowledge (Du, Johnson, & Keil, 2004; PMBOK, 2000). New projects present opportunities for identifying and selecting employees with leadership potential to undertake roles as program managers. Nurses often possess the interpersonal and organizational skills that are critical to the success of projects, and many nurses have found exciting career opportunities as project managers or as members of project teams. These opportunities will continue to increase.

Several other chapters of this book have dealt with the knowledge, processes, and skills that are important in effective project management. As explained in Chapter 8, projects are temporary matrix structures that are introduced to achieve horizontal coordination or forward momentum for specific, time-limited initiatives or planned changes and innovations. This may include initiatives to introduce evidence-based practice at the level of a nursing unit or program as discussed in Chapter 17. Project management has become a widely accepted approach for implementing organization-wide change, and the specific techniques of project management provide a mechanism through which planned change as discussed in Chapter 22 can be implemented (Söderlund, 2004).

Projects are implemented through teamwork, both within the project team and between the project team and organizational stakeholders. Project managers must have highly developed skills of team leadership and collaboration, and these are discussed in greater detail in Chapter 21. Throughout the life of a project, there is an ongoing need for negotiation and conflict resolution among organizational stakeholders affected by the project. These skills are discussed in Chapter 27.

Once an idea or issue has been defined as a project of the unit, program or organization, it usually receives support from one or more leaders in the organization and will usually have resources committed to it. This, in turn, enhances the likelihood that the project will be successful. To be successful, projects originating at the grassroots of organizations will need broader support. Issues and skills involved in developing intraorganizational support were discussed in Chapter 23. In the final chapter of this book, there is a discussion of how issues get onto the "policy agenda" of organizations and governments.

Projects can be undertaken to develop and gain organizational support for policies or to implement them once they have been approved; therefore, they provide a way for nurses and nurse leaders to define and pursue their goals. By defining their goals in the practical terms necessary to describe the objectives and obtain the resources in order to implement a project, nurses who possess skills of effective communication, planning, teamwork, and collaboration can achieve greater influence and power in their workplaces.

Summary

- Projects are temporary management structures that are usually implemented when there is a need to diffuse an innovation rapidly or to make a major organizational change within a specified period of time.
- Projects can be initiated in a variety of ways and at various levels of an organization. To be successful, most projects will need approval or support from the senior level of the organization as well as from key stakeholders.
- The structural elements of a project include a sponsorship and reporting mechanism, a committee for planning and monitoring, a project manager, project team, objectives, and a work plan that usually includes some means of evaluating the project.
- An executive champion and broadly based organizational support can be critical to the success of projects.
- Projects require a clear mandate in the form of goals, objectives, and deliverables.
- Project management requires many operational management skills, but it is particularly dependent upon the interpersonal, conceptual, and organizational skills of the project manager.
- The work plan of a project is a tool for scheduling project activities, assigning responsibility for tasks, allocating resources, monitoring achievements, and identifying issues and problems. Planning and scheduling are of critical importance to most projects and can often be facilitated by the use of computer software designed to support project management.
- Projects usually develop a unique culture. A key feature of this culture is the acceptance of ambiguity and uncertainty as unavoidable within the project and the organization. To be successful, projects must often be freed from the usual procedures and reporting channels of an organization. Organizations that hope to be successful in diffusing innovations and initiating change will need to develop a project culture that takes this requirement into account.
- Projects are an important means of legitimizing and implementing planned change.
- Registered nurses who have highly developed interpersonal, conceptual, and planning skills often make successful project managers. The role of project manager provides unique career and professional development opportunities.

Applying the Knowledge in this Chapter

Exercise

1. Select an activity for which you are responsible in your work or your personal life. Develop a simple project management plan for this activity specifying the following:
   a) Goals
   b) Deliverables
   c) Time period for completion
   d) Resources required
      ✔ Person-hours/cost
      ✔ Supplies
      ✔ Consultation
      ✔ Other

2. Identify the main activities required to implement the project you have described, and depict these in the form of a Gantt chart.

Activity	Start Date	Completion Date	Person Responsible

3. Are there any factors that will be critical to the success of the project you have described? What are these critical success factors?

Resources

evolve Internet Resources

A Guide to the Project Management Body of Knowledge (PMBOK® Guide), 2004 edition excerpts:
   www.pmi.org/prod/groups/public/documents/info/1pp_pmbokguidethirdexcerpts.pdf
Project Management Institute (PMI):
   www.pmi.org
   The Project Management Institute (PMI) is a not-for-profit project management professional association for individuals from many different industry areas who are studying or practicing project management. The PMI offers its members professional standards, certification, research, publications, education and training, a knowledge and wisdom centre, professional development, PMI professional awards program, PMI educational foundation, and component organizations.

Project Management Journal:

www.pmi.org/info/PIR_PMJournal.asp

This journal publishes articles on subjects that span the field of project management within the areas of research, techniques, theory, and practice.

Further Reading

International Journal of Project Management

This journal offers comprehensive coverage of all facets of project management, including project concepts, project evaluation, team building and training, communication, project start up, risk analysis and allocation, quality assurance, project systems, project planning, project methods, tools and techniques, cost and time allocation, estimating and tendering, scheduling, monitoring, updating and control, contracts, contract law, project finance, project management software, motivation and incentives, resolution of disputes, procurement methods, organization systems, decision-making processes, and investment appraisal.

Turner, J.R., & Miller, R. (2003). On the nature of the project as a temporary organization. *International Journal of Project Management, 21*(1), 1–8.

This article utilizes organizational theory as a basis for exploring the nature of the project as a temporary organization. This exploration leads to a contemporary reassessment of the definition of a project that suggests that classical definitions are not wrong but rather are incomplete.

References

Bishop, S.K. (1999). Cross-functional project teams in functionally aligned organizations. *Project Management Journal, 30*(3), 6–7.

Du, S. M., Johnson, R.D., & Keil, M. (2004). Project management courses in IS graduate programs: What is being taught? *Journal of Information Systems Education, 15*(2), 181–187.

Galbraith, J. (1982, Summer). Designing the innovating organization. *Organizational Dynamics, 10,* 5–25.

Glaser, J. (2004). Back to basics: Managing IT projects. *Healthcare Financial Management, 58*(7), 34–38.

Glasser, J.J. (1963). Critical path method. In C. Heyel (Ed.), *The Encyclopaedia of Management* (pp. 142–144). New York: Reinhold.

Hartman, F.T. (2000). *Don't park your brain outside: A practical guide to improving shareholder value with SMART management.* Newtown Square, PA: Project Management Institute.

Hermann, M.K., Alexander, J.S., & Kiely, J.T. (1992). Leadership and project management. In. P.J. Decker & E.J. Sullivan (Eds.), *Nursing administration: A micro/macro approach for effective nurse executives* (pp. 569–590). East Norwalk, CT: Appleton & Lange.

Kanter, R.M. (1989). *When giants learn to dance.* New York: Simon & Schuster.

Kerzner, H. (1984). Matrix information: Obstacles, problems, questions, and answers. In D.I. Cleland (Ed.), *Matrix management systems handbook* (pp. 307–329). Toronto, ON: Van Nostrand Reinhold.

Loo, R. (2003). Project management: A core competency for professional nurses and nurse managers. *Journal for Nurses in Staff Development, 19*(4), 187–193.

Meredith, J.R., & Mantel, S.J. (2000). *Project management: A managerial approach* (4th ed.). New York: John Wiley & Sons.

Nordqvist, S., Hovmark, S., & Zika-Viktorsson, A. (2004). Perceived time pressure and social processes in project teams. *International Journal of Project Management, 22*(6), 463–468.

PMBOK (Project Management Body of Knowledge). (2000). *A guide to the project management body of knowledge: PMBOK guide.* Newtown Square, PA: Project Management Institute.

Salesse, M. (2002). *Workforce redesign in a multisite continuing care organization: Implementing a planned change.* Unpublished report of Nursing 900 Project Faculty of Nursing, University of Alberta, Edmonton.

Scholtes, P.R., Joiner, B.L., & Streibel, B.J. (1996). *The team handbook* (2nd ed.). Madison, WI: Oriel Incorporated.

Söderlund, J. (2004). Building theories of project management: Past research, questions for the future. *International Journal of Project Management, 22*(3), 183–191.

Thamhain, H.J. (2004). 15 rules for consulting in support of a client project. *Consulting to Management, 15*(2), 42–46.

Turner, J.R. (2004). Five necessary conditions for project success. *International Journal of Project Management, 22*(5), 349–350.

DEVELOPING HUMAN RESOURCES IN HEALTH AGENCIES

Greta Cummings, Marianne McLennan, and Ardene Robinson Vollman

Learning Objectives

In this chapter, you will learn:

- The important role leaders have in creating a positive work environment in which employees will be healthy, satisfied, and able to achieve organizational and professional goals

- How the individual is fundamental to work performance management, and the importance of matching individuals to their positions in organizations

- How individual performance feedback, goal setting, and career planning can be enhanced by leadership, coaching, mentoring, and staff development activities

- The building blocks for effective human resource management, including clear position descriptions, performance standards, personnel policies, and performance feedback

- About assessing work performance by collecting data about employee behaviour and achievements from several sources, including supervisory observation, peer review, and self-appraisal

- About compiling work performance information into a performance appraisal (evaluation), which forms the basis for management decisions regarding salary, promotion, and whether to retain or release probationary employees

- The performance appraisal process, which provides an opportunity for employees and managers to work together to achieve common goals

The field of health care is labour intensive. According to the Canadian Institute for Health Information (CIHI), the nursing workforce accounts for more than half of all health care workers in Canada and for 3% of all workers in the Canadian labour force (CIHI, 2003). Competition for funding in today's environment is intense, and health care organizations face the challenge of assuring that all employees are competent and able to provide quality service that leads to positive patient outcomes. Within the overall context of organizational goals and values, sound human resources and performance management processes are required to meet this challenge. This chapter is not intended to be an exhaustive discussion of these processes, but rather, to introduce readers to some key concepts and issues in this specialized field.

Recruiting and retaining qualified professionals require the efforts and talents of all organizational leaders. Nurse managers cannot undertake this task alone; however, their participation is integral to its success. To be successful, managers must ensure that there is an appropriate skill mix of professional and support staff in order to deliver the program or service within the overall mission, values, and goals of the organization and to achieve the agreed-upon service levels with the available resources.

Nursing Work Environments

The nature of the nursing workplace as a factor in nursing retention came to light in the 1980s with the magnet hospital study, which examined the traits of hospitals that had less difficulty recruiting and retaining registered nurses (Kramer & Schmalenberg, 1988; McClure, Poulin, Sovie, & Wandelt, 1983). These traits included the visibility and accessibility of the nursing leader, relationships with physicians, sufficient resources to support professional practice and ongoing nursing development, and opportunities to participate in policy and decision making about professional practice. Several contemporary studies have confirmed the findings of this original work (Aiken, Havens, & Sloane, 2000; Havens & Aiken, 1999; Lacey, 2003; Scott, Sochalski, & Aiken, 1999), and detailed recommendations for improving nurses' work environments are the substance of several recent policy papers, including one from the Canadian Nursing Advisory Committee (Advisory Committee, 2001) and two from the Canadian Policy Research Networks (Koehoorn, Lowe, Rondeau, Schellenberg, & Wagar, 2002; Lowe & Schellenberg, 2001).

High turnover is expensive and can have a negative impact on morale, job satisfaction, and the future recruitment efforts of the organization. Therefore, it is necessary to focus on the factors that are important in retaining registered nurses (RNs) and other health care workers by examining the current work environment, analyzing reasons for turnover (i.e., through exit interviews and employment data systems), and implementing initiatives to foster positive work places based on this feedback. Providing developmental opportunities or adapting work for existing staff through remediation, in-service, or education programs are avenues that can be explored within the context of staff development. Job modification and restructuring are others. The way work is designed affects personal health, job satisfaction, and, ultimately, patient care outcomes. The psychological health of employees can be improved if they are able to assume greater control and influence over their own work, if information is provided to them to reduce uncertainty, and if conflicts are managed constructively. When managers organize work so that it is meaningful, by providing feedback and encouraging shared ownership for work outcomes, they help workers improve their performance.

By maintaining relationships with staff, listening and responding to their concerns, and investing in their ongoing development, leaders build trust and resonance that lead to improved staff health, well-being, and, ultimately, to improved quality of care (Cummings, 2003). Leaders play a key role in shaping the way work is designed and operationalized.

Key success factors for creating and maintaining a healthy work environment are supports and opportunities for individual and group learning. Senge (1990, 1999) suggests that three levels of learning support are required—individual needs for mental stimulation and personal mastery, group processes that foster a shared vision and collaborative effects, and organizational systems that promote systems thinking. Several recognized approaches to foster learning will be outlined in the next section: coaching, mentoring, and preceptorships.

A Conceptual Framework for Performance Management

Contemporary organizations formally define their corporate vision, mission, values, goals, and objectives. These form the basis for organizational structures that are represented by organizational charts and statements of departmental roles, functions, and responsibilities. Ideally, through effective human resource management, the roles and work performance of individual workers are aligned with organizational objectives so that workers can develop professionally while carrying out their work. Figure 25.1 illustrates four main areas of focus for organizational leaders: personnel, finances, materials, and services or programs. There are usually standardized procedures to guide managers in each of these areas.

The personnel, or human resource, management system (Figure 25.1) is now examined in more detail with emphasis on the manager's role in helping workers become and remain successful in their positions.

The term *performance management* is used to describe the process of ensuring that each worker contributes to the successful achievement of the organization's strategic goals. Performance management means deploying a comprehensive, strategy-linked framework for measuring performance across the entire enterprise and then using the results to make informed, evidence-based decisions about important issues and addressing areas where structural or process changes are needed. The ultimate goals of performance management are to develop, sustain, and amplify service quality over the long term in order to achieve the mission of the health agency, that is, positive patient outcomes.

Six key elements of successful performance management are strong executive support, linkages between performance measures and strategic goals, measures that cross traditional work boundaries, reward schemes to reinforce cooperation, performance measures tailored to the

Figure 25.1 Performance Management System

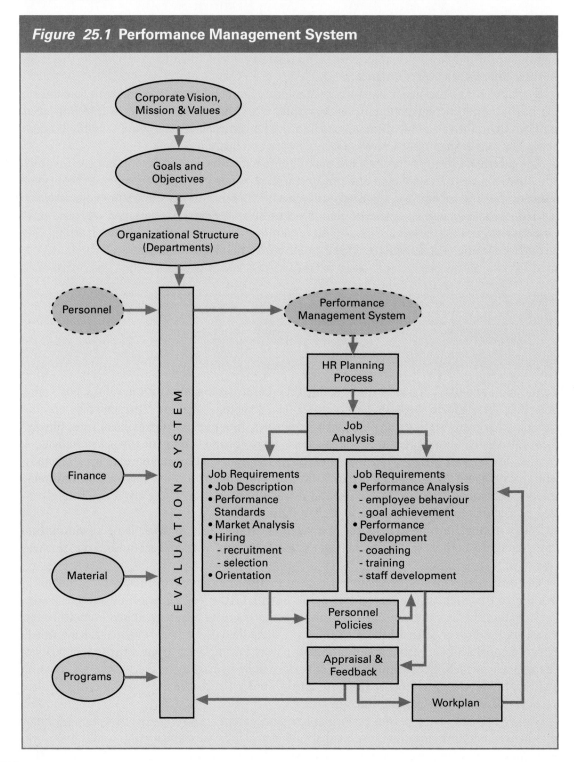

special roles of each unit/program, and information focused on the user, not the technology (Kruzner & Trollinger, 1996). These elements are key to staff recruitment, selection, appraisal, and development functions. Together, they comprise the "human resource (HR) planning process," which is a complex operation to carry out in this rapidly changing health care environment.

Before any staffing action can be initiated, a manager must review the work requirements so that position descriptions accurately reflect the knowledge, skills, and values required to perform the role and also reflect what employees will be expected to do in the foreseeable future. This step is always important but is particularly so when health settings are in transition. The HR department can help the manager determine if the position descriptions and care setting requirements "fit" with the performance standards supplied by professional organizations, legislation, and collective agreements because these often have employment contract and legal implications. Table 25.1 lists the steps of the human resource planning process. This analysis provides the foundation for selection and hiring activities as well as for staff performance appraisals, which are supported by the personnel policies of the organization.

Hiring

Finding and selecting the best employees for the positions available is an important leadership responsibility. Managers have many responsibilities in the hiring process: screening applicants, managing the interview process and team input, developing interview questions and/or practice scenarios, selecting and orienting members of the interview panel, organizing interview schedules and team meetings, checking references, and following up with all applicants, successful or not. Most HR departments have standardized guidelines for conducting interviews to assure that best practices are maintained in accordance with applicable legislation, and it is often standard practice for a person from that department to participate in selection interviews. Although the manager shares responsibility for the selection process by involving others, accountability for the hiring decision should not be delegated. Decisions are important as errors in judgment can have a negative impact on the work, goals, and, ultimately, the survival of the organization.

The process of hiring staff includes both recruiting applicants and selecting those who best match the needs of the workplace. Every newly hired staff member has the potential to affect patient outcomes as well as the success of the work team and the organization; therefore, the manager's investment of time and diligence as employees are hired and orientated will pay off if performance problems can be averted and a stable work team developed.

Recruitment

Recruitment can be viewed as a marketing process whereby well-qualified candidates are attracted to the organization for employment. Recruitment is particularly challenging when several organizations are vying for the same few candidates during times of shortage. Human resource professionals frequently conduct market analyses and can assist in effectively targeting and implementing recruitment activities. As part of a long-term recruitment program, applicant sources outside the organization must be developed. Besides advertising to attract those nurses

Table 25.1 Human Resource Planning Process

1. Set the organizational context.	• Review organizational and departmental documents, economic and job forecasts, and trends in service delivery. • Survey the literature regularly. • Maintain an active professional network to use in benchmarking and planning activities. (Vaziri, 1992)
2. Analyze the job.	• Describe what the work seeks to accomplish. • Describe the necessary employee activities or behaviour required by the job. • List the equipment used to perform the job. • Determine factors in the work environment deemed essential for acceptable job performance. (Dolan & Schuler, 1987)
3. Determine job requirements.	• Collate and review job descriptions in light of the job analysis, provincial standards of practice, and special professional interest groups' recommended guidelines. • Articulate the human requirements necessary to perform the functions of the job. • Assess the efficacy of the systems internal to the organization that disseminate information and communicate expected standards.
4. Examine environmental influences.	• Review policies, regulations, procedures, and standards of care. • Ensure that they are current, relevant, realistic, and readily available to staff. • Inspect facilities, resources, and equipment to ensure they are maintained and available for staff to fulfil their roles effectively. • Assess whether staff have opportunities to learn. • Review staff development and training processes.
5. Consider legal implications.	• Review and understand the employment contracts, labour codes, and other relevant regulations. • Ensure that the components of the performance management system are written, job-related, objective, easily understood, and up-to-date, with provision for staff input at all stages. (Martin & Bartol, 1991)

who are currently not in the work force or who are employed elsewhere, university and college nursing programs should be regarded as important sources of new nurses. The clinical placement of students in a care setting provides an opportunity for managers to observe and assess students' interaction with other team members and their potential as future employees. Other external sources include professional conferences, where word-of-mouth and direct recruitment can be effective strategies. Finally, current employees may be encouraged to use their personal and professional contacts to recruit new staff members.

Recruitment efforts can be evaluated by asking two basic questions: Does the recruitment program attract good applicants? Do the individuals selected become good employees? When interviewing applicants, it is useful to ask them how they heard about the organization. Reviewing this information can provide insights into which recruitment strategies have been effective and how the nurses recruited by them fared in terms of work performance and satisfaction.

Selection

Once a pool of applicants is available, the selection process begins to choose a candidate for a particular position. This is a focal point of the HR planning process and represents one of the most visible outcomes. Selection processes are intended to investigate applicants' skills, knowledge, attitudes, and values to see if these are congruent with the professional practice environment and the available position.

Pre-screening, the first stage of the selection process, begins with a thorough review of résumés, application forms, and biographical data. Using a consistent set of criteria that match the position description and job advertisement (or internal posting information), managers develop a preliminary short list of the most qualified applicants. Large amounts of complex information may be generated during this stage, and electronic checklists, spreadsheets, and databases (in increasing order of technological complexity) can be useful for collecting and analyzing such information (Bowles, 1995). Pre-screening interviews may be useful to obtain additional information about the candidates and also provide the candidates with the opportunity to obtain information about the role and expectations prior to a formal interview.

A preliminary check of references may also be done to narrow the short list to applicants who will go on to a formal interview. Reference checking is increasingly done by phone and requires skill and intuition on the part of the manager. Since the applicant provides the references, it can be assumed that these people generally will be favourable to the applicant. Managers can phrase questions in a way that encourages the referee to go beyond the surface of clichés and standard responses. A checklist of standard questions such as those in Box 25.1 should be used. It is generally not acceptable practice to contact references other than those provided. If an applicant requests that his or her current employer not be contacted, this request should be respected. Organizations and individuals who respond to reference inquiries are increasingly aware of the legal consequences of dishonesty (e.g., giving an excellent reference to rid themselves of a problem employee can lead to a lawsuit for negligence). As a result, HR departments rarely disclose more than dates of employment; therefore, personal references become a most valuable source of information for the manager.

Box 25.1

Common Questions for Checking References

1. How long have you known [the candidate] and what was your relationship with this individual?

2. Can you provide an example of how [the candidate] approached new assignments?

3. How would you describe the interactions of [the candidate] with (a) colleagues, (b) patients, (c) others?

4. How often was [the candidate] absent from work?

5. How frequently was sick time taken? Were there any noticeable patterns in absences?

6. What types of on-the-job education and development did [the candidate] undertake while employed by you? Was this at [the candidate's] initiative or at the suggestion of the supervisor? Who bore the costs?

7. What were the reasons why [the candidate] left your employ? Would you rehire this person?

8. Is there anything you would like to add to what you've already told me?

By carefully preparing to conduct interviews, managers ensure that important dimensions from the position description and work team input are considered as the interview questions are developed and the candidates' responses evaluated. A common set of questions should be used for all candidates so comparisons and ratings can be fairly assessed; however, there is usually latitude to add questions or follow up on areas that arise from each candidate's responses. It is wise to use a team approach to interview candidates, both to engage the team members in making decisions that affect them and to allow candidates the opportunity to meet their potential future team members. The selection team should be comprised of members that represent relevant disciplines, position categories, and experienced and new staff. A pre-meeting of the selection team is often held to finalize interview questions and decide on roles during the interview. If the final decision about whether to offer a position will remain with the manager, it is important that the interview team understands this in advance. The team must also understand that an interview is a two-way process and that the candidate will evaluate the organization based, in part, on the interview experience.

After the candidate is welcomed and members of the interview team are introduced, it is usual practice to invite the candidate to describe how their background, education, and experience prepare him or her for the position. Team members then usually take turns asking questions. Often, the candidate is asked to give or respond to practice examples because these responses provide insight into the candidate's problem-solving abilities, communication style, and potential future behaviours. Careful listening is required to determine how the applicant may approach her or his work, where true talents lie, and how well the person is likely to work with the current team members. When interviewing, it is important to be aware of cues so that follow-up questions can be used to solicit more information or specific examples of practice. Asking for examples is a way of finding out about an applicant's characteristic responses in workplace situations. Time should be reserved at the end of the interview for the candidate to ask questions; such questions sometimes reveal the extent of the candidate's preparation for the interview.

Effective interviewers create an open atmosphere for communication, deliver standardized questions consistently, avoid questions or conversation not related to the applicant's ability to do the job (e.g., marital status, religion), maintain control over the interview, listen attentively, take good notes, keep conversations flowing without leading the candidate, appropriately interpret non-verbal cues, and ask good follow-up questions to evaluate the use of higher level cognitive skills (Norton & Crissman, 1992). Interviewer bias can be minimized by using an interview panel and standardized questions and by scoring the applicant against predetermined criteria that are consistent with the job description (Bowles, 1995).

Each candidate should be rated immediately following the interview. After all the interviews are completed, the selection team will discuss their ratings, rank all applicants, and suggest any special points they want raised in any further reference checks about a particular candidate. A decision to offer a position should not be made until the references for the two or three top candidates have been reviewed. Once a decision has been made, the manager collaborates with the HR department to conclude the procedural steps for offering a position in the organization. When the preferred candidate has formally accepted the position, unsuccessful candidates can be advised of the decision. Those not offered a position may want feedback about their performance during the interview process. The manager should be prepared to offer some examples of what they did well and how they might strengthen their presentation in a future competition.

Orientation

A complete introduction to the organization and the work unit are essential to ensure that a new employee will be both productive and satisfied. Orientation is more than a schedule of meetings, seminars, and work-relevant activities—it sets the stage for future workplace success. A good orientation will reduce the possibility of errors, save time, and present clear and realistic expectations. The new employee will begin to understand the technical, social, and cultural aspects of the organization and the work setting.

Most organizations offer a general orientation under the auspices of the HR department to present the mission, vision, goals, and objectives of the organization to all new employees. The organizational structure and the members of the senior administration are generally introduced. Physical facilities, regulations, policies, and procedures are presented, and employees are often given a handbook to keep. New employees are informed about HR management procedures such as employee benefits, pay issues, vacations, and probationary periods.

Once the new employee is introduced to co-workers, the on-the-job orientation begins. The manager is ultimately responsible for overseeing this process. The position responsibilities should be explained, the new employee's current knowledge and skills should be assessed, and developmental opportunities should be provided in a manner consistent with the principles of adult education. Pairing the new employee with an experienced worker complements the supervisor's orientation and begins the development of preceptoring relationships within the team.

There is often a defined "probationary period" for new employees. During this time, the manager should monitor the orientation process and the new employee's response to it by taking time to answer questions, provide feedback, and offer relevant information or support. This process involves more than rushing past a new employee and asking, "Is everything okay?" The manager must set time aside to build rapport and listen to questions and suggestions. If problems become evident during this period, they should be dealt with promptly and directly so that the new employee has the best possible chance of being successful and is able to use feedback to correct any performance deficits.

An experienced manager knows that developing effective relationships with new employees during their early employment is important to their successful transition into the team; regular feedback on work performance further optimizes learning and confidence. As with all aspects of management, an evaluation process should be in place to ensure that the new employee has all the information needed to do the job well. Sometimes, information given at formal orientation meetings in the early phases is not recalled; it may have seemed unimportant or irrelevant at the time. An orientation survey should be used once new staff are settled into their roles to determine if the process went smoothly, if the information provided was complete and relevant, if they were satisfied with their orientation, and if they have any ongoing learning needs. Findings from this evaluation should be incorporated into future orientation procedures.

Monitoring Work Performance Over Time

In addition to attracting and hiring new staff, managers work with new and continuing employees to help them maintain and improve their work performance on an ongoing basis. This process is illustrated on the right side of Figure 25.1. The characteristics of an effective performance appraisal system are validity, reliability, responsiveness, flexibility, and equitableness (Nelson & Quick, 1997). Managers enhance the validity of the performance appraisal process when they consider the multiple dimensions of the work being done. It is important to collect information from several relevant sources such as peers, patients, and family members as well as from the employee. When information is collected in a similar manner for all workers and at different times over the assessment period, one incident does not predominate in the manager's assessment, and reliability is enhanced. Responsiveness can be achieved by finding ways that enable the employee to have an active role in the performance appraisal process. Managers and systems must demonstrate flexibility by modifying expectations in response to changing conditions in the organization. For example, if there is a staff shortage, it may not be possible for workers to meet the same performance standards as when there is a full complement of staff. Equitableness is demonstrated when similar levels of performance are acknowledged in the same way. This is easier to accomplish when explicit work standards and assessment criteria are used as reference points in the performance appraisal process.

Performance Appraisal

Performance appraisals are conducted to identify areas for employee growth and educational development in order to nurture optimal employee performance. The leader works in partnership with the staff member using personalized coaching techniques to identify and discuss individual and organizational goals. Effective interpersonal communication is the foundation of the performance appraisal process.

Managerial expectations and established standards of practice are also considered in the performance appraisal process. Performance standards for the organization are updated as information about the performance of individual workers is collected and compared. Across the organization, performance data assist managers in planning for resource and education requirements, in determining staff mix needs, in identifying areas for quality improvement, and in strategic planning for future service capacity. Sometimes, the performance appraisal process is a mechanism for identifying and working with employees whose work is below acceptable standards. The manager and the employee share the responsibility for making the performance appraisal a constructive experience.

Analysis of job performance is required for all employees, not just new staff; however, feedback and evaluation for new workers usually takes place more frequently during the orientation and probationary phases of employment. The process of monitoring work performance includes gathering, analyzing, evaluating, and communicating information about an employee's behaviours and how they contribute to achieving the goals of the work team, service setting, and organization. When goals and expectations for improvement are presented to workers in clear and unambiguous terms, it is more likely that they will be able to improve their work performance. When objectives are clear and mutually understood, it is easier for the worker to know what is expected and for the manager to assess improvement. On the other hand, when goals and tasks are described ambiguously, conflict and disagreement can result. Workers need to know what they are expected to do, how soon they must demonstrate improvement, and how their performance is being assessed. Realistically, work performance can be affected by factors such as the time lag between a nursing intervention and patient outcome, the involvement of many different staff members, and the social characteristics of the environment. For example, a single task may entail many activities and have several outcomes. Therefore, documenting patterns in work performance is sometimes more important than single incidents. Performance analysis strategies can be devised to meet the needs of the organization, to recognize and reward outstanding work, to identify performance gaps, and to plan development strategies for individuals and the team.

Getting input from multiple sources enhances the reliability and credibility of the performance appraisal process. Four sources of information that can be used in appraising work performance are discussed briefly below:

1. In many health institutions, information systems are used to collect quantitative information such as attendance and sick time usage. Other employee-specific information, such as changes in educational qualifications, is also collected. At an individual level, information of this nature can contribute to certain dimensions of the performance appraisal process. When compiled and reported for particular work settings or for the organization as a

whole, workforce trends can be monitored and programs can be planned and evaluated.

2. Patient satisfaction and unsolicited "beefs and bouquets" from professional colleagues within and external to the workgroup are helpful data sources. Depending on the work area, documents such as nursing care plans, patient teaching records, and patient assessments may be reviewed.

3. Self-appraisal has become a common component of performance analysis and a key component of participatory management. When staff are asked to prepare a written self-appraisal prior to the performance review, their involvement in and commitment to performance improvement is enhanced. Self-appraisal is most beneficial when the performance appraisal process in the organization focuses on professional development and personal growth. Managers can ensure the success of a self-appraisal process by fostering a climate of frequent feedback in which constructive criticism is seen as useful for improvement and focuses on development and linkage to organizational goals. Mentoring, coaching, and role modelling can also emphasize self-appraisal and instill realism into staff opinions of their skills, capabilities, and contributions. Provincial nursing associations expect registered members to take ownership for ensuring and documenting their own competence to practice, often through a self-appraisal process of reflective practice. Given the current work structures wherein managers may have an extraordinary number of individuals to supervise and appraise, it makes sense for professionals to take a more active role in the appraisal process through self-appraisal and through input into the appraisals of peers.

4. Peer review is the process of having work performance analyzed and evaluated by co-workers or colleagues of equal rank against established criteria or competencies. It is based on the principles of professional autonomy, accountability, and collegiality. Peer review in nursing can be an excellent method of quality control and consumer protection (Gerstner, McAllister, Wagner, & Kraus, 1988). The degree to which staff members are comfortable with the peer-review process depends upon the history of the work unit, the extent to which it has developed as a team, and the level of trust staff members have in each other and in their supervisor. Although the potential advantages of peer and self-ratings have been well documented in the literature, they have not been highly utilized as tools for responding to ongoing performance pressures (Bader & Bloom, 1992; Buhalo, 1991). In unionized workplaces, there are sometimes structural barriers to peer review, but it is usually possible to design processes for peer input that allow colleagues to contribute information without making final judgments about the performance of team members.

In general, managers need to assess two aspects of performance: employee behaviour and achievement of goals (Goodale, 1992). The manager should determine not merely what took place, but what challenges the worker had to deal with and what actions were taken to try to overcome them (Burdett, 1988). This allows goals, objectives, and actual work performance to be understood and assessed in context. Employees may be measured or compared against themselves, other employees, or some absolute standard depending on the organization's performance management system (Dolan & Schuler, 1987). When a manager states, *"Ms. Jones* is an excellent employee," it means that *Ms. Jones* is being compared with others; *"Mr. Brown* has improved himself" means that *Mr. Brown* has performed better on a specific criterion than he did during the last performance appraisal period; "*Ms. Miller* meets the job requirements" means that, compared to the established standard for that task or role, *Ms. Miller* meets the criteria. These statements reflect different dimensions of work performance and require different methods of measurement. In most organizations, a combination of methods is used. In health care settings, using a multi-faceted approach makes it easier for managers to provide staff with reliable and valid performance assessments that address most dimensions of the complex and dynamic nature of their work.

Feedback

Feedback on performance needs to be frequent, especially when an employee has not managed a situation as well as expected. Critical feedback requires special skill and attention by the manager. The following process can be followed:

1. Check the facts and make direct observations.
2. Provide an opportunity for the employee to describe their views of the situation and circumstances as soon as possible in a private place. Allow adequate time.
3. Share specific feedback that focuses on the desired behaviour, ensuring that there is a clear understanding of the expected level of future performance.
4. Determine if education or other support is needed to achieve improvement.

Effective managers view this process as an opportunity to work collaboratively with employees to help them be successful. They perceive that employees are motivated to improve their performance, not to simply meet minimum expectations. There are occasions when performance problems are repetitive or have serious consequence, and a more formal review of the situation with the employee is required to determine the causes of the problem and appropriate next steps (see Chapter 26). The manager records instances where positive or critical feedback was given, the behaviour of the employee, and how it relates to the expectations of the position. Such documentation is needed to identify patterns or to recall specific examples that substantiate judgments made in the formal appraisals.

The performance management process must be documented appropriately and in a standard fashion for all employees. This becomes particularly important if a staff member challenges a performance-related issue (Scholtes, 1993). Employers' use of performance analysis data to make significant human resource decisions creates the potential for conflict and misunderstanding between employer and staff and has been a factor in increasing litigation (Martin & Bartol, 1991). In general, employers are better able to make convincing arguments for the legitimacy of their actions when they have performance documentation on file. Employers can also be legally challenged on the basis of what nurse managers write in staff members' performance appraisals. Problems can be avoided when statements refer to specific performance expectations that are concise, objective, and easily understood by all parties involved (Saxe, 1988). The manager's written comments must reflect an objective and precise analysis of the staff member's performance strengths and weaknesses. Generalizations can take weaknesses out of context and overemphasize them; ambiguous wording can lead to an inaccurate and incomplete summary of performance. When a behaviour occurs once, it is an incident; twice is a coincidence, and three times is a pattern (Smith, 1993). The behaviour, task, or responsibility under discussion should be part of an observed pattern, not an isolated incident or a one-time uncharacteristic behaviour (Ilgen & Feldman, 1990).

When regular performance feedback is provided, there are not usually surprises in the formal appraisal sessions at the end of the probation period or during annual reviews. Meaningful feedback close to the time of an incident provides well-deserved recognition or facilitates growth and learning. When frequent and regular feedback has been given during the year, it is possible to quickly review progress and focus on developmental and longer-range goals during the more formal process of an annual review. Ideally, a personalized work plan is jointly developed to provide a road map for ongoing development and the basis for future performance reviews. The manager uses coaching skills to facilitate performance planning with a focus on setting goals and identifying activities and supports necessary for success.

Performance Development

Performance development is the process of enhancing employee productivity and work quality through motivation and education in response to the strategic needs of specific workplaces and the organization as a whole. Leaders in progressive work settings use performance management systems to help individuals understand themselves better, build upon their strengths, and optimize their contributions to the organization's mission and goals. An effective performance development system will incorporate the following principles advocated by Buckingham and Coffman (1999):

- Employees take an active role in directing, recording, and making progress toward their development goals.
- Leaders assist individuals to develop in their careers and be successful in their roles.
- Joint goal setting and dialogue result in clear role understanding and shared expectations.
- Outcomes are specified and measurable, allowing for feedback from a variety of perspectives.
- The process is simple, allowing for frequent interaction, a focus on the future, and flexibility to respond to the needs of the individual.

This learning approach to performance improvement encourages change, a willingness to try new things, and the confidence to explore new practice options. In the prevailing climate of fiscal constraint and continual change, this approach is particularly important. Blitzer, Petersen, and Rogers (1993) identified several benefits of a development-oriented improvement system that helps to improve individual and organizational performance. Such a system values individuals, supports their learning and goals, and fosters an open collaborative relationship with their manager and peers. This connects people and the organization in ways that support respect, excellence, and commitment.

Short-term development or education is usually founded on building knowledge, skill, and expertise, while longer-term development responds to an individual's career goals and aspirations as well as to the institution's anticipated strategic requirements. One example of short-term development is in-service education and on-the-job coaching for nurses who will be working with new technology introduced into a hospital's critical care unit. New employees are provided with on-the-job education as part of orientation; regular employees may need to show proof of ongoing competence of specific knowledge or procedures by going through a recertification procedure. Other types of staff development designed to meet organizational goals would be considered longer-term. For example, if a hospital recognizes the need for advanced practice nurses to meet changing patient care requirements, the financial support of nurses wishing to continue their education at the master's level may be seen as a sensible investment.

Education and development may be formal or informal. Learning can take the form of lectures, courses (local or distance), rounds, or books, and it is often delivered by audiovisual and electronic means (e.g., the Internet or interactive CD-ROMs). Experiential development through on-the-job coaching and job rotation can be informal or formal, depending on the mentorship available and the degree of formality of such programs. Education and development should focus on the employee's strengths and interests, as well as on areas that need improvement in order to achieve the organization's goals and objectives. Work assignments designed to allow and encourage the performance of new skills and competencies are an integral component of the development process. A transfer of learning from theory to practice can be fostered through appropriate recognition, monitoring, evaluation, and reward of positive performance. Evaluation of education and development must be a continuous process, not a one-time terminal event, if effective learning is to be facilitated.

Managers who are purchasing or planning to develop an education program must assure that the content and delivery methods are appropriate to the employees and the organizational context. Among the components to be considered are goals and objectives, breadth and depth of content, education methods, sequencing of activities, evaluation procedures, monitoring and feedback systems, resources required, cost, and time.

Employee development needs can also be supported through a mentorship program. Mentors are seasoned leaders who voluntarily work with less experienced staff to assist them in meeting their career goals. A formal mentorship program may be established, or matching can occur informally upon request when both parties share a commitment to work together. Mentors can help make connections between theoretical learning and practical applications, and they can provide workable solutions to problems and valuable insight into the culture and social politics of the organization. External mentors can provide a unique perspective not biased by organizational history. The most successful relationships are built on mutual respect and trust where two-way feedback and learning occurs. Honest assessments of work events and talents serve as a way to pass on the knowledge and experience of senior leaders and grow future leaders for the organization.

Leadership Implications

Every nurse and employee should be familiar with the human resources policies and practices of their employing agency that affect them. Human resources management is an important area of competence and can be particularly challenging to newly appointed managers. The information in this chapter is relevant to nurses who are seeking to develop management careers or who have recently been appointed to a management position.

Nurses who become managers have an advantage in this area because they develop knowledge and skills in interpersonal relations, teaching and coaching, problem solving, and conflict resolution as part of their basic educational preparation. As managers, nurses apply their interpersonal knowledge and skills within the context of the mission, goals, and human resources policies and procedures of the agency. Through organizational learning opportunities, collegial relationships with other managers, and discussion with specialists from the HR Department, a newly appointed nurse manager can learn and develop confidence in this important dimension of the leadership role. Consistency in the application of human resources policies and procedures is important and provides one way of showing respect for all employees. However, the manager has the opportunity to encourage, motivate, and acknowledge the contributions of individual employees, and it is through this process that the goals for coaching and mentoring often become clear. Managers who view themselves as helping individual employees to achieve their career aspirations make contributions that extend beyond their own program or unit to the organization and even the health system as a while. Employees who feel acknowledged and valued represent themselves and their organization to other disciplines, departments, and the public in positive ways.

Most employees are willing to learn and want to do a good job in their work. Human resources policies and procedures are intended to support both individual employees and managers in making this possible. A small proportion of employees are unable or unwilling to respond to standard processes of performance planning, education, coaching, mentoring, and performance appraisal in order to competently perform their work and improve their performance as necessary. Human resources policies and procedures and the requirements of collective agreements provide structure for working with these employees. Consultation with senior managers and HR specialists becomes important in assuring that the performance problems of such employees are promptly and objectively identified and managed. Ideally, managers, educators, and, sometimes, employee assistance programs are able to help these employees to become contributing members of the work team. In the relatively small number of situations in which this is not possible, professionalism and managerial competence are required to manage corrective or disciplinary processes so that the morale of the work team as a whole is not affected by the behaviour or inadequate work performance of a small number of people.

Human resources management is an area of leadership in which individual contact between the manager and employees can benefit both individuals and the organization. It consumes a significant portion of time for managers in operational roles and has a direct effect on important organizational outcomes. Nurses who become managers can excel in this area because of their professional grounding in interpersonal and teaching skills and their understanding of the importance of teamwork and collaboration.

Summary

- Providing health services is an inherently human endeavour, with nurses accounting for more than half of the health care workforce in Canada.
- Human resource management is a specialized field. Front-line leaders and middle managers in the health system have important responsibilities for certain aspects of human resource management, and particularly for performance management process.
- Leaders and managers must devote time and energy to building relationships with their staff in order to foster optimal work performance by all team members.
- Investing in the development of individual employees is a way for front-line leaders to have a positive and direct impact on clinical and organizational outcomes.
- Performance management is a shared responsibility of managers and employees and can benefit individual workers as well as the organization. When employees are successfully matched to their work settings and responsibilities, they can remain healthy and improve their performance over time, thus making a difference to the health outcomes for patients.

Applying the Knowledge in this Chapter

Exercise

In this year's budget request, you have outlined the need to add two new categories of staff to your patient care team. You have received funding to add one aide position and one advanced nurse practitioner. Your literature search and consultations with experts in the field have given you confidence that you have set accurate job descriptions and clear performance indicators consistent with the philosophy of professional nursing practice.

1. Outline an implementation plan that captures key activities related to recruitment, selection, orientation, and performance management for these two different roles.

2. Describe how these new roles will have an impact on the existing roles of your patient care team and how you will integrate them into your implementation plan.

3. Detail who should be involved and in what components of the implementation plan.

4. What indicators will you use to gauge your success in this initiative?

Resources

evolve Internet Resources

Canadian Nursing Advisory Report:

www.hc-sc.gc.ca/english/for_you/nursing/cnac_report/index.html

Canadian Policy Research Networks:

www.cprn.org

Further Reading

Brooks, S.B., Olsen, P., Reiger-Kligys, S., & Mooney, L. (1995). Peer review: An approach to performance evaluation in a professional practice model. *Critical Care Nursing Quarterly*, *18*(3), 36–47.

Role expectations of staff nurses are changing, and nurses must become empowered and actively involved in facilitating change, rather than having change foisted on them. This article provides graphic representation of a practice model as well as suggested forms to use in performance evaluation.

Dunn, M.G., Norby, R., Cournoyer, P., Hudec, S., O'Donnell, J., & Snider, M.D. (1995). Expert panel method for nurse staffing and management. *Journal of Nursing Administration*, *25*(10), 61–67.

The method described in this article represents a bold new approach for the identification of nurse staffing requirements and the management of resources.

References

Advisory Committee on Health Human Resources. (2001). *Our health, our future: Creating quality workplaces for Canadian nurses. Final report of the Canadian Nursing Advisory Committee*. Retrieved October 2, 2002, from http://www.chsrf.ca/docs/finalrpts/prcomcare_e.pdf

Aiken, L.H., Havens, D.S., & Sloane, D.M. (2000). The magnet nursing services recognition program: A comparison of two groups of magnet hospitals. *American Journal of Nursing*, *100*(3), 26–36.

Bader, G.E., & Bloom, A.E. (1992). How to do peer review. *Training & Development*, *46*(6), 61–62, 64–66.

Blitzer, R.J., Petersen, C., & Rogers, L. (1993). How to build self-esteem. *Training & Development, 47*(2), 58–60.

Bowles, N. (1995). Methods of nurse selection: A review. *Nursing Standard, 9*(15), 25–29.

Buckingham, M., & Coffman, C. (1999). *First, break all the rules: What the world's greatest managers do differently.* New York: Simon & Schuster.

Buhalo, I.H. (1991). You sign my report card I'll sign yours. *Personnel, 68*, 23.

Burdett, J. (1988). Results driven performance appraisal. *The Human Resource, 5*(1), 19–21.

Canadian Institute for Health Information. (2003). *Health human resources databases.* Retrieved May 26, 2003, from http://secure.cihi.ca/cihiweb/dispPage.jsp?cw_page=hhrdata_e

Cummings, G.G. (2003). *An examination of the effects of hospital restructuring on nurses: How emotionally intelligent leadership styles mitigate these effects*. Unpublished doctoral thesis, University of Alberta, Edmonton, Alberta, Canada.

Dolan, S.L., & Schuler, R.S. (1987). *Personnel and human resource management in Canada.* St. Paul, MN: West.

Gerstner, M., McAllister, L., Wagner, P.L., & Kraus, C. (1988). Peer review. In S.E. Pinkerton & P. Schroeder (Eds.), *Commitment to excellence: Developing a professional nursing staff* (pp. 199–209). Rockville, MD: Aspen.

Goodale, J.G. (1992). Improving performance appraisal. *Business Quarterly, 57*(2), 65–70.

Havens, D.S., & Aiken, L.H. (1999). Shaping systems to promote desired outcomes: The magnet hospital model. *Journal of Nursing Administration, 29*(2), 14–20.

Ilgen, D.R., & Feldman, J.M. (1990). Performance appraisal: A process focus. In L.L. Cummings & B.M. Staw (Eds.), *Evaluation and employment in organizations* (pp. 1–57). Greenwich, CT: JAI Press.

Koehoorn, M., Lowe, G.S., Rondeau, K.V., Schellenberg, G., & Wagar, T.H. (2002). *Creating high-quality health care workplaces.* Canadian Policy Research Networks Inc. (Document No. 18127). Retrieved December 4, 2004, from http://www.cprn.org/en/doc.cfm?doc=112

Kramer, M., & Schmalenberg, C. (1988). Magnet hospitals: Part I, institutions of excellence. *Journal of Nursing Administration, 18*(1), 1324.

Kruzner, D., & Trollinger, R. (1996, November 11). Performance management vital in implementing new strategies. *Oil and Gas Journal, 94*, 66–72.

Lacey, L.M. (2003). Recruitment & retention report. Called into question: What nurses want. *Nursing Management, 34*(2 part 1), 25–26.

Lowe, G., & Schellenberg, G. (2001). *What's a good job? The importance of employment relationships.* (Study No. W05). Ottawa, ON: Canadian Policy Research Networks.

Martin, D.C., & Bartol, K.M. (1991). The legal ramifications of performance appraisal: An update. *Employee Relations Law Journal, 17*(2), 257–286.

McClure, M., Poulin, M., Sovie, M., & Wandelt, M. (1983). *Magnet hospitals: Attraction and retention of professional nurses.* Kansas City, MO: American Nurses Association.

Nelson, D.L., & Quick, J.C. (1997). *Organizational behavior: Foundations, realities and challenges* (2nd ed.). St. Paul, MN: West Publishing Company.

Norton, S.D., & Crissman, S. (1992). Staffing, recruiting, and selecting. In P.J. Decker & E.J. Sullivan (Eds.), *Nursing administration: A micro/macro approach for effective nurse executives* (pp. 257–280). East Norwalk, CT: Appleton & Lange.

Saxe, S.D. (1988). Do performance appraisals violate the Human Rights Code? *The Human Resource, 5*(2), 18–19.

Scholtes, P.R. (1993, Summer). Total quality or performance appraisal: Choose one. *National Productivity Review, 13*, 349–363.

Scott, J.G., Sochalski, J., & Aiken, L. (1999). Review of magnet hospital research. *Journal of Nursing Administration, 29*(1), 9–19.

Senge, P. (1999). *The dance of change.* New York: Doubleday Currency.

Senge, P. (1990). *The fifth discipline.* New York: Doubleday Currency.

Smith, M.L. (1993, February). Give feedback, not criticism. *Supervisory Management, 38*, 4.

Vaziri, H.K. (1992, October). Using competitive benchmarking to set goals. *Quality Progress*, 81–85.

HUMAN RESOURCE ALLOCATION: STAFFING AND SCHEDULING

Germaine M. Dechant

Learning Objectives

In this chapter, you will learn:

- About the staffing of patient care units and the critical variables to be considered

- The elements of a basic staffing plan

- The manager's role in scheduling

- The objectives of staff schedules and three approaches to scheduling: traditional, cyclical, and self-scheduling

- Creative approaches to scheduling

- The potential of automated scheduling software

- How managers analyze existing staffing elements and work schedules

- Legal and ethical issues pertaining to staffing and scheduling

"If not properly staffed and managed, 24/7 operations are critically vulnerable to human errors and accidents, sickness and absenteeism, low morale, labour strife and increased employee turnover" (Moore & Kerin, 2002, p. 21). Mastery of resource allocation and financial management is clearly among the conditions of survival for first-level managers in the current health care environment, with its flattened organizations and philosophy of decentralized decisions. Two key functions of the first-level manager are allocating and managing resources of all kinds, including equipment, supplies, services, and human resources. The manager sets the standards and direction for practice and is directly responsible for managing all aspects of service delivery. This represents a significant change in the role of the first-level manager; managers now must have a skill set that was once only required of directors of nursing services and other senior administrative personnel. This new direction presents challenges, both intimidating and exciting, and enriches the role of the first-level manager.

Work scheduling is a complex task. However, an excellent work schedule can benefit staff morale and the quality of patient care. Nevertheless, current resources for staffing and scheduling are hard to find. Learning tools, support resources (e.g., printed materials about work schedule design), and training for managers are almost non-existent, and exchanges of schedule-related information among organizations, even among organizations within the same region, occur rarely. As a result, managers often approach staffing and scheduling haphazardly, without an understanding of the underlying principles and procedures. There is a critical need, largely unaddressed by senior administrative personnel, for initial and ongoing education, support, and mentoring for first-level managers in the area of staffing and scheduling.

Human resources represent the largest portion of the total operating budget in any health care organization. Successful fiscal management begins with managers understanding that expertise in staffing and scheduling is essential for human resource allocation. Managers also must understand that manipulating a variable in one of these areas has an impact on variables in the other area. Scheduling issues have long been recognized as having significant productivity impacts. Adverse outcomes in patient care (e.g., pressure ulcers, pneumonia, fractures from falls, urinary tract and postoperative infections) have been correlated with the level of nursing staffing and skill mix (American Nurses Association, 1997). Few of the many challenges confronting the nursing profession today cause a more intense response from nurses than the issue of staffing adequacy. Canadian nurses are concerned that quality of patient care and patient safety are being jeopardized by pervasive changes in staffing practices. These changes generally include:

- Greater part-time to full-time ratios
- Increased use of casual employees
- Excessive use of overtime, linked with an unprecedented rate of absenteeism
- Substitution of registered nurses (RNs) with licensed practical nurses (LPNs) or unregulated nursing personnel
- Increasingly rare use of patient classification systems for acuity-based staffing, even though data are available for use

The complex issues of staffing and scheduling are presented in this chapter. Without being a mathematical wizard, the reader can develop basic skills in this area in order to begin to build a comprehensive approach to human resource allocation. The approach to staffing and scheduling that is presented is both systematic and practical.

Staffing and Its Critical Variables

Staffing is the process of determining the acceptable number and skill mix of personnel needed to meet patients' treatment and care needs. Staffing is required in all programs or units in any care setting, whether hospital based (e.g., an emergency department) or community based (e.g., a home care agency). An ongoing challenge for managers is to match appropriately skilled staff with patient needs for quality care—and to do so within the parameters of available resources. When developing the staffing plan, the manager must consider the following key variables and understand their interdependence: (a) the philosophical framework for practice, (b) characteristics of the patient population, (c) environmental factors, and (d) personnel characteristics.

Philosophical Framework for Practice

A unit or program's vision, mission, values, philosophy, goals, and objectives directly affect the staffing plan. These need to be stated precisely because they guide quality standards, policies, procedures, and service delivery strategies. They also guide the patient by clarifying the service standards that should be expected. For example, a statement of vision will indicate the type and scope of nursing activities required in a particular unit or program. A mission statement that includes patient and family education and a focus on health promotion will have workload implications for unit personnel. So will a management philosophy that promotes continuous service improvement, staff development, decentralized decision making, or staff participation in such activities as clinical research and community liaison.

The philosophical framework of the unit will also guide the choice of service delivery model. The model will, in turn, have a tremendous impact on the approach to decisions regarding staff mix; for example, a patient-focused care model will need different types and numbers of professionals than will primary nursing, team nursing, or functional nursing models. Similarly, medical models (where physicians are in control of all aspects of care) and interdisciplinary team models (where physicians serve as team members and consultants) have different staffing requirements. Teaching units that are affiliated with a college or university also have unique staffing needs that must be considered, such as the types and levels of students and the extent of staff involvement with student teaching and supervision.

The unique blend of history and traditions—the unit's culture—may also influence the unit's approaches to service delivery. Knowledge of the unit's culture is very useful, and in some cases, a change in paradigm may be needed to simplify practice and lead to adjustments in staffing mix.

Characteristics of the Patient Population

The type of patient admitted to a unit is obviously an important factor in the development of a staffing plan. Collecting and analyzing data about the patient population is an essential first step in the staffing process. This can be accomplished by reviewing relevant literature, consulting with similar units, or checking data from previous years' experience. Managers must identify the following elements:

- Number of patients and demand for service (unit average occupancy)
- Patterns and trends in census
- Admission and discharge rates in a unit, or, in the case of a clinic, the number and length of visits
- Average length of stay (ALOS)
- The conditions or illnesses experienced by patients (e.g., medical, surgical, psychiatric, oncological)
- Level or complexity of treatment needs, as well as direct and indirect care requirements (patient classification)
- Patient demographics: age; education level; socioeconomic factors influencing health care needs; physical, psychological, spiritual, cultural, and recreational needs
- Patient expectations for services (patient satisfaction results)
- Needs of patients' families and significant others

Environmental Factors

It is well known that management decision making is influenced by the environmental factors affecting a unit or program. The following environmental factors must be considered when developing a staffing plan:

- The number of patient beds or clinic spaces
- The number of hours the unit or clinic is open
- The design of the unit (e.g., a medical unit made up exclusively of private rooms may be preferable from the patient's perspective, but will affect workload and staff assignment patterns)
- The unit's role within the organization (e.g., a stand-alone unit, isolated clinic, or one of several units within a large organization where human resources are supported and shared)
- The physical design of units or the distance between units where safety of staff and patients is an issue (i.e., will more caregivers be required than the census indicates?)
- The unit's fit within the community (i.e., is the unit functioning within an integrated network of agencies that support each other?)
- Availability of equipment and supplies (e.g., the need to share equipment among teams on the same unit or among several units will affect planning for staff allocation)
- Technological advances
- New medications or treatment approaches
- Number of staff physicians and residents on the unit, their expectations, and their approaches to practice

- Legal considerations (e.g., collective agreements)
- The organization's personnel policies and management practices (e.g., policies on employee leaves of absence, vacations, staff development)
- Service boundaries; services for which the unit is responsible (e.g., traditional laboratory functions such as blood collection, covering dietary and pharmacy services on evening or night shifts)

Personnel Characteristics

The personal characteristics of the unit's caregivers are another factor affecting staffing. A unit's ability to meet service delivery requirements rests to a great extent on the individual competence of the caregivers—competence that results from education, experience, motivation, health, attitude, and perhaps a variety of other personal factors. In practice, individual differences in competence among caregivers in the same classification are extremely important and cannot be ignored. A comprehensive personnel inventory should account for the following factors:

- Skill mixes available
- Role functions and professional mandate of each group
- Competitive markets for staff in the larger community, and the unit's potential for success in recruitment
- Education
- Classification
- Experience
- Length of service
- Individual aspirations, goals, and objectives
- Level of expertise
- Age
- Gender
- Social and ethnic background and languages spoken
- Use of staff positions such as clinical specialists or senior therapists
- Access to staff resources from other departments, such as physiotherapy and respiratory therapy

The Staffing Plan

Having analyzed the critical staff variables, the first-level manager now has the information needed to develop a staffing plan. The staffing plan includes the basic number of staff in each discipline required to adequately staff the unit on each shift. The staff may be all RNs, RNs working with LPNs, or a combination of several types of professionals working together as a multidisciplinary team.

Where a workload measurement system is in place, the manager must consider its results as a guide in the process of developing a staffing plan. Workload measurement systems first emerged in the 1960s as patient classification systems were developed, and they were used primarily to identify the patients' nursing care needs and the nursing resources necessary to meet those needs. Workload measurement systems typically identify the following: (a) direct nursing care requirements of patients (often referred to as levels of patient acuity), (b) indirect nursing care (i.e., care activities carried out on behalf of patients but not in their presence, such as charting), and (c) activities that are unit related but not necessarily patient-contact related, such as the narcotic count. Patients are assigned to categories of care, and staffing is then determined according to specific decision rules.

A large body of literature is available on the topic of workload measurement systems (see, for example, Giovannetti, 1994). Although a first-level manager cannot rely exclusively on the organization's workload measurement system to generate a staffing plan, workload indicators of nursing care requirements and indirect staff activities provide useful information. Managers should know their organization's workload measurement system and decide whether it would be useful in predicting workload and staffing requirements.

Table 26.1 presents a staffing plan for a residential treatment centre for adolescents with mental illness. This tertiary care centre in Edmonton is a community-based program offered through the Child and Adolescent Services Association (CASA).

The staffing plan in Table 26.1 shows the number and classification of staff needed for all three shifts. What this plan does not show, however, is the number of employees who must be hired in order to fulfill these staffing requirements; for example, how many nurses need to be hired so that four nurses will be in attendance on days and one on evenings? The key question is this: "How many individuals must be hired in order to have one individual in attendance 24 hours per day, 365 days per year?" To answer this question, the first-level manager must understand the difference between benefit hours, effective hours, and paid hours.

Benefit hours are the number of hours spent on sick days, vacation days, statutory holidays, education days, and leaves with pay, such as bereavement leave. Benefit hours are determined by the organization's personnel policies and the terms of the applicable collective agreement.

Table 26.1 Basic Staffing Plan for a 12-Bed Residential Treatment Centre for Adolescents

Staff Classification	SHIFT		
	Day	Evening	Night
Registered Psychiatric Nurse (RPN)/RN	4	1	0
Childcare Counsellors	1	3	2
Senior Therapist	1	0	0
Secretary	1	0	0
Total Staff	7	4	2

In an organization where there are no collective agreements, personnel policies guide the decision making. Historical patterns of use (e.g., sick time) must also be taken into consideration. Table 26.2 lists typical benefit hours that are applicable to the 12-bed residential treatment centre.

Effective hours is another term for *worked hours*. Effective hours are the number of hours during which the employee is either (a) providing direct care to patients or (b) engaged in indirect activities. Direct care generally is time spent with the patient (e.g., in group therapy), and indirect care is time spent preparing for or following up on a direct activity (e.g., post-group debriefing). Agencies differ in what they consider direct and indirect activities, so the manager must be familiar with organizational policy or practice. Effective hours are determined by subtracting the benefit hours from the paid hours. Box 26.1 provides a detailed explanation of how to calculate effective hours, using the treatment centre for adolescents as an example.

Table 26.2 **Typical Benefit Hours for a 12-Bed Residential Treatment Centre for Adolescents**

Benefit Hours	Days per Year	Hours per Day	Hours per Year
Vacation	15	7.75	116.25
Statutory Holidays	11	7.75	85.25
Paid Education Days	2	7.75	15.50
Average Paid Sick Days	4	7.75	31.00
Total	32	7.75	248.00

Box 26.1

Calculating Effective Hours

Effective hours can be calculated in two ways, using either benefit days or benefit hours. Consider the residential treatment centre for adolescents. Using the information presented in Table 26.2, effective hours can be calculated as follows:

Using Benefit Days		Using Benefit Hours	
Total days per year	365	Total hours per year	2828.75
		(365 × 7.75)	
Less total benefit days per year	− 32	Less total benefit hours per year	− 248.00
	333		2580.75
Less total number of days off		Less total number of hours off	
per year (2 × 52 weeks)	− 104	per year (104 × 7.75)	− 806.00
days:	229		
hrs/day:	× 7.75		
Effective Hours	1774.75	Effective Hours	1774.75

Paid hours are the number of hours for which the employee is remunerated; paid hours include (a) worked hours, (b) benefit hours, and (c) hours spent doing work activities while away from the work place. Box 26.2 shows how to calculate paid hours for the residential treatment centre for adolescents.

Box 26.2

Calculating Paid Hours

Paid hours include effective hours plus benefit hours. In the residential treatment centre example, the number of paid hours can be calculated as follows:

Effective hours	1774.75
Benefit hours	+ 248.00
Paid hours	2022.75

An employee in this residential treatment centre is therefore paid for 2022.75 hours while actually working 1774.75 hours.

Calculating Number of Staff Members Needed

A clinical unit that is open 24 hours a day, every day of the year, requires 8760 hours (365 days × 24 hours) of coverage per year. If one employee provides 1774.75 hours per year, a simple process of division shows that 4.94 (8760 ÷ 1774.75) staff members are needed for one staff member to be available 24 hours a day, 365 days of the year. The residential treatment centre, however, is closed on weekends; therefore, only 6264 hours (261 days × 24 hours) of coverage are needed. Once again, a simple process of division shows that, for this centre, 3.53 (6264 ÷ 1774.75) staff members are needed in order for one staff member to be available 24 hours a day, 261 days of the year. It is essential at this stage to calculate staffing requirements for each staff classification, applying the reality of each particular unit. In the 12-bed residential treatment centre, four nurses are needed on days and one on evenings.

In an environment where a combination of full-time and part-time employment is common, the terminology used to describe staff totals can be confusing. To minimize confusion, staff positions are usually expressed as full-time equivalents (FTEs). A full-time equivalent represents the paid hours of work for a full-time position. In the example used above, one FTE = 2022.75 paid hours. For this same example, then, the following calculation is applied to determine the number of FTEs required:

Minimum Staff Requirement	5.00 FTE
Relief Staff (1240 ÷ 2022.75)	+ 0.61 FTE
(See Table 26.3 for relief hours)	
Total RPN/RN FTE Requirement	5.61 FTE

These 5.61 FTEs could be comprised of any combination of full- and part-time staff. The mix of full- and part-time positions should be decided based on the configuration that best meets the operational needs of the unit. Table 26.3 illustrates how the RPN/RN staffing requirements for the residential treatment centre are calculated. Note that the manager who completes this calculation process for all classifications in a specific unit has also completed the fundamental work required for budget preparation:

$$5.61 \text{ FTEs } (5.61 \times 2022.75) \times \text{Average Hourly Rate} = \text{Budget Required}$$

Table 26.3 Staffing Requirement for a 12-Bed Residential Treatment Centre for Adolescents

Staff	Shift	M	T	W	R	F	S	S	Total
RPN/RN	Days	4	4	4	4	4	0	0	20
	Evenings	1	1	1	1	0	0	1	5
	Nights	0	0	0	0	0	0	0	0
								Total	25
	Each nurse has 2 days off, therefore								÷ 5
	Minimum staff requirement								5 RPN/RN
	Convert to effective hours								× 1774.75
	Total effective hours								8873.75
	Paid hours (5 × 2002.75)								10,113.75
	Relief hours (10,113.75 − 8873.75)								1240.00

Staff Scheduling

Staff scheduling is the process of distributing budgeted personnel work days and days off according to the basic staffing plan so that patient care needs are met on all shifts. Scheduling is time-consuming and can be fraught with frustration; however, it is also an important process that deserves attention and effort. The objectives of a staff schedule are to

- meet patient care requirements,
- operate within the parameters of the allocated budget,
- maintain fairness, flexibility, and quality of work life, and
- consider the personal needs of individual staff members.

Many factors influence staff scheduling and how it is approached; for example, a unit's staff schedules must accommodate the requirements of local collective agreements, reflect personnel policies and procedures, and be responsive to varying workload demands on the unit. Scheduling is, without question, a complex and challenging process for the first-level manager. Box 26.3 provides a comprehensive list of factors that should be considered when making staff scheduling decisions. Many are driven by the requirements of the collective agreement. Where there is no collective agreement, local personnel policies and labour laws can provide guidance.

For every shift, first-level managers must consider many factors when determining workload and staffing requirements. Successfully achieving this goal is an admirable accomplishment, especially considering the number of unexpected events that can occur in any clinical environment. There are a variety of approaches to staff scheduling that can simplify this process while ensuring quality of care, good staff morale, and efficiency. The three major approaches to staff scheduling are the traditional approach, cyclical scheduling, and self-scheduling. All three approaches may be assisted or supported by the range of scheduling software that is now available.

Box 26.3

Factors to Consider when Making Staff Scheduling Decisions

Staff Factors
Availability
Mix needed:
- Discipline mix (e.g., RN/LPN ratio)
- Male/female ratio
- Full time/part time
- Temporary positions

Expertise needed
Supervisory needs
Continuity-of-care requirements

Staff Special Requests
Procedure for shift trades, leaves of absence, vacation, and paid holidays:
- Requests
- Response to requests
- Approval guidelines
- Time frame

Unusual Staff Occurrences
Procedure for:
- Tardiness
- Absenteeism without notice
- Absenteeism program in the organization

Scheduling Model
Eight hours, extended, or mixed shifts
Hours worked per schedule
Weekends worked per schedule
Maximum number of days worked before days off
Length of cycle rotation
Posting time requirements

Casual or Float Pool
Guidelines regarding:
- Structure of pool: central or unit-based
- Availability requirements
- Assignment method
- Orientation requirements
- Supervision and performance review
- Compensation

Irregular Hours of Work
On-call and overtime guidelines for:
- Availability
- Authorization
Guidelines for:
- Being called after shift begins
- Returning staff home after they have reported to work
- Split shifts
- Call back

Temporary Reassignment
Guidelines for:
- Equity in deciding who will float
- Assignment method
- Orientation
- Supervision and performance review
- Feedback and recognition

Traditional Approach

The traditional approach to staff scheduling means that the manager develops a new schedule from scratch each month, taking all appropriate factors into consideration. The major advantage of this approach is its flexibility—it allows for the impacts of changes to be addressed. However, the traditional approach has major disadvantages, including being extremely time-consuming for the manager and therefore costly. Most managers have opted for more effective and efficient approaches. Those who have not, should.

Cyclical Scheduling

In the cyclical scheduling approach, the manager develops a schedule for a certain number of weeks. Six weeks is a typical time frame. The schedule then repeats itself in cycles. A cyclical schedule must meet collective agreement requirements and accommodate rotating, permanent, or mixed shifts, as well as fixed days off, such as four- or five-day weekends. Its design will vary depending on whether the unit uses regular or extended hours of work, or a combination of the two. Figure 26.1 presents an example of a simple cyclical schedule used in the residential treatment centre for adolescents discussed earlier.

Advantages of cyclical scheduling include (a) stability (once it is set up, it undergoes only minor changes); (b) lower cost (a result of the manager not starting over each month); and (c) predictability (staff members appreciate knowing their schedule weeks or months in advance

Figure 26.1 Sample Cyclical Schedule for the 12-Bed Residential Treatment Centre

	S	M	T	W	R	F	S	S	M	T	W	R	F	S
Senior Therapist (RN)	X	P	S	P-T	P	S	X	X	P	P	P-T	P	S	X
Primary Therapist	X	D	D	D	D	D	X	X	D	D	D	D	D	X
Primary Therapist	X	D	D	D	D	D	X	X	D	D	D	D	D	X
Primary Therapist	X	S	S	S	S	S	X	X	S	S	S	S	S	X
Charge Nurse	B	E	E	K	I	X	X	B	E	E	K	I	X	X
CCC (Childcare Counsellor)	B	E	I	K	E	X	X	B	E	I	K	E	X	X
CCC	B	E	I	K	E	X	X	B	E	I	K	E	X	X
Recreation	B	E	E	K	I	X	X	B	E	E	K	I	X	X
CCC	X	N	N	N	N	N	X	X	N	N	N	N	N	X
CCC	X	N	N	N	N	N	X	X	N	N	N	N	N	X
Cook	X	C	C	C	C	W	X	X	C	C	C	C	W	X
Secretary	X	S	S	S	Y	S	X	X	S	S	Y	S	X	X

Key

B = 1900 to 2315	C = 0845 to 1715	D = 0700 to 1515	E = 1400 to 2315
I = 1430 to 2315	K = 1430 to 2315	N = 2300 to 0700	P = 0845 to 1515
S = 0815 to 1630	T = 1800 to 2100	W = 0845 to 1600	Y = 0900 to 1715
P-T = Split Shift	X = Days Off		

Note: Every person repeats the same two-week schedule continually. This two-week schedule averages 38.75 hours per week per person. The longest work span is 5 days. Individuals in a unit-based casual pool cover long weekends, special leaves, vacation, and other absences.

Source: Twelve-Bed Residential Treatment Centre for Adolescents, Child and Adolescent Services Association (CASA), Edmonton, Alberta.

so that they can make personal plans). The major disadvantage of cyclical schedules is that they are inflexible—days on and off are fixed, and the changing workload requirements that characterize most patient care environments are not easily accommodated. Managers can minimize this inflexibility by establishing a protocol that allows staff to exchange shifts and permits staffing to be adjusted as workload requirements dictate.

Self-Scheduling

The self-scheduling approach allows staff members on a unit to develop and implement the work schedule themselves. This enables staff to solve problems and make decisions without having to seek approval from their manager. Self-scheduling first began in hospitals because work schedules had been a major source of discontent among nurses. The approach is designed to provide staff with control over decisions that have a significant impact on their professional and personal lives. The goals of self-scheduling are to

- increase staff autonomy through control over the work schedule,
- promote staff retention by providing increased flexibility and creativity in scheduling,
- decrease absenteeism by introducing a self-coverage plan for illness, and
- support team development by requiring staff members to negotiate among themselves, thus enhancing their sense of accountability to one another.

For self-scheduling to succeed, unit staff must be committed to this approach. Ideally, the staff provides the impetus for implementing self-scheduling. The manager and staff need time to learn the approach before deciding to move ahead with implementation. The manager and union must strongly support this approach, and the staff must participate in every aspect of the changeover. A fair pilot should be at least six months long. The first three months are demanding because of the magnitude of the change and the intensive teaching and coaching required. Developing a plan of the entire implementation process enables staff to better understand what to expect. An implementation plan also allows the manager to plan, monitor, and evaluate the change process very carefully (Dechant, 1989).

The impact of this approach on the first-level manager is considerable. The manager in this scenario becomes a facilitator of the process—a mentor or coach rather than a supervisor, empowering staff to make effective choices as members of a self-directed team (Teahan, 1998). This approach is consistent with modern principles of leadership and with a philosophy of decentralized decision making and shared governance.

Despite its potential benefits, self-scheduling is rarely used, possibly because it is very time-consuming to implement. As well, staff might be unwilling to add to their already onerous workloads and may consider scheduling to be the manager's responsibility. Because staff members are responsible for resolving the inevitable conflicts, some might worry about not being assertive enough to get a fair schedule.

Self-scheduling has proven to be a very creative way to increase staff dignity and job satisfaction. It reflects a change not only in how we do things, but also in how we think about staff and the role of the manager. Self-scheduling may be considered a "power strategy": it empowers staff by allocating them the responsibility, authority, and accountability to gain and retain control over an aspect of their work that is vitally important to their lives. This approach is well worth the manager's consideration.

Automated Scheduling Software

Technological advances have always affected the workplace, changing the way jobs are done. Some would say that managing staff scheduling today with pen and paper is an antiquated method of operational management; computerized staffing methods handle this complex task faster, with great accuracy and increased efficiency. Software enables managers to schedule and track global and individual rotations, callbacks, on-call priorities, and all scheduling issues vital to operating an effective unit.

Several factors must be considered when choosing scheduling software. See, for example, the guide in McConnell (2000) for an excellent overview of factors to consider and questions to ask. Organizations should consider whether the software is designed, or can be customized, to meet the unique staffing requirements of diverse departments (e.g., pharmacy, respiratory therapy) so that it can be of substantial benefit throughout the organization rather than to inpatient units exclusively.

Some organizations have introduced scheduling software as a pilot for a small number of units or for a single program. These organizations found that, despite some clear benefits, the associated costs were too great to further expand the application. Box 26.4 presents a case study of the Calgary Health Region's wide-scale application of an automated staff scheduling system. Before emulating this case study, however, it would be important to look at the evaluation results of this operation.

Of course, ultimately, automated scheduling software is a useful tool only if the manager is knowledgeable and skilled in the basic practices of staffing and scheduling.

Staffing Adjustments

Patient care needs vary from shift to shift, and unfortunately, such variations often cannot be anticipated. This generates a need for staffing adjustments. Staffing adjustments should not be confused with regular staff scheduling. Staff scheduling involves planning for staff allocation throughout the year on the basis of predictable factors, whereas staffing adjustments involve changing staff allocation in response to unexpected conditions that caused either over- or under-staffing. The staff adjustment process occurs by means of various approaches, of which perhaps the best known is the float pool.

Float pools consist of casual or relief staff members employed by an organization to work on an as-needed basis. Expectations of these float staff members vary from one organization to another. The parameters in most cases are defined by the collective agreement. The structure of float pools also varies. In some organizations, float personnel are unit-based and managed by the first-level manager. In others, float personnel are based in a centralized pool that is managed by a staffing coordinator. The advantages of a unit-based, relief staff structure are that it

Box 26.4

Case Example: Calgary Health Region's Automated Scheduling System

The Calgary Health Region is a large, fully integrated Canadian health care organization that provides health services to more than 1.5 million people. The four acute care hospitals, Care in the Community (home care and long-term care), and Healthy Communities (public health) portfolios employ more than 22,000 staff and over 320 first-level managers. Since the year 2000, managers have been assisted with the complex processes of staffing and scheduling through a central Staff Scheduling Department. First-level managers retain the responsibility and accountability for the allocation and management of staff, but the Staff Scheduling Department provides a large component of the clerical processes related to staffing and scheduling. In this role, the scheduling staff contact and schedule approximately 11,000 nursing and allied health employees. Schedulers use an automated staff scheduling software system to record schedules, worked shifts, and overtime. Managers and staff have "view and print" access to their schedules at any time in their workplace. Information related to time and labour is electronically exported from the staff scheduling information system directly to the automated payroll system.

Close collaboration and frequent communication between managers and the schedulers promote accurate staffing and payment of staff, as well as consistent application of collective agreements and regional guidelines and policies. Cyclical rotation and self-scheduling information is maintained in the software, making substantial amounts of data available to managers. This data may assist with decision making, budgeting, and planning. Standardization of staff scheduling processes across all sectors of regional services has been achieved. The delivery of the scheduling service can be customized to accommodate the unique and varied business of each service area. The staff scheduling office administers the staff float pools.

The partnership between the manager and the scheduling office is strengthened by frequent evaluation and feedback. Processes continue to evolve in order to improve staff scheduling services to managers and staff. Future plans include developing education and assistance for managers with cyclical rotation and exploring integration of workload measurement information with the staffing information.

Source: Contributed by Shirley Meyer, Director, Integrated Nursing Systems, Calgary Health Region, Alberta.

includes a small number of flexible staff under the direct supervision of a manager, and it develops within this staff a high level of commitment to the unit. Relief staff members are expected to have the same performance standards and ongoing professional development as full-time staff. In many organizations, unit-based relief staff also work through the centralized float pool when their commitment to their unit of origin is fulfilled and they desire extra work.

Cross-utilization is an enhancement of the historical approach of floating. *Floating* occurs when nurses who had been assigned to one unit are reassigned to another unit or department with which they may not be familiar. Floating occurs shift by shift, in response to patient needs.

Cross-utilization partners groups or units with similar patient populations requiring similar nursing skills (American Organization of Nurse Executives, 1993). Because individual units in the group experience variations in census and acuity, skilled staff move from one unit to the other. This process benefits both patients and staff—patients receive care from personnel with the appropriate skill mix, and nursing staff become familiar with colleagues in the group and feel more inclined to include these "floating" nurses in unit and social activities. In cross-utilization, the nurse manager must ensure that there are appropriate supports through policies and standards of care and that there is a clear structure for accountability and decision making.

The management of overstaffing is a challenge. It is imperative that staff-reduction strategies be developed in advance of need. Managers must understand the process and the financial and other implications of, for example, sending a staff member home after the start of a shift. These strategies must also be consistent with collective agreement requirements and be supported by the organization.

Most staffing schedules must be revised or redesigned periodically as a result of any of the following:

- Change in patient demographics
- Start of a new service
- Change in the hours during which the service is offered
- Change in workforce availability and demographics (e.g., the aging of the nursing workforce)
- Change in professional education or skill set
- Legislated changes (e.g., change in the number of hours in the average work week)
- Change in the collective agreement
- Change in workload patterns
- Change in patient acuity and support services available in the community
- Increased knowledge and expectations of service recipients

First-level managers need to be alert to extraneous factors that affect staffing. They also must be aware of the impact these changes have on service delivery and the need to adjust staffing accordingly.

Job Sharing

Job sharing refers to two or more part-time staff members filling one full-time equivalent position. These individuals provide coverage on the shifts required for a full-time position and cover for each other's vacations and absences. Today's managers generally stay away from traditional job sharing contracts and address the need for scheduling flexibility by developing a balance of full- and part-time positions in their complement of FTEs. The manager must be aware of the increased benefit costs associated with part-time positions.

Analyzing Existing Staffing Elements and Work Schedules

Rarely do managers have the opportunity to open a new unit and be the first to develop its staffing requirements and work schedule. Most often, managers assume an existing unit with entrenched staffing and scheduling practices. Managers not yet knowledgeable and proficient in staffing and scheduling could be overwhelmed by these responsibilities. Poor staffing and scheduling can decrease employee morale and the quality of patient care, while also increasing costs and liabilities. Although the manager may be tempted to import practices and procedures from another unit, staffing and scheduling must be highly individualized to a particular setting—staffing and scheduling practices used in one area can rarely be used in another area without adjustments.

As discussed earlier in this chapter, a critical first step for the manager is to understand the unit's philosophical framework for practice, characteristics of its patient population, environmental factors affecting the unit, and characteristics of the personnel staffing the unit. With this understanding, the manager can analyze or audit the staffing and scheduling realities of the unit. Box 26.5 lists questions to ask when performing a staffing and scheduling audit.

Box 26.5

Staffing and Scheduling Audit: Identifying the Existing Staffing Elements and Work Schedules

Staffing Elements
Refer to staff factors, Box 26.3, and understand each element. Identify:
- Number of classifications
- Number of FTEs, full-time, and part-time
- Temporary and casual staff
- Novice and expert staff

Is staffing uniform each day? Is it variable by time of day, day of the week, or both?
What is the unit's
- Use of flex-time?
- Number of staff who are job sharing?
- Use of overtime?
- Approach to assignment of breaks?
- Experience of
  - Absenteeism?
  - Staff retention and turnover?
  - Accident rates?
  - Patient and staff injury rates?

Is employee fatigue an issue?

Are employees asking for a change?

Are your supervisors indicating a need for change?

How are these staff factors impacted by the collective agreement?

Work Schedule

Refer to scheduling, Box 26.3, and understand each element.

Not all units operate 24/7. Examine the schedule.

Identify the shift configuration:
- Number of shifts per day
- Shift length
- Shift start and end times
- Use of overlapping shifts
- Use of split shifts (shifts interrupted by a period of off-duty time)

Identify the shift assignments:
- Are they permanent or rotating?
- If rotating, do employees change shifts at regular intervals?
- In what order are employees assigned to shifts? For example, are they rotating from days to evenings to nights, which has been shown to allow the body to more easily adapt to a new schedule?
- Are the shifts eight hours, extended, or mixed?
- Does the assigned shift rotation accurately reflect the employment status of the individual? For example, is the 0.74 FTE working at, more, or less than the 0.74? The answer to this question has implications for your budget.

Identify the pattern of the shift cycle:
- Length of the cycle (speed of shift rotation): weekly, monthly, every 2 weeks?
- Length of consecutive days of work
- Pattern of days off duty
- Day of the week that the schedule begins
- Frequency of weekends off
- Days off before and after shift changes

Identify schedule simplicity/complexity:
- Can the staff easily understand the schedule?
- What is the process for assignment changes, vacation requests, and trading of days off?
- What is the approach to conflict resolution?
- What is the process for handling absenteeism with and without notice?
- What is the role of the nursing office?
- Are employees hired for a specific unit or can they request a transfer to another unit? What is the process for requesting a unit transfer?

Identify:
- How staffing levels and individual employee skills are matched with fluctuating workloads
- How the patient classification system works
- The constraints that limit responsiveness to individual employee needs
- If written policies and procedures provide a means for consistency and fairness
- If the schedule in place meets all the requirements of the collective agreement; this process cannot be successfully completed without an in-depth understanding of your collective agreement

Having completed these steps, the manager will have a substantial understanding of the unit's staffing and scheduling and will be prepared to either leave these unchanged or to propose changes. Remember the "Golden Rule of Employee Involvement": involve staff in decisions that have an impact on the quality of their work life. Therefore, involve staff in scheduling and staffing decisions. Also, after the changes have been implemented, remember to evaluate whether or not the new schedule has met design objectives.

Ethical and Legal Issues in Staffing and Scheduling

First-level managers are legally and ethically obligated to plan staffing and scheduling so that patient care will be safely delivered according to professional standards and policies. This underscores the need for the manager to have an excellent understanding of all the variables highlighted in this chapter and an ability to integrate these variables into an effective staffing plan and scheduling practices. When scheduling, the first-level manager is legally bound to integrate the requirements of the collective agreement and is not free to negotiate with individual staff members any special arrangements that would be in breach of the collective agreement.

In addition to the patient care imperative, first-level managers must recognize their obligation to continually strive for improvement and to examine, analyze, and shape the work environment. Nevertheless, nothing in the collective agreement prevents a manager from seeking staff input and feedback in the process of staffing and scheduling. Such staff consultation promotes individual autonomy, trust, collegiality, and opportunities for professional contribution. Continued learning and growth are hallmarks of the professional.

The first-level manager also has an ethical imperative to optimize outcomes in patient care and staff satisfaction, while balancing these with judicious use of the unit's limited resources or the program budget. Dilemmas may arise, for example, in striving for fairness in the allocation of evening and night shifts while ensuring the adequacy of staffing to meet patient care needs. There is considerable research evidence to suggest that, for some individuals, there are physiological, emotional, and social consequences of working shifts. The subject of shift work and its implications for staff are beyond the scope of this chapter, but managers need to be knowledgeable about this topic and understand staff tolerance for shift work because it is yet another variable to consider in the planning and maintenance of schedules. Finally, the manager has an ethical responsibility to advocate when necessary for the resources required to deliver the unit's mission.

Leadership Implications

Allocating human resources is an integral part of the first-level manager's role. To be an effective leader, the manager must demonstrate vision and sensitivity to workforce issues. The manager must also be able to integrate and manipulate many interrelated variables. This is accomplished through a complex process that presents many leadership opportunities and challenges. Managers are successful at this task when they know the unit or program for which they are accountable, recognize that they can influence this environment by their approach to staffing and scheduling, and are committed to excellence in staffing and scheduling as a means of ensuring a satisfying and productive workplace.

Managers with leadership skills, commitment to excellence, and expertise in human resource allocation can create effective teams and implement flexible strategies that cope with rapidly changing and unpredictable work environments. The manager's success in this area has a positive impact on the quality of patient care. Successful staffing and scheduling also fosters a healthy environment for caregivers. These are important outcomes, and the manager who achieves them is an expert role model and deserves respect. The first-level manager's role is integral to the success of the patient care unit. Senior administrative leadership is imperative to address the current gap in education, support resources, and mentoring for first-level managers in the area of staffing and scheduling. Administrative attention to this need would facilitate optimal patient care outcomes, staff satisfaction and retention, and efficient resource utilization.

Summary

- Staffing is the process used to determine the acceptable number and skill mix of personnel needed to meet the treatment and care requirements of patients in a program or unit in any health care setting.
- Key variables that directly affect a program or unit's staffing plan include the philosophical framework for practice, the characteristics of the patient population, environmental factors, and personnel characteristics.
- To develop a basic staffing plan, the first-level manager must be able to calculate paid hours, effective hours (also called worked hours), and benefit hours.
- Staff scheduling is the process of distributing budgeted personnel days of work and days off in the pattern identified in the basic staffing plan in order to meet the requisite patient care needs on all shifts.
- Many complex factors influence staff scheduling decisions and choice of approaches. The objectives of the staff schedule are to meet patient care requirements; operate within the parameters of the allocated budget; and maintain fairness, flexibility, and consideration of workers' needs.
- Key factors to consider in staff scheduling decisions include staff factors, the scheduling

model in use, special requests by the staff, casual or float pool availability, structure and guidelines, unusual staff occurrences, irregular hours of work, shift work, and guidelines for temporary reassignments.

- The most commonly used approach to staff scheduling is the cyclical schedule, which provides the desired coverage over a number of weeks and then repeats itself in cycles.

- Automated scheduling software may serve as a powerful tool for staffing and scheduling. Thoughtful consideration should be given to its use in the complex labour environments typical of health care settings.

- Patient care managers rarely have an opportunity to open a new unit. Typically, they are hired into a unit with a staffing and scheduling approach already in place. For these managers, knowing how to analyze existing staffing elements and work schedules is imperative.

- The primary legal and ethical obligation of the first-level manager in relation to staffing and scheduling is to provide safe patient care within professionally defined clinical standards, standards of practice, and organizational policies and procedures. Managers must have an excellent understanding of all the variables highlighted in this chapter and must have the ability to integrate these variables in an effective staffing plan and scheduling practices.

Applying the Knowledge in this Chapter

Case Study

A regional health authority has just released its business plan for the next three years. This new business plan reflects the recent expansion of the health region to include a large adjoining suburban community with a population of just over 60,000 people, a great number of whom are retired older adults. Recognizing the importance of promoting health and preventing hospitalization in this population, the health region decided to include in the business plan an ambulatory health clinic for older adults. This clinic is modelled on a very successful existing clinic in the greater region. It is to be integrated in the local geriatric program, which includes home care services, a 30-bed sub-acute care unit, and a 28-bed acute care unit co-located in the community hospital.

Lorie Girard, BScN, an experienced manager with an impressive background in health care services for older adults, has just been hired to implement this new initiative and to fill the vacant management position for the existing two units. Lorie understands that no new funding is available for this initiative and that her mandate includes redistribution of resources for the implementation of this clinic through closure of beds in the current units.

1. What key variables will Lorie need to understand thoroughly as she begins to develop a plan of action?

2. Lorie will need to identify the staffing requirements of the ambulatory clinic before she can determine the impact of the change on the two existing units. What factors must she consider when developing a staffing plan?

3. Identify the factors Lorie should take into account in designing a staff schedule for this clinic.

4. As the new manager of the two existing units, Lorie should analyze the existing staffing elements and work schedule. Discuss how she might approach this task.

5. The changes to the existing units' staffing and scheduling will be difficult for the staff and challenging for Lorie. What is the golden rule that Lorie must follow in this process?

6. What are some of the built-in constraints that might have an impact on the success of this change?

Resources

evolve Internet Resource

International Council of Nurses:
   Position Statement: Nurses and Shift Work
   www.icn.ch/psshiftwork00.htm

Further Reading

Readers interested in learning more about the effects of shift work might start with the three references below. Each offers an excellent review of the literature on shift work.

Fitzpatrick, J.M., While, A.E., & Roberts, J.D. (1999). Shift work and its impact upon nurse performance: Current knowledge and research issues. *Journal of Advanced Nursing, 29*(1), 18–27.
   This is a report of a small study of 34 staff nurses using participant observation. The primary aim of the study was to refine and validate a performance scale. As the authors say, generalizations should not be made from this study (nurses on 8-hour shifts scored significantly higher on the performance scale than those working 12.5-hour shifts), but the paper contains an excellent review of the literature, and the authors discuss several research issues as well.

Poissonnet, C.M., & Véron, M. (2000). Health effects of work schedules in healthcare professions. *Journal of Clinical Nursing, 9,* 13–23.
   This paper is a systematic review of the research literature on the effects of irregular schedules on health care professionals. The authors, two Parisian physicians, report findings in relation to physical and mental health, sleep and performance, and risks specific to women, and they make six recommendations.

Wilson, J.L. (2002). The impact of shift patterns on healthcare professionals. *Journal of Nursing Management, 10,* 211–219.

The author's primary interest was in finding evidence of those factors associated with shift work that have been identified as detrimental, for example, problems with eating, sleeping, and social disruption. She identified several consequences of shift work, including some compensatory behaviours that employees use in adapting to shift work.

In addition to the annotated references above, three recent works are listed below as further readings on staffing, scheduling, and shift work.

Hader, R., & Claudio. T. (2002). Seven methods to effectively manage patient care labor resources. *Journal of Nursing Administration, 32,* 66–68.

Moore, M., & Kerin, K. (2002). *Circadian Technologies: Shiftwork practices survey, 2002.* Lexington, MA: Circadian Technologies.

Shaver, K., & Lacey, L. (2003). Job career satisfaction among staff nurses: Effects of job setting and environment. *Journal of Nursing Administration, 33,* 166–172.

References

American Nurses Association. (1997). *Implementing nursing's report card: A study of RN staffing, length of stay and patient outcomes.* Washington, DC: Author.

American Organization of Nurse Executives. (1993). Cross-utilization of nursing staff. *Nursing Management, 13*(7), 38–39.

Dechant, G. (1989). Self-scheduling for nursing staff. *AARN Newsletter, 46*(5), 4, 6, 8.

Giovannetti, P. (1994). Measurement of nursing workload. In J.M. Hibberd & M.E. Kyle (Eds.), *Nursing management in Canada* (pp. 331–349). Toronto, ON: W.B. Saunders.

McConnell, E. (2000). Staffing and scheduling at your fingertips. *Journal of Nursing Management, 31*(3), 52–53.

Moore, M., & Kerin, K. (2002). *Shift pattern.* Lexington, MA: Circadian Technologies.

Teahan, M. (1998). Implementation of a self-scheduling system: A solution to more than just schedules! *Journal of Nursing Management, 6*(6), 361–369.

CONFLICT RESOLUTION AND NEGOTIATION

Judith M. Hibberd, Patricia E.B. Valentine, and Lana Clark

Learning Objectives

In this chapter, you will learn:

- Theory and concepts related to conflict and negotiation

- Conflict resolution strategies

- Typical responses to conflict by staff nurses and nurse managers

- Differences between day-to-day negotiations and collective bargaining

- Key principles of the negotiating process

- Four phases in the negotiating process

- Common negotiating tactics and the rationale for using them

- Mediation between individuals or groups in conflict

- Gender as an issue in conflict resolution and negotiation

In the face of rapid changes and shrinking resources in the health care system, conflict is inevitable. Differences in beliefs, values, opinions, strategies, and goals are part of the every day experiences of health care workers, and people no longer consider conflict as unusual or necessarily harmful. Indeed, the occurrence of conflict between individuals or groups often leads to new ways of dealing with problems and the introduction of important changes. Once conflict has been identified and assessed, the next question faced by managers is whether and how, to intervene. Negotiating skills are essential if managers are to find effective ways of coping with conflicts and disputes. As Saner (2000) indicated, negotiations and conflict belong together like conjoined twins because their combination is irrefutably part of our existence. We all experience conflicts in our personal and professional lives, and we all use various forms of negotiation when we choose to confront conflict. People differ in their approaches to the resolution of personal conflict, but managers have a responsibility to monitor workplace conflict and to address it if it threatens to interfere with the safety and effectiveness of patient care, the efficiency of work, or the quality of the working environment.

This chapter is about conflict, conflict management, negotiations, and mediation. Strategies and tactics for negotiating and dealing with conflict situations are offered. This information is useful for all nurses, whether or not they occupy leadership or management positions. Conflicts that arise from the process of negotiating and administering collective agreements are not discussed in detail because it is an extensive subject and beyond the scope of this chapter.

Definitions

There is no single definition of *conflict*, but the one used in this chapter is by Thomas (1992). He defined conflict as "the process that begins when one party perceives that the other [party] has negatively affected, or is about to negatively affect, something that he or she cares about" (p. 653). Conflict stems from differences in thoughts, beliefs, attitudes, feelings, or behaviour of two or more parties.

Conflict resolution refers to the various ways in which people or institutions deal with social conflict (Barsky, 2000). As Barsky noted, conflict is neither good nor bad, but the way in which we deal with it determines whether it is constructive or destructive. Some intractable conflicts, in which the parties adopt inflexible polar positions, may never be fully resolved and may require ongoing management. In this chapter, the terms *conflict resolution* and *conflict management* are used synonymously.

Negotiation is "a process whereby two or more parties seek an agreement to establish what each shall give or take, or perform and receive in a transaction between them" (Saner, 2000, p. 15). Negotiation occurs on many levels: among individuals, groups, corporations, governments, or countries. Negotiations are not necessarily confined to two opposing parties; they are often multilateral, as are, for example, the negotiations among coalitions of member countries of the United Nations.

Forms of Conflict

There are three forms of conflict: intrapersonal, interpersonal, and intergroup. In all three, tension is produced within an individual or party because of unmet needs, goals, or expectations. Intrapersonal conflict occurs within an individual and may manifest itself as role conflict. A typical example is the nurse in charge of a unit who faces two competing demands—the desire to provide care to patients and the obligation to attend to unit administrative tasks. Nurse managers may sometimes experience ethical dilemmas when their positions involve the implementation of policies that violate their professional values and beliefs (Gaudine & Beaton, 2002).

Interpersonal conflict occurs among two or more individuals or parties, for example, when health care professionals disagree over treatment plans for specific patients or over ethical dilemmas concerning advance directives for seriously ill patients. Intergroup conflict occurs among two or more groups; it often involves patient care issues and personnel policies or procedures. For example, two groups, such as nurses and physicians, vie for the same funds—the nurses may want the money to increase staffing to improve the delivery of patient care, while the physicians may want to use the money to purchase the latest technological innovation.

Models for Understanding Conflict

Two frequently cited models for understanding conflict are the structural model and the process model (Thomas, 1976). The structural model is useful because is suggests that conflict can be understood by viewing the underlying conditions that shape it, such as rules, roles, and relations. On the other hand, the process model focuses on the internal dynamics of specific conflict events and situations. The two models are complementary: the structural model is useful for suggesting systemic changes, and the process model is useful for managing an ongoing system and coping with crises.

Structural Model

The structural model takes into account the context and its influences on the process of conflict and conflict management. This model is comprised of four factors that influence how conflict is managed in organizations: behavioural predispositions of the parties involved, social pressure, incentive structure of the organization, and rules and procedures. Parties in conflict have behavioural predispositions based on their motives and abilities; pressures in the immediate social environment influence both parties; both parties respond to conflict incentives in the situation, such as conflict of interest between them and their investment in the relationship; and both parties interact in a context of rules and procedures that constrain their behaviour.

Process Model

In the process model, conflict is described as a dynamic process with several stages that result in an episode of conflict. Researchers often begin describing conflict situations by using Thomas's model (1992), which includes five stages: awareness, thoughts and emotions, intentions, behaviour, and outcomes (Figure 27.1).

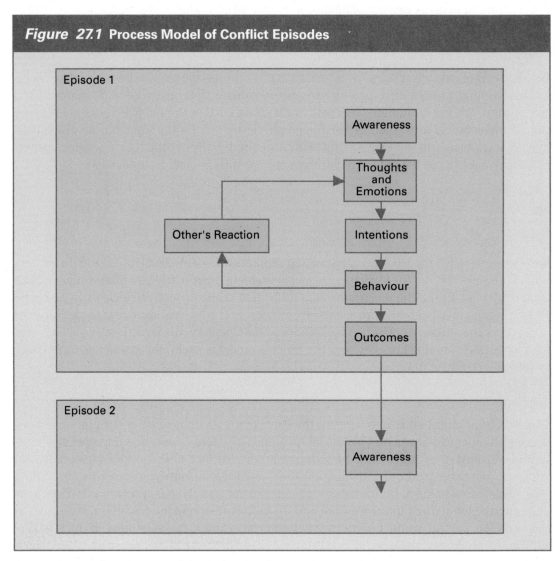

Figure 27.1 Process Model of Conflict Episodes

Source: Adapted from *Handbook of Industrial and Organizational Psychology* 2nd ed., Vol. 3 (p. 658), edited by M.D. Dunnette and L.M. Hough, 1992, Palo Alto, CA: Consulting Psychologists Press, Inc. Copyright 1992 by CPP, Inc. Reproduced by special permission of the publisher. All rights reserved. Further reproduction is prohibited without the publisher's written consent.

An episode of conflict starts with one party's awareness of the conflict. Awareness leads to a variety of thoughts and emotions about the conflict episode and potential responses to it. The thoughts and emotions are based on normative reasoning and rational/instrumental reasoning that result in the development of intentions. These intentions, which are related to trying to cope with the conflict situation, result in some type of observable behaviour that evokes a reaction from another person (other's reaction). The interaction may be prolonged because each party's behaviour stimulates the other party's response. As the interaction progresses, each party's thoughts and feelings about the conflict issue may change, affecting their behaviour accordingly. When interaction on the issue stops, outcomes are produced. The outcomes have consequences for both parties, such as mutual agreement, mutual avoidance, control by one party, or no resolution. The outcomes of a given situation determine whether a subsequent episode on the same issue will recur in the future.

Aspects of Conflict

Initially, organizational conflict was considered destructive to organizational life. Managers were expected to control it at all costs by having rules or procedures for governing all situations (Etzioni, 1961; Fayol, 1949; Lewin, 1948; Weber, 1946). If conflict occurred, it was thought that a manager should confront it openly. During the 1950s and 1960s, the management literature began to suggest that conflict was not necessarily dysfunctional but could serve positive functions (Blake & Mouton, 1964; Coser, 1956), although there has not been much research to support this contention (Johnson, 1994). Currently, conflict is considered to be neither intrinsically good nor bad; it need not necessarily be eliminated, but it must be effectively managed. An optimal level of conflict seems to be necessary for effective functioning of an organization.

Those who take a negative view argue that too much conflict can interfere with the climate of the organization, decrease staff performance by dissipating energy, impact negatively on morale, and interfere with teamwork. Negative effects can produce ineffectiveness and inefficiency and eventually result in organizational stagnation.

On the other hand, viewed positively, optimal conflict can unite a group by setting boundaries and strengthening the group's identity, unify a group by distributing power, help to balance a group by acting as a testing ground for contrary interests, and forge crucial relationships and teams (Huber, 1996). Growth, creativity, innovation, and change are stimulated by conflict (Coser, 1956).

Conflict Management Strategies

Since conflict first began to be studied, various conflict management strategies have been delineated. Follett (1926/1940) described three main ways of dealing with conflict: domination, compromise, and integration. Blake and Mouton (1964) developed a conceptual model that classifies styles for handling interpersonal conflicts into five types based on managers' attitudes toward production and people. Thomas (1976) honed this system by separating the conflict from the behaviours people used for handling it. Using different terms and slightly different meanings, Thomas identified five strategies for handling conflict: competing, compromising, avoiding, collaborating, and accommodating. The strategies were based on the intentions of a party; for example, these intentions could represent assertiveness (i.e., attempting to satisfy one's own concerns) or cooperativeness (i.e., attempting to satisfy another's concerns).

The Thomas-Kilmann conflict mode instrument (TKI) was developed to measure five ways of handling conflict (Thomas & Kilmann, 1974). Although several other conflict-handling instruments have been developed, the TKI has been the most widely used to measure nurses' strategies for handling conflict. Therefore, Thomas and Kilmann's five strategies, their uses, and the specific outcomes produced by them will be described:

1. *Competing* (also known as *dominating, coercing, forcing,* and *telling*) is a mode that results in one party winning and another losing. It involves high concern for self and low concern for others (Rahim, 1986). Competing is power-oriented, with one party strongly defending its own stance and believing it to be the right one. Often, an issue is forced onto the table through direct orders and voted on, with the minority losing. Competing is used when dealing with unpopular causes, aggressive people, and issues requiring quick decisions. It is also used when one has expertise that enables better decision making and as a defense against others who exploit non-competing behaviour (Hightower, 1986; Marriner, 1982; Rahim & Bonoma, 1979). Winning may be the goal. People who successfully use competing often avoid the truth, others' disagreement, or being challenged, even if they are wrong. They often respond aggressively when challenged. Decisions that are forced often produce unsatisfactory resolutions.

2. *Compromising* (also known as *sharing* and *negotiating*) is a mode used when each party relinquishes something to produce a decision acceptable to both (Rahim, 1986). Compromising, the "staple" (Huber, 1996, p. 422) of conflict management, involves democratic values. Compromising means taking a middle position, and it can often result in a quick fix. It is frequently used for temporary resolution of complex issues, for inconsequential issues, when emotions have reached such a pitch that they require diffusion, and when goals are important but not worth major disruption. Compromising is often used as a backup when collaborating and competing fail.

3. *Avoiding* is a mode used when one party does not pursue his or her own concerns or those of the other party. Avoiders may deny the existence of conflict either consciously or subconsciously, or if they acknowledge conflict, they may avert it or withdraw from it (Barsky, 2000). Avoiding often results in issues being postponed or completely withdrawn. It is used as a "cool-down" mechanism or for dealing with issues in which the impact of confronting the other party is perceived to be more negative than attaining resolution of conflict (Rahim & Bonoma, 1979). It is also used when more information is needed; when issues are tactical, trivial, or pressing (Thomas, 1977); or when there is no chance of resolution.

4. *Collaborating* (also known as *integrating* and *problem solving*) is a mode used when one party works with another party to find a mutually satisfying resolution. Collaborating

includes cooperation between parties, candidness, and information sharing (especially differences) to reach consensus. Confronting and problem solving are part of this strategy and lead to creative solutions to issues (Rahim, 1986). Collaborating is used to (a) develop an integrative solution to issues considered too crucial for compromise, (b) merge insights from different perspectives, (c) increase understanding by testing out various perspectives, (d) gain commitment to change, (e) work through disruptive emotional issues, and (f) spread responsibility while reducing risk taking. It is especially useful when time is not a consideration and long-term resolution of conflict is desired.

5. *Accommodating* (also known as *obliging* and *smoothing*) is a mode used when one party deliberately neglects his or her own concerns to satisfy the concerns of the other. It involves focusing on similarities between parties while minimizing differences and being self-sacrificing (Rahim, 1986). Accommodating may be used when one party realizes an error, the issue is more important to the other party, one party decides to relinquish a point in order to gain another point later on, one party is outmatched, harmony must be preserved, or when others need to learn from their mistakes. It is often considered appropriate for routine issues; however, its overuse may result in disappointment and resentment, especially if there is lack of reciprocation.

Table 27.1 summarizes these five strategies, their outcomes, and how nurses use them.

Research suggests that the modes of competing, compromising, avoiding, and accommodating usually result in temporary conflict management, but some frustration often remains in one or both parties (Thomas, 1976). In one study, subordinates perceived that supervisors handled conflict constructively when they used accommodative or collaborative techniques; competing and avoiding techniques were perceived to be the least constructive (Burke, 1970). Johnson (1994) suggested that collaborating is rarely used when a wide power differential exists between parties in conflict. Compromising and accommodating are frequently used when differences in power permit one party to predominate.

Although competing is considered to be one of the more ineffective conflict management strategies, its infrequent use by staff nurses and nurse managers may suggest they feel powerless or have trouble taking a firm stand. The infrequent use of this strategy also suggests that women (nursing is still a female-dominated profession) may view competition differently than how men view it. Does concern for others stop nurses from using this mode?

The frequent use of compromising by nurse managers suggests that they focus more on practicalities rather than larger issues. The merits of crucial issues may be deflected by the gamesmanship of trading and bargaining. Nurse managers may think they have to compromise because of their hierarchical position between the traditional decision makers (administrators, boards, physicians), who are mostly men, and the subordinate workers (staff nurses, other health care workers), who are mostly women.

Staff nurses' strong propensity to use avoiding suggests they may be reluctant to provide input into decisions. Overuse of avoiding may result in decisions on crucial nursing issues being arrived at by default. The frequent use of this mode may also indicate that nurses feel powerless or think that conflict is incompatible with the caring ideology of nursing.

Table 27.1 Conflict-Management Strategies, Outcomes, and Research Findings

Strategies	Outcomes	Nursing Research Findings
Competing	win-lose assertive, uncooperative short-term resolution	• used infrequently by all nurses • *not* competing was strategy of choice used by nurse educators in one study
Compromising	no win-no lose moderately assertive, cooperative short-term resolution	• used predominantly by nurse managers
Avoiding	lose-lose unassertive, uncooperative short-term resolution	• used predominantly by staff nurses • used often by nurse managers
Collaborating	win-win fully assertive, cooperative long-term resolution	• no distinct pattern in usage by nurse managers • used infrequently by staff nurses
Accommodating	lose-win unassertive, cooperative short-term resolution	• used infrequently by nurse managers

The research on ways of handling conflict by nurses, nurse managers, and nurse educators suggests that nurses prefer non-assertive methods. Although there may be a number of explanations for these findings, one reason may be the lack of formal knowledge and skill, and indeed, confidence, in the art of negotiation. Although negotiating is recognized as an important skill for case managers, undergraduate curricula may not emphasize negotiating as a necessary interpersonal skill. Moreover, nurses may associate negotiating with union activities. It is only a few of the members of nurses' unions who become sufficiently involved in the collective bargaining process to acquire experience in resolving contentious issues.

Assessment of Conflict Situations

When conflict occurs, the process for management or resolution needs to be identified and understood. Critical thinking, information gathering, and a clear definition of the problem are important initial stages before intervening. Just as staff nurses assess patient situations, nurse managers need to assess organizational conflict situations. It is helpful for them to recognize their usual conflict management strategies and to know the five strategies for handling conflict. Because specific modes for handling conflict are useful in specific situations, nurse managers must be aware of the outcome of each strategy. Nurse managers need to choose conflict management strategies that produce positive outcomes.

When conflict is identified, the following steps may be used to manage the situation:
1. Diffuse strong feelings associated with the issue.
2. Gather all facts before defining the issue.
3. Be aware of past personal approaches to conflict management.
4. Determine whether the situation requires intervention.
5. Determine whether intervention requires long- or short-term resolution.
6. Be aware of research literature on effective conflict management strategies.
7. Intervene using the appropriate mode.
8. Evaluate the outcome.

Negotiation

Once the conflict situation has been assessed and the problems identified, a decision will be made as to the most appropriate approach to take. Regardless of which approach to resolving conflict is selected, negotiating skills are essential. Nursing leaders must learn the principles and process underlying the art and science of negotiation. Although they may have opportunities to take part in formal negotiations such as collective bargaining, they are more likely to become involved in less formal, everyday types of negotiation, such as advocating for additional staff for a busy shift or helping individual staff members settle disputes over patient care. Not only are managers increasingly required to engage in negotiations in various contexts, they are also expected to serve as mediators and to work with third parties using alternative dispute resolution processes, thus creating innovative and less formal ways of resolving conflict (Grant, 1995).

Negotiation is replacing the traditional authority of the leader's coercive power (Biggerstaff & Syre, 1991) and is recognized as a key strategy in successful conflict resolution (Smeltzer, 1991; Snyder-Halpern & Cannon, 1993). Defined as "a process of communicating back and forth for the purpose of reaching a joint decision" (Fisher, Ury, & Patton, 1991, p. 32), negotiation has moved from a rarely used technique to a basic survival skill for nurse managers.

Day-to-Day Negotiation versus Collective Bargaining

Day-to-day negotiation is a process that emphasizes the need to maintain long-term interpersonal relationships. It is an ongoing process built on trust, creativity, and cooperative decision making. Going beyond the traditional win-lose conflict resolution style (i.e., competing) and even the contemporary win-win style (i.e., collaborating), day-to-day negotiation attempts to resolve conflict through communication, exchange of ideas, and commitment to a course of action.

In contrast, negotiation associated with collective bargaining has an identifiable time frame characterized by start and completion dates. Moreover, rules, often specified in labour laws and associated regulations, govern the process. In collective bargaining, the parties are essentially required to negotiate together, and even if talks break off, they know that at some point they must return to the bargaining table. In this process, the objective is to attain a settlement, and there is little emphasis on maintaining long-term relationships. Indeed, the atmosphere tends to be one that emphasizes the "we-they" component of the relationship, in contrast to the collaborative problem-solving environment associated with the daily negotiation style.

In collective bargaining, it is possible that any or all of the Thomas and Kilmann (1974) strategies might be observed during the process of negotiation. However, too much avoiding, competing, compromising, or accommodating, to the exclusion of collaboration, will not produce a result satisfactory to both parties. For example, employers usually want to avoid discussing salaries when bargaining with nurses until the rest of the contract is settled; at that time, they can no longer avoid the issue. In the end, there must be a willingness to collaborate, however brief or reluctant, if agreement is to be reached.

Why Negotiate?

As already mentioned, conflict in the Canadian health care system is inevitable. Nurse managers increasingly encounter conflict situations, and the need to resolve these situations has become a significant challenge (Collyer, 1989). Contemporary management theorists view conflict resolution as a critical process in searching for new methods or solutions to problems (Jones, 1993).

Industrial research has found that the collaborative approach to conflict resolution is most likely to achieve successful outcomes (Citron, 1981). Marriner (1982) found that nurses who used collaborating or compromising approaches were more likely to have successful conflict resolution than nurses who used avoiding or competing approaches. A collaborative approach has been associated with the search for integrated solutions and empowerment of others, two outcomes that are highly valued within successful health care organizations (Kouzes & Posner, 1987).

Negotiation in day-to-day practice is an effective interactive strategy that allows for the sharing of power and control (Barton, 1991) and emphasizes the need to maintain ongoing relationships (Fisher et al., 1991). Because it promotes an environment that emphasizes collaboration, negotiation becomes a strategy for conflict resolution. Increasingly, managers use negotiation for securing the resources needed to support the effective delivery of health services. In addition, successful use of negotiation skills may enhance nursing team spirit and benefit the organization, the patient, the nurse, and the nursing profession (Smeltzer, 1991). Kritek argued that negotiating is a central aspect of nurses' work because nurses not only provide care to patients, but they also manage the context of that work, "synchronizing the diverse components that impinge on outcomes, coordinating the people who provide nursing care, and integrating the multiple dimensions of quality patient care" (1995, p. 207). She noted that negotiation is so much a part of nursing that this skill is rarely recognized or valued.

When to Negotiate?

Negotiation is required in many facets of life (Fisher & Ury, 1983). It can be used in any situation where there is a desire to affect the behaviour of others (Cohen, 1982). Whether it is used to determine the price of a new car, a teenager's curfew, or the details of a salary increment, negotiation can help to ensure an effective outcome for all parties. In their national best-seller, *Getting to Yes*, Fisher and Ury (1983) dismissed the belief that negotiation is used only for collective bargaining, and they helped to bring daily negotiation to the forefront in conflict resolution and into the daily professional and home life of individuals and groups. Although every negotiation is different, the basic principles are the same. Once the skill is learned, the daily negotiation process becomes easier with experience (Fisher et al., 1991).

Negotiating Style

The actual "how to" of negotiation consists of two interrelated components: negotiating style and negotiating process.

A negotiating style is a method or manner of approach. The well-known, traditional negotiating style is described by Fisher and colleagues (1991) as hard positional negotiation. Using this style in collective bargaining, each party takes a position on certain issues. There is generally a contest of wills in which each side, through sheer power, attempts to change the other party's position (i.e., competing). Hard negotiation tends to strain relationships and may even destroy them during the bargaining process.

An alternative to hard positional bargaining is a style referred to as soft bargaining (Fisher et al., 1991). In this style, positions are still taken, but there is an emphasis on being friendly, trusting the other side, making offers and concessions, and avoiding confrontation. Although this style emphasizes the building and maintaining of relationships, it often falls short of providing the best outcome for all parties.

A third negotiation style (Fisher et al., 1991) is known as principled bargaining. The elements of principled bargaining are (a) separating the people from the problem, (b) establishing precise goals at the start of negotiations, (c) working together to create options that are satisfactory to both parties, and (d) negotiating successfully with opponents who are more powerful, refuse to play by the rules, or who resort to "dirty tricks." This style is based on a collaborative process that looks beyond the problem to the interests and mutual gains. The situation of concern becomes depersonalized, and energies are focused on issues rather than on defending positions. Because this style emphasizes the need to maintain ongoing relationships and promotes trust and collaborative decision making, principled bargaining is generally the style of choice for nurse managers.

Negotiating Process

Principles are the foundation for all negotiation activities, whether they involve individuals or groups. In the literature on negotiation (Fisher et al., 1991; Jones, 1993; Roberts & Krouse, 1988; Smeltzer, 1991; Snyder-Halpern & Cannon, 1993), the following key principles have been identified:

- Focus on the problem and not the individual or the individual's behaviour;
- Build rapport and maintain communication;
- Build trust;
- Explore interests and gather information;
- Maintain an open mind by searching for creative options (techniques such as brainstorming or the Delphi strategy may assist in this process);
- Focus on issues rather than taking positions; once a position is taken, there is a tendency to defend the position rather than explore the underlying reason for the problem;
- Use facts and objective standards to shape solutions;
- Be aware of your own values and motives, and attempt to understand the perspective of the other party;
- Emphasize mutual benefits rather than costs;
- Avoid blaming statements, such as "You are late, as usual"; blaming tends to result in defensive behaviour;
- Promote cooperation instead of competition.

These principles are inherent in each of the four phases of the negotiation process: analyzing, planning, negotiating, and following up.

Phase 1: Analyzing

Before initiating negotiation activities, it is imperative that the manager analyzes the context of the conflict situation or problem. A thorough analysis will enhance the possibility of achieving a successful outcome in the shortest period of time. Six major components of the analysis include the following:

1. *Delineating the underlying conflict*, problem, or issue. Separate personal characteristics and behaviour from the issues, and identify factors that contribute directly or indirectly to the problem.
2. *Identifying the individuals involved in the situation*. Who is directly involved, and who are the other stakeholders? Who is in conflict with whom? This information helps to ensure that the right people are involved in negotiation and that stakeholders are kept informed.
3. *Determining personal factors that may affect the process*. Because trust is a major component in the success of negotiation (Fisher et al., 1991), the nurse manager needs to determine the previous working relationships of the parties involved.
4. *Identifying the power distribution of both parties*. Power is of major consideration in any negotiation because an unequal balance of power may set up a win-lose outcome. Two key

goals of daily negotiation are to strive for collaborative decisions and to maintain relationships. Win-lose situations do not generally facilitate these outcomes.

5. *Collecting all necessary information.* The negotiation will be enhanced if all information is compiled in advance.

6. *Identifying the environment where negotiation will occur.* An individual's or group's power is enhanced when negotiation occurs in their territories. Selecting a neutral location will eliminate this possibility.

Identifying the power distribution (component 4) is essential to the analysis phase. One way to determine the power distribution of parties is known as Best Alternative to Negotiated Agreement (BATNA) and has been described by Fisher and colleagues (1991) and Keeney and Raiffa (1991). Simply stated, BATNA is a cut-off point—below that point, there is no agreement, and above it, there is agreement (Keeney & Raiffa, 1991). Negotiating power related to BATNA depends primarily on how attractive the option of not reaching an agreement is to each party (Fisher et al., 1991). For example, consider the situation where the nurse manager and a staff nurse are negotiating the nurse's request for a leave of absence when there is a shortage of qualified nurses. In this scenario, the nurse manager's BATNA is high and the staff member's is low. The alternative to a negotiated agreement is less critical to the nurse manager than it is to the staff member. However, the nurse manager who is aware of this unequal power distribution and who wishes to avoid a win-lose solution will need to approach this negotiation so that the outcome is not solely attributed to the manager's power.

Those who take the time to identify their own BATNA and determine the BATNA of the other side are better prepared for negotiation. In situations of low BATNA, the nurse manager should make every effort to develop greater negotiating power. Developing BATNA may be accomplished through the exploration and refinement of options other than a negotiated agreement (Fisher & Ury, 1983).

Phase 2: Planning

During the planning phase, both parties determine a proposed course of action for negotiation. There may be joint discussions to determine meeting times and to arrive at a decision regarding the general approach to negotiation. In addition, individuals plan their specific strategy and style based on the completed analysis of the problem. It would be foolhardy to attempt to negotiate an important objective without a well–thought-out plan and some ideas about the negotiating techniques to employ.

Phase 3: Negotiating

In Phase 3, the actions of negotiation are implemented. In any negotiation, some techniques enhance the process and some inhibit it. The manager needs to optimize enhancing techniques and minimize or eliminate restrictive techniques. Techniques that enhance negotiation include the following:

- *Communicating openly:* This encourages participation by all involved in the process and allows for an interchange of ideas.

- *Focusing on the task or situation:* This technique promotes communication and collaboration while minimizing power struggles; an environment of trust is likely to develop, which, in turn, facilitates more open discussion of options to resolve the problem at hand.
- *Focusing on the benefits rather than the costs:* This reinforces a sense of mutual responsibility; communication that requires people to exchange ideas reinforces the belief that the participants can attain resolutions.

Techniques that impede negotiation include the following:

- *Dividing and conquering:* Discourages group problem solving and curtails open communication.
- *Pretending differences do not exist (suppression):* Does little to promote collaborative decision making or trust.
- *Setting up competition for votes (majority rule):* Does not generally enhance successful resolution of differences.
- *Blaming the other party, or implying that the participants lack objectivity and rationality.*
- *Withdrawing before resolution is achieved.*

In addition to these techniques, there is a range of tactics inherent in the negotiating process. Tactics are behaviours that can be used individually or in combination to influence negotiation. Either party may use them. The advantages and disadvantages of each tactic need to be considered carefully before it is used so as not to compromise the negotiation process. Table 27.2 lists common negotiating tactics compiled from various sources (Cohen, 1982; Dolan, 1988; Fisher & Ury, 1983; Snyder-Halpern & Cannon, 1993).

Throughout the negotiating phase, there should be an exhaustive search for solutions or alternatives. The ultimate goal is to reach an agreement that satisfies those involved while also maintaining interpersonal relationships.

Phase 4: Following Up

Once an agreement has been reached, the final phase involves a process of evaluation to ensure the problem has been successfully resolved. The uniqueness of each negotiation process means that the follow-up needs to be tailored to the specific situation. In this phase, there is a need to ensure that the plan of action successfully addresses the problem and that no further intervention is required.

What to Negotiate?

Day-to-day negotiation can be used in any situation where two or more individuals need to reach an agreement on a particular issue. The negotiation process may be informal, such as discussing changes to uniform style, deciding the content of an orientation program, or choosing the topics of a six-month in-service program. A more formal style in daily negotiation may be required in situations such as a grievance meeting or when the nurse manager needs to attain an increased operating budget.

Table 27.2 Negotiating Tactics and Their Uses

Tactic	Rationale for Use
Silence	Encourages the other party to continue to talk, thus revealing more information
Answers that don't answer	Used to buy time or to subtly evade the need to answer a question directly
Good guy/bad guy	Used to attain a specific result; there is a staged quarrel between two members on the same side, in which one member takes a tough stand and the other appears to do a favour to the other side by intervening
Limited authority	A means of avoiding agreement by indicating that others with greater authority need to be involved in the solution
Dumb may be smart	Used to buy time or to have the other side further articulate its perspective/concerns; involves role playing and appearing not to understand the other party's point
Nibbling	A means of getting more by breaking a large request into small parts so that it is easier to sell to the other side
Package deal	Used to achieve concessions by grouping items together in a single offer
Deadlines	A way to force the other party to make a decision by a designated time
Trial balloon	Used to generate feedback by suggesting a position or idea without expressing commitment to the idea; usually prefaced with a question such as "What if...?"
Change of pace	A means to postpone the need for a decision or to give the impression of a need to escalate the process
Extreme demands	An attempt to eventually attain what is really wanted by beginning with options that are known to be extreme

Regardless of the situation, the negotiating process described in this chapter provides a guide to help maximize the chance of a collaborative outcome and maintain the integrity of relationships. Although the steps are consistent, the formality and intensity of the negotiation meeting will vary with the situation.

Mediation

Sometimes, individuals or groups in conflict are not able to settle their differences without assistance and may be helped by mediation. Mediation is a process of assisted negotiations, and it generally has the following characteristics: (a) it is a voluntary process, (b) it is non-adversarial, (c) it is facilitated by a neutral third party, (d) it requires the parties to have equal bargaining power, and (d) it is guided by a mediator who helps the parties reach a mutually satisfying agreement (Barsky, 2000).

Although there are many forms of mediation, mediation for workplace conflicts in which the parties are stuck in their polarized positions can begin on a very informal basis. The mediator must be someone whom the parties can trust, must be skilled in problem solving and interpersonal communication techniques, and must be able to remain unbiased. More importantly, the parties must perceive the mediator as being unbiased throughout the process. For this reason, the manager of the department may not the best person to mediate a dispute between subordinate individuals, and selecting an independent mediator to help the parties reach an agreement is an intelligent alternative.

Leadership Implications

Nurses in leadership and management positions can do much to promote a good working environment where staff can provide a high quality of patient care. Such workplaces are likely to minimize the stress of unresolved conflict and to provide support for appropriate approaches to managing it. Research suggests that when nurses and nurse managers use mostly avoidance and compromise to deal with conflicts, the goals of nursing may be compromised (Valentine, 2001). Thus, nurses in leadership positions need to encourage approaches that are more effective in handling conflict (e.g., collaborative approaches). Continuing education to improve the skills and confidence needed for successful conflict resolution, negotiation, and mediation would be a valuable investment of organizational resources because these skills are readily transferable to direct patient care situations.

Leaders should consider gender differences between men and women in their approaches to conflict resolution and negotiation. Valentine (2001) suggested that nurses tend to adopt passive roles when faced with conflict because most nurses are female, and, therefore, their early childhood socialization and professional education emphasized caring for others. Men generally engage in confrontational approaches to conflict, possibly because of their socialization and society's expectations. Differences in the approach to negotiating have also been observed between men and women. According to Wyatt (1999), women negotiate for what is fair, and men tend to be more competitive and play to win. Given that conflict is a common occurrence in nurses' workplaces, nurses need to be supported and encouraged to develop conflict resolution skills. Their concerns about patient care and their goals for nursing require constructive approaches to workplace conflicts.

Summary

- Conflict is inevitable in all health care organizations.
- Knowledge of the five conflict handling strategies (competing, compromising, avoiding, collaborating, and accommodating) and their outcomes is essential to produce positive outcomes of conflict episodes.
- The modes of handling conflict most frequently used by nurse managers are compromising and avoiding, and the mode most frequently used by staff nurses is avoiding.
- Negotiating has become a basic survival skill for contemporary nurses and health care managers.
- Negotiating is an interactive skill for resolving conflict or making joint decisions. It can be used in any setting, with individuals or groups, and as an approach to personal or professional problem solving.
- The negotiation process has four phases (analyzing, planning, negotiating, and following up) and involves principles, strategies, and tactics.
- Nurse managers prefer principled bargaining because it emphasizes maintenance of relationships, promotion of trust, and collaborative decision making.
- Men and women tend to differ in their approaches to conflict resolution and negotiation.

Applying the Knowledge in this Chapter

Case Study

For several months, Jocelyn Brown, the nurse manager responsible for children's services in a community hospital, has been aware of tensions between the two designated team leaders of the inpatient pediatric unit. These two registered nurses, Michelle Fontaine and Cheryl Booker, are both competent and have equal seniority on this unit. However, they differ in their leadership styles and in their attitudes towards the role of parents in the care of their own children. They rarely work on the same shifts as team leaders, and, therefore, their direct contact with each other is restricted to the 15-minute period when the shifts change.

Their different styles of leadership and their attitudes regarding parents are confusing for the staff and upsetting for parents. For example, Michelle insists on only two visitors at a time for each child, and she restricts what mothers may do for their infants and toddlers. Cheryl is more relaxed about the role of parents: she allows extended families into the children's rooms and encourages parents to be involved in all aspects of their children's care. Michelle monitors the unit clerk very closely, whereas Cheryl is content to delegate all clerical duties with little supervision. As a result, directives are often given to staff on one shift and then counteracted on the next shift. The tension between the two team leaders is generally tolerated by the medical staff, although several have voiced their preference for one or the other.

Michelle and Cheryl tend to undermine each other's decisions about nursing care in their progress reports and interactions with attending physicians. Within the last week, Jocelyn has had a tearful unit clerk in her office threatening to resign and two sets of parents complaining about their children's care. Jocelyn has spoken to both team leaders about their responsibility to work together cooperatively. However, she now realizes that it is time to take a different approach to this ongoing conflict.

1. What types of conflict are evident in this case, and what approach or approaches has Jocelyn taken in addressing the problem?

2. What appears to be the problem, and what goals should Jocelyn set for herself in dealing with the problem?

3. Draw up a plan for Jocelyn's intervention, and discuss the approaches most likely to be effective in managing this conflict.

4. Recognizing that there will be negotiations between the parties, what strategies would you recommend to Jocelyn? Who should be involved in the negotiations?

5. Are there any organizational or administrative changes that Jocelyn might consider as a means of improving the quality of the working environment on this unit?

Resources

evolve Internet Resources

Canadian Healthcare Association (CHA):

www.cha.ca/documents/joint.htm
Here you can find the joint statement issued by the Boards of Directors of the Canadian Healthcare Association, Canadian Medical Association, Canadian Nurses Association, and Catholic Health Association of Canada on preventing and resolving ethical conflicts involving health care providers and persons receiving care.

Conflict Management Group:

www.cmgroup.org/home.html
Conflict Resolution Network:

www.crnetwork.ca/

References

Barsky, A.E. (2000). *Conflict resolution for the helping professions*. Scarborough, ON: Brooks/Cole, Thomson Learning.

Barton, A. (1991). Conflict resolution by nurse managers. *Nursing Management, 22*(5), 83-84, 86.

Biggerstaff, R.P., & Syre, T.R. (1991). The dynamics of hospital leadership. *Hospital Topics, 69*(1), 36–39.

Blake, R., & Mouton, J. (1964). *The managerial grid*. Houston, TX: Gulf Publications.

Burke, R. (1970, April). Methods of managing superior-subordinate conflict: Their effectiveness and consequences. *Canadian Journal of Behavioural Science, 2,* 124–135.

Citron, D. (1981). Facing up to conflict. *Nursing Life, 1*(1), 47–49.

Cohen, H. (1982). *You can negotiate anything*. New York: Bantam Books.

Collyer, M.E. (1989). Resolving conflicts: Leadership style sets the strategy. *Nursing Management, 20*(9), 77–80.

Coser, L. (1956). *The functions of social conflict*. New York: Free Press.

Dolan, J. (1988). *Negotiating skills for attorneys: Workbook*. Boulder, CO: Career Track.

Dunnette, M.D., & Hiugh, L.M. (1992). *Handbook of Industrial and Organizational Psychology* (2nd ed., Vol. 3, p. 658). Palo Alto, CA: Consulting Psychologists Press, Inc.

Etzioni, A. (1961). *A comparative analysis of complex organizations*. New York: Free Press.

Fayol, H. (1949). *General and industrial management*. London: Sir Isaac Pitman.

Fisher, R., & Ury, W. (1983). *Getting to yes: Negotiating agreement without giving in*. New York: Penguin Books.

Fisher, R., Ury, W., & Patton, B. (1991). *Getting to yes: Negotiating agreement without giving in* (2nd ed.). New York: Penguin Books.

Follett, M. (1940). Constructive conflict. In H. Metcalf & L. Urwick (Eds.), *Dynamic administration: The collected papers of Mary Follett Parker* (pp. 30–49). New York: Harper. (Original work published 1926)

Gaudine, A.P., & Beaton, M.R. (2002). Employed to go against one's values: Nurse managers' accounts of ethical conflict with their organizations. *Canadian Journal of Nursing Research, 34*(2), 17–34.

Grant, A. (1995). Alternative dispute resolution. *Canadian Nurse, 91*(7), 53–54.

Hightower, T. (1986). Subordinate choice of conflict handling modes. *Nursing Administration Quarterly, 11*(1), 29–34.

Huber, D. (1996). *Leadership and nursing care management*. Philadelphia: W.B. Saunders.

Johnson, M. (1994). Conflict and nursing professionalization. In J. McCloskey & H. Grace (Eds.), *Current issues in nursing* (pp. 643–649). St. Louis, MO: Mosby.

Jones, K. (1993). Confrontation: Methods and skills. *Nursing Management, 24*(5), 68–70.

Keeney, R.L., & Raiffa, H. (1991). Structuring and analysing values for multiple-issue negotiation. In H.P. Young (Ed.), *Negotiation analysis* (pp. 131–152). Ann Arbor, MI: University of Michigan Press.

Kouzes, J.M., & Posner, B.Z. (1987). *The leadership challenge*. San Francisco: Jossey-Bass.

Kritek, P.B. (1995). Nursing: Negotiating at an uneven table. In L.J. Marcus (Ed.), *Renegotiating health care: Resolving conflict to build collaboration*. San Francisco: Jossey-Bass.

Lewin, K. (1948). *Field theory in social science*. New York: Harper and Bros.

Marriner, A. (1982). Comparing strategies and their use managing conflict. *Nursing Management, 13*(6), 29–31.

Rahim, A. (1986). *Managing conflict in organizations*. New York: Praeger.

Rahim, A., & Bonoma, T. (1979). Managing organizational conflict: A model for diagnosis and intervention. *Psychological Reports, 44,* 1323–1344.

Roberts, S.J., & Krouse, H.J. (1988). Enhancing self care through active negotiation. *Nurse Practitioner: American Journal of Primary Health Care, 13*(8), 44–52.

Saner, R. (2000). *The expert negotiator: Strategy, tactics, motivation, behaviour, leadership.* The Hague, The Netherlands: Kluwer Law International.

Smeltzer, C.H. (1991). The art of negotiation: An everyday experience. *Journal of Nursing Administration, 21*(7/8), 26–30.

Snyder-Halpern, R., & Cannon, M.E. (1993). A framework for the development of nurse manager negotiation skills. *Journal of Nursing Staff Development, 9*(1), 14–19.

Thomas, K. (1976). Conflict and conflict management. In M. Dunnette (Ed.), *Handbook of organizational psychology* (pp. 889–935). Chicago: Rand McNally College Publishing.

Thomas, K. (1977, July). Toward multi-dimensional values in teaching: The example of conflict. *Academy of Management Review, 22,* 142–149.

Thomas, K. (1992). Conflict and negotiation processes in organizations. In M.D. Dunnette & L.M. Hough (Eds.), *Handbook of industrial and organizational psychology* (pp. 651–717). Palo Alto, CA: Consulting Psychologists Press.

Thomas, K., & Kilmann, R. (1974). *Thomas-Kilmann conflict mode instrument*. Tuxedo, NY: XICOM.

Valentine, P.E.B. (2001). A gender perspective on conflict management strategies of nurses. *Journal of Nursing Scholarship, 33*(1), 69–74.

Weber, M. (1946). *From Max Weber: Essays in sociology*. (H. Gerth & C. Wright Mills, Eds. & Trans.). New York: Oxford University Press.

Wyatt, D. (1999). Negotiating strategies for men and women. *Nursing Management, 30*(1), 22–26.

Judith M. Hibberd

Learning Objectives

In this chapter, you will learn:

- Major components of the system in which union-management relations operate, including collective bargaining

- Rights and obligations of employers and employees

- Typical terms and conditions of employment contained in a collective agreement

- The grievance procedure

- Steps managers may take to discipline an employee

- Issues related to union-management relations, including bumping and professional responsibility committees

- Ways of promoting effective employment relations

Most non-managerial health care workers in Canada belong to unions; therefore, administration of collective agreements is a key responsibility of managers. In a typical patient care area, a manager may administer several union contracts because labour board rules often require that health care workers belong to pre-designated categories for collective bargaining purposes. As a result, several unions may be operating independently in a hospital or community agency.

Effective administration of union contracts requires a basic understanding of the labour relations system and how collective agreements are reached. Managers should also understand the goals and objectives of unions, the nature of the employment relations, and the procedures for resolving union-management conflicts, especially grievance and disciplinary procedures. The purpose of this chapter, then, is to address these issues. With knowledge of these topics, managers should be able to develop appropriate skills and attitudes needed to establish constructive relations with union representatives.

Because nurses, who are local union representatives, often attend workshops and labour schools sponsored by their unions, managers need to be just as well informed in the area of labour relations so that they may deal intelligently with union officials. Although there is a tendency to think of nurses' unions as somehow different from traditional blue-collar unions, the main difference is that nurses are apt to bring a broader range of issues to the bargaining table, including problems that focus on patient care. Nurses who are members of unions should understand that there is a legal framework governing relations between unions and employers, and that precedent and past practices play an important role in shaping the outcomes of disputes between their unions and employers. As unions are self-governing democratic organizations, nurses should inform themselves of how their union represents them and how decisions are made, even if they choose not to take an active role in the union.

Framework for Understanding Collective Bargaining by Nurses

A collective agreement is a contract of employment. To understand the processes by which such a contract is reached, nurse managers need basic knowledge of the industrial relations system. Scholars frequently view the field of industrial relations from a systems perspective (e.g., Anderson, Gunderson, & Ponak, 1989; Craig, 1996). The Canadian industrial relations system is decentralized, somewhat like the health care system, in that responsibility for employment relations rests with the provinces. Although the federal government has enacted the *Canada Labour Code* to regulate and set standards for its own employees and interprovincial enterprises such as shipping, banks, and railways, each province establishes its own labour legislation. Consequently, there are both federal and provincial labour relations systems in the country, which means that procedures relative to collective bargaining tend to vary from province to province and among the territories. This explains why nurses are entitled to strike in some provinces but not in others.

Environmental factors, such as the state of the economy and the legal system, can influence the goals of the parties in collective bargaining. For example, during a recession, unions are more likely to give priority to job security demands than to wage demands, and employers may try to secure wage concessions from unions, as Alberta's nurses discovered in 1988 (Hibberd, 1992). Although environmental factors vary from province to province, there are common elements in their industrial relations systems. Figure 28.1 shows components of these systems that directly or indirectly influence nurses' collective bargaining.

In the model shown in Figure 28.1, the principal participants in collective bargaining are the employers, their organizations, nurses, and the nurses' unions. However, governments play a major part in labour relations in the health field; not only do they fund hospitals and community health care agencies, they also make the rules governing collective bargaining (i.e., the labour laws) and are responsible for protecting the public interest. Third parties include such

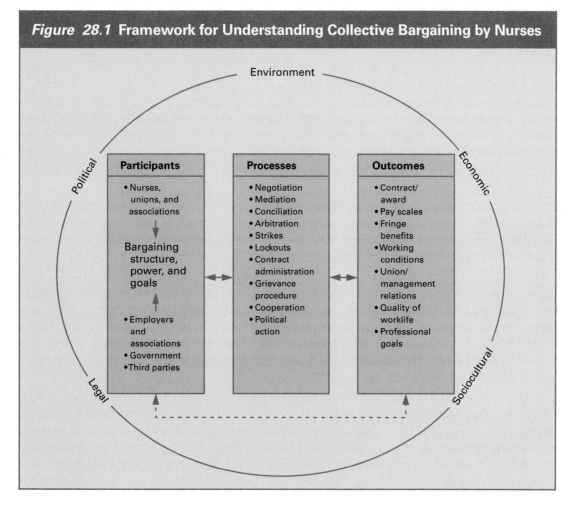

Figure 28.1 Framework for Understanding Collective Bargaining by Nurses

people as conciliators, arbitrators, and lawyers called in to assist the main parties with processes. All parties at the collective bargaining table have goals and special interests, and each party draws on its own power resources to influence the process and outcomes.

The principal participants pursue their goals through a series of processes in which conflict, cooperation, and compromise are anticipated. Figure 28.1 includes various processes and procedures that may be employed in reaching a collective agreement, such as negotiation, mediation, arbitration, strikes, lockouts, and the grievance procedure, to name a few. In the vast majority of cases, collective bargaining results in an agreement without conflict (Craig, 1996), and the main outcome of these procedures is an employment contract, whether negotiated with or without third-party assistance or imposed by an arbitrator.

In addition to this contract between the parties with all its terms and conditions of employment, there are consequences to continuing relations between the union and employer. A long and bitter strike, for example, may have a lingering and negative impact on relations in the workplace and can influence the goals that the parties pursue at the next round of bargaining. Because collective bargaining recurs at periodic intervals, this framework is a dynamic system in which component parts influence each other on a continuing basis. (Systems theory is discussed more fully in Chapter 8.)

Union-Management Relations

The nature of relations between employers and employees has been defined historically by past practices, common law, and labour statutes. Over the years, total employer domination over employees has been replaced with increasingly progressive laws protecting the rights of employees. All provinces have passed employment standards acts, which establish minimum terms and conditions of work for all employees, and labour relations acts, which govern union-management relations (Morris, 1991). Labour relations boards (or, in the case of Quebec, labour courts), administer labour statutes. The role of labour relations boards (and Quebec's labour courts) is to oversee certification procedures, interpret the law, make decisions, and provide third-party assistance in disputes between the parties. The law further protects employees' rights in the areas of occupational health and safety, human rights, pay equity, workers' compensation, unemployment insurance, and tax and pension provisions.

Union-management relations are formalized through the process of certification. The union applies to the labour relations board for the exclusive right to represent a defined group of employees. The union must file its constitution and bylaws, together with evidence that it represents a majority of a group of employees. Employers are entitled to submit contrary evidence to the labour boards, but they are prohibited from resisting legitimate unionizing activities. Once certified, the union notifies the employer of its intention to negotiate terms and conditions of employment, and the employer must then recognize the collective bargaining relationship.

Successful union-management relations will depend a great deal upon how the parties view each other. If they operate from a conflict viewpoint, then the collective agreement will be perceived as merely a temporary "peace treaty" (Giles & Jain, 1989). A more enlightened perspective is to recognize collective bargaining as "a joint decision-making process for determining terms and conditions of employment and spelling them out in collective agreements. It is grounded on a dependence or symbiotic relationship between employees and employers" (Fisher

& Williams, 1989, p. 185). Such a definition implies a legitimate role for unions in framing the rules by which the parties relate to each other, and it is more in keeping with the consultative approach to labour relations taken by professional employees such as nurses and teachers.

Terms and Conditions of Employment

Collective agreements in the health care field are becoming more complex. Nevertheless, some standard provisions are common to most agreements, and these are listed in Box 28.1. The contract usually begins with a preamble in which the parties recognize each other and state their intention to work together for the common purpose of providing health care services. Each category of worker covered by the agreement is then defined. In many jurisdictions, first-level nurse managers may be excluded from the bargaining unit (i.e., they are considered out-of-scope) by virtue of their managerial responsibilities. Where nurse managers are in-scope, they may face conflicts of interest, as in the case of a grievance over the application of disciplinary measures. Unions have policies to deal with such situations that generally favour the grievor, although there may be informal discussions between the union and nurse manager about the case.

It is important to keep in mind that the parties jointly agree to the provisions in the contract—albeit reluctantly in some cases and often in emotion-laden, marathon bargaining sessions. Nevertheless, if parties have ratified the agreement, they have a duty to honour it until such time that the contract is renegotiated.

Box 28.1

Standard Provisions of Nurses' Collective Agreements
1. Recognition of the parties and purpose of agreement
2. Definitions: nursing personnel covered by agreement
3. Union security: deduction of union dues or the Rand Formula*
4. Management rights
5. Grievance procedure
6. Seniority, promotion, layoff, and recall
7. Hours of work, shift schedules, holidays, vacations
8. Fringe benefits: health care benefits, sick leave
9. Compensation and premium payments
10. Committees: professional responsibility, occupational health and safety
11. Term of agreement: expiry date of contract
12. Appendices: letters of understanding, salary schedules

*A contractual arrangement in which the employer makes a payroll deduction of an amount equal to union dues from each member of the bargaining unit, whether or not the employee is a member of the union.

Management Rights–Implied and Expressed

Historically, employers have gone to great lengths to protect their common law prerogatives, and almost all collective agreements contain a management rights clause. The clause (or clauses) may take the form of a broad general statement or a detailed list of specific rights (Cohen, 1989); in either case, the nurse manager must be familiar with these express management rights. There is considerable debate in the labour relations literature on management rights. Unions argue that once parties enter a union-management relationship, unilateral discretion by the employer ceases and all decisions become negotiable. On the other hand, employers prefer a residual rights theory "based on management's assertion that all the rights and privileges that employers exercised before unionization must be considered to be reserved to them afterwards except for those specifically limited by the collective agreement" (Giles & Jain, 1989, p. 323).

Much of what goes on in the workplace, however, is not governed by union contracts because, as Giles and Jain (1989) stated, "collective agreements cannot possibly regulate even a small proportion of the issues, tensions, and relationships that spring from the social and physical setting[s]" (p. 340). Therefore, managers need to be aware of the implied rights and duties derived from common law and past employment practices; these underlie all employment contracts, whether or not expressed in written contracts (McPhillips & England, 1989). Implied rights and duties, some of which are outlined in Table 28.1, serve as a guide to management practices when the collective agreement is silent on an issue, and they also influence arbitrators' decisions when interpreting a collective agreement or judging the merits of a grievance.

Employment relations are fiduciary; in other words, they are based on good faith and trust (McPhillips & England, 1989). While the employer retains the right to run the health care agency, the employee has an obligation to cooperate with the employer. Any failure to fulfill these rights and responsibilities constitutes a breach of the employment contract.

Conflict between unions and management during the term of the collective agreement, whether or not over the question of management rights, may be resolved informally. Disputes that are more serious may need to be formally resolved through the grievance procedure. Strikes

Table 28.1 Implied Employment Rights and Duties	
Employer	**Employee**
• Provides work and pays compensation for labour • Responsible for safe workplace • Responsible for employees' conduct at work • Gives reasonable notice of termination in absence of just cause	• Cooperates with employer • Exercises reasonable skill and care • Obeys lawful directives • Is not excessively absent from work • Behaves in good faith and does not disseminate confidential information

Source: Adapted from The Contract of Employment at Common Law, by H.J. Glasbeek. In *Union Management Relations in Canada* (pp. 47–77), edited by J. Anderson and M. Gunderson, 1982. Don Mills, ON: Addison-Wesley.

and lockouts are dispute resolution processes (see Figure 28.1), but in Canada, they are not allowed during the term of the collective agreement (Sethi & MacNeil, 1989); for this reason, collective agreements must contain a grievance procedure.

Grievance Procedure

A grievance is not only an allegation that one or more provisions of an agreement have been violated, it is also a claim for redress (Gandz & Whitehead, 1989). There are three types of grievances: individual, group, and policy. The type of grievance determines the level at which it can be initiated in the grievance procedure. A policy grievance affecting the union itself, for example, is usually filed directly with the chief executive officer of the agency, whereas an individual or group grievance must first be discussed with immediate supervisors. In Canada, the subject of a grievance is confined to the contents of the collective agreement; in other words, there must be at least one clause in the union contract that relates to the complaint.

Although it is almost impossible to know the entire contract in detail, nurse managers must be thoroughly familiar with the grievance procedure. They must also know the scope of their authority in handling grievances; for example, they need to know at what stage human resources personnel are to become involved in the process. A typical grievance procedure is presented in Table 28.2.

Not much research exists on the incidence and pattern of nurses' union grievances. Research in other fields suggests that grievances may serve many functions: (a) they are a means by which unions may communicate with employers, (b) they permit one of the parties to challenge the rights or actions of the other party, (c) they may be a form of continuous bargaining (i.e., a way of forcing a concession that could not be obtained through collective bargaining), or (d) they may be politically motivated by self-serving individuals or groups, either within the union or managerial ranks (Gandz, 1982).

Arbitrators have recognized the powerlessness and vulnerability of individuals who choose to challenge an employer's authority, and they uphold the principle of natural justice underlying the grievance procedure. A grievance allows a union member to appeal a manager's negative decision to increasingly higher levels of administrative authority and ultimately to an independent arbitrator or arbitration board, without fear of punishment or dismissal. Even with the protection that a collective agreement affords, a nurse may feel too intimidated to complain. This is why unions have fought for the right to accompany their members throughout the grievance procedure and to receive copies of all written communications about grievances.

The first-level manager plays a critical role in the first step of the grievance procedure. This step is an informal discussion during which the nurse (or grievor) and manager determine if a problem exists. This is where the facts of the situation are carefully and thoroughly investigated, where consultation is sought, and, ideally, where the problem is solved. If the decision is well founded at this point, the nurse manager can expect to be supported by senior administrators should the grievance advance through subsequent steps. To avoid the demoralizing experience of having a decision overturned at a more senior level of the organization, the manager should consult the human resources department and the next level of management before dismissing or allowing a grievance. Senior administrators bring a broader perspective to bear on the

Table 28.2 A Typical Grievance Procedure	
Complaint	A nurse discusses a complaint or concern informally with the immediate supervisor, and the complaint is satisfied or dismissed within seven working days.
Step 1	The complaint becomes a grievance and is written on the union's grievance form, specifying (a) the nature of the grievance, (b) the articles in the collective agreement allegedly violated, and (c) the remedy sought. It is then submitted to the first-level manager within seven working days of the initial discussion. A meeting may be held with the grievor, union representative, and manager. The nurse manager delivers a response in writing to the nurse within seven working days and sends a copy to the union.
Step 2	If the grievance has not been settled, it may be submitted in writing to the department head within seven working days. A meeting of all parties may be convened to discuss the grievance. The director's decision is communicated in writing to the grievor (copy to the union) within seven working days.
Step 3	If the grievance has not been settled, it may be submitted in writing to the chief executive officer within seven working days. A meeting of all parties may be convened. The chief executive officer's decision is communicated in writing to the grievor (copy to the union) within seven working days.
Step 4	If the grievance is not settled, either party may consider whether to proceed to arbitration or to abandon the grievance. The decision to proceed to arbitration is communicated in writing to the other party, together with the name of a nominee to the arbitration board, within seven working days.
Arbitration	The final, binding decision is made.

procedure and may have handled similar grievances in the past. Nevertheless, what seems like a clear-cut case to unions and employers may be seen in a totally different light by an arbitration board. Indeed, it is often difficult to predict the outcome of arbitration.

Grievance Arbitration

At step four of the grievance procedure (see Table 28.2), either party may refer the dispute to an external arbitration board. Grievance arbitration should not be confused with interest arbitration, which is used to settle disputes arising out of collective bargaining. The two procedures are similar, but they deal with different types of disputes. Grievance arbitration deals with disputes arising out of the interpretation, application, or alleged violation of the terms of an existing collective agreement.

According to Gandz and Whitehead (1989), fewer than 2% of written grievances proceed to arbitration, so nurse managers rarely take part in arbitration proceedings. However, if a grievance does go to arbitration, union and management each select a nominee to serve on the arbitration board. The nominees jointly select the chair, but if they cannot agree on this person, the provincial minister of labour will appoint the arbitrator. In some cases, the board consists of a sole arbitrator. A hearing is held, at which the parties may be represented by legal counsel. Witnesses may be called and cross-examined, and the parties formally present their arguments (Gandz & Whitehead, 1989).

Arbitration is time-consuming and expensive; the parties are responsible for the expenses of their respective nominees and witnesses, and they share the arbitrator's fee. By the time a grievance goes to arbitration, the parties are usually entrenched in their opposing positions and determined to win the case. The arbitration board's decision is final and binding on the parties, and it can only be appealed under specific circumstances, such as if the arbitrator exceeds his or her jurisdiction or makes an error of law (Craig, 1996).

Appearing at an arbitration hearing is much like attending court, except that rules of evidence and procedure are not as rigorous and the hearing may be held in a less formal setting than a law court. In preparation for serving as a witness for management, the manager and other witnesses must be well briefed on their roles at the arbitration hearing, preferably at a meeting with the lawyer or person presenting the case. Because of the potential for every grievance to become an arbitration case, managers must keep meticulous notes on each phase of the grievance process, noting who attended each meeting, what main points were discussed, what decisions were made, and the underlying reasons for allowing or disallowing the grievance. Moreover, care must be taken with the content and language used in all written communications to the grievor because these will undoubtedly be filed as exhibits at the arbitration hearing. Even past performance appraisals may be submitted as an exhibit if the grievance involves the discipline of a nurse.

Progressive Discipline

Occasionally, disciplining a staff member is necessary, and arbitrators in the past have expected employers to apply discipline in a progressive manner (Pearlman, 1991). One might well ask, as Eden (1992) did, whether applying negative sanctions is an appropriate corporate response to employee misconduct in light of contemporary trends in human resource management. The objective of progressive discipline should be to correct behaviour, not to punish it (Cannon, 1980). Nevertheless, if the employee fails to respond to repeated warnings, the ultimate penalty could be dismissal. A typical disciplinary procedure appears in Table 28.3.

Discipline should be used to correct patterns of unsatisfactory behaviour, not to deal with occasional errors or misjudgments. On the other hand, gross misconduct (e.g., physical abuse of a patient) requires immediate suspension so that an investigation can take place. Where a staff member has demonstrated unsatisfactory behaviour in more than one area

Table 28.3 Progressive Discipline	
Step 1	Informal discussion. A private meeting is held between the nurse manager and nurse to identify the problem, discuss it, and coach or counsel the nurse.
Step 2	Verbal warning. Assuming no improvement in behaviour, another meeting is held between the nurse manager and nurse. Three points are made: (a) the problem is identified and the desired change in behaviour stated, (b) a time limit is set during which improvement is to occur, and (c) the consequences of failure to improve are stated. The nurse must also understand that he or she has received a verbal warning.
Step 3	Written warning. At least 24 hours' notice of a meeting is given to the nurse, who may be accompanied by a union representative. Discussion of the problem follows, with reference to previous verbal warnings. A letter is given to the nurse containing the same three points outlined in Step 2. Copies are filed in the employee's personnel record and with the union.
Step 4	Suspension. The procedures in Step 3 are repeated, but the letter states the length of the suspension and whether it is to be with or without pay. The nurse must understand that the ultimate consequence of not responding to discipline in the specified amount of time will be dismissal. Copies are filed in the employee's personnel record and with the union.
Step 5	Dismissal. A final meeting is held, which includes representatives from the human resources department and the union. The letter terminating the nurse's employment contains a final pay cheque and relevant severance papers. Copies of the letter are filed in the employee's personnel record and with the union.

Note: The level at which discipline begins will depend upon the severity of the employee's misconduct or problem and the situation. Steps in the procedure may be repeated. A union representative may be present at each step of the procedure.

(e.g., absenteeism and failure to chart narcotic drugs), it would be necessary to apply discipline progressively to both problems. Moreover, a nurse manager has discretion to repeat a step or to begin the procedure again if there has been a significant time lapse since an earlier disciplinary step. Whatever the situation, the problem must be communicated to the staff member immediately and in private, never in hallways or within hearing distance of patients or other staff. Discipline that is loudly applied in public is humiliating for the employee and unprofessional on the part of the manager. It also undermines its objective, namely, to effect a positive change in behaviour.

At every step of the disciplinary procedure, the manager should be prepared for a grievance. The grievance procedure and the disciplinary procedure are similar processes in which increasing pressure is placed on the other party to bring about a change in thinking or behaviour. The disciplinary procedure, however, is the prerogative of management and is not usually spelled out in detail in the collective agreement. Even so, should the case go to arbitration, the employer will be required to show that there was sufficient cause to discipline the nurse, that the nurse understood the problem and was given opportunities and assistance to improve his or her performance, that there were no extenuating circumstances, and that the discipline was not arbitrary or unreasonable.

As in the grievance procedure, careful documentation is absolutely essential. All evidence that led to the discipline and relevant details of discussions and interviews must be recorded in the employee's file. Such data will likely be used at arbitration. Unions often negotiate time periods beyond which such documentation must be purged from the employee's file.

Few managers look forward to using disciplinary measures, but if handled thoughtfully, objectively, and in a timely manner, both parties should emerge with their self-respect intact and with respect for each other.

Insubordination

As shown in Table 28.1, an implied duty of employees, whether unionized or not, is to cooperate with lawful directives of the employer. Willful refusal to obey a lawful order is known as *insubordination*; employers consider insubordination a serious breach of the employment contract and just cause for discipline. Effective management is impossible if the nursing staff no longer respect legitimate orders from the person in charge of a unit.

To be successful in disciplining a person for insubordination, a nurse manager has to prove that

- a valid order was given to the employee,
- the order was clearly communicated by a person having the authority to direct the employee, and
- the employee failed to comply with the order (Mrazek & Tumbach, 1990).

It is important to note that failing to comply with physicians' orders relative to patient care is not considered insubordination. Nurses are obligated under professional practice acts to question and, if necessary, refuse to carry out a physician's order that they know to be erroneous and harmful to patients. Such disputes between professional colleagues fall outside the meaning and definition of insubordination because nurses do not normally report to physicians but to someone in a line position in the formal structure of the health agency. Insubordination is failing to comply with orders given by an immediate supervisor, such as a nurse manager (as the employer's designate), including patient care assignments that an individual nurse might consider intolerable and unsafe.

Whether or not a nurse can refuse a legitimate order to care for patients is a complex question (Creighton, 1986; Huerta & Oddi, 1992; Northrop, 1987; Wahn, 1979), and nurse managers need to be clear where they stand in such situations. More importantly, a nurse manager must decide if the refusal to obey is serious enough to be defined as insubordination. For example, a nurse may try to avoid working with a particularly difficult client or may simply forget to carry out a delegated task, neither of which really constitutes insubordination. A nurse manager's most reasonable response would be to try to negotiate an acceptable compromise with the unwilling nurse, but the problems with this response are that it can set a precedent and other staff members may resent manipulative employees. The nurse manager must be sure of the facts before alleging insubordination.

Nurses need to know what their rights are in relation to a supervisor's order with which they seriously disagree. An employee is entitled to refuse a supervisor's order when compliance (a) constitutes an illegal act, (b) endangers the health or safety of the employee or co-workers, or (c) causes irreparable damage to the interest of other employees (Mrazek & Tumbach, 1990), for instance, refusing to grant leave of absence to a union representative resulting in the loss of a union member's job at grievance arbitration. Refusing a supervisor's orders under one of these circumstances does not mean that the employee would necessarily escape discipline; rather, it means that arbitrators likely would rule in favour of the employee. However, the employee who invokes any of these exceptional circumstances bears the onus of proving the case to the arbitrator; therefore, when refusing the order, the employee must explain the reason for refusal. Because most employees would not be able to articulate their rights and obligations in a case of insubordination, the nurse manager, before administering discipline, must explain the seriousness of refusing to comply with a legitimate order and help staff articulate their reasons for refusing.

Nurses' refusal to undertake patient care assignments has created some interesting jurisprudence. In the Mount Sinai case, in which three nurses were disciplined for refusing to take an additional patient into an intensive care unit (Sklar, 1979a, 1979b), arbitrators found the discipline to be justified because—notwithstanding the professional judgment and legal liability of the nurses relative to patient safety—the health and safety exemption listed above applies only to employees and co-workers, not to patients. In other words, "heavy or excessive patient workloads alone cannot be used as a basis for refusal to carry out an assignment" (Mrazek & Tumbach, 1990, p. 19) because the employer (including the nurse manager) is vicariously liable for any injuries to patients arising out of a nurse's inability or failure to provide safe care to patients. However, many nurses' collective agreements now contain mechanisms for addressing disputes that arise from heavy workloads, staffing issues, and patient care safety. Nevertheless, employees should generally observe the principle of obey now, grieve later, which reflects the duty of the employee to cooperate with the employer.

Of course, it does not solve the dilemma of the nurse who wishes to refuse a patient assignment on moral and ethical grounds. Such situations can be avoided in part by frank discussions with nurses at the time they are hired, but there appears to be little to protect the conscientious objector (see Creighton, 1986; *Peterborough Civic Hospital,* 1982). Similarly, nurses who whistle-blow are largely unprotected at the present time, but there seems to be some movement toward policy changes in this area (Canadian Nurses Association, 1999; Fiesta, 1990; McKenna, 1989). Currently, nurses who expose unlawful or hazardous working conditions to the media risk being disciplined by their employer. Nevertheless, when all internal avenues of protest have been exhausted, professional employees have a duty to their clients to ensure that their safety and interests are properly served. Under such circumstances, the first step would be to consult the professional nurses' association.

Developing Constructive Union-Management Relations

First-level managers, whether or not they are nurses, play key roles in promoting good relations between union and management. Although they may regard the collective agreement as limiting their freedom to make decisions and introduce change, the existence of a union contract requires managers to be fair and impartial when supervising employees. Dealing with staff in an equitable manner is essential if teamwork and cooperation are to flourish in the work setting. The contract provides a clear set of rules guiding decisions about such issues as allocation of unpopular shifts and vacation times. If properly administered, the collective agreement ensures standard treatment of staff throughout the health care agency, not solely on a particular unit. If any clause in the collective agreement is unclear or unworkable, it may become the subject of a grievance in order to obtain clarification. Alternatively, at the next round of collective bargaining, the employer can propose new wording for the clause. Collective agreements eventually expire, and although terms and conditions continue until a new contract is signed, this open period allows both parties to negotiate improvements to the contract.

Effective Management

Employment relations are more likely to be cooperative when there is effective management. On the whole, unions have little respect for ineffective managers and can readily find ways to create a hostile climate on a unit. For example, they might challenge all management decisions (whether related to the contract or not), file grievances, spend inordinate amounts of time on complaints, or file "professional responsibility forms." Under such circumstances, creating positive relations with a union representative is challenging, especially if that person has leadership aspirations and is intent upon demonstrating militancy and developing a power base within the union. Most nurses promoted to a management position have at one time been members of unions, so they are likely to understand the goals, values, beliefs, and internal organization of the nurses' union. An open-minded attitude toward unions will be a distinct advantage when working with union representatives, as will a willingness to listen to problems, investigate them, and negotiate solutions.

Collective agreements for nurses have become so complex that solving problems arising from their interpretation and administration should not be attempted without assistance. Health care agencies have access to labour relations specialists, whether on site in the human resources department, externally from the health care agency's legal firm, or from the provincial regional health authorities' association. Managers need to find out what the scope of their authority is with respect to contract administration and the grievance procedure in their own agency. Most health care agencies have policies about reporting complaints and potential grievances, so it is important for managers to be aware of such internal guidelines.

Role of Union Representatives

Program areas or patient care units typically have a local shop steward, or union representative. Indeed, representing colleagues as a union representative is an opportunity for a nurse to learn and exercise leadership skills. Many nurses have gone on to lifelong careers as union leaders. Union representatives within health agencies may be elected, but usually they volunteer for these unpaid jobs within the union organization. They work closely with the union's employment relations officers and leaders. Their role includes ensuring that rights of union members are enforced, being available to union members during disputes, attending grievance or disciplinary meetings, helping to write out grievances, preparing cases for arbitration, and collecting information for the union (American Nurses Association, 1985). Requests by the local union representative to leave the clinical area during a workday must not be unreasonably denied; nevertheless, such requests are negotiable, and the needs of patients and clients remain the prime factor in granting permission to leave a clinical area.

There is great variability in the degree to which union representatives pursue their roles and responsibilities. Some are aggressive in their approach to their duties, while others seem to be reluctant volunteers with little aptitude or enthusiasm for their roles. Nevertheless, unions have a duty to provide fair representation, that is, to represent all members of the bargaining unit fairly and without discrimination (Craig, 1996). Human rights legislation applies equally to employers and unions. In all but the most hostile cases, managers and union representatives are able to work out a mutually respectful and constructive relationship.

Professional Responsibility Committees

In the late 1970s, nurses began to demand ways and means of discussing their concerns about patient care with employers. After two major strikes in Alberta, nurses there obtained a clause in their collective agreement entitled "Professional Responsibility Committees" (PRCs). These committees meet regularly and are made up of equal numbers of managers and nurses. The committees provide a means for nurses to initiate needed changes affecting their work. They also provide a forum for the free flow of communication, ideas, and debate about nursing issues, problems, and events in the health care agency in general.

In a study of the effectiveness of these committees (Hibberd, 1996), the majority of the managers and union members from the 19 hospitals surveyed said that their PRCs were operating effectively. Nurses' concerns, rather than management concerns, dominated the agendas, and the type of problems referred to the PRCs included security issues, staffing levels, clinical protocols, and patient safety. Participants identified many concrete results from PRC meetings, such as new or revised policies (e.g., policies related to "do not resuscitate" procedures, smoking, or staff abuse), systems improvement (e.g., security, parking, paging), and staffing improvements (e.g., float staff, job descriptions). Many of the participants commented that PRCs had improved the communication between management and union. Thus, PRCs have much potential as a forum for fostering union-management relations. Since then, unions have negotiated other joint working committees for discussing a range of issues, including workload and staffing issues.

Regionalization and Staffing Issues

In the last few years, one of the most stressful aspects of being a manager has been dealing with the human consequences of regionalization and restructuring. Unions have also been affected by these trends because regionalization has led to changes in bargaining units and the merger of previously competing unions (see Pedersen, 1997). In hospitals, restructuring and downsizing have led to widespread layoffs of health care workers, especially registered nurses. Unions have a stake in how health care agencies go about laying off their members because of their highly cherished principle of seniority. Unions argue that because seniority is the most objective criterion for making decisions about employees' jobs, it should be the only criterion for determining who gets laid off. Seniority means that the longer an employee works for an employer, the greater the job security; therefore, if there are to be layoffs, the seniority principle ensures that members with the least seniority will be the first to be laid off and the last to be recalled to work. Applying the seniority principle results in bumping, with many associated stresses and strains for employers and unions, as well as many grievances.

Bumping is defined as "the procedure by which the employee with the greatest seniority who is about to be laid off is allowed to invoke her [or his] seniority rights so as to displace, or bump, a more junior employee from a job unaffected by the lay-off" (Brown & Beatty, 1994, 6:2330). This procedure can set off a chain of bumps. Generally, the senior employee must possess the skills and ability to do the desired job of the more junior employee. Ability to perform the work is a contentious issue between managers (who try to protect the integrity of workgroups, particularly in highly specialized areas) and union leaders (who want to defend the bumping rights of their members). Whether or not an employer can refuse a nurse's request to bump depends on the specific wording in the collective agreement and on precedents set in previous arbitration rulings. Employers are generally expected to familiarize (i.e., provide orientation to) staff exercising bumping rights, but not necessarily to provide training where new knowledge and skills may be needed. For example, where hospital policy requires nurses to have qualifications beyond basic nursing preparation (e.g., in areas such as neonatal intensive care or coronary care units), an employer may be entitled to restrict bumping just to nurses possessing those qualifications.

The turmoil created by downsizing and restructuring during the 1990s has had unintentional consequences for the nursing workforce. There is evidence of a growing shortage of registered nurses, and this shortage is expected to worsen as the nursing workforce ages and retires (Canadian Nurses Association, 2002). Employers' strategies to counteract the scarcity of professional nurses while keeping labour costs down include increasing part-time positions, decreasing full-time positions, employing non-regulated patient care workers, and changing the nursing skill mix. Such managerial responses do not necessarily create good working environments, as is well documented by the Canadian Nursing Advisory Committee (2002) and the Auditor General of British Columbia (2004) in his report *In Sickness and in Health*. The leading workforce management issue at the present time is the promotion of healthy working environments that are conducive to achieving the best possible patient care outcomes and the retention of a professional nursing workforce. Other issues currently of concern to nurses include nurse-to-patient ratios and workload, contingency staffing, counteracting violence and abuse in the workplace, and the prohibition of mandatory overtime. Nurses' unions will continue to press for these quality of work life issues at the bargaining table along with their socioeconomic demands.

Leadership Implications

There is a saying in the labour relations field that "management gets the union it deserves." In other words, failure by management to treat union leaders and their goals respectfully and with integrity may lead to ongoing conflict and hostile relations. Few relations in the health care system are as highly structured as the employment relationship between health agency boards and their employee unions. Nurses in management positions must be well informed of the provisions in nurses' collective agreements and must ensure that the contract is honoured consistently and fairly. When contracts are renewed, it is important that a senior nurse be included in the employers' negotiating team, whether at the agency, regional, or provincial level. Nurses on the management team have an important role to play in advising other team members, such as the finance and human resources personnel, of the implications of service delivery and patient care issues that are brought to the negotiating table by nurses. Many additional channels exist through which nursing leaders can advocate for healthy working environments for nurses, including health agency boards, professional nursing associations, and provincial governments.

Summary

- Nurse leaders, managers, and nurses working in a unionized environment should have a basic understanding of the labour relations system.
- The collective agreement is a contract between employer and employees that outlines terms and conditions of employment and the rules that govern relations between them.
- Employers and employees have common law rights and responsibilities toward each other.
- Grievances provide the means by which employees, without fear of reprisal, may lodge complaints against employers who allegedly violate the collective agreement.
- Discipline is the means by which employers may deal with employees who fail to fulfill their employment obligations.
- An employee who refuses to follow a manager's direction may be disciplined; however, arbitrators would likely rule in favour of the employee if he or she refuses to follow direction because doing so would (a) be illegal, (b) endanger the health or safety of the employee and co-workers, or (c) cause irreparable damage to the interest of other employees.

- Nurse managers can promote constructive union-management relations by becoming knowledgeable about the purpose of unions and the role of union representatives, by serving on professional responsibility committees, and by providing effective leadership and management.

- Laying off unionized staff results in bumping. Managers need to develop strategies for minimizing the disruption and distress created by the relocation of nursing staff.

- Restructuring and regionalization in the health care system have been accompanied by major issues in the nursing workforce and work life. Nurse leaders can address these issues through organizational and political channels, and nurses' unions can address them through collective bargaining.

Applying the Knowledge in this Chapter

Case Study

Maureen Anderson is scheduled to attend an arbitration hearing next week. She is a nurse and the manager of a busy home care program. The agency receives referrals from several hospitals and physicians' offices as well as direct referrals from the community; the clients are assigned to any one of six programs. Her staff consists of 45 registered nurses, 12 of whom function as case managers. She also is responsible for licensed practical nurses (LPNs), home health aides, occupational therapists (OTs), physiotherapists (PTs), social workers, respiratory therapists, an administrative assistant, and several clerical staff.

The home care program has an excellent reputation in the community, and Maureen is respected as a leader and manager. She has a motivated staff that works well together. Two regional unions represent her staff—one for the professional staff, and the other for auxiliary and clerical staff. In general, relations with these unions have been mutually respectful, that is, until Martina Scott filed a grievance 18 months ago.

Martina is an LPN who had completed her probationary period in this agency without incident and became a permanent member of the staff. Not long after, Martina's case manager noticed a marked change in her attitude, attendance, and willingness to take direction. A PT and an OT both complained about Martina's lack of cooperation and abrasive manner. Maureen met with Martina on several occasions and then assigned a senior staff nurse, Ginny Beckham, to work with Martina, identify her performance difficulties, and offer remedial help.

Several weeks later, the daughter of an elderly client claimed that Martina had physically abused her mother. Ginny and Maureen both were involved in the investigation of this complaint. The agency has a policy of zero tolerance for any kind of abuse, and following the investigation, Martina was dismissed. Martina's union filed a grievance on her behalf, requesting that she be immediately reinstated with full retroactive compensation and that all documentation relative to the investigation be removed from her personnel file. Maureen denied the grievance at every step in the grievance procedure, and subsequently, the board of the home care agency also denied the grievance.

The union decided to take the dispute to arbitration, the parties selected their nominees, and they in turn agreed upon the arbitrator. This three-person panel will hear evidence and argument from management and union personnel, and both sides of the dispute will bring witnesses. It may be many months before the arbitrator hands down his decision. Maureen feels she has handled this case fairly and objectively. She has spent many hours over the past few months meeting with Martina and coaching her, and now that the case is going to arbitration, she expects to spend more time away from her regular work with the region's Human Resources Department. Martina feels she has been harassed by management and was "framed" during the client abuse investigation. She is a single parent and needs her job to support two children. She is happy to have the representation of her union.

1. Given the time-consuming and costly process of arbitration, suggest reasons why the board of the home care agency and the union are referring this conflict to a third party for resolution. Why can they not settle this dispute between themselves?

2. What can Maureen do to prepare herself for the arbitration hearing?

3. What is Maureen's role in preparing her staff as witnesses for management (e.g., the role of Ginny Beckham, senior staff nurse)?

4. Identify the main points that the parties are likely to emphasize in their presentation to the arbitration board.

5. List a few of the exhibits (documentary evidence) that the parties are likely to submit to the arbitrator in support of their positions.

6. The arbitrator will find in favour of one of the parties. If you were the arbitrator, what would your decision be? Explain why.

Resources

evolve Internet Resources

Canada Labour Code (R.S. 1985, c. L-2):
   http://laws.justice.gc.ca/en/L-2/text.html
Canadian Nurses Association:
   www.cna-nurses.ca/
Health Canada:
   www.hc-sc.gc.ca/
International Council of Nurses:
   1999 Position Statement on Strike Policy
   www.icn.ch/psstrike.htm

Province	Provincial Employers' Association	Nurses' Union
Alberta	Provincial Health Authorities of Alberta www.phaa.com/	United Nurses of Alberta (UNA) www.una.ab.ca/
British Columbia	Health Employers Association of British Columbia (HEABC) www.heabc.bc.ca/	British Columbia Nurses' Union (BCNU) www.bcnu.org/
Manitoba	Regional Health Authorities of Manitoba (RHAM) www.rham.mb.ca/	Manitoba Nurses Union (MNU) www.nursesunion.mb.ca/
New Brunswick	New Brunswick Healthcare Association (NBHA) Web site under construction	New Brunswick Nurses' Union (NBNU) www.nbnu-siinb.nb.ca/
Newfoundland and Labrador	Newfoundland and Labrador Health Boards Association (NLHBA) www.nlhba.nf.ca/	Newfoundland and Labrador Nurses' Union (NLNU) www.nlnu.nf.ca/
Nova Scotia	Nova Scotia Association of Health Organizations (NSAHO) www.nsaho.ns.ca/	Nova Scotia Nurses' Union (NSNU) www.nsnu.ns.ca/
Ontario	Ontario Hospital Association (OHA) www.oha.com/	Ontario Nurses' Association (ONA) www.ona.org/
PEI	Health Association of PEI (HAPEI) (no Web site)	Prince Edward Island Nurses' Union (PEINU) (no Web site)
Quebec	Association des hôpitaux du Québec (AHQ) www.ahq.org/	Federation des Infirmieres et Infirmiers du Quebec (FIIQ) www.fiiq.qc.ca/
Saskatchewan	Saskatchewan Association of Health Organizations (SAHO) www.saho.org/	Saskatchewan Union of Nurses (SUN) www.sun-nurses.sk.ca/
Canada	Canadian Healthcare Association www.canadian-healthcare.org/	Canadian Federation of Nurses Unions www.nursesunions.ca/

References

American Nurses Association. (1985). *The grievance procedure*. Kansas City, MO: Author.

Anderson, J.C., Gunderson, M., & Ponak, A. (1989). *Union-management relations in Canada* (2nd ed.). Don Mills, ON: Addison-Wesley.

Auditor General of British Columbia. (2004). *In sickness and in health: Healthy workplaces for British Columbia's health care workers*. Victoria, BC: Office of the Auditor General of British Columbia. Retrieved August 25, 2004, from http://www.bcauditor.com/AuditorGeneral.htm

Brown, D.J.M., & Beatty, D.M. (1994). *Canadian labour arbitration* (3rd ed.). Aurora, ON: Canadian Law Book.

Canadian Nurses Association. (1999). *I see and am silent/I see and speak out: The ethical dilemma of whistleblowing*. Ottawa, ON: Author.

Canadian Nurses Association. (2002). *Planning for the future: Nursing human resource projections*. Ottawa, ON: Author.

Canadian Nursing Advisory Committee. (2002). *Our health, our future: Creating quality workplaces for Canadian nurses*. Final report. Ottawa, ON: Health Canada.

Cannon, P. (1980). Administering the contract. *Journal of Nursing Administration, 10*(10), 13–19.

Cohen, A. (1989). The management rights clause in collective bargaining. *Nursing Management, 20*(11), 24–34.

Craig, A.W.J. (1996). *The system of industrial relations in Canada* (5th ed.). Scarborough, ON: Prentice-Hall.

Creighton, H. (1986). When can a nurse refuse to give care? *Nursing Management, 17*(3), 16–20.

Eden, G. (1992). Progressive discipline: An oxymoron? *Relations Industrielles, 47*(3), 511–528.

Fiesta, J. (1990). Whistleblowers: Retaliation or protection? Part 2. *Nursing Management, 21*(7), 38.

Fisher, E.G., & Williams, C.B. (1989). Negotiating the union-management agreement. In J.C. Anderson, M. Gunderson, & A. Ponak (Eds.), *Union-management relations in Canada* (2nd ed., pp. 185–207). Don Mills, ON: Addison-Wesley.

Gandz, J. (1982). Grievances and their resolution. In J. Anderson & M. Gunderson (Eds.), *Union-management relations in Canada* (pp. 289–315). Don Mills, ON: Addison-Wesley.

Gandz, J., & Whitehead, J.D. (1989). Grievances and their resolution. In J.C. Anderson, M. Gunderson, & A. Ponak (Eds.), *Union-management relations in Canada* (2nd ed., pp. 235–260). Don Mills, ON: Addison-Wesley.

Giles, A., & Jain, H.C. (1989). The collective agreement. In J.C. Anderson, M. Gunderson, & A. Ponak (Eds.), *Union-management relations in Canada* (2nd ed., pp. 317–345). Don Mills, ON: Addison-Wesley.

Glasbeek, H.J. (1982). The contract of employment at common law. In J. Anderson & M. Gunderson (Eds.), *Union management relations in Canada* (pp. 47–77). Don Mills, ON: Addison-Wesley.

Hibberd, J.M. (1992). Strikes by nurses. Part 2: Incidence, trends and issues. *Canadian Nurse, 88*(3), 26–31.

Hibberd, J.M. (1996). *Effectiveness of nurses' labour-management committees*. Final report to the Alberta Foundation for Nursing Research, Edmonton, Alberta.

Huerta, S.R., & Oddi, L.F. (1992). Refusal to care for patients with human immunodeficiency virus/acquired immunodeficiency syndrome: Issues and responses. *Journal of Professional Nursing, 8*(4), 221–230.

McKenna, I. (1989). Whistleblowing and criticism of employers by employees: The case for reform in Canada. In *Papers presented at the Conference on Labour Relations into the 1990s*. School of Management, University of Lethbridge, September 10–12, 1987 (pp. 141–184). Don Mills, ON: CCH Canadian.

McPhillips, D., & England, G. (1989). Employment legislation in Canada. In J.C. Anderson, M. Gunderson, & A. Ponak (Eds.), *Union-management relations in Canada* (2nd ed., pp. 43–69). Don Mills, ON: Addison-Wesley.

Morris, J.J. (1991). *Canadian nurses and the law*. Toronto, ON: Butterworths.

Mrazek, M., & Tumbach, D. (1990). Insubordination and incompetence: A nurse's dilemma. *AARN Newsletter, 46*(10), 18–l9.

Northrop, C.E. (1987). Refusing unsafe work assignments. *Nursing Outlook, 36*(6), 302.

Pearlman, D. (1991). Progressive discipline: The grievance and arbitration process. In S.A. Ziebarth (Ed.), *Pinched: A management guide to the Canadian health care archipelago* (pp. 185–191). Ottawa, ON: Canadian Hospital Association.

Pedersen, R. (1997, September 26). Nursing unions unite for "stronger voice." *Edmonton Journal*, p. B5.

Peterborough Civic Hospital v. Ontario Nurses' Association (1982), 3 L.A.C. (3d) 21.

Sethi, A.S., & MacNeil, M. (1989). Issues in contract administration and human rights. In A.S. Sethi (Ed.), *Collective bargaining in Canada* (pp. 317–340). Scarborough, ON: Nelson.

Sklar, C.L. (1979a). Saints or sinners? The legal perspective: Part I. *Canadian Nurse, 75*(10), 14–16.

Sklar, C.L. (1979b). Saints or sinners? The legal perspective: Part II. *Canadian Nurse, 75*(11), 16, 18, 20–21.

Wahn, E.V. (1979). The dilemma of the disobedient nurse. *Health Care in Canada, 21*(2), 43–46.

BUSINESS PLANNING AND BUDGET PREPARATION

Judith M. Hibberd, Linda M. Doody, and Moira Hennessey

Learning Objectives

In this chapter, you will learn:

- How budgeting is part of the business plan approach to health services management

- Key budgeting concepts, including how capital and operating budgets work

- How to develop and manage an operating budget for a 24-bed nursing unit

- The importance of financial controls and reporting at the middle management level in a health organization

- Cost containment initiatives and resource management

It is estimated that health care spending reached 10.1% of Canada's gross domestic product in 2004. In dollar terms, this amounts to approximately $130.3 billion, representing a 5.9% increase over the previous year (Canadian Institute for Health Information, 2004). Barely a day goes by when the cost of health care is not featured in the Canadian media, most likely because expenditures on health care consume a large portion of provincial governments' budgets. The health care system is a highly valued social program and generates great public debate whenever it is the subject of federal and provincial discussions. The provision of health services is a provincial responsibility under the *British North America Act,* but both federal and provincial governments contribute financially to the system. The proportion of funding flowing from the federal government has declined in recent years, placing increasing fiscal pressure on provincial governments and often generating friction between the two levels of government. In order to preserve and maintain the health care system within available financial resources, provincial governments have found it necessary to restructure health care services. This restructuring has placed increased emphasis on regionalization and the devolution of service authority to the local level.

Provincial governments have established broad directions and guiding principles for the comprehensive and effective delivery of health programs and services, consistent with the tenets of the *Canada Health Act.* Guiding principles for the provision of reasonable access to primary, secondary, and tertiary services for all residents have been developed. Implementation of these principles varies from province to province, depending on population size and geography. In most provinces, regional health authorities (RHAs) or regional boards have been formed to administer programs and services to residents within defined geographic areas. These organizations have adopted a business approach to managing health services, based on the development of business plans, or blueprints, for the future delivery of programs and services.

In this chapter, budget preparation is discussed as an integral element of overall business planning for health organizations and regions. The responsibilities of managers of nursing services are discussed with respect to matching the health needs of clients with available financial resources. To assist managers in applying the basic concepts of budgeting for capital and operating expenditures, a sample budget for a 24-bed general medical and surgical unit is developed and discussed in this chapter. Variance reporting and cost containment initiatives are outlined in relation to the provision of high quality health services and the need to be accountable for the use of scarce financial resources. A glossary of budgeting terms is provided in Box 29.1.

Box 29.1

Glossary of Budgeting Terms

Budget	A detailed financial plan for achieving organizational goals and objectives within a specific period of time. It exemplifies the managerial functions of planning and controlling.

Capital budget	A financial plan for purchasing major equipment expected to have a useful lifespan of more than one year (e.g., beds, computers). Also included are alterations (renovations) to the physical plant.
Cost	The sum of resources used to provide a service, a specific intervention, or to achieve an objective.
Cost accounting	A process of recording, measuring, and reporting information about the cost of a service or program.
Cost benefit analysis	A procedure for identifying the total costs and benefits of a specific project or intervention. It answers the question "Is this project worthwhile?"
Cost centre	An organizational unit or program for which costs can be identified and allocated, sometimes known as a responsibility centre (e.g., a patient care unit).
Cost effectiveness	An analysis of expenditures for a particular project or intervention to determine if the same results can be achieved with fewer resources.
Expense	A cost charged against revenue within an accounting period; often used as a synonym for cost.
Fixed costs	Costs that remain the same regardless of changes in volume of service or activity (e.g., rent, telephone service).
Labour costs	Expenditures on employee salaries and benefits.
Operating budget	A financial plan for the day-to-day activities of a service, including income (revenue, if any) and expenses (labour, supplies, minor equipment).
Program budget	A financial plan for all aspects of a particular service (e.g., a diabetic teaching program). It usually includes both fixed and variable costs, overhead (e.g., lighting, heating), labour expenses, revenues, and it sometimes extends beyond a single fiscal period.
Revenue	Money flowing into, or generated by, a cost centre regardless of source (e.g., government funds, donations, service charges, parking).
Variable costs	Costs that fluctuate in accordance with the volume of service or activity (e.g., surgical supplies, drugs).
Variance	The difference between a budgeted amount and the actual amount spent to achieve a service or activity. Variances can be positive (budget surplus) or negative (budget deficit).
Zero-based budget	An approach to program budgeting that requires an examination and justification of all costs rather than just incremental costs (Finkler & Kovner, 2000). It proceeds as if there is a zero balance and requires examination of alternatives for achieving service objectives.

The Business Plan

A business plan has been defined as a set of statements about the mission, goals, and strategies of an organization that are accomplished within a set period of time (Oberg & Wagner, 1994). The plan must be based on the strategic directions established by the province and must provide a seamless continuum of health services. Ideally, a health business plan will have input from consumers and key stakeholders. It must ensure that core health services are available, accessible, and affordable, and it must meet the financial targets established for the region by the department of health. A business plan generally includes the following elements:

- Health care needs assessment
- Vision, mission, and values
- Guiding principles
- Goals, objectives, priorities, and strategies for service delivery
- Human, structural, and financial resources

Health Care Needs Assessment

The health care needs assessment includes (a) an inventory of current health programs and services offered in the region, (b) a demographic and health status profile of the catchment population, (c) consumer expectations regarding health services, and (d) gaps in programs and service delivery. This information can be obtained from sources such as Statistics Canada census data and Canadian Institute for Health Information (CIHI) data, proposals for new health services submitted by special interest groups, customer satisfaction surveys, and focus groups and community meetings.

As part of the senior management team, the top nurse executive is actively involved in conducting the health care needs assessment by collecting and analyzing data and by participating in focus groups and community meetings. Managers in charge of nursing at the unit level provide data to the senior nursing executive, and they are involved in discussing the program or services they manage from utilization, consumer demand, human, and financial perspectives. For example, the nurse in charge of an eight-station dialysis unit notes that patients are not being dialyzed properly—some patients who need three treatments weekly are receiving only two treatments because the patient workload has increased beyond the available capacity. There is also a waiting list for this service, and residents who require dialysis treatments are relocating to other areas that provide renal dialysis services. A review of five years' historical workload data indicates that the number of patients receiving the treatment has doubled. The manager's responsibility in contributing to the health business plan might be to lead or work with a team of colleagues to develop a proposal to expand the renal dialysis service to meet the health needs of the population in the region.

Vision, Mission, and Values

The vision statement considers the health care needs assessment and states health ideals for the organization. It reflects the values of the organization and provides a common direction for the provision of health services. A vision statement might include a goal such as the following: "To assist communities and individuals to achieve the highest level of health possible."

The mission statement describes how the organization will fulfill its vision. It is the driving force for all actions within the organization. It should be brief, succinct, and clear. The following is an example of a mission statement: "Working in partnership with other health service providers, communities, individuals, families, groups, and organizations, the regional health authority is responsible for the delivery of institutional acute and long-term care services."

To assist in achieving the mission and interpreting the vision for the organization, the board may affirm a set of values. These values assist the organization in decision making and other relevant activities. Some common values are respect for persons, a caring community, justice and fairness, collaboration, and the pursuit of excellence. One of the value statements of the Health Care Corporation of St. John's (1996), for example, focuses on respect for persons:

> The Corporation respects the needs and rights of clients/patients and their families, staff members including physicians, volunteers and others. We believe in keeping client information confidential and in providing the client with information to make informed choices. We value the needs of the whole person and we place the clients and their families at the centre of our service.

The vision, mission, and value statements provide broad policy directions and a framework for choosing, developing, and evaluating programs and services. The nurse manager must be cognizant of these ideals and reflect them in the delivery of services at the unit level.

Guiding Principles

Guiding principles are derived from the vision and mission statements. Examples of some guiding principles for an RHA include the following:
- To ensure that the RHA, in collaboration with other health providers, delivers comprehensive health care services for individuals and groups of clients as part of a health continuum
- To be accountable to the community and government for the delivery of effective programs and services within available financial resources

Goals, Objectives, and Strategies for Service Delivery

The organization must establish goals consistent with its mission and vision. Goals are usually stated in more specific terms than guiding principles:
- To provide a continuum of affordable, accessible, and appropriate quality care
- To enable the consumer to lead a healthy and independent life.

Objectives are the key to achieving goals, and strategies are the means by which the objectives are accomplished. In terms of the first goal, providing a continuum of quality care, a specific objective might be the development of lower cost ambulatory care programs. A strategy that the board might use to achieve this objective would be to close inpatient beds and enhance outpatient and community support services within the current approved budget. Extending this example to the nursing unit level, a strategy that the nurse manager could use would be piloting a pre-admission clinic to reduce lengths of stay and improve accessibility to the fewer inpatient beds.

Another example that shows the relationship between goals and objectives concerns a comprehensive mental health program that has inpatient and daycare activities. The patient census for the daycare program is low, and staffing costs are high. Because the organization has a mandate to provide a comprehensive mental health program, the nurse manager cannot unilaterally make a decision to discontinue the daycare program. However, she or he can review the utilization data and the mental health needs of the catchment population to make recommendations to the senior administration regarding proposed changes for the daycare service. These might include discontinuing the program, extending services to residents of another region, or changing the types of activities offered in the daycare program to better address actual needs.

In terms of the second goal, enabling the consumer to adopt a healthier lifestyle, a board objective might be to offer educational services to the consumer regarding healthy living habits in order to cope with factors affecting their health, such as obesity, stress, or diabetes. In this example, a strategy for the nurse manager would be to facilitate the development of a teaching program, pamphlets, and other educational materials on these subjects.

Human, Structural, and Financial Resources

In this element of the business plan, the vision, mission, objectives, and strategies are translated into concrete tangible terms such as staffing, facilities, and finances.

Human Resources

The organization must develop a workforce plan that includes the number and type of staff required to carry out its service delivery plan. In health organizations, salaries and related costs represent about 80% of the total operating budget. The human resources plan identifies management personnel and staff who provide direct care and support services. It may also forecast needs for certain types of personnel and incorporate strategies for recruiting and training them.

Structural Resources

Structural resources include equipment and physical facilities. In developing the business plan, the organization must identify the need for new equipment and the areas where new facilities are needed or where existing facilities require upgrading or renovation. In times of financial scarcity, facility renovations and redevelopment are normally limited to those projects that address safety issues or improve service delivery.

Financial Resources

The majority of the money allocated for operating hospitals, nursing homes, health units, and community services comes from the general revenues of provincial governments. There are three provinces still raising money specifically for the health system by levying individual and family health care premiums, namely Alberta, British Columbia, and Ontario. Other sources of revenue for hospitals include insurance companies and workers' compensation boards, and many of the large urban facilities raise money through such on-site services as parking fees and cafeteria sales. The allocation of public monies to health facilities is preceded by the submission of detailed business plans and budgets months in advance of the fiscal year. Approval of budgets often does not occur until the health facilities are well into the time period for which the budget has been prepared. It should be clear that a budget is an instrument for planning and controlling financial resources.

Budget Definition

The budget is a detailed financial plan for achieving organizational goals and objectives within a specific period of time. Budgeting is the process whereby objectives and plans are translated into financial terms and evaluated using financial and statistical criteria (Swansburg, 2002). Evaluation involves monitoring actual expenditures and comparing them against financial targets or predicted expenditures. The budget is often a basis for evaluation of organizational effectiveness as it is an indicator of how well resources are used.

Many health organizations take a participatory approach to the budgeting process. Although the coordination and assembly of a range of input takes considerable time and effort, this approach is well worth the effort. McConnell (1993) cites the following advantages associated with a participatory budgeting process:

- The end result is a more realistic and workable budget because front-line supervisors are familiar with the day-to-day operations and the financial resources needed to manage programs and services.
- There is increased commitment to and ownership for managing the budget due to active involvement in its preparation.
- Interdepartmental and intradepartmental relationships improve because front-line supervisors obtain a better understanding of the total picture and the various responsibilities of the individual players.
- A team spirit is created whereby all managers are working together for a common goal.

Budgets are usually prepared for the fiscal year, which begins April 1 and ends March 31. They are based on a combination of past activity, current trends, and whatever knowledge is available regarding future situations. The budget is the best estimate of the financial resources needed to carry out the projected work activity for the fiscal year. It must be realistic and reflective of the economic and political environment. The board of the organization is ultimately responsible for the budget. It does not prepare the budget, but it must understand, support, and approve financial proposals developed by the executive team.

The Budget Process

The process of developing a budget, whether for a whole region or an individual hospital or health unit, follows a predictable annual pattern. It begins with a communication from the provincial health department announcing general guidelines by which regional health authorities must prepare their budgets. There is an indication of the limit to which budgets may exceed the previous fiscal year's allocation. For example, the government may determine that budget increases be restricted to an amount equal to the consumer price index for the area. Alternatively, the government may require all budgets to be cut back by a given percentage. Health care spending has been increasing around the world, and in Canada it is estimated that it rose by a real (inflation adjusted) 4.6% in 2003 over the previous year (CIHI, 2003). Health care institutions are familiar with requests from governments to cut back on financial demands and to contain costs. The budget process is an important instrument both for planning the economic delivery of health services and for controlling necessary expenditures. Within the RHA, the budget process is delegated to the finance director, who identifies and communicates with the people responsible for the various cost centres.

Cost Centres

A cost centre is the smallest organizational unit for which a budget is prepared (McConnell, 1993). It can be a unit or a program for which costs can be identified and allocated, and it is often known as a responsibility centre. A 24-bed surgical patient care unit and a walk-in outpatient clinic are examples of cost centres. Budgets for individual cost centres are prepared by supervisors or managers and assembled by senior level administrators for their overall areas of responsibility; for example, all individual budgets for each surgical patient care unit may be amalgamated and submitted as a single surgical services budget. Thus, the organizational chart is a guide to the general distribution of cost centres throughout the institution and illustrates the structures for producing the agency's overall budget.

Some budgets are organized functionally, as in the case of the laboratories and housekeeping services, while others may be organized as programs. Cancer services might be budgeted as a program because it is multidisciplinary in nature and operates across departmental boundaries. In order to identify the cost of such services, it may be planned and budgeted as a facility-wide program. The budgets for all functional departments and programs are then compiled and summarized into an overall budget for the hospital or agency, and ultimately, the RHA consolidates all budgets for institutions, programs, and services in the region.

Types of Budget

There are two basic types of budget—capital and operating. The capital budget deals with fixed assets such as equipment, furnishings, land, and buildings. The operating budget includes all revenue and expenses related to the day-to-day operations of the programs and services offered by the organization.

Capital Budgets

There are two components to capital budgeting in health institutions: capital equipment and capital projects. Capital equipment includes large items such as CT scanners, ventilators, dialysis stations, or electric beds. Items that cost more than $1000 or have an expected lifespan longer than three to five years are included in the capital equipment budget. Smaller items, such as intravenous (IV) poles and medical trays, that normally cost less than $1000 and have shorter lifespans are included as part of supplies in an operating budget. The actual dollar amounts and lifespan criteria for capital equipment may differ from province to province. Capital equipment can be either purchased or leased. If the equipment is purchased, the cost is included in the capital equipment budget. If the equipment is leased, as IV pumps may be, the annual lease payments are included in the operating budget.

Sometimes, organizations will enter into cost-sharing arrangements with the provincial government for equipment that requires a large investment of money. These cost-sharing arrangements may extend over three to five years. For example, the organization may cost-share the replacement of standard beds with electric beds over a three-year period in a long-term care facility.

Managers of programs or patient care units are usually involved in preparing capital equipment budgets. Requests for capital equipment frequently exceed available financial resources. Managers in nursing may receive individual requests for equipment from the medical staff and allied health professionals working on the unit. Some requests to replace or purchase new equipment are essential to the safe operation of the program or service, whereas other requests may be less oriented to safety than to an interest in having the most recent technology.

Development of a capital equipment budget should include short- and long-range plans for equipment. The process requires the preparation of a capital equipment inventory, which includes the age, condition, and life expectancy of each piece of equipment. A three-year capital equipment plan should be developed that outlines equipment purchases in order of priority. This plan should include costs of inflation and a contingency factor for unexpected replacement of equipment. In most health organizations, this process is coordinated through one division of the organization, such as materials management (also known as purchasing) or biomedical engineering. Increasingly, nurses participate in formal product evaluation or technology assessment committees and can influence the actual models of equipment purchased.

Capital projects include renovations to existing buildings or the construction of new buildings, for example, renovations to an existing nursing unit to include rehabilitative space, upgrading electrical equipment to specifications defined by the Canadian Standards Association (CSA), or replacement of windows or even a roof. Program and first-level managers are not usually involved in preparing cost estimates for capital projects, but as members of planning or user groups, they contribute to the identification of needs and operational requirements.

Operating Budgets

An operating budget is the financial plan for the day-to-day activities of a unit or program and consists of statements of revenues and expenses. Revenue includes money from provincial governments, third-party payers such as Veterans Affairs Canada or the RCMP, private room accommodation premiums, and other sources. Expenses include compensation in the form of salaries, employee benefits, and supplies, including medical and surgical items, drugs, oxygen, and food.

Guidelines for the development of operating budgets were drawn up through the cooperative effort of provincial and national governments and health care associations. These guidelines are known as management information systems (MIS) and are followed by many health institutions. The MIS guidelines reflect management information principles and provide a conceptual framework for the collection, integration, and reporting of financial, statistical, and clinical data. They specify what data to collect, how to group and process the data, and how to use the data to support management functions of decision making, planning, budgeting, controlling, and evaluating (CIHI, 1994).

Data can be reported at global and/or departmental levels when using the MIS guidelines. The global approach identifies the resources used to provide a specific service to a specific group of patients, for example, all cardiopulmonary patients. Global costs for such a group include staffing and supplies for all aspects of patient care, not just nursing care, including dietetics, social work, and housekeeping. In a global reporting system, the total cost of a surgical procedure such as a coronary artery bypass graft can be determined.

The departmental approach is the system typically used in Canadian health facilities. It includes all resources used to provide a specific service within a specific functional centre, for example, surgery as a part of nursing inpatient services. Key components of departmental reporting comprise financial data, statistical data, indicators, and variances. Financial data consist of all revenues and expenses associated with a service or program. There is not usually very much revenue generated in nursing units, but the main source would likely be private and semi-private accommodation *per diem* charges. There is no out-of-pocket charge for public accommodation. Expenses on a nursing unit include direct operating costs such as salaries, employee benefits, and supplies. There are also indirect operating costs such as housekeeping and laundry services, but these may be reported on a global basis.

Statistical Budget

Statistics always accompany an operational budget; indeed, they may comprise what is referred to as the statistical budget. Managers must compile and summarize data from the previous 12 months and make projections for the next financial year. Some common statistics include patient activity (e.g., patient days, clinical visits), workload data, and staffing figures. Patient activity on a nursing unit may include average occupancy, total patient days, and the number of admissions, discharges, and transfers, as well as a summary of workload measurement.

Workload measurement and patient classification systems are tools that assist the manager in providing an appropriate level of staffing to meet the expected demand for nursing care. Prior to the development of patient classification systems, staffing levels were determined by global standards; for example, 2.5 hours of direct nursing care were estimated to be required per patient per day, or one registered nurse (RN) to care for three patients. These global standards did not reflect variations in the care requirements of the patients; therefore, patient classification systems were designed to provide a more accurate estimate of nursing workloads by using critical indicators of care, such as bathing, ambulation, and feeding. Workload measurement systems, if well designed and maintained, often provide a reliable and valid assessment of patient care needs, which can then be used to help the nurse manager efficiently allocate staff to patients. Data generated by a workload measurement system should be part of the permanent clinical record and should be summarized and reviewed from time to time to assess changing trends in patient care requirements. These systems are often referred to as "acuity systems," but the measurement of workload tells us little about how acutely ill the patients are.

The MIS guidelines permit the use of indicators for managers to evaluate and control current operations and to plan for the future. Indicators are calculated using financial and statistical data, which produce various ratios and percentages. For example, an outpatient visit may be considered a unit of service for which the direct cost can be calculated. If the direct cost per unit of service is known (e.g., $60.50 per clinic visit), it can be monitored over time and compared with other similar units of service. Such indicators assist managers in controlling expenditures.

Another example of an indicator is the productivity of nursing staff. Productivity is calculated by dividing the required hours of care (as estimated by the workload measurement system) by the actual hours of care provided (from payroll data) and multiplying the quotient by 100. A productivity rate of 100% indicates that the actual hours of care match the required hours of care. A rate greater than 100% indicates that the actual hours provided were less than required, while a rate less than 100% indicates that more hours of care were provided than were necessary. If health institutions use productivity indices, acceptable productivity ranges would range from approximately 85% to 115%.

Variances

The final key component of the MIS departmental reporting system is variances. A variance refers to the difference between the budgeted cost and the actual cost of an item. Variances can be positive or negative. For example, if a manager budgeted for 1000 hours of overtime but actually paid for 1200 hours of overtime, the budget report would show a negative variance for the cost of overtime hours (i.e., 200 $\times$ the hourly rate of overtime pay for an RN). Variances will be discussed in more detail later in this chapter.

Developing a Budget for a Patient Care Unit

To apply the concepts discussed thus far, a step-by-step procedure is now described for developing an operating budget. The case study to be used is a 24-bed general medical/surgical patient care unit, which, for the sake of illustration, has a permanent, full-time nurse manager and a unit clerk in addition to full- and part-time nursing staff. This is a departmental approach because it will not include any of the services supplied to the unit by social work, dietary, pharmacy, or rehabilitation services, or even housekeeping or transportation services. The characteristics of this unit are summarized in Box 29.2. The tasks for the manager are (a) to determine what it will cost to provide human resources (nursing services) and medical/surgical supplies in order to operate this unit over the next fiscal year and (b) to identify sources of revenue, if any.

Box 29.2

Characteristics of the 24-Bed Medical/Surgical Unit

Bed Allocation
4 private (4 beds), 4 semi-private (2 beds each = 8 beds), and 3 public wards (4 beds each = 12 beds)

Most Common Medical Diagnoses
cardiac and pulmonary disorders (including chronic obstructive lung disease, myocardial infarction, angina, pneumonia, and peripheral vascular disease) and diabetes

Most Common Surgical Diagnoses
gynecological procedures such as hysterectomies and ovarian cysts; mastectomies; abdominal peritoneal resections; cholecystectomies

Other Characteristics
In the year prior to the budget year, there were 8322 patient days.
The average patient requires 5.0 hours of nursing care per 24 hours.

Performance Summary for Previous Budget Year

The first step in preparing an operating budget is to review the performance figures and statistics for the current budget year and compare them against actual performance. Unless a zero-based budget approach is being taken (see glossary in Box 29.1), a review of past experience will be regarded as the place to start planning for the upcoming year. One problem is that next year's budget is generally planned before the current year has ended, so predictions must also be made about the remainder of the current period. Assuming there will be a total of 8322 patient days (see Box 29.2) in the current year, the manager must consider if this is likely to be the same or different for next year. Similar factors to consider might include the following:

- Has the type of patient admitted to this unit changed in the past 12 months?
- Has there been a change in medical staff practices during the year?
- Is the average length of patient stay decreasing/increasing?
- Has the workload index increased/decreased?
- Has there been any staff turnover?
- Has the amount of sick leave taken by staff exceeded estimates?
- Have nurses' overtime hours increased?

If the answer to any of these questions is "yes," then the manager must consider if this is evidence of real change and whether the budget needs to be adjusted accordingly for next year. Therefore, it can be seen that budgeting is a rather imprecise managerial function that is dependent on a systematic review of past experience and a careful estimate of future performance.

Costs Associated with Staffing

The bed allocation, patient days, and average hours of nursing care are used to determine the cost of human resources or staffing needed to care for patients on this nursing unit, as shown in Box 29.3.

Staffing consists of management and operational support and unit producing personnel (UPP). Management and operational support personnel refer to nurse managers and the unit clerks. This category might also include a ward aide or porter, although the trend has been to centralize such operational support under housekeeping or even to contract it out to the private sector. The UPP are RNs and registered nursing assistants (RNAs), whose primary function is to carry out activities directly related to the care of patients, in other words, they are the caregivers. Other types of nursing staff in the UPP category might include a clinical nurse specialist or nurse educator, although such positions are mainly found in large teaching hospitals.

In preparing the budget, managerial and operational support and UPP are expressed as full-time equivalent (FTE) positions. One FTE refers to a full-time position in which the employee works for an entire year (Finkler & Kovner, 2000). In other words, a nurse occupying a full-time position would work 7.5 hours daily, or 37.5 hours per week, for a total of 1950 earned hours per year. These earned hours include worked hours (the hours a nurse actually works) plus benefit hours, such as sick leave and vacation leave. The FTE concept is useful because it is divisible, allowing the manager to summarize the hours worked by the growing cadre of part-time nurses. For example, one full-time position may be worked by two or three staff members who, together, are paid for 1950 hours per year. FTEs may be determined in terms of hours or shifts; for example, a person who works half time, or 975 hours per year, is 0.5 FTE, a person who works

Box 29.3

Human Resources / Staffing Characteristics

- Management and operational support personnel consist of one nurse manager and one unit clerk.
- The unit producing personnel include registered nurses and registered nursing assistants.
- The average annual salary for the nurse manager is $68,250.
- The average hourly rates for remaining staff are as follows:

Registered Nurse	$28.51
Registered Nursing Assistant	$19.82
Unit Clerk	$15.26

- The skill mix for the unit producing personnel is 70% RNs and 30% RNAs.
- Benefit salaries are 20% of regular salaries.
- The benefit contribution expense is 19.5% of regular salaries plus benefit salaries.

800 hours per year is 0.4 FTE, and a person working one shift per week, or 7.5 hours, is 0.2 FTE. The total number of FTEs is not usually the same as the total number of staff; for example, a nursing budget may have 16.4 FTEs but may consist of 21 individuals. The total number of hours making up one FTE may vary from province to province, depending on collective agreements and provincial labour laws. (See Chapter 26 for more on FTEs.)

Regular Salaries: Unit Producing Personnel

To calculate the required UPP, or caregivers, for this 24-bed unit, the nurse manager must first determine the occupancy rate. The occupancy rate is the ratio of occupied beds to the total number of beds on the unit. This 24-bed unit has the potential for 8760 patient days (24 beds × 365 days) per year. In this case, however, there were 8322 patient days in 2002/2003. To calculate the occupancy rate, the following formula is used:

$$\text{Occupancy Rate} = \frac{\text{Actual patient days}}{\text{No. of beds} \times 365 \text{ days}} = \frac{8322}{24 \times 365} = 95\%$$

A 95% occupancy rate for this unit means that there is an average of only 22.8 beds occupied each day.

To determine the total number of unit producing FTEs required for this 24-bed nursing unit, the occupancy rate or number of beds occupied is used in conjunction with the average hours of care per patient per 24-hour period. The figure used for average hours of care per patient in the following formula is derived from the workload measurement system employed in the facility. In some jurisdictions, this figure may be arbitrarily set by the funding or government agency. The formula is as follows:

$$\text{FTEs} = \frac{\text{No. of beds occupied} \times \text{hours of care per patient per 24 hrs.} \times 365}{\text{Earned hours per FTE}}$$

$$= \frac{22.8 \times 5.0 \text{ hours} \times 365}{1950 \text{ hours}}$$

$$= 21.3$$

This number of FTEs (21.3) is not the full complement of staff because no allowance has yet been made for relief staff to cover for vacations, sick leave, and other leaves of absence (to be calculated later).

Based on a skill mix of 70% RNs and 30% RNAs, the 21.3 FTEs would consist of 14.9 RNs and 6.4 RNAs. Regular salaries for nursing personnel are based on a salary scale negotiated through collective agreements. Based on an average hourly rate of $28.51 for RNs and $19.82 for RNAs, regular salaries are calculated as follows:

```
14.9 RNs  @ $28.51/hour × 1950 hours/year  =  $   828,358
6.4 RNAs  @ $19.82/hour × 1950 hours/year  =  $   247,354
                                              $1,075,712
```

Note: All calculations are rounded to the nearest dollar.

Benefits: Unit Producing Personnel

Direct benefits are referred to as benefit salaries (i.e., benefits linked to salaries) and include relief for vacation, sick leave, and statutory holidays, as well as overtime, in-charge pay, shift differential, and educational allowances, to list a few. These benefits are generally negotiated through the collective bargaining process and vary from province to province. In recent years, fiscal realities have led to minimum staffing levels on many nursing units. Minimum staffing levels mean that units are unable to absorb the occasional absence of staff and must routinely replace the absent person adding to the benefit salary costs. Benefit salary costs may be calculated individually or estimated as a percentage of regular salaries. For the purpose of this exercise, benefit salaries are estimated at 20% of regular salaries. Accordingly, regular salaries are $1,075,712 and benefit salaries are $215,142 (1,075,712 × 0.20). Regular salaries and benefit salaries must be added together before calculating the total direct wage expense.

Indirect benefits are referred to as the benefit contribution expense, and they represent the facility's contribution to employee benefits such as the Canada Pension Plan (CPP), Employment Insurance (EI), provincial pension, and health insurance schemes. Benefits such as CPP and EI are constant among the provinces; other benefits may vary slightly. Benefit contribution expense is calculated as a percentage of regular salaries plus benefit salaries. In this case, the benefit contribution expense is estimated at 19.5% of these costs or $251,717 [(1,075,712 + 215,142) × 0.195].

Regular Salaries and Benefits: Management and Operational Support Personnel

To calculate the management and operational support personnel costs for this 24-bed unit, the nurse manager's salary and the unit clerk's salary are added together. Based on an average salary of $68,250 for the nurse manager and an average hourly wage of $15.26 for the unit clerk, regular salaries for these personnel are calculated as follows:

Nurse Manager	= $68,250
Unit Clerk @ $15.26/hour × 1950 hours	= $29,757
	$98,007

The manager is not usually replaced when absent for vacation or sickness, so there are no benefit salaries associated with the position. The unit clerk may be replaced depending on the health agency's personnel policies, so the benefit salary for the unit clerk would be $5951 (29,757 × 0.20).

Employee benefit contributions amount to 19.5% of regular salaries (plus benefit salary for unit clerk) or $20,272 [(98,007 + 5951) × 0.195].

Other Compensation Considerations

When calculating regular salaries for all personnel working on the unit, the nurse manager must be aware of future changes such as step progressions (i.e., increments on the salary scale) and wage increases. Step progressions will vary from employee to employee on an annual basis;

wage increases may vary by job classification. Occasionally, an employee who is entitled to accumulated annual leave and/or severance pay will leave or retire. Severance pay is a termination bonus based on years of service and is a benefit accrued in some provinces. The funding allocated for these benefits is a one-time cost that should be included in budget projections in the year the cost will be incurred.

The total compensation expense for management and operational support as well as unit producing personnel for this 24-bed nursing unit is calculated in Table 29.1.

Supplies

According to the MIS guidelines, supplies are divided into various categories such as medical and surgical supplies, drugs, medical gases, printing and office supplies, laundry, and linen. Supplies usually represent about 20% of the total operating budget. In many cases, nurse managers are responsible only for determining the budget allocation for supplies that are used directly for patient care, such as medical/surgical supplies, drugs, and medical gases. Medical/surgical supplies include items such as dressings, catheters, needles, syringes, and gloves. Drugs are subdivided into categories such as IV solutions, anti-neoplastics, total parenteral nutrition, and antibiotics. Medical gases include anesthetic gases and oxygen. Other supply costs include laundry and linen, which may be determined by other departmental managers.

In determining the current year's budget for supplies, the nurse manager should review actual costs for the previous year and adjust these amounts for inflation and workload changes caused by such factors as bed closures, a new physician, or increased patient acuity. Such changes may be interdependent. For example, a new physician can effect a change in the patient profile by performing more complicated surgeries or admitting patients who require higher levels of

Table 29.1 Calculating Compensation Expenses

Management and Operational Support Personnel	
Regular Salaries	98,007
Benefit Salaries	5,951
Employee Benefit Contributions	20,272
Subtotal	$124,230
Unit Producing Personnel	
Regular Salaries	1,075,712
Benefit Salaries	215,142
Employee Benefit Contributions	251,717
Subtotal	$1,542,571
Total Compensation Expense	**$1,666,801**

care, thereby increasing the intensity of care. The change in intensity of care will result in increased usage of more costly medical/surgical supplies and drugs.

To calculate the supply costs in this case example, the nurse manager must make an adjustment only for inflation, if all other factors remain constant, including number of beds, occupancy rate, and other factors. Inflation is based on the Consumer Price Index and is provided on an annual basis by Statistics Canada. If the inflation rate for the budget year is estimated at 3%, and the actual cost for the previous year was $282,000, the projected costs for the budget year's supplies would be $290,460 (282,000 × 1.03). The allocation of these supply costs is shown in Table 29.2.

The personnel and supplies components of the budget are known as variable costs since they are affected by the volume of work. As the intensity of patient care increases, one can expect more staffing and an increase in expenditure on supplies, and vice versa. Fixed costs are those expenditures that do not vary in relation to the volume of work, such as lighting and heating (refer to Box 29.1 for definitions of fixed and variable costs). Agency policy determines whether a manager must include fixed costs in unit budgets. For our purposes, there are no fixed costs to be included in the budget of the 24-bed unit as these are calculated on an agency-wide basis and not assigned to individual cost centres.

Revenue

Revenue for this 24-bed nursing unit is limited to income from patients in the private and semi-private rooms. The daily rates that patients are charged for these rooms are usually established by the province. In this example, revenue is generated from the four private and four semi-private rooms; the room rates are $80 for a private room and $60 for each patient in a semi-private room. Based on the 95% occupancy rate on this nursing unit, the revenue is calculated as follows:

Private:	4 rooms @ $80/day × 365 days × 0.95	= $110,960
Semi-private:	4 rooms × 2 people @ $60/day × 365 days × 0.95	= $166,440
		$277,400

Table 29.2 **Calculating Supply Costs**

Supply Item	Previous Year	Budget Year
Medical Surgical Supplies	109,000	112,270
Drugs	146,000	150,380
Medical Gases	27,000	27,810
Total	**$282,000**	**$290,460**

The invoices for recovering this revenue are usually generated by the accounting office and given to patients upon discharge. As revenue calculations are completed by staff in the finance department, the nurse manager is not usually involved in the revenue recovery process.

A summary of the whole operating budget appears in Table 29.3.

Table 29.3 One Year Operating Budget

Compensation

Management and Operational Support Personnel		
Regular Salaries	98,007	
Benefit Salaries	5,951	
Employee Benefit Contributions	20,272	
Subtotal	$124,230	$124,230
Unit Producing Personnel		
Regular Salaries	1,075,712	
Benefit Salaries	215,142	
Employee Benefit Contributions	251,717	
Subtotal	$1,542,571	$1,542,571
Total Compensation Expense		**$1,666,801**

Supplies

Medical and Surgical Supplies	112,270	
Drugs	150,380	
Medical Gases	27,810	
Total Supplies Expense	**$290,460**	**$290,460**
Total Expenses		**$1,957,261**
Less Revenue		
Accommodations		
Private	110,960	
Semi-Private	166,440	
Total Revenue		**– $277,400**
Total Operating Budget		**$1,679,861**

Financial Control and Reporting

While reviewing the monthly budget reports, managers should seek clarification from accounting staff regarding areas of concern or instances where details seem to be unclear. Developing a good working relationship with accounting staff will assist the nurse manager in becoming more knowledgeable about variance reporting, and it will enable the manager to alter expenditure patterns to address unfavourable trends that may be developing.

Variances are the differences between budgeted or expected performance and actual performance. Under a participative budgeting process, managers are provided with a monthly report that shows a comparison of budget projections and operating results for the month, and a variance column displays the differences between actual and budget projections. A negative variance occurs if actual costs are greater than budgeted costs; a positive variance occurs if actual costs are less than budgeted costs. Negative variances are sometimes indicated in parentheses. Both negative and positive variances are demonstrated in the simplified example of a budget report for the month of August in Table 29.4.

Budget reports also provide a year-to-date summary of actual and budget expenditures, and they sometimes include information about workload and patient activity. Managers should examine these monthly reports and be able to justify variances outside the expected range. Ongoing negative variances may indicate trends that require the intervention of a more senior manager. For instance, if the volume of work is increasing and the worked hours remain constant, the manager may need to make a temporary increase in the number of staff for peak periods. Note that, in Table 29.4, there is a negative variance for unit producing personnel for both the month of August and the year to date. If the variance continues much longer, a permanent staffing adjustment may need to be made.

Table 29.4 Budget Report for the Month of August

Item	August Budget	Actual	Variance	Year to Date Budget	Actual	Variance
Compensation						
Management/support	6,772	6,772	—	33,860	33,860	—
UPP	90,331	93,000	(2,669)	451,655	476,200	(24,545)
Supplies						
Medical/surgical	8,933	9,000	(67)	44,665	42,600	2,065
Drugs	11,675	10,700	975	56,375	60,725	(4,350)
Medical gases	1,841	1,500	341	9,455	8,050	1,405
Total	$119,552	$120,972	$(1,420)	$596,010	$621,435	$(25,425)

Managers are usually expected to answer to their immediate supervisors for budget variances. According to McConnell (1993), "answering to variances under budget is almost as important as answering to variances over budget" (p. 327). Being under budget may be due to a seasonal variation in expenses and does not necessarily mean a cost savings. For example, the vacation relief budget for nursing staff may be distributed equally over a 12-month period, but there may not be any actual expenses incurred for vacation relief during the winter months.

Resource Management

According to Buchan (1992), "cost containment is the key concept that nurses must grasp in this time of shrinking budgets and growing demands for health care. As health-care budgets come under increased scrutiny, nurses must prove their cost effectiveness" (p. 117). If nurses ignore this issue, important decisions on resource allocation will be made by administrators who have a strong knowledge of costing but a weak appreciation of the impact of cost containment strategies on the quality of nursing care.

Nurse managers need to be aware of the costs of staffing, supplies, and equipment used to provide health services. The most costly input in the provision of nursing care is staffing, which represents approximately 70% of the operating budget. As noted earlier, workload measurement systems can be used to control staffing costs by assigning staff according to the actual demand for nursing care. However, patient care requirements often fluctuate, and the nurse manager must monitor these changes in patient acuity and adjust the staffing levels accordingly. This may be done by calling in casual staff to meet increased demands or by floating excess staff to understaffed units. If nurses are transferred to another nursing unit for relief reasons, the unit manager must ensure that costs are allocated to the receiving unit where the staff actually perform the work.

It is important that the mix of nursing skills matches patient care requirements. Nursing workload measurement systems do not solve the question of what category of nursing staff to assign to patients—that decision requires nursing judgment. In general, work should be assigned to the least costly personnel capable of doing the work. Professional staff should be assigned to work that requires their expertise; for example, the registration function in an outpatient clinic should be assigned to clerks rather than RNAs, while patient assessment is the function of RNs. The skill mix of nursing staff differs from unit to unit. Some specialized areas like obstetrics, emergency, and critical care are generally staffed by RNs only, whereas general medical surgical units may have a mix of RNs and RNAs. Nurse managers must be constantly monitoring the profiles of patients on the unit and adjusting the staffing complement and skill mix to match patient need.

Managers can also control input costs through the judicious use of supplies and equipment and by selecting products that have the desired qualities at the lowest price. Most facilities have a product evaluation committee that considers new products from quality and cost perspectives. The committee's findings regarding various products will assist the manager in choosing quality supplies and equipment at a reasonable price. Supply costs can also be controlled by closely monitoring the amount used. Managers should encourage practices that control waste and prevent pilferage; for example, equipment that is reusable should not be treated as if it were disposable.

McKay, cited by Edwardson (1988) suggests that increasing the cost sensitivity among nursing personnel is another means of controlling supply costs. McKay further states that "one nurse manager was able to produce large savings by simply placing price tags on chargeable supplies. Nurses in the study hospital discovered that they could substitute less costly items with no untoward effects and avoid using some items altogether" (Edwardson, 1988, p. 84).

Nurse managers must also look at utilization indicators as a way to monitor costs while providing quality care. A review of indicators such as occupancy and average length of stay over a specified time period will reveal trends that can assist the nurse manager in making decisions regarding appropriate bed utilization. The use of care maps, for instance, allows managers to monitor the average length of stay for selected diagnostic groups of patients.

To manage resources effectively, nurse managers must also examine the process used in providing care. A nurse manager should ask, for example, whether some of the routine tests and procedures for patients could be done more efficiently. Raising such questions often leads to important changes in the delivery of services. For example, pre-admission clinics and same-day admission programs have become common practice, allowing elective patients to receive their diagnostic tests as outpatients one or two days before admission to hospital. Pre-admission clinics reduce the average length of stay for patients and improve their quality of life by reducing their time spent away from home. It is worth noting, however, that while pre-admission programs increase the number of patients who can be admitted, the patients who are admitted to hospital are, on average, more acutely ill while in hospital and will therefore likely increase the overall cost of care provided by the facility.

Managers of nursing services must work closely with other health care providers, including medical staff and allied health professionals, to assess the utilization of services. Working as a team, these individuals can determine whether services and programs should be introduced, continued, or discontinued. Efforts should be made to ensure that more effective use of resources is accompanied by an improvement in the quality of care provided.

Leadership Implications

The budget is a potent instrument for introducing important changes because of the necessity to plan and evaluate patient care services on an annual basis. The requirement to develop persuasive arguments, not only for retaining existing services at current levels, but also for implementing new or improved services, provides many leadership challenges. Leaders will not hesitate to propose changes that have budgetary ramifications, even in tight economic circumstances. Indeed, if there are unmet health care needs, operational inefficiencies, or quality of work life problems, it is the responsibility of leaders and managers to bring these issues forward at budget time, if not before. Once articulated, new proposals can be subsequently revived if they do not at first succeed. Skilled leadership is required to handle the less desirable aspects of budgeting, for example, when cuts have to be made and staff must be laid off. Such times are difficult enough for staff whose jobs are at risk during cutbacks, but they also create anxiety for people in leadership positions who must implement the bad news and interpret the reasons for unpopular administrative decisions to a vulnerable staff. The exercise of sensitive leadership during these times is essential for maintaining effective health services during periods of cost containment.

Preparing budgets often requires attending meetings with finance and human resource personnel who generally know much more about finance than they do about nursing. As nursing services consume such a large proportion of hospital budgets, the nursing budget is apt to come under heavy scrutiny as a target for economizing. This is why it is imperative that nurses be represented at executive levels of health agencies by professional nurse leaders who can interpret the nature of patient care requirements and justify the nursing resources requested in the budget. The findings of research with respect to professional nurse staffing and patient outcomes (see Chapters 18 and 19) are providing a good source of information to support the case for professional nursing resources. As well, it can still be argued that patients are not generally admitted to hospitals unless they need nursing care.

Summary

- Fiscal restraint has resulted in the restructuring of health care organizations throughout Canada, and health agencies are adopting business strategies to deliver services to patients and clients.
- A business plan is a set of statements about the mission, goals, and strategies of an organization that are to be accomplished within a set period of time.
- Budgeting and financial management are integral components of a business plan.
- Nursing services generally consume approximately 70% of the total operating budgets of hospitals.
- Managers are responsible for two types of budgets, capital budgets and operating budgets.
- Management information systems (MIS) guidelines are used across Canada to standardize financial reporting and statistics related to health care costs.
- Budget reports are used to provide managers with the means for controlling costs through regular monitoring of variances. Comparing the difference between expected performance and actual performance will reveal both positive (under budget) and negative (over budget) variances, allowing corrective action to be taken, if necessary.
- Cost containment is the responsibility of managers and staff and can be achieved by re-examining all aspects of patient care delivery to ensure efficient use of human and material resources.

Applying the Knowledge in this Chapter

Case Study

Using the concepts discussed in this chapter for calculating staffing and medical/surgical supplies, draw up an operating budget for a pre-admission clinic having the characteristics listed below.

Human Resources:

0.2 FTE Manager whose annual salary is $65,000*

1.5 FTE Registered nurses each at the 4th level of the salary scale ($27.55 per hour)

0.75 FTE Receptionist at entry level salary ($13.25 per hour)

0.5 FTE Ward aide ($12.00/hour)

0.5 FTE Transportation aide ($12.00/hour)

*The manager is responsible for four other outpatient clinics.

Medical and Office Supplies:

Stationery	$1500.00
Photocopy	$ 500.00
Laundry	$1200.00
Miscellaneous medical	$ 850.00

Revenue:

Donations	$175.00

The current year's budget was calculated using the rates above. You expect a 2% increase in the cost of living by the end of the current year. The clinic operates 220 days per year with an average of 40 patients per day.

1. What assumptions will you need to make? For example, what assumption will you make about the hours that make up one FTE position? If you make assumptions, you must state them.

2. Identify the fixed and variable costs of this clinic. If there are fixed costs, decide if they should be added to your budget.

3. What proportion of the manager's salary will you allocate to this clinic?

4. The finance director has asked you to calculate the cost per visit. How would you calculate this item?

Resources

𝑒𝑣𝑜𝑙𝑣𝑒 Internet Resources

Canadian Institute of Health Information:
  http://secure.cihi.ca/cihiweb/splash.html
The Management Information System Guidelines:
  http://secure.cihi.ca/cihiweb/dispPage.jsp?cw_page=mis_e

References

Buchan, J. (1992). Cost effective caring. *International Nursing Review*, *39*(4), 117–120.

Canadian Institute for Health Information. (2004). *Healthcare spending to reach $130 billion this year; per capita spending to hit $4,000*. Retrieved January 17, 2005, from http://secure.cihi.ca/cihiweb/dispPage.jsp?cw_page=media_17dec2003_e

Canadian Institute for Health Information. (2003). *Health spending expected to reach 10% of GDP in 2003, reports CIHI*. Retrieved August19, 2003, from http://secure.cihi.ca/cihiweb/dispPage.jsp?cw_page=media_17dec2003_e

Canadian Institute for Health Information. (1994). Nursing inpatient services. In *Guidelines for management information systems in Canadian health care facilities*. Ottawa, ON: Canadian Institute for Health Information.

Edwardson, S.R. (1988). Productivity. In E.J. Sullivan & P.J. Decker (Eds.), *Effective management in nursing* (2nd ed., pp. 71–92). Menlo Park, CA: Addison-Wesley.

Finkler, S.A., & Kovner, C.T. (2000). *Financial management for nurse managers and executives*. Philadelphia: W.B. Saunders.

Health Care Corporation of St. John's. (1996). *Mission statement*. [Mimeograph]. St. John's, NF: Author.

McConnell, C.R. (1993). The *effective health care supervisor*. Gaithersburg, MD: Aspen.

Oberg, L., & Wagner, N. (1994). *Getting started II: Health business plan guidebook*. Edmonton, AB: Alberta Health.

Swansburg, R.C. (2002). Principles of budgeting. In R.C. Swansburg & R.J. Swansburg (Eds.), *Introduction to management and leadership for nurse managers* (3rd ed., pp. 179–226). Boston: Jones and Bartlett.

Judith M. Hibberd

Learning Objectives

In this chapter, you will learn:

- The importance of effective writing skills for influencing decisions in health care agencies

- Basic principles of successful business writing

- Common types of administrative documents and the general purpose of each

- Resources and strategies for improving writing skills

- Practical guidelines for communicating with electronic technology

Nurses spend much of their time documenting clinical information, completing forms, and recording data from interviews with patients and colleagues. This type of writing is highly structured and repetitive, and although clinically and legally important, it often does not require composition of a complete sentence, much less a whole paragraph. However, increasingly nurses are required to prepare other types of documents such as formal letters, memoranda, minutes, reports, evaluations, briefs, and proposals. Producing such documents requires planning, collecting information, working with various formats, writing, and rewriting. Some documents written by managers may serve as evidence in a courtroom or arbitration hearing, for example, investigative reports or dismissal letters.

Despite extensive preparation, many health professionals do not write well and lack the confidence to compose an original report. This is also true of many managers, who may have difficulty putting ideas onto paper or into a word processor. Effective writing is a complex skill and an important professional and managerial responsibility. A well-written memorandum or report submitted in a timely manner can be a powerful means of influencing policy decisions in health care agencies.

When views, facts, arguments, and decisions are committed to paper, they become part of the permanent administrative record of a health care agency. Because institutional memories may be short and vague, written materials serve as a reliable historical record of events and are available to managers contemplating future organizational changes. If a written document is poorly constructed and the ideas not clearly developed, it will not direct or inform the reader, and it may stand as a lasting testimony to the writer's carelessness or lack of skill; ultimately, it could undermine the writer's credibility, professional reputation, and influence.

The purpose of this chapter is to provide practical advice on writing the most common types of administrative documents; to examine the most common types of documents that staff write, receive, and review; and to discuss the impact that electronic technology has had on written communications.

For those who are already good writers, this chapter will serve as a quick reference. For those who find writing difficult and time-consuming and want to do something about it, this chapter may provide encouragement and tips on how to improve this essential skill. Writing skills can be improved, and for many professionals, writing becomes a routine process of self-assessment, trial, error, and continuous learning.

Practical Guidelines for Writing Administrative Documents

Some general guidelines apply to all types of administrative writing, regardless of the type of document or method of transmission. These guidelines cover issues relating to style, writing resources, organization, and communications technology.

Style

The style of writing in administrative documents tends to be more formal than that used in personal letters and notes, and less formal than that used in term papers or journal articles. The writer should review memoranda (or memos), reports, and other documents in the workplace to determine the level of formality generally adopted because it varies among institutions. In fact, much can be learned about the culture of an organization from the standard of writing displayed in memoranda and communications posted on bulletin boards. For example, the tone of a memorandum and the way in which it gives direction may reveal the writer's values and management style; they may even reflect the writer's mood at the time of writing. When composing a memorandum, writers must think about the impression they wish to leave with the reader and the extent to which their directives and communications are consistent with the organization's mission and culture.

A fundamental rule in writing is to make the tone sound genuine; you will sound genuine by simply being yourself (Zinsser, 1985). It is possible to write in a formal manner without seeming pretentious or stuffy (Stewart & Kowler, 1991). Your personal standards will undoubtedly be reflected in your writing and will be a model for your staff. Business writing should be direct, simply expressed, and without clutter. Shorter sentences are better than longer ones. Language should be chosen carefully to promote uniform interpretation by your readers. Jargon and rhetoric should be avoided, and emotional undertones such as innuendoes and euphemisms should be rejected.

Zinsser (1985) was highly critical of most business writing, saying that we "are a society strangling in unnecessary words, circular constructions, pompous frills and meaningless jargon" (p. 7). He suggested that every sentence should be stripped to its cleanest components. Remove words that serve no function, replace long words with shorter words, eliminate redundancies, and substitute the active case for the passive. Such plain writing may be difficult to adopt at first, but it is essential for expressing your ideas clearly. When giving direction to staff, for example, there is no room for ambiguity. If a communication is unclear and confusing, staff will waste time trying to interpret the message and may even be misled by it.

The principle of unambiguous writing is especially true when issuing a policy (in which the reader is being told what to do) or a procedure (in which the reader is being told how to do it). In the case of policy and procedure manuals, "the writer must pay particular attention to the needs of the reader and use every technique available to communicate with accuracy, clarity, [and] brevity so that the material can be readily understood. True sophistication in manual writing lies in expressing complex ideas in a simple manner" (Cryderman, 1996, p. 209). Thus, efficiency and effectiveness will be enhanced when the rules and directives that guide decision making are written with clarity.

Writing Resources

Effective writing cannot be achieved without a good grasp of the basic rules and writing techniques. When drafting an administrative document, it is important to use proper grammar, syntax, spelling, and punctuation. One might expect such rules to be applied automatically in institutional writing, but common errors can often be found in all but the most highly scrutinized documents. Many excellent handbooks on style and grammar are available if you need to review basic elements of grammar.

Few people can write effectively without some basic tools, such as a dictionary, style guide, and thesaurus. These resources are standard office equipment for any manager. They also are incorporated into word processing packages and are available on the Internet. Some resources are listed at the end of this chapter. Consult these tools frequently, and keep hard-copy versions within reach of your desks at work and at home; they will help you avoid embarrassing errors and may stimulate creative writing. The spell-check function on computers is useful, but it is not infallible and cannot detect errors such as a wrong date, time, or place of a meeting.

It may sometimes be tempting to dictate a letter and ask a clerical assistant to sign it on your behalf. With the widespread use of computers, a person may draft a dozen letters at home, then hand a disk containing the files to an assistant to be formatted, printed, signed, and dispatched. With routine letters, this is an effective time management strategy; however, in non-routine letters that convey significant messages or announcements to key people in an organization, failing to include your personal signature may offend the recipients and diminish the impact of the message. Moreover, you should read these important messages over again; there may be mistakes, misinterpretations, or just plain bad writing that a clerical assistant has not questioned.

If a report is lengthy and has undergone many drafts and changes, hiring an editor may be money well invested. An editor will review consistency of style and format and give the document a final polish. It is common practice for scholars to write multiple drafts of a single journal article and then obtain several reviews and editorial assistance before submitting it for publication.

Organizing the Content

The format of the document is the way in which the text is laid out on the page and the ideas and points are organized. Standardized formats exist for memoranda, letters, incident reports, and other short reports. Most hospitals, nursing homes, and community health agencies use printed letterhead and printed forms for these communications. Non-routine reports and proposals are generally not as structured, so creativity and imagination will be needed when organizing ideas and recommendations in these less standardized forms of writing.

A variety of software programs are available to help writers organize their ideas in an attractive manner. Word processing programs often include a range of templates for standard business documents such as memoranda, letters, and reports. Health care agencies (especially the smaller ones) generally ensure that at least one clerical employee has the skills needed to handle graphics and produce professional looking documents without incurring a great deal of expense and effort. Such people can help produce a well-designed title page for a report, discussion paper, or proposal. An attractive title page is likely to catch the reader's attention in much the same way that a succinct abstract or executive summary will determine whether the reader will read the full report or not. Such fine tuning lends credibility to documents and makes the job of the reader much easier. Even those who do not possess graphics software can produce a document that is neatly formatted and well spaced on the page or even attractively handwritten, if necessary. The overall appearance of any written document is important; it creates a supportive framework for the arguments, ideas, and information contained within the message.

Students often underestimate the importance of the appearance of their papers and resist producing their written assignments in the prescribed formats. Many are frustrated when professors insist on fine details, such as requiring them to follow APA style as described by the American Psychological Association (APA, 2001). However, attending to the seemingly minor details is essential for creating a well-written document. According to Harris and McDougall (1958), a grammatical error is a barrier to effective communication because it undermines the writer's authority. So does a carelessly prepared manuscript. They also noted that

> If the writer has chosen the wrong kind of paper, has failed to provide adequate margins, has not numbered his [or her] pages, or has neglected to place the title of the essay in the appropriate position on the first page, the reader is likely to feel either that the writer is ignorant of what constitutes a well prepared page or that he [or she] is not willing to take the necessary pains. To antagonize the reader at the outset is certainly not going to improve our chances of convincing him [or her] that what we have to say is sound (Harris & McDougall, p. 100).

The final point in this excerpt is particularly true if the reader happens to be a teacher, or worse, an employer whom you want to influence or, at least, impress. Try to avoid the gender-biased writing demonstrated in the quotation above. Such writing was prevalent until the 1950s, but it is not tolerated today in professional writing. Most reputable handbooks on style contain advice on how to keep your writing free of gender bias and other types of bias (see, for example, APA, 2001, pp. 66–67).

Communications Technology

There is little doubt that communications technology has quickened the pace of managerial work. Written information that would have taken days or even weeks to transmit a few years ago can now be obtained within minutes by fax or e-mail. A letter can be sent instantaneously to hundreds of names on a mailing list all around the world. Responses to such communications are often immediate. You can also transmit lengthy documents by attaching files to e-mails, saving reams of paper in the process. Individuals can set up personal Web sites on the Internet and communicate daily with people they may never meet in person. Groups of managers may be connected to a local area network or may join newsgroups for communication and exchange of information.

Communications technology has changed our work lives—and not always for the better. People have come to expect instant information when needed. If the technology breaks down or cannot be accessed, stress may be created in the workplace, and routine operations may be seriously affected. Also, one can easily become a slave to e-mail. After a few days away from work, managers may find a hundred or more e-mail messages (to say nothing about copious junk mail) awaiting their attention, as well as the customary pile of hard copy items in their in-baskets. Responding to such a deluge of information can be time-consuming. Managers need to establish ways to control the torrent of information before it controls them. Nevertheless, when used wisely, this technology improves efficiency and saves a great deal of time.

E-mail messages should be written with the same kind of care as a hard-copy letter or memorandum in all but the most informal of messages. They can be printed out and filed for future reference and can be used by lawyers as evidence in legal proceedings. Because access to e-mail is so quick and easy, messages can be fired off rapidly before collecting one's thoughts. This can be particularly devastating if a person writes in anger or frustration. After you hit the send button, the message cannot be retrieved, and the consequences may be regrettable and even harmful to individuals.

It is important to proofread e-mail messages before sending them because people expect high standards from professional workers. Blicq and Moretto (2000) suggested that choosing e-mail over a written letter should always be a conscious decision. They also say that e-mail does not give you permission to write snippets of disconnected information, write incorrectly constructed sentences, forget about using proper punctuation, ignore misspelled words, or be abrupt or impolite.

Health care agencies should issue written policies clearly stating the expectations of employees with respect to the use of e-mail. E-mail should not be used to transmit patient information because security and confidentiality cannot be guaranteed, thus raising risk management and privacy concerns. It also should not be used for personal communications. Employees have been disciplined for using employers' e-mail for personal reasons (Tapp, 2001). There are similar problems and legal risks related to the use of the Internet at work, and again, employers should develop written policies about this issue (Tapp, 2002).

Right Type of Document

There are often no guidelines for helping a nurse select an appropriate type of written document, and there seems to be little in the nursing management literature on forms of writing. How does a person decide whether an issue or problem can be addressed with a memorandum, a letter, or a report, or whether it can be dealt with simply by a telephone call or an e-mail? Much will depend on the recipient of the document, the nature of the problem or issue, whether or not the matter is routine, and the ultimate distribution of the document. If the recipient is an individual staff member and the subject is related to performance, a future career, or a specific assignment, the document most likely should be a letter. If the recipient is someone who has sent you a letter that requires a response—for example, a request for a reference—then you should certainly reply with a letter. On the other hand, if the recipient was your entire staff, a memorandum would be the most appropriate choice, especially if your purpose is to make an announcement or communicate new information.

Routine reports to senior management generally follow a standard organization and may even be submitted on a form specifically designed for the purpose. However, if a manager wishes to propose an operational activity, such as a major change in staffing or programming for clients, a less standardized document will be required. An executive secretary can provide examples of proposals, discussion papers, and position statements; experienced executive secretaries handle dozens of types of written documents, and they can offer advice on how documents should be written and presented and what form they should take.

The remainder of this chapter is devoted to describing some of the most common administrative documents encountered by nurses, the purposes of these documents, and how they may be written to achieve the health care agency's goals.

Minutes of Meetings

In health agencies, as in most organizations, much time is spent at meetings where many administrative decisions are made. Permanent records of such decision making are kept as minutes. Minutes are a kind of report of what happened at a meeting and what action was taken (Zilm & Entwistle, 2002).

Few people like "taking the minutes," for various reasons; for example, some may find that contributing to the discussion is difficult when one is responsible for recording it. Moreover, not every manager has secretarial support; these managers must take time after the meeting to finalize the document before circulating it to the participants. Despite these problems, taking the minutes might be a good opportunity to start developing reporting skills.

Minutes should be recorded accurately and concisely, and they should be organized in the same order as the agenda that was approved at the meeting. The structure and formality of meetings varies enormously; for example, health agency board meetings will most likely follow *Robert's Rules of Order* (Robert, 1967), and the minutes will include names of movers and seconders of motions, the motion itself, and some of the principal arguments in favour of or in opposition to the motion. At the other end of the formality spectrum, unit staff meetings are likely to be informal and consist primarily of information giving. Decisions may be made by consensus rather than by formal motion and vote. The minutes may be typed, printed, and filed in a manual, or they may be as brief as a few handwritten notes in a communications book. Novice minute takers should check previous minutes to determine the expected standard of recording. The recording of decisions in the minutes can provide indisputable evidence that an issue or problem has been addressed, which can be influential in settling disputes and questions.

Business Letters

Writing letters is a common task for nurses but particularly for managers. For example, reference letters may be written on behalf of staff or former employees who are applying for jobs or research grants. References generally are written as letters unless, of course, you have been requested to complete a specific form. Letters are written also to document disciplinary problems, and copies are sent to the union (if any) and to the employee's file. Letters are also the document of choice when answering a job advertisement for a senior position, when making complaints about patient services or treatment, or when writing to the editor of a newspaper.

A "covering" letter almost always accompanies such documents as discussion papers, reports, and briefs. In other words, written communications that are sent outside the agency are most likely to be in the form of letters. If for no other reason than for good public relations, letters should be well written and look presentable.

Business letters follow a standard format, are written on agency letterhead, and consist of the following elements:

- Logo, address, and telephone/fax number of sender (usually part of the letterhead)
- Date
- Recipient's name, title, and address
- Salutation
- Text of the letter
- Complimentary closure
- Signature (with the sender's name and title, typed)

In addition to these elements, business letters may include a file number, placed under the date, which respondents are expected to quote when replying. The abbreviation "encl." placed under the sender's signature indicates that another document is enclosed with the letter; the abbreviation "cc:" (which stands for "carbon copy") followed by a name or names indicates who received copies of the letter. Letters written on word processors usually include the name of the file in fine print in the bottom left-hand corner. A sample letter responding to an applicant for a registered nurse position appears in Box 30.1.

Memoranda

Memoranda, or memos, are documents used exclusively for communicating information, announcements, instructions, policies, and decisions to employees within organizations. They are therefore internal documents, and nurses are likely to write memoranda more than any other type of administrative document. A memorandum is often shorter and less formal than a letter, and because it may be disseminated to a wide audience, it must be accurate, concise, coherent, and focus on only one topic. For example, it would not be helpful to write about an upcoming fire drill in the same memorandum announcing the date of the next accreditation survey; the two events are unrelated, and memoranda often are filed by subject matter.

As with letters, there is a standard format for memoranda. Health care agencies often have a printed form, with the name of the hospital, nursing home, or clinic at the top. Because memoranda are used internally, they do not record the recipients' address. Individual departments may use specially printed memoranda that indicate the departmental telephone and fax numbers. The elements of any memorandum are as follows:

- Date (date the memorandum is sent)
- To (person, group, or department)
- From (name and title of sender)

Box 30.1

Sample Letter

WELL KNOWN HOSPITAL
54321 Major Drive
Well Known City, BC V4Z 6X3
Telephone (604) 555-1234
Fax (604) 555-5678

December 18, 2005

File: 02:30

Ms. Anne Applicant, RN
1234 Urban Ave.
Well Known City, SK S7R 8K0

Re: Application for RN position

Dear Ms. Applicant:

The Personnel Office has given me your letter of application. You expressed interest in a position in Extended Care, and I will have an opening at the end of January. Our unit has 46 long-term female residents, mainly elderly, but also has a few young women with severe physical and mobility disabilities. I have looked over your letter and résumé, and I believe you may have the skills we need for our unit's team of nurses.

I will be holding interviews with two other possible applicants in early January. If you would like an interview, please telephone me as soon as possible so that we can schedule a time.

The best times to reach me are weekday afternoons between 1300 and 1500 hours. Telephone the hospital number above and ask for local 305.

Sincerely,

K. Smithers

Kerin Smithers, RN, BSN
Unit Care Manager
Westbrook Unit

KS/at
cc: Personnel Office, T.K. Paterson

Source: Adapted from *The SMART Way: An Introduction to Writing for Nurses* (2nd ed., p. 136), by G. Zilm and C. Entwistle, 2002, Toronto, ON: Elsevier. Reprinted with permission.

- Subject (concise description of subject)
- Message
- Signature (optional).

The first four elements are grouped together at the top of the page. The subject is given prominence, usually in bold type and underlined, and represents the title of the memorandum. The message, or body, of the memorandum consists of an introduction or a statement of the purpose of the memorandum, a discussion or explanation of the main points, and a conclusion and/or instructions. Box 30.2 is an example of a memorandum.

It is important to attract and retain the reader's attention in the first few sentences of a memorandum. Zinsser's (1985) advice to those writing articles applies equally well to memoranda. He stated that the first sentence is the most important: "If it doesn't induce the reader to proceed to the second sentence, your [memo] is dead. And if the second sentence doesn't induce [the reader] to continue to the third sentence, it's equally dead" (Zinsser, 1985, p. 65). Memoranda should be logically constructed so that each sentence leads directly into the next, "tugging" readers forward until they are safely "hooked" (Zinsser, 1985). In the sample memorandum in Box 30.2, the first sentence will undoubtedly catch people's attention because the incidence of severe acute respiratory syndrome (SARS) is a serious concern.

Unlike letters, memoranda do not need any form of greeting, salutation, or complimentary closure. Some people sign memoranda; others simply initial by their names at the top of the page. Like letters, memoranda may include abbreviations related to enclosures (encl.), copies (cc:), or filing information in the bottom left-hand corner of the page.

Most memoranda are no longer than a page, but this type of document is flexible and can also be used for short reports, investigations, or even proposals and recommendations.

Proposals

Proposals are often written to obtain approval and funding for research, but they also are written for other reasons, such as requesting approval for projects or even new pieces of equipment. Because almost any new program or procedure is likely to have financial implications not encompassed in the current budget, nurses should develop the skills required to write a good proposal. Proposals are often the end product of much discussion among staff and managers about a problem or an idea, and they may involve a preliminary investigation to collect information, review the literature, and survey similar health care agencies.

There is no standard format for proposal writing because much will depend on the nature of the plan, the audience, and the resources required to carry out the project. If research is planned, the proposal must be prepared in the format required by review bodies, namely ethics committees and internal or external funding agencies. Guidelines for preparing a research proposal may be found in introductory research textbooks. Examples of research proposals can usually be obtained from agency files or people who have joint appointments with universities.

Box 30.2

Sample Memorandum

PLAINS REGIONAL HEALTH AUTHORITY
Memorandum

Date: April 2, 2003

To: Clinical Directors and Program Managers
          All staff

From: James Hinton, RN, MN
          Infection Control Coordinator

Subject: **Severe Acute Respiratory Syndrome (SARS): Lecture Series**

As a result of the recent outbreak of SARS in Toronto, the Plains Regional Health Authority (PRHA) has authorized a plan to prepare for the admission of patients with SARS. Although there have been no reported cases of SARS in this province, we must be ready to provide the necessary services should a patient with suspected SARS arrive in the Emergency Department. Over the next two weeks, we are offering a series of lectures on what is currently known about this new disease, its origin, transmission, signs, symptoms, duration, treatment, and care. The requirement for quarantine for persons exposed to people with suspected SARS will be explained.

All lectures will be held in the Louis Riel Auditorium from 1100–1200 hours. Dr. W. A. Williams, Medical Officer of Health, will give the first lecture on Monday, April 7, 2003, at 1100 hours, and his topic is "SARS: Overview of a new infectious disease." There will be an opportunity for the staff to ask questions, so as many of you as possible should attend these lectures.

Each lecture will be videotaped, and the videos will be available through the Continuing Education Office (Room 101.2, Main Building) to any member of the staff who is unable to attend. The schedule of lectures will be posted on main Notice Boards and on the PRHA's Infolink by Friday, April 4, 2003. In the meantime, up-to-date information on SARS can be found on the Health Canada (www.hc.gc.ca/) and the World Health Organization (www.who.int/) Web sites.

tel: ext. 6243
e-mail: james.hinton@PRHA.mb.ca
cc: Katrina Korechka, BA, MEd
          Director, Continuing Education
          PRHA Infolink

To obtain approval for innovative ideas, you must present a good argument. Arguing in this sense is not to disagree about something, but "to offer a set of reasons or evidence in support of a conclusion" (Weston, 1992, p. x). A proposal usually starts with a problem statement, for example: "With the marked increase in clients attending outpatient clinics, the existing waiting room area and washroom facilities are now inadequate." The proposal in this example would include supporting evidence, such as figures on clinic attendance, to illustrate the problem. It also might include client comments about lack of privacy and waiting in line for the washrooms. Several possible solutions would then be suggested, with a specific recommendation. The cost of this specific recommendation, and possibly the comparative costs of other options, would be itemized.

In short, a proposal is a plan for addressing a problem or suggesting an innovative idea. It includes reasons why senior management should support the plan, the methods to be used, the human and financial resources required, the necessary time period, and the implications for the health care agency. A proposal is thus a forward-looking document.

Written Reports

Once a proposal's plan is implemented, there usually will be progress reports and a final report to write. Reports, therefore, are retrospective documents that account for events or projects that have already taken place.

There are many kinds of reports, but they all have two characteristics in common: they are based on factual information that has been collected and presented in an organized form, and they supply needed information to the person or institution requesting the report (Stewart & Kowler, 1991). In all cases, the information reported is used as a basis for decision making. A report is an impartial objective account of events, activities, or investigations. Topics of reports may range from information as simple and routine as a narcotic count, to periodic summaries of operations or highly complex confidential inquiries.

The majority of reports that nurses write are of a routine nature. Many are written on specially designed forms, ensuring consistency of reporting and adequacy of information. An incident report used for reporting medication errors is an example. Facts from this kind of report may be entered into databases for legal or accounting purposes. For example, the manager of an intensive care unit (ICU) may be required to submit a monthly report summarizing all codes responded to within the hospital. These reports may be used to calculate costs associated per code and may ultimately assist with resource planning for the ICU. Similarly, a manager may occasionally be required to explain variances between actual and budgeted expenditures so that total expenditures for a health care agency can be closely monitored.

Other routine reports include personnel performance appraisals, for which specially designed forms may be used. These forms usually do not require the manager to plan or organize the information but merely to write short answer and narrative responses to questions. On the other hand, if a special report is requested on the performance of a staff member who has been in some kind of difficulty, then the manager may have to plan and organize an original document.

It is generally true that the less routine the report, the fewer the guidelines for writing it. However, most non-routine reports contain the following items in this order:

- Title page
- Executive summary
- Introduction and background, including review of relevant reports and literature
- Methods used to collect data and sources of information
- Presentation of findings, analysis, and discussion
- Conclusions and recommendations (may be separate sections)
- Reference list
- Appendices (may include terms of reference or authorization, letters, charts, data sheets, or cost implications of various options recommended).

In summary, a report is an account of an investigation, event, or problem. Many reports are made verbally, leaving no permanent record, but written reports usually become part of the organization's archives. The nature and scope of the subject and the person or group commissioning the report will determine the formality and detail to be included in the document. Whatever the nature of the subject, all written reports, whether a single page or more than 100 pages, consist of four main elements: an introduction, an investigation, a discussion, and conclusions.

Literature Reviews

A literature review is a written summary of the current literature on a topic. It involves an extensive, thorough, and systematic examination of publications relevant to the project (Seaman, 1987). Obviously, managers need to subscribe to some key journals so that they can keep current with trends and issues in their field. They also need to have access to libraries and databases so they can review literature on various aspects of their work. The rate at which both administrative and clinical changes are occurring requires that managers demonstrate skill in assessing current literature. Moreover, there is a need to read the literature critically, weigh the strengths and weaknesses of the research methods, and evaluate the findings of published research. For example, in developing care maps, professional staff need to be aware of the latest approaches to care and treatment of clients in a particular diagnostic category; one of the first tasks would be to see what is being reported in the professional and research literature.

Reviewing literature is a complex intellectual skill that takes much time to develop. Most undergraduate textbooks on research contain whole chapters on how to review the literature. A brief literature review is an integral part of any research article, and sometimes, journals include literature reviews as complete articles (see, for example, Hall & Donner, 1997). Whether writing a report, brief, or discussion paper, a manager's effectiveness in influencing decisions will be enhanced if these documents reflect a careful analysis of recent literature on the topic being addressed.

Briefs

A brief is a short report, usually recommending some kind of action (Zilm & Entwistle, 2002). It may be delivered verbally or in writing. In the political world, one might read in the newspaper that the minister of some federal department has been "briefed" on the latest developments in the portfolio. In this situation, an aide or advisor has investigated the issue or problem, summarized the information, and identified options open to the minister for his or her public statement. Briefs in the health care system are more likely to be written, and due to their nature, are often biased toward a particular position. Indeed, they may also include a formal position statement on the topic. Briefs are written with the intention of influencing decisions or public policy. To be effective, they should be written clearly, persuasively, and succinctly, and they should stick to the point, avoiding rhetorical digressions. Nurses' professional associations and unions often write briefs to governments to inform the public policy process and express their perspectives and recommendations on a variety of issues affecting either nursing services to the public or the work of nurses.

Nurses in leadership and management positions may write briefs to influence policy decisions in their agency. They may write a brief individually or in collaboration with colleagues in other disciplines. With the disappearance of functional departments, a brief can, for example, be a useful way to inform administrators of the potential impact of organizational decisions on the practice of nursing. Hence, the brief can be written from a nursing perspective or any other perspective. It must provide supporting evidence to strengthen whatever position is being taken; for instance, if an agency has no policy statement about physical or verbal abuse from staff and clients, a brief could be written pointing out the need for such a policy. Evidence of recent abusive incidents in the agency could be cited, together with information on the policies that exist in other agencies. Again, reference to trends reported in the literature on institutional policies advocating zero tolerance of abuse in health care agencies would strengthen the brief.

A brief can be written as a memorandum or as a mini-report. Like all reports, it should have an introduction that includes a clear statement of purpose, a body of information, and arguments, conclusions, and recommendations. Unless its subject is confidential, the brief can be circulated among the staff as a means of informing them and securing their assistance and support.

Notes to File

The myriad of problems, issues, decisions, and events that nurses deal with on a daily basis places great demands on individual memories. Some of these decisions and events should be stored as written documents or electronic files, and this is particularly important in the case of management personnel. Over time, relying solely on memory can lead to disagreements about facts. Should a problem wind up in court or arbitration, evidence drawn from "notes to file" is likely to be more credible than evidence drawn from memory alone.

Managers can avoid the failure of their memories, besieged as they are with a great deal of daily minutiae, by dictating or entering a note to the relevant file. Notes to file are informal personal records of events, decisions, discussions, or telephone conversations. They are frequently confidential and thus kept in a locked filing cabinet or drawer. A note to file must be made when a manager gives an individual staff member a verbal warning. The date, time, incident, what was said, and the staff member's response will all be recorded in such a note along with plans for future follow-up. Depending on agency policy, such notes to file would also appear in the personnel file in the human resources department. Similarly, if the manager receives a complaint from a patient or patient's relative, the manager should create a file and document the conversation. Thus, managers should create a diary of events about situations that have the potential to become significant problems later on. Investing in a "day timer," or electronic diary, is probably the most efficient means of keeping track of items that require a note to file. Notes to file can be of great assistance in recalling events and a great source of historical data when justifying decisions or writing more formal and public documents.

Policy Issue Papers

Nurses are more likely to receive policy issue or discussion papers than they are to write them. Such documents are common in the health care system, and they may require an individual to formulate a response to the points raised in the discussion. The subject of these documents is often an emerging issue or proposed public policy.

Unlike briefs, policy issue or discussion papers are often lengthy and do not fall under a clear or universal format. Because the topics addressed are often new, one of the purposes of the paper may be to educate the reader. Hence, the body of the document may be didactic in tone, and careful attention may be given to defining the terms being used. For example, in a discussion paper released by the Alberta Association of Registered Nurses (AARN) on professional boundaries (1997), the introduction is devoted entirely to explaining what is meant by professional boundaries. In the body of the paper, the nurse-client relationship is examined. It uses case studies to illustrate many aspects of the issue, such as non-professional relationships, recognizing boundary signs, crossing professional boundaries, violations of professional boundaries, ethical implications, solutions, and options. After reading this paper, nurses should be able to discuss this subject with colleagues and describe professional boundary problems or concerns. Subsequently, they could be expected to develop the standards that would guide their practice in the work setting.

Because the topic of a policy issue or discussion paper is usually new, there are often many attachments or appendices. In the AARN paper, a glossary of terms is provided, followed by references, a review of the literature, a summary of what is happening in other jurisdictions, and a list of various teaching resources. Examples of policy issue papers, position statements, and reports can be found on the Canadian Nurses Association's Web site provided in Internet Resources at the end of the chapter.

Leadership Implications

Nurses aspiring to leadership and management positions in the health care system are expected to be effective writers and skilled users of information and computer technology. Career development may include writing articles for publication in professional journals, which contributes to the advancement of nursing as a discipline and provides a service to the public (Zilm, 2002). Nurse leaders should identify potential scholars on the staff and encourage them to co-author or take part in writing briefs, reports, and other types of papers. For this, they will need to be familiar with the Internet and finding reliable information.

Recent nursing graduates are computer literate and are used to searching the Web for information; however, senior staff nurses who were educated before the universal use of computers may not be confident using computer technology for communicating and obtaining information. Studies suggest that many factors mitigate the effective use of online resources by nurses, including anxiety or computer phobia, lack of time to experiment, problems of access, outdated hardware, lack of compatibility between work and home systems, poor technical support, and lack of writing and typing skills (Hughes & Pakieser, 1999; Scollin, 2001). With the availability of Web-based instruction, many nurses are taking advantage of this learning medium. Clearly, nurses in leadership positions can do much to help the staff identify, evaluate, and take advantage of Internet resources. They also can provide working environments that promote confidence and success in professional writing.

Summary

- Effective writing skills are essential for professional nurses and contemporary managers who spend much of their time documenting events and responding to requests for information.
- Well-written documents are likely to be more effective in influencing agency policies.
- Writing is a complex intellectual skill that can be developed with practice and critical self-appraisal.
- The most common administrative documents nurses will write are letters, memoranda, proposals, and reports.
- Electronic messages speed up the process of communicating, but the principles of effective writing are no less important than when using traditional media.
- Nurse leaders and managers serve as exemplars and teachers in identifying reliable Internet resources that will contribute information in support of clinical practice and professional writing.

Applying the Knowledge in this Chapter

Case Study

John Tarrant, BScN, has been appointed as the case manager for the Acquired Head Injury Rehabilitation Program of a large home care agency in a metropolitan area. This is an internal promotion and will take effect in a few weeks. Although he is well qualified to work with this client population, it has been four years since John has cared for a patient with a head injury or consulted the literature in this area. Consequently, John is anxious to update his knowledge of trends and practices in this clinical field. After finding a workshop that seems highly relevant to his continuing education needs, he discusses his need for financial support with his department head. She advises him to write a memorandum explaining his request for educational funding and send it as an attachment by e-mail to the chair of the Educational Fund Committee. John's expenses will include $350 for tuition (registration fee), $500 for travel, $425 for accommodation for three nights, and the standard $50 per diem allowance for meals and sundry expenses.

1. Compose John's memorandum to the chair of the Educational Fund Committee outlining his need.

2. Compose the e-mail communication explaining this request.

Resources

evolve Internet Resources

The Canadian Encyclopedia:
   www.thecanadianencyclopedia.com

Canadian Health Network:
   www.canadian-health-network.ca/

Canadian Nurses Association:
   www.cna-nurses.ca

Nursing Information:
   www.NurseLinx.com

US National Institutes of Health:
   www.health.nih.gov/

Webster's Dictionary and Thesaurus:
   www.m-w.com/home.htm

References

Alberta Association of Registered Nurses. (1997). *Professional boundaries: A discussion paper on expectations for nurse-client relationships.* Edmonton, AB: Author.

American Psychological Association. (2001). *Publication manual of the American Psychological Association* (5th ed.). Washington, DC: Author.

Blicq, R., & Moretto, L. (2000). *Get to the point! Writing effective email, letters, reports, and proposals.* Scarborough, ON: Prentice-Hall.

Cryderman, P. (1996). Manuals that work: A focus on writing and regionalisation. In S.A. Ziebarth (Ed.), *Pinched: A management guide to the Canadian health care archipelago* (pp. 207–219). Nepean, ON: Pinched Press.

Hall, L.M., & Donner, G.J. (1997). The changing role of hospital nurse managers: A literature review. *Canadian Journal of Nursing Administration, 10*(2), 14–39.

Harris, R.S., & McDougall, R.L. (1958). *The undergraduate essay.* Toronto, ON: University of Toronto Press.

Hughes, J.A., & Pakieser, R.A. (1999). Factors that impact nurses' use of electronic mail (E-mail). *Computers in Nursing, 17,* 251–258.

Robert, H.M. (1967). *Robert's rules of order.* New York: Jove Publications.

Scollin, P. (2001). A study of factors related to the use of online resources by nurse educators. *Computers in Nursing, 19,* 249–256.

Seaman, C.H.C. (1987). *Research methods: Principles, practice and theory for nursing* (3rd ed.). Norwalk, CT: Appleton & Lange.

Stewart, K.L., & Kowler, M.E. (1991). *Forms of writing: A brief guide and handbook.* Scarborough, ON: Prentice-Hall.

Tapp, A. (2001). The legal risks of e-mail. *Canadian Nurse, 97*(3), 35–36.

Tapp, A. (2002). Cyberlaw. *Canadian Nurse, 98*(4), 30–31.

Weston, A. (1992). *A rulebook for arguments* (2nd ed.). Indianapolis, IN: Hackett.

Zilm, G. (2002). The write time. *Canadian Journal of Nursing Leadership, 15*(2), 25–30.

Zilm, G., & Entwistle, C. (2002). *The SMART way: An introduction to writing for nurses* (2nd ed.). Toronto, ON: Elsevier.

Zinsser, W. (1985). *On writing well: An informed guide to writing nonfiction* (3rd ed.). New York: Harper & Row.

Donna Lynn Smith and John Church

Learning Objectives

In this chapter, you will learn:

- ■ Terminology relevant to an understanding of the policy process

- ■ The roles and influence of the environment and stakeholders in the policy process

- ■ A model of problem-centred policy analysis

- ■ How issues and trends become identified as policy problems needing to be acted upon

- ■ Models of policy and decision making

- ■ About the relationship between policy and strategy

- ■ How policy analysis is organized and conducted in large organizations

- ■ Skills of the policy analyst

There is a large and growing stream of nursing literature that emphasizes the importance of nursing contributions to public policy discourse, instances in which nursing has successfully influenced policy formation, and concern about the exclusion of nursing and nursing issues from mainstream health care decision making (Cheek & Gibson, 1997; Clarke, 2003; Dannemiller & Jacobs, 1992; Helms, Anderson, & Hanson, 1996; Hewison, 1999; Prescott, 1993; Shamian, Skelton-Green, & Villeneuve, 2003; Skelton-Green, 1996; Valentine, 2000; West & Scott, 2000). This emphasis upon the importance and skills of *policy advocacy* is valuable to all registered nurses (RNs); however, this chapter focuses on the skills associated with *policy analysis*, which often occurs in organizational settings where opportunities for policy advocacy are more limited.

Since politics and public policy are inseparable, we begin this chapter with a brief discussion of these two concepts. This sets the stage for a more detailed discussion of models and analytical approaches for understanding and analyzing health policy in an applied setting.

What Is Politics?

At its very heart, politics is about power—the ability to control and manipulate one's environment and everything in it. An important means of doing this is by deciding which set of societal values will be given priority (Easton, 1965). When politicians are deciding which values will receive greater priority, they are also deciding how public resources, often taxpayers' money, will be allocated, or more to the point, "who gets what, when and how" (Lasswell, 1958). Public policy, then, is what government chooses to do or not to do (Dye, 1972), and as the contemporary rock band Rush once noted, "If you choose not to decide, you still have made a choice" (Rush, 1980).

What Is Public Policy?

Public policy decision making is rarely a single event (Lomas, 2000). More realistically, as Jenkins (1978) points out, it is a set of interrelated decisions about what the policy goals are and how best to achieve them. In principle, at least, whatever is decided should be within the power of the decision makers to achieve.

The noted management theorist and researcher Henry Mintzberg (Mintzberg & Waters, 1985) has described policy as "pattern in action," emphasizing the point that policies rarely tackle single problems. Rather, they face clusters of entangled problems that have complex and contradictory solutions (Pal, 1997). When we observe how governments respond to large and complex issues, such as poverty, we see that they often address certain specific issues (e.g., nutrition for young children) with fairly narrow policy responses (e.g., school lunch program). In directing resources toward a partial solution, the government hopes that, over time, the larger problem will be diminished. The government response is intended to demonstrate to voters that politicians are aware of the problem that needs attention and they have done what they can within the limits of available public resources.

However, the public policy process is not as straightforward as the above example might imply. Figure 31.1 provides a framework for understanding the context within which public policy decisions are made. This figure helps to explain why the policy process is so complex, and it illustrates some of the many individuals and groups who may be involved in public policy decision making.

At the centre of the diagram are the structures and processes of government, including who has authority to make decisions, who will have a say in the process of making those decisions, and how those decisions will be made. Aside from the actual organizations of government and related processes, the institutional structure also includes the "rules of the game" for public policy decision making. These are usually fleshed out through government policy statements, legislation and related regulations, and informal understandings among government and non-government actors (interest groups, private organizations, and individuals) about what is

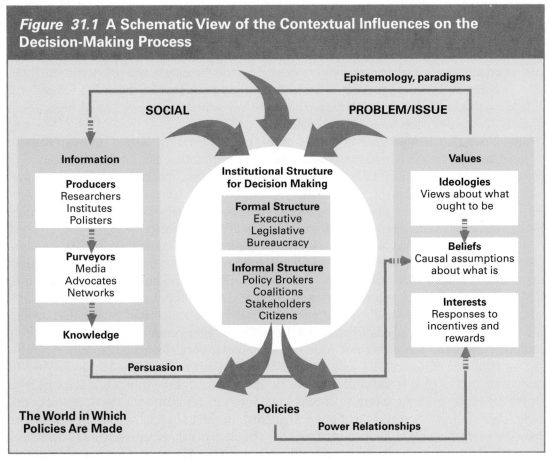

Figure 31.1 **A Schematic View of the Contextual Influences on the Decision-Making Process**

Source: From Connecting Research and Policy, by J. Lomas, 2000, *ISUMA: Canadian Journal of Policy Research*, *1*(1), p. 143.

acceptable behaviour. Policy issues arise within the context and structure of relationships and the division of power and accountability between federal, provincial, and local governments and the legislated mandates of other organizations (Brooks, 1993; Doern & Phidd, 1983). The role and prerogatives of the elected government, and the responsibilities of the courts and the bureaucracy responsible for carrying out government policy through departments and agencies, are key elements of the institutional framework.

In Canada, the constitutional division of power between the federal and provincial/territorial governments dictates that the provinces have the primary responsibility for making policy in the area of health care. The Constitution also assigns a major role for the federal government in raising money for public purposes. Thus, institutions in the Canadian federal system have created a situation in which one level of government is responsible for the provision of services but is reliant on another level of government for (in some cases) a significant part of the funding in order to provide those services.

Informal structures also play a key role in public policy making. Stakeholders are individuals or groups who have an interest in a particular issue, policy, or organization. A variety of internal and external stakeholders influence the process of policy formation and implementation in the health sector. Identifying key stakeholder groups and analyzing their interests and agendas is therefore a critical activity for policy makers. As noted in Chapter 8 on structure in health service organizations, certain stakeholder groups have traditionally held disproportionate influence in policy and decision making in the health care system. This is reflected in the national legislation that created the publicly funded health system, which emphasized payment for physician services and services provided in hospitals.

In the past two decades, the supremacy of these groups and the lack of transparency and accountability in the governance and management of health care organizations have been challenged by unions, individual citizens, consumer organizations, special interest groups representing particular religious views, and other organizations. It has now become necessary for health service organizations to develop processes to manage stakeholder participation or, more positively, to foster citizen engagement in policy and decision making.

In general, policies that are developed without the input of affected stakeholders are resisted and may not be successfully implemented. Therefore, the policy process typically includes an analysis of stakeholder groups and various consultation and communication activities designed to inform them, secure their cooperation, and, if this is not possible, at least to identify and plan for the areas and issues of resistance that can be anticipated. Stakeholder groups are sometimes called *policy audiences*, and the ability to tailor communications appropriately to these multiple audiences is now considered an important organizational capacity.

The right side of Figure 31.1 lists values, which are a mix of our individual and collective understandings of what is and what ought to be, and interests, those things that serve us best. At the collective level, the interplay of values and interests feeds into the development of differing views of how the world functions (paradigms). In the Canadian health care system, we have two overriding sets of competing paradigms. The clash of values between those who believe in a limited role for government in the health care market and those who see a significant role for government is often characterized as the debate over "privatization." A second debate revolves around the purpose of health care. Some interests view health care as primarily about the treatment of disease; others argue that, above all else, health care is about preventing disease and promoting health. Arguably, a third clash of values occurs around the role of federal, provincial, and territorial governments in the financing and delivery of health care. Some interests see the role of the federal government as limited to transferring money to the provinces and territories. Others see a strong role for the federal government in maintaining and enforcing some sort of uniform national standards.

On the left side of Figure 31.1 are the various sources and processes of information that feed into both values and the formal and institutional structures. These might include academic research, public opinion polls, reports from private think-tank organizations, government statistics, anecdotal stories, and reports in the media. All of these types of information are used in the public policy process. Significant resources are spent on getting and manipulating information by government and interest groups. The media (e.g., newspapers, books, magazines, radio, television) is a major lens through which most of us, including politicians, view the rest of the world.

Beyond the elements illustrated in Figure 31.1 are the larger environmental influences, such as economic, technological, and environmental change, that interact with institutions, interests, and ideas in the policy process (Weller, 1980). All health care organizations are affected by threats and opportunities in their environments, and these, in turn, influence organizational structure and strategies (Longest, 1996). Senior managers bear the ultimate responsibility for the analysis of public policy environments, but they typically rely on staff within policy and planning departments to implement the analyses and develop policy proposals and strategic plans. This is done frequently through a systematic process of environmental scanning (Longest, 1996). From this, alternative courses of action (policy options) are identified and presented to decision makers who then must make a choice. The remainder of this chapter focuses on understanding various ways in which policy decisions are made and the role of the policy analyst.

Models of Decision Making

While recognizing that most modern decision making is structured roughly around the rational model, we acknowledge that there is an element of truth in all of the models described.

The *rational model* and approach to policy analysis is one that assumes decisions can or should be "driven by information and by the careful and systematic comparison of alternatives and consequences" (Pal, 1997, p. 24). When the rational model is applied, objectives are chosen, and various alternatives or options for achieving the objectives are identified. The impacts of each alternative are analyzed in terms of their ability to achieve the objectives. Criteria for ranking the alternatives are made explicit. These may include consideration of financial issues and also the need for congruence with the opinions and preferences of key stakeholders and the public in general. Once a preferred alternative or set of alternatives is chosen, further analysis may be conducted to model the anticipated costs and consequences of implementing the preferred policy. An implementation strategy (usually including specific communications strategies) is then developed and the policy is implemented, either through existing operational departments of the organization or through a specially created project management structure or team. Ideally, both the implementation process and the outcomes of the policy are monitored and evaluated to determine what happened as the consequence of the policy decision and whether the predicted outcomes were achieved.

There are obvious benefits of bringing evidence and objectivity to bear on policy decisions. However, as Pal (1997) has explained, "rational decision-making models work best, if they work at all, when there is a single decision-maker with a clear and ordered set of priorities, and objectives, plentiful information, and comfortable timelines" (p. 20). Policy making occurs in contexts where political factors, ideology, and belief systems; the relative power of interest groups and public opinion; and financial constraints influence decision-making processes. Thus, most scholars and public administrators acknowledge that the policy process is inherently political and seldom operates in the linear fashion exemplified in the rational model.

Whereas the rational model is based on the assumption that decision makers will want to make decisions based on the best available information, other explanatory models have been proposed to explain the way policy and decision making actually occur (Brooks, 1993; Longest, 1996; Plumptre, 1990). In a classic paper entitled "The Science of 'Muddling Through'," Lindblom (1959) described an opportunistic approach to policy formation in which decision makers make "successive limited comparisons" of one alternative with another to see which is most likely to meet their objectives. Wrapp (1979) explains that it is neither practical nor desirable to have a policy statement to cover every possible eventuality; rather, he contends that policies can be inferred from an "indescribable mix" of operating decisions that evolve over time and which have discernable patterns. While specific goals may be appropriate for managers at lower levels of the organization, they may have the effect of limiting the opportunity for, and scope of, decision making at the top of the organization where there is a great deal of ambiguity and uncertainty.

Another description of the policy process is the *garbage can model*, which is based on an assumption that political realities and individual inclinations are the dominant elements in policy and decision-making processes. The model acknowledges the reality that decision making is a complex and unpredictable process that involves high levels of ambiguity, the need for pragmatism and compromise among stakeholder interests, political factors, and matters of expediency and timing. In descriptions of this model, problems are said to be "dumped" into a "garbage can" to be retrieved by decision makers at a time and in the manner best calculated to achieve the goals of decision makers on a given day (Cohen, March, & Olsen, 1979).

One final approach, the *Applied Problem Solving Model* (Howlett & Ramesh, 1995), focuses on the notion that decision making in the policy process occurs in a cyclical pattern through identifiable stages. A model of problem-centred policy analysis developed by Dunn (2004) is used to structure the discussion that follows. This model is presented in Figure 31.2.

Dunn's approach emphasizes the *process of policy inquiry* and the *methodology of policy analysis*. It is not always possible to apply a formal analytical approach to solving practical problems in organizations. However, government departments and most larger public sector organizations recognize the need to develop capacity for strategic planning and policy making. This is usually achieved by creating designated positions or organizational units devoted to policy or strategic planning, an issue to which we will return later in the chapter.

Figure 31.2 Problem-Centred Policy Analysis

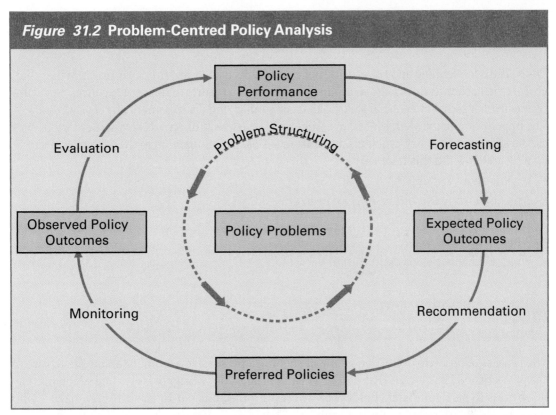

Source: Adapted from *Public Policy Analysis: An Introduction* (3rd ed.) (p. 56), by W.N. Dunn, 2004, Upper Saddle River, NJ: Prentice-Hall. Reprinted with permission.

The Policy Process

As already noted, the rational model, which is systematic and information-driven, underpins the modern public policy process. Within this, *policy analysis* is "the disciplined application of intellect to public problems" (Pal, 1992, p. 16) and is a collective activity that takes place within complex political contexts. *Policy analytic procedures* include activities such as problem structuring; forecasting; drafting policy papers, briefing notes, and policy recommendations; and monitoring and evaluating policy implementation and outcomes. *Policy analysis methods* are procedures for producing and transforming policy relevant information for use by decision makers in various contexts. They include specific techniques such as cost-benefit analysis, time series analysis, and knowledge synthesis (including meta-analysis). All of these techniques may be used by the policy analyst when responding to the demands of the policy cycle.

Policy Issues and Problems

The impetus for defining and structuring policy problems usually arises from changes in the policy environment, such as a decrease in funding, unfavourable reports in the media, concerns or complaints from internal or external stakeholders, or conflict and disagreement among stakeholders. The impetus for acknowledging policy issues and for defining or structuring issues so that they can be addressed as policy problems arises from simple questions such as the following:

- Why and how did this happen?
- What is about to happen?
- Who and how many will be or have been affected?
- Why is this important?
- What do we need to do?
- What will happen if we do nothing?

Problem Structuring and Agenda Setting

The process of problem definition is one of shaping a persuasive argument about the nature of the problem and its solution (Pal, 1997). The importance or priority of issues and problems may be obvious to particular stakeholders or interest groups, but not to the decision makers who have the authority to act upon the problem. Therefore, it is necessary to structure or frame the problem in a way that will capture the attention of decision makers, shifting their focus from the problems of the day to a new issue, or causing them to take a new look at an old problem. In the problem structuring process, conceptual and communication skills are applied to defining and structuring policy issues in a manner and format that are understandable and manageable by the individuals and groups who have the authority to make decisions.

Some policy problems are identified and structured through regular monitoring and reporting processes. For example, through the balanced scorecard process described in Chapter 13, the board of a health region may be alerted to hot spots by variances in indicators of quality or costs from one site or time period to another. The analysis of administrative information and the interpretation of indicators are critical if decision makers are to understand and focus on policy issues that are identified through routine reporting.

A sense of urgency and publicity often directs the attention of decision makers to particular problems, events, or catastrophes. A receptive public mood, media reporting, and the agendas of individual politicians or political parties intensify the impact of single focusing events (Pal, 1997). Various aspects of problem definition are discussed by Rochefort and Cobb (1993) and include the following:

- Cause (whether intentional or accidental, simple or complex)
- Severity
- Novelty (new or unexpected problem)

- Proximity (how close to home is the problem)
- Crisis (whether or not the problem presents a crisis)
- Populations affected
- Incidence
- Solutions available.

Whether the problem is about ends or goals (*instrumental orientation*), the means of achieving them (*expressive orientation*) is also important. This aspect is sometimes referred to as the "optics" of a problem, that is, the way the problem or the proposed solution looks to the various stakeholders or audiences concerned about it. Policies, decisions, and communications strategies for damage control often are determined by an assessment of how taking action, or not taking action, will be perceived or how they may increase or decrease liability for damages. Table 31.1 summarizes these aspects of problem definition.

Table 31.1 Defining a Policy Problem

Dimensions of a Problem	Options
Causality	Personal – Impersonal Intended – Accidental Blame allocated – Blame avoided Simple – Complex
Severity	Degrees of severity
Incidence	Growing, stable, or declining Social patterns: by class Population, cohort, age, etc.
Novelty	Unprecedented – Familiar
Proximity	Personally relevant – A general social issue
Crisis	Crisis – Non-crisis Emergency – Non-emergency
Problem Populations	Worthy – Unworthy Deserving – Undeserving Familiar – Strange
Ends-Means Orientation of Problem Definer	Instrumental – Expressive
Nature of Solution	Available – Nonexistent Acceptable – Objectionable Affordable – Unaffordable

Source: From Problem Definition, Agenda Access, and Policy Choice, by A.D. Rochefort and W.R. Cobb, 1993, *Policy Studies Journal, 21*(1), p. 62.

A case example illustrating how a recurring administrative problem was redefined as a policy problem that needed to be solved was documented by Anderson (1999) and is summarized in Box 31.1. This description of the development and implementation of a new regional ambulance diversion policy illustrates several aspects of the policy analysis process.

Box 31.1

Development and Implementation of a Regional Ambulance Diversion Policy

A case example of how an administrative issue was redefined as a policy problem in a large metropolitan health region was documented by Anderson (1999).

In this situation, as in many other hospitals (Mintzberg, 1997), problems of overcrowding of emergency room (ER) departments had been an ongoing operational issue and the subject of discussion in a variety of committees. A system of diverting ambulances from one hospital to another had evolved, and problems of access and inconvenience for patients had been reported frequently in the press. Thus, the senior administrative committee of the region took ownership of the problem by establishing an Ambulance Diversion Task Force under the direction of the Vice-President of Medicine to develop a new ambulance diversion policy.

Policy-relevant information was obtained through a telephone survey of hospitals in various parts of Canada to understand how they dealt with this problem. The policies of other hospitals were obtained and analyzed. A selective review of literature was also undertaken. It became evident through these activities that specific strategies for improving ER efficiency could only be effective if there were appropriate supporting strategies throughout the entire institution. This information was presented to members of the task force. Extensive consultation involved many internal stakeholders within the various hospital sites in the region. External consultation activities involved the ambulance service providers who were organized under the auspices of the municipal Fire Department. A variety of internal communication strategies were devised to engage all stakeholders and involve them in a process for reaching consensus on a policy.

Options were considered, and eventually, the preferred option was drafted into a "Request for Decision" format used within the region as the basis for formal discussion and executive-level policy decision making. A senior representative of the municipal emergency medical services agency was invited to participate in the presentation given by the task force to the senior executive committee. The policy was formally approved, and a further series of communications activities began in preparation for implementation.

A formal policy implementation plan described as "a living document which was constantly being revised" (Anderson, 1999, p. 36) was developed. This included the development of an information system to support the operation and evaluation of ambulance diversions and a training plan for the ER staff who would use this system. Implementing hospital-wide strategies in each of the sites and related staff training were other key elements of implementation. A detailed plan was developed to assure that there would be a smooth transition to the new approach to ambulance diversion on the day the new policy was implemented. A project manager was assigned to conduct and coordinate this work and to assure that the implementation schedule was maintained. A simulation exercise was conducted to test the new policy and information system. A formal evaluation plan was developed to monitor compliance with the new policy and the quality indicators deemed to be important.

Source: Adapted from *The Analysis of a Policy Problem in a Large Metropolitan Health Region,* by E. Anderson, 1999, unpublished master's project, University of Alberta, Edmonton, Alberta.

Policy-Relevant Information

Policy and decision makers require information of various kinds to determine a course of action and assure the successful implementation of policies and programs. As in research, the use of information from multiple sources improves the validity and reliability of decisions. Ideally, facts, opinions, and research findings will inform the way policies are developed, implemented, evaluated, communicated, changed, and advocated.

The term *critical multiplism* describes a technique that involves looking for common overlapping themes from information collected through a variety of ways; however, this ideal approach to policy analysis may be limited by constraints on both time and money (Dunn, 2004).

Development of Policy Options

After consideration of policy-relevant information, one or more policy options or alternatives is usually proposed. Policy options are sometimes developed as scenarios so that the costs, benefits, and predictable consequences of their underlying assumptions can be assessed and compared. The organizational culture and preferences of the chief executive officer (CEO) and senior management team will influence the way policy options are presented and evaluated. The input of key stakeholders is often solicited at this stage to assess the feasibility of proposed policy options. The time available, or perceived to be available, for decision making often determines the depth of analysis that is carried out.

Policy Recommendations

In some situations, policy recommendations are made in an informal and verbal fashion, based on personal or political beliefs and ideology. However, in environments where policy analysis or policy research is formally conducted by specialists, significant policy recommendations are brought forward to senior management through a specified process. Recommendations would usually be accompanied by a rationale or justification for why one policy is being recommended over other alternatives that have been analysed and considered. Often, these recommendations will be presented in the format of a *briefing note*. Prior to this, a *request for decision* may be used to notify key stakeholders that a policy recommendation is being brought forward and to provide opportunity for final comment before a decision is made.

Writing an effective briefing note requires both good literary skills and a mastery of computer presentation software. The past approach of crafting long exhaustively researched documents has given way to shorter written and oral presentations (Quiney, 1991). A good policy analyst tasked with creating a briefing note must take several key things into consideration. The briefing material must be oriented to the needs of the customer. This means being timely and succinct in the presentation of the issue. Senior decision makers are busy people and must process a large amount of information on any given day. Often, they will be brought up to speed on an issue while riding in a taxi or sitting on an airplane in between meetings. Thus, whatever they read or hear will have to fit into a short and often hectic time period. Although individual decision makers will have different preferences for processing information (learning styles), research has shown that most top CEOs receive key information orally (Mintzberg, 1973).

A second consideration is the context within which an issue is occurring. The decision maker will need to have a very clear understanding of the context within which a decision is to be made; therefore, an accurate and complete description of the policy problem is essential. Included in this would be an overview of stakeholder positions on the particular issue. Normally, a briefing note would begin with a summary of the issue and follow with an overview of the context. Once the problem and the context have been described, possible policy responses and their consequences should be discussed.

Where public decision makers are involved, the potential public impact of policy options will always be a primary consideration—will this choice of action generate positive or negative publicity? Other considerations relate to the potential financial and social impact on individuals and society in general. How all of this is viewed may relate back to how the issue is framed. (See the previous discussion of Rochefort & Cobb's (1993) aspects of problem definition.)

Although many possible courses of action are theoretically available, some policy options are not worth pursuing because of resource constraints (e.g., insufficient money or expertise), timelines, ideological positions, or likely, stakeholder response. Some policy ideas are not viewed as legitimate by major stakeholders and are thus not considered to be "ideas in good currency" (Schon, 1971). For example, while the option of putting all physicians on salary is sometimes discussed, no political decision maker in Canada has ever seriously considered choosing that option. Anticipation of the negative reaction from the medical profession and the possibility of public backlash make this rational policy option a non-starter. Overall, policy makers are most likely to choose options that are the least complicated and disruptive to the existing environment.

A briefing note should conclude with a good summary of the issue, options, and recommendations. While, on the surface, the structure of the briefing note seems straightforward, the trick is to include all of this information in a very small amount of space, possibly two pages. Given the complex nature of many problems, delivering all of this in two pages or 10 minutes is no small feat.

Policy Adoption

Policies are formally adopted when an accountable body or individual makes a decision. Accountable bodies may be legislatures or government committees that are sometimes empowered to approve legally binding regulations. They may also include governing boards, committees of senior officials within agencies, and sometimes approved individuals in positions of formal authority. In the Canadian parliamentary system, final decision making authority rests with the legislature (provincial or federal), although, in practice, the Cabinet, which is made up of the various ministers of government departments, is responsible and accountable for the decisions of the government.

Policy Implementation

It seems obvious to say that, once policies have been accepted or adopted, they must be implemented. Experts differ as to the degree of overlap between policy development and policy implementation processes. However, implementation has been described as a "dismal science" (Pal, 1997, p. 149) because it is a complex process often not successfully achieved. Studies of implementation have highlighted the multi-dimensionality, difficulty, and ambiguity of the process, as well as the growing realization of its importance. Factors that determine whether or not a particular policy choice is likely to succeed are summarized in Box 31.2.

Box 31.2

Factors Determining Success of Policy Choices

Perfect Implementation
1. No insurmountable external constraints
2. Adequate time and sufficient resources
3. Required combination of resources is available
4. Policy is based on a valid theory
5. Cause and effect relationships are direct and uncluttered
6. Dependency relationships are minimal
7. Objectives are agreed upon and understood
8. Tasks are specified in correct sequence
9. Perfect communication and coordination
10. Power and compliance

Problems in Assessing Policy Goals
1. Stated goals may be imprecise
2. True policy and goals may be deliberately hidden
3. Few policies have a single overriding objective
4. Limitations of measuring impacts

Source: Adapted from *Policy Analysis for the Real World* (pp. Chapter 11), by B.W. Hogwood and L.A. Gunn, 1984, Oxford, UK: Oxford University Press, as cited in Pal, 1992.

As policy analysis is conducted, efforts are often directed to involving stakeholders and attempting to gain their cooperation by means of consultation and communication activities. Wrapp (1979) noted the importance of the power structure in organizations, suggesting that the successful manager must "plot the position of the various individuals and units in the organization on a scale ranging from complete, outspoken support, to determined, sometimes bitter, and often-times well cloaked opposition" (p. 76). To implement a new initiative, Wrapp advised managers to identify and analyze the "corridors of comparative indifference" because it is in this middle ground of opinion and behaviour that individuals and groups can be influenced to cooperate with the new strategy. When Wrapp coined this insightful term, the external environments of most organizations were much less complex than they now are. Instability and rapid change in global economic conditions, government policies and funding, public opinion, and the attitudes and behaviours of previously compliant employees and patients have all added complexity to the process of policy implementation. Studies have shown that interest group agendas become prominent during the process of policy implementation, and "agencies originally established to serve the public interest end up as the compliant tools of the private interests they were supposed to regulate" (Brooks, 1993, p. 122) in a process that has been termed *co-optation*.

Policies are usually implemented by introducing new processes or programs. In some organizations, there is a clear separation between the activities of policy development and planning and implementation. One justification for this is that planners in staff departments may not be sufficiently knowledgeable about operational aspects of the organization or system to design successful implementation strategies. However, operational managers tend to be occupied with operational matters, and even those with good intentions often find that they have limited time for planning and implementing innovations.

When implementation strategies are successful, it is usually because resistance from particular stakeholder groups was anticipated accurately and dealt with. In some cases, resistance is directed to maintaining the status quo; in other situations, it may be a signal that an adaptation to the implementation strategy or policy is needed. In responsive organizations, issues and concerns raised by stakeholder groups during implementation are carefully and respectfully analyzed to add any necessary refinements to the policy or program and its implementation.

When organizational decision makers have decided to adopt a policy or to advocate for a particular policy, there is more detailed planning for the development of an implementation strategy. A new team or project management structure may be created for this task. Public relations and communications specialists are often engaged at this point to develop key messages and to package them in ways that are aligned with the communication preferences of various policy audiences. For example, governments have carefully weighed evidence and stakeholder input on the relationship between smoking, disease, and health system costs. In many Western countries, policies of various kinds have been adopted to discourage individuals from smoking. Some implementation activities for these policies fall within the domain of public health and are implemented through social marketing initiatives such as anti-smoking campaigns, health education, and the development of services to assist people who want to stop smoking.

Evaluation of Policy Performance

Ideally, clear objectives and indicators of success are identified prior to policy implementation and then monitored to assess whether the policy achieved the intended or expected results. Policies may be evaluated informally or by using rigorous research methodologies.

Program evaluation is widely used to assess policy performance and program outcomes. When new funding from external agencies is involved, there may be a requirement for a formal evaluation conducted by independent evaluators. Some organizations have an internal capacity for evaluation and voluntarily initiate monitoring and evaluation activities as a matter of course in the organizational culture. Pressures to conduct evaluation within a specified period of time can lead to premature or incorrect conclusions about the outcomes of a policy or program. Preferably, the outcomes of the implementation process and early outcomes of new policies and programs are assessed through *formative evaluation* studies, which occur as an initiative is unfolding. *Summative evaluations* assess policy and program outcomes and are best conducted after new policies and programs have stabilized and the effects of the new interventions can be distinguished from the confounding effects resulting from change management strategies and other contextual influences. Often, due to the need to be seen as objective or because of a relative lack of expertise within the organization, evaluations are conducted by management consulting firms and are designed to meet the minimum requirements of the funding agency.

There is an extensive professional and methodological literature in the field of program evaluation. Professional associations, standards, and journals have developed in this field. The merits of individual evaluation projects must be considered when assessing whether a program evaluation meets research standards. In *evaluation research*, the questions and methodology are formally specified at the outset and would be subject to other generally accepted standards of research, including ethics review. As Wood (1989) has noted, evaluation research often uses methods and tools from more than one level of research but "applies them in an action setting that may not always fit with the assumptions and principles of traditional research" (p. 223). Program evaluation methods encompass a range of approaches, from descriptive case studies to quasi-experimental and experimental designs. External validity is a matter of particular concern in evaluation research, but it can be improved by the use of multiple methods, replication, and the involvement of decision-making partners who can assist in identifying and interpreting contextual factors (Ferguson, 2004; Wood, 1989).

A case example illustrating the rational model and the policy cycle, including the implementation and evaluation phases, is presented in Box 31.3. The evaluation team for the provincial adult day programs described in this example was led by Dr. Janet Ross Kerr from the Faculty of Nursing at the University of Alberta. A number of peer-reviewed conference presentations and two peer-reviewed publications have resulted from this evaluation, which was completed in 1995 (Ross Kerr, Warren, Schalm, Smith, & Godkin, 2003; Warren, Ross Kerr, Smith, Godkin, & Schalm, 2003).

Box 31.3

Case Example: Policy, Demonstration, and Evaluation of Adult Day Programs in Alberta

Following a series of broadly based public policy consultations that took place over a 10-year period, the Alberta Ministry of Health established a Long Term Care Branch in 1978. The mandate of the newly created branch included responsibility to develop, implement, and evaluate a series of special programs located in key settings throughout the province to serve the needs of specific continuing or community care populations. An *Operational Plan for Long Term Care and Geriatric Programs* (Alberta Health, 1990b) was approved by the Minister and disseminated to stakeholder groups. The Program Development Section within the Long Term Care Branch was assigned the responsibility for developing policy implementation and evaluation strategies.

One of the special programs to be initiated under this mandate was the Adult Day Program Demonstration Project. Policy for the programs was defined and widely disseminated through a document entitled *Adult Day Support and Day Hospital Program: Background and Standards* (Alberta Health, 1990a). Two program models were described in this document: Day Hospitals, which were to offer an intensive physical and rehabilitation program for clients who would participate for no more than a few months, and Day Support Programs, which were to address the socialization needs of clients and respite care for informal caregivers over longer periods of time.

A group of programs representing each model and various regions of the province was selected for funding through a competitive process in which organizations responded to a *Request for Proposal: Adult Day Program Demonstration Project* (Alberta Health, 1991) issued by the Long Term Care Branch.

Evaluation was an integral part of the Demonstration Project, and consultants and academic investigators were invited to respond to a separate Request for Proposals in order to win the right to conduct the funded evaluation. The proposals were evaluated through a competitive process against predetermined criteria. An academic team was selected.

Results of the evaluation were initially reported in a technical document entitled *Evaluation of Adult Day Programs in Alberta: Final Report* (Kerr, Warren, & Godkin, 1995). (This and other Ministry of Health documents referred to in this case example are available from the library of Alberta Health.)

Knowledge from the evaluation has been widely disseminated through presentations at conferences of professional and scholarly organizations associations in Canada and abroad. Reports of the evaluation have also been published in peer-reviewed journals (Ross Kerr, Warren, Schalm, Smith, & Godkin, 2003; Warren, Ross Kerr, Smith, Godkin, & Schalm, 2003).

Policy in a Changing Environment

Arguably, the *incremental model* is one that accounts for the familiar situation in which policy positions are arrived at through bargaining and compromise between key decision makers. Feasibility and acceptability to stakeholders are thus the key criteria for policy adoption, and changes are made in small incremental steps so that new policies are not dramatically different from the status quo. For example, by 2004, most Canadian provinces had adopted some form of regional governance structure for the health system. Before regionalization began in the early 1990s, policy analytical activities within government departments and professional organizations had resulted in recommendations that regional structures be adopted to reduce competition for funds and to promote integrated planning and delivery of all health services. Governments in various provinces encouraged a "bottom-up" approach (Sabatier, 1986) in which stakeholders would work together to recommend strategies for collaboration and integration. In Ontario, health planning councils were formed and funded by government. However, the traditional financial incentives and communication structures in the health system had not been designed to reward collaboration, and individual health boards continued to use their direct communication with the health minister to advocate for the specific needs of their individual communities, organizations, and programs. In the early 1990s, the governments of Alberta and Saskatchewan ended the period of incrementalism and adopted a "top-down" approach (Sabatier, 1986) by passing legislation that dissolved most existing health boards and created health regions.

In the incremental approach to policy development, it is often difficult to distinguish between what Plumptre (1990) has called the "policy" and the "administrative or managerial" (1990) aspects of a new initiative. Since most policy problems have many administrative implications, "to be responsible for policy does not constitute a leave of absence from the realm of administration" (Plumptre, 1990, p. 112). The ownership of a policy problem and the policy decision-making process may therefore shift from politicians and senior leaders to administrative officials, and back again. Policy is then pragmatically defined as "anything you want to decide yourself" and administration as "anything you don't want to be bothered with" (Plumptre, 1990, p. 112).

Policy issues do not occur in a vacuum and are usually multi-dimensional. Quinn and Voyer (1996) point out that a body of literature has emphasized multiple goal structures, the politics of strategic decisions, bargaining and negotiation processes, "satisficing" in decision making, the role of coalitions, and the practice of muddling in public sector management. They (Quinn & Voyer, 1996) contrast this "power-behavioral" approach with the rational model of "formal systems planning" and point out that neither approach adequately describes strategic approaches. These authors (Quinn & Voyer, 1996) offer persuasive arguments for the use of "logical incrementalism" as an approach to improving and integrating both the analytical and behavioural aspects of strategy formation. Mintzberg and Waters (1985) offer further support for this approach, pointing out that strategies are both plans for the future and patterns from the past.

To aid in this task, the Canadian Health Services Research Foundation was created with a mandate to encourage closer partnerships between researchers and decision makers so that there will be greater receptivity to evidence and more context-sensitive evidence available to inform decision making in the health system. A model depicting a contemporary view of the complex processes through which information and evidence enter the decision-making process is illustrated in Figure 31.3. The role of knowledge purveyors or knowledge brokers in translating and synthesizing various kinds of knowledge into formats that can be used and applied in the fast-paced world of health care decision-making can be understood as a variation or specialization of more traditional policy and planning roles.

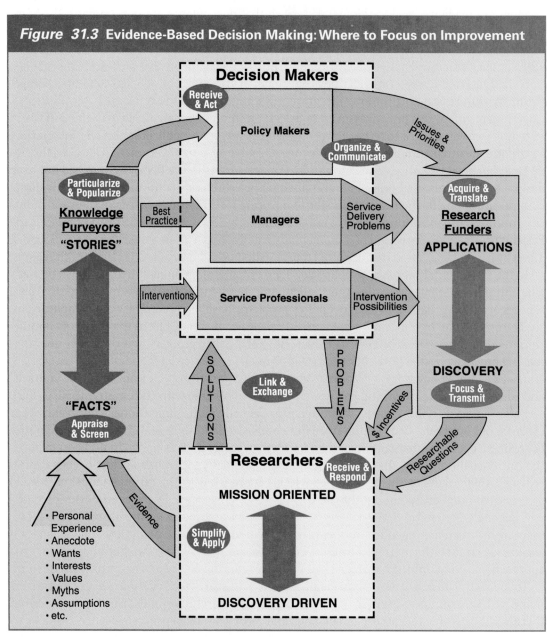

Figure 31.3 Evidence-Based Decision Making: Where to Focus on Improvement

Source: From *Health Services Research and Evidence-Based Decision-Making* (p. 7), by Canadian Health Services Research Foundation, 2000, Ottawa, ON: Author.

The Professsional Field of Policy Analysis

Policy analysis is a specialized field. It has been described as "the application of scientific methods to problems of public policy, choice and implementation," (Plumptre, 1990, p. 300) dependent upon familiarity with the social sciences, economics, and the physical sciences; upon competence in a number of analytical techniques; and upon the ability and confidence to move across interdisciplinary lines. Policy research draws upon multiple data sources and is conducted using a variety of methods. Policy analysis also has been described as "a process of multidisciplinary inquiry designed to create, critically assess and communicate information that is useful in understanding and improving policies" (Dunn, 2004, p. 2). The purpose of this process is to collect, analyze, synthesize, and formally present information from multiple sources for consideration by decision makers.

Policy analysis can take a number of forms. *Retrospective analysis* can be conducted to gain an understanding of past events. *Prospective analysis* is a process of synthesizing information to objectively develop and compare policy alternatives. Analysis may be directed to finding and structuring problems or to solving problems that have already been identified (Dunn, 2004).

As Table 31.2 demonstrates, *academic policy analysis* can be distinguished from *applied policy analysis* in terms of its goals, methods of analysis, independence, duration, and objectivity. Academic research is characterized by a focus on "big questions" and theory development and is designed to explain and understand policies. The research agenda is determined independently by the researcher, who adopts an objective or value neutral position to the extent possible. Whereas policy analysis is undertaken to achieve goals within a political mandate or to solve organizational problems (Pal, 1992), policy research is a more lengthy process intended to add to the body of knowledge about the policy process.

Experts in health service research methodology have advocated the use of a combination of qualitative and quantitative methods to account for the importance of contextual factors in

Table 31.2 Summary of Differences, Academic and Applied Policy Analysis

	Academic Policy Analysis	Applied Policy Analysis
Focus	theory; "big questions"	specific policy; specific problems
Mode of Analysis	explanation	evaluation
Goal	understand policies	change policies
Research Agenda	independent	client determined
Duration of Analysis	lengthy	short
Value Orientation	strive for objectivity; neutrality; "improvements"	accept client values; advocate

Source: From *Public Policy Analysis: An Introduction* (p. 25), by L.A. Pal, 1992, Toronto, ON: Methuen.

studies of health interventions and outcomes and to account for the impacts of policy and management innovations in the health system (Isaacs, 1993; McCloskey et al., 1996; Morse, Penrod, & Hupcey, 2000; Rowe & Jacobs, 1998; Sandelowski, 1996; Schein, 1993; Sidani, 1996).

An example of economically oriented health policy research is presented in Box 31.4. In this example, administrative data sets were compiled and analyzed to identify actual costs of health services and to model alternative scenarios using different combinations of services with different costs. This case example can be contrasted with a comparative case study conducted by Paras (2004) in which the problem structuring process in two cases of unexpected infant deaths at the Hospital for Sick Children in Toronto and the Winnipeg Health Sciences Centre were examined. In this retrospective policy analysis, documentary evidence from judicial reports,

Box 31.4

Modelling Alternatives for Financial Sustainability in the Canadian Health System

Sustainable Health Care for Canada is the synthesis report of a project undertaken to examine the outcomes and costs of treatments and to determine if there are less expensive but equally effective alternatives. Secondary goals were to enhance public understanding of the health care system and to provide policy makers with better frameworks and tools with which to make decisions on resource allocation. Researchers at Queen's University and the University of Ottawa conducted the project, which was funded by 16 public, private, and professional organizations.

This quantitative economic analysis required pioneer work to develop integrated data sets for each sector of the Canadian health system. The new data set was developed from existing administrative data collected at national, provincial, and local levels. Data were consolidated into a systematic framework of cost accounting called the Resource Allocation Framework. The actual costs of encounters between patients and health care interventions were documented in relation to health outcomes. Formal accounting procedures were used to estimate the costs and calculate the relative contributions of cost increases in each of the following sectors of the health system.

1. *Costs of hospitals* accounted for 38% of health care expenditures and increased because of general wage and price inflation, increased service intensity, and more outpatient care.

2. *Costs of physician services* per patient increased 153% over a 10-year period, at an annual rate of 10%.

3. *Costs of residential care facilities* remained relatively constant, and increases were attributed to wage and price inflation.

4. *Costs of home care* accounted for about 2% of overall health costs, and increases were a result of providing more resources per client.

5. *Costs of pharmaceuticals* rose by 90%, or 15% per year during the 1980s, and represented the third largest expenditure in total health care costs.

Information about actual costs in these sectors was used as the basis for testing or modelling a series of alternative scenarios for which costs and outcomes could be compared. The scenarios were the following:

1. Reducing acute care beds by 20% and length of stay by 20%;

2. Substituting continuing care for acute inpatient care (acute care substitution model);

3. Reducing rate variation for selected medical and surgical activities, and substituting day surgery for inpatient surgery for designated cases; and

4. Facility substitution and de-institutionalization (long-term care substitution model).

The researchers concluded that wage and price inflation accounted for over 50% of cost increases. Population growth added 10%, but the aging of the population had a marginal overall effect and little influence on hospital costs. Most cost increases came from more intensive hospital care and more physician visits and prescriptions. Therefore, strategies to shift emphasis away from hospital costs, to control variations and costs of physician services, and to control the costs of pharmaceuticals could produce significant savings for the system as a whole. A significant limitation of the study was that it did not account for the contributions of unpaid caregivers. The authors note that the role of unpaid caregivers is rapidly increasing with shifts to ambulatory and community-based care, and some estimates of the value of family care suggest that it exceeds the value of formal services by three or four times.

Source: Adapted from *Sustainable Health Care for Canada. Synthesis Report*, by D.E. Angus, L. Auer, J.E. Cloutier, and T. Albert, 1995, Ottawa, ON: Queen's University–University of Ottawa Economic Projects.

published professional commentary, and media reports were analyzed using confirmable and replicable procedures. Similarities and differences in the problem structuring process in the two hospitals were identified, and administrative behaviour was described and evaluated with reference to normative standards.

On the basis of personal experience and interviews with senior officials in the Canadian public service, Plumptre (1990) concluded that the key skills of a policy analyst include the following:

• Ability to see to the heart of an issue;

• Ability to describe complex issues in ways that make them understandable to people who are not "insiders" or experts in the area; and

• Ability to listen to and consult with stakeholders, including internal stakeholders who are the managers of operational programs and whose insight, cooperation, and leadership may be necessary to correctly define policy problems and implement approved policies.

Clearly, this requires a combination of intellectual and interpersonal skills. Since policy is made of language, policy argument in written or verbal form is central to all stages of the policy process (Majone, 1989, as cited in Dunn, 2004, p. 20). Policy arguments are developed from policy-relevant information and include proposals and their justification or rationale. Thus, as previously discussed, a key skill of the policy analyst is the ability to speak and write well in a language and style that are appropriate to the various audiences concerned with the content and implementation of a policy.

Government departments and large organizations typically have designated positions or organizational units whose role it is to conduct policy analysis and related activities such as planning. This has been termed the "policy development capacity" of the organization. At one time in public service organizations, managers were content experts who were able to offer informal advice to senior officials based on their knowledge of the programs administered by particular departments, the stakeholders typically dealt with, and the relationships with other sectors of the public service that were key to the successful acceptance and implementation of policies (Plumptre, 1990). Management philosophies in many sectors of public service have now changed so that professionals are valued less for their content knowledge and more for their generic abilities to manage processes and people.

During the 1970s, policy analysis activities began to be formalized through the creation of policy analysis units, sometimes called "policy shops," formed in government departments and some larger organizations (Brooks, 1993; Hollander & Prince, 1993; Hollander, Shapiro, & Nahmiash, 1989; Plumptre, 1990). In organizational contexts, policy analysis activities are conducted by individuals with position titles such as "policy analyst," "policy officer," or "policy advisor."

Leadership Implications

Problems may be identified and structured at any level within an organization or from outside of an organization. As Pal (1992) has emphasized, policy analysis is a cognitive activity; it is about learning and thinking critically. Individuals, departments, and stakeholder groups can, and often do, identify issues which they feel should be considered by senior decision makers. Often, however, issues remain in circulation and do not reach the agendas of decision makers. For example, many specific instances and issues are documented on the reporting forms associated with the professional responsibility committees that are mandated in the collective agreements between registered nurses and their employers. Often, the information produced through such routine procedures and reporting systems is never synthesized and framed in terms of the larger organizational context or in a manner that will enable or assure it to move forward to the decision-making agenda of the organization. The conceptual and process skills of policy analysis could be used to align these themes and issues with (a) various existing organizational messages and policies, such as the overall mission statements, (b) with specific human resources policies, such as those requiring a respectful workplace, or (c) with clinical policies, such as the requirement that physicians sign verbal orders within a certain time. Skills in oral and written communication must then be applied to conduct targeted stakeholder consultations and to create succinct briefing memos or short briefing papers that can be readily understood by senior decision makers and that provide clarity as to the magnitude or significance of issues and problems. A factual and unemotional discussion of two pages or less will be necessary to elevate an issue to the policy agenda of senior decision makers. This type of "issue alert" briefing memorandum should contain a description of the background or context of the issue, the current situation, and specific recommendations for short term action by organizational leaders. Once an issue or problem has been presented in this type of written format to individuals in positions of authority, it will usually require some sort of formal response. At this stage, more extensive briefing will likely be needed to carry the issues forward; it is sometimes possible to bring forward other policy-relevant information from previous studies or reports or from external reports of policy statements, practice in other organizations, public relations, or legal implications of the issue. Again, skillful synthesis and succinct presentation will be necessary to continue to introduce new information and perspectives to the decision-making process.

Senior leaders are usually responsible for approving policies; however, the knowledge required to successfully implement policies usually resides nearer to the grass roots of the organization. Therefore, first-line and middle managers and individuals with specialized knowledge who occupy staff positions have critical roles to play in policy implementation.

Opportunities to act as a project manager in the implementation of policies or programs sometimes arise and present nurses with opportunities for career development in which they can apply their extensive knowledge of organizational processes and interrelationships and their interpersonal and conceptual skills. Skills in written communication are essential in all aspects of policy analysis and implementation. More broadly, insights into the perspectives of various stakeholders and their preferred styles of receiving communication are required to achieve the necessary degree of consensus and collaboration required to define policy problems and implement new policy initiatives. As Pal (1997) has noted: "New ideas do not completely displace old ones in public discourse, and indeed some of the older ones float in a purgatory of lost causes, to ascend again to political heaven when the time is propitious" (p. 88).

Summary

- Public policy decision making involves a complex interplay of ideas, people, and institutions in the pursuit of solutions to problems of public concern. Within this environment, the role of the policy analyst in processing and synthesizing information, defining issues, and formulating solutions is crucial.

- Associated with this important function is a distinctive set of skills, including the ability to think systematically and critically about complex policy problems; the ability to translate this complexity into something that major stakeholders can understand; the ability to synthesize existing knowledge about the problem and translate it into potential solutions; and the ability to develop solutions that are workable within the context of a complex environment that is in a constant state of flux.

- In recognition of this key role, most public sector agencies have developed structures and processes to facilitate the work of policy analysts. In addition, a distinct body of knowledge and techniques has developed around the functions of the policy analyst. Given the increasingly complex nature of public policy, the need for this type of expertise will increase in the future.

- Politics is about power and the allocation of societal values and resources.

- Public policy is about the structures and processes through which collective decisions are made about often complex societal issues.

- Policy analysis supports public policy decision making.
- Policy analysis has evolved as a specialized field requiring advanced skills in research, critical thinking, and oral and written communication.
- Policy analysis involves the combination of a variety of approaches to information gathering, synthesis, and analysis.

Applying the Knowledge in this Chapter

Exercise

Introductory Exercise: Select a policy issue or a formal policy in your organization and answer the following questions:

1. Who are the policy stakeholders and what are their interests?
2. Is the policy formally stated? If so, in what forms and to which audiences or stakeholders?
3. Describe the context or environment in which this policy was created or is applied.
4. What national, provincial, regional, and organizational factors influence the policy?
5. How and why would this policy have reached the policy agenda of senior managers or government?
6. What types/fields/domains of knowledge are relevant to the policy and why?
7. What analytical and research strategies can be used to locate or generate policy-relevant knowledge?
8. How was the policy implementation process structured? How was it managed?
9. Where there incentives involved in the policy? If so, to whom do these apply?
10. Has there been an evaluation of the policy outcomes or impact? If so, what evaluation approaches were used?

Advanced Exercise:

1. The Situation and Problem
   - John Fog, RN, BScN, has recently been hired as a planner in the policy and planning department of the Big Blizzard Regional Health Authority. He reports to Martha Firestone, the Director of Policy and Planning. She is a Chartered Accountant who branched out into total quality management during a successful career in a public utilities company before being recruited to the health region. There are two other employees in the planning department. One is a planner who is dedicated to work on the new capital project being developed in the region. The other is an analyst who has been seconded to a provincial costing project and is only available in the regional office for a day and a half per week.

- Martha Firestone recently attended a conference where she heard a presentation referring to a study by the Health Services Utilization and Research Commission of Saskatchewan entitled: *The Impact of Preventive Home Care and Seniors Housing on Health Outcomes*. This presentation led her to wonder whether preventive home care services could be reduced or eliminated, thereby saving money that could be allocated to other programs in the region. She has asked John to analyze the report and prepare recommendations for her by the end of the week.
- John has not had a work assignment quite like this before. He quickly reads the report. It worries him a little, and he is not quite sure where to start with his assignment. He decides to consult one of his former university professors and sends the following message:

Hi Dr. Blatherskate,

I hope you remember me from your class last year.

I have been asked to provide recommendations on the report of a study entitled *The Impact of Preventive Home Care and Seniors Housing on Health Outcomes* (available at: http://www.ocsa.on.ca/PDF/Impact_of_preventive_home_care_and_seniors_ho using_on_health_outcomes.pdf)

I hope you may be able to discuss this report with me and offer some advice on possible recommendations. Could I call you to discuss? I have some concerns about the implications of the findings for home care. Thanks.

John

- His professor's reply is as follows:

Hi John,

I haven't had time to read the article you referenced and am away from the office. However, I am aware of a large national study on the cost-effectiveness of home care that may be of help to you. It is available at: http://www.home-carestudy.com/reports/index.html

Dr. B.

---

2. The Policy Analysis Task

- You are John Fog and will respond to your Director's request for a briefing memo.
- Your response should take the form of a transmittal memorandum (1–2 pages) and a short discussion paper (3–5 pages).

- Both the transmittal memorandum and discussion paper should contain your recommendations.

3. The Deliverables

- The *transmittal memorandum* should briefly refer to the assignment you have been given and describe how you have gone about it (this material should also appear at the beginning of the discussion paper).
- The *discussion paper* should open with a summary of the task you have been given and how you went about it. You should then include the following:
  - A summary of the research report you have been asked to review;
  - A discussion of the main issues raised by the report and other information on the subject that you may have reviewed, such as the other research on a similar subject recommended to you by your former professor; and
  - Your recommendations and the rationale for each. Remember that you are responding to a concrete inquiry: should changes be made to the current home care program on the basis of the study you have been asked to review? Why, or why not? If not, what, if anything else, should be done? In writing the recommendations, give thought to the time frame and activities that would be required to implement them. Consider developing at least one immediate or short-range recommendation and other mid-range and longer-range recommendations.

4. Resources

- Specialized forms of policy communication are discussed in this chapter.
- Refer also to Chapter 30 for guidance on writing memos and discussion papers.
- The reports referred to in this case are as follows:
  - The Impact of Preventive Home Care and Seniors Housing on Health Outcomes (www.ocsa.on.ca/PDF/Impact_of_preventive_home_care_and_seniors_housing_on_health_outcomes.pdf)
  - The National Evaluation of the Cost-Effectiveness of Home Care (www.homecarestudy.com/reports/index.html)
    - ✓ Overall synthesis report www.homecarestudy.com/reports/full-text/synthesis.pdf
    - ✓ Substudy 1: Final Report of the Study on the Comparative Cost Analysis of Home Care and Residential Care Services (www.homecarestudy.com/reports/full-text/substudy-01-final_report.pdf)
    - ✓ Substudy 5: Study of the Costs and Outcomes of Home Care and Residential Long Term Care Services (www.homecarestudy.com/reports/full-text/substudy-05-final_report.pdf)

5. Factors the Director of Policy and Planning Will Assess

- Were the memo and discussion paper professionally presented and on time?
- Did the planner or policy analyst carry out the right task?

- Were professional knowledge of the health system and skills of policy analysis applied in completing the task?
- Were key issues identified and, if necessary, prioritized?
- Were realistic recommendations presented?
- Was there appropriate and objective justification and rationale for the recommendations presented?
- Is the style and tone of the memorandum and discussion paper sensitive to the reader and culture (i.e., avoiding jargon or insider language and suitable for a variety of readers with different backgrounds and experience)?

Resources

evolve Internet Resource

Canadian Health Services Research Foundation (CHSRF):
www.chsrf.ca/home_e.php

Further Reading

Health Services Utilization and Research Commission. (2000, May). *The impact of preventive home care and seniors housing on health outcomes* (Summary report no. 14). Saskatoon, SK: Author.

Hollander, M.J. (2001, April). *Substudy 1: Final report of the study on the comparative cost analysis of home care and residential care services*. Victoria, BC: National Evaluation of the Cost-Effectiveness of Home Care.

Hollander, M.J., & Chappell, N. (2002, March). *Synthesis report: Final report of the national evaluation of the cost-effectiveness of home care*. Victoria, BC: National Evaluation of the Cost-Effectiveness of Home Care.

Hollander, M.J., Chappell, N., Havens, B., & McWilliam, C. (2002, February). *Substudy 5: Study of the costs and outcomes of home care and residential long term care services*. Victoria, BC: National Evaluation of the Cost-Effectiveness of Home Care.

References

Alberta Health. (1990a). *Adult day support and day hospital program: Background and standards*. Edmonton, AB: Author.

Alberta Health. (1990b). *Operational plan for long term care and geriatric programs*. Edmonton, AB: Author.

Alberta Health. (1991). *Request for proposal: Adult day program demonstration project*. Edmonton, AB: Author.

Anderson, E. (1999). *The analysis of a policy problem in a large metropolitan health region*. Unpublished master's project, University of Alberta, Edmonton, Alberta, Canada.

Angus, D.E., Auer, L. Cloutier, J.E., & Albert, T. (1995). *Sustainable health care for Canada. Synthesis report.* Ottawa, ON: Queen's University.

Brooks, S. (1993). *Public policy in Canada: An introduction* (2nd ed.). Toronto, ON: McClelland & Stewart Inc.

Canadian Health Services Research Foundation. (2000). *Health services research and evidence-based decision-making.* Ottawa, ON: Author.

Cheek, J., & Gibson, T. (1997). Policy matters: Critical policy analysis and nursing. *Journal of Advanced Nursing, 25*(4), 668–672.

Clarke, H.F. (2003). Health and nursing policy: A matter of politics, power, and professionalism. In M. McIntyre & E. Thomlinson (Eds.), *Realities of Canadian nursing: Professional, practice and power issues* (pp. 61–82). Philadelphia: Lippincott Williams & Wilkins.

Cohen, M., March, J., & Olsen, J. (1979). People, problems and solutions and the ambiguity of relevance. In J. March & J. Olsen (Eds.), *Ambiguity and choice in organizations.* Bergen, Norway: Universitetsforlaget.

Dannemiller, K.D., & Jacobs, R.W. (1992). Changing the way organizations change: A revolution of common sense. *The Journal of Applied Behavioral Science, 28*(4), 480–498.

Doern, G.B. & Phidd, R.W. (1983). *Canadian public policy: Ideas, structure, process.* Agincourt, ON: Methuen Publications.

Dunn, W.N. (2004). *Public policy analysis: An introduction* (3rd ed.). Upper Saddle River, NJ: Prentice-Hall.

Dye, T.R. (1972). *Understanding public policy* (3rd ed). Englewood Cliffs, NJ: Prentice-Hall.

Easton, D. (1965). *A framework for political analysis.* Englewood Cliffs, NJ: Prentice-Hall.

Ferguson, L. (2004). External validity, generalizability, and knowledge utilization. *Journal of Nursing Scholarship, 36*(1), 16–22.

Helms, L.B., Anderson, M.A., & Hanson, K. (1996). "Doin' politics": Linking policy and politics in nursing. *Nursing Administration Quarterly, 20*(3), 312–321.

Hewison, A. (1999). The new public management and the new nursing: Related by rhetoric? Some reflections on the policy process and nursing. *Journal of Advanced Nursing, 29*(7), 1377–1384.

Hogwood, B.W., & Gunn, L.A. (1984). *Policy analysis for the real world.* Oxford, UK: Oxford University Press.

Hollander, M.J. & Prince, M.J. (1993). Analytical units in federal and provincial governments: Origins, functions and suggestions for effectiveness. *Canadian Public Administration, 36*(2), 191–224.

Hollander, M.J., Shapiro, E., & Nahmiash, D. (1989). The analytical manager: Integrating research and service delivery to build a better tomorrow. *Healthcare Management Forum, 2*(4), special supplement, 29–35.

Howlett, M., & Ramesh, M. (1995). *Studying public policy: Policy cycles and policy subsystems.* Toronto, ON: Oxford University Press.

Isaacs, W.N. (1993). Taking flight: Dialogue, collective thinking and organizational learning. *Organizational Dynamics, 22*(2), 24–39.

Jenkins, W.I. (1978). *Policy analysis: A political and organizational perspective.* London: Martin Robertson.

Kerr, J.C., Warren, S., & Godkin, M.D. (1995). *Evaluation of adult day programs in Alberta. Final report.* Edmonton, AB: Alberta Health, Long Term Care Branch.

Lasswell, H. (1958). *Politics: Who gets what, when, how.* Cleveland, OH: World Publishing Company.

Lindblom, C. (1959). The science of "muddling through." *Public Administration Review, 19*(2), 79–88.

Lomas, J. (2000). Connecting research and policy. ISUMA: *Canadian Journal of Policy Research, 1*(1), 140–144.

Longest, B.B., Jr. (1996). *Seeking strategic advantage through health policy analysis.* Chicago: Health Administration Press.

McCloskey, J.C., Maas, M.L., Huber, D.G., Kasparek, A., Specht, J.P., Ramler, C.L., et al. (1996). Nursing management innovations: A need for systematic evaluation. In K. Kelly & M.L. Maas (Eds.), *Outcomes of effective management practice, SONA 8: Series on nursing administration* (pp. 3–19). London: Sage Publications.

Mintzberg, H. (1973). *The nature of managerial work.* New York: Harper & Row.

Mintzberg, H. (1997). Toward healthier hospitals. *Health Care Management Review, 22*(4), 9–18.

Mintzberg, H., & Waters, J.A. (1985). Of strategies, deliberate and emergent. *Strategic Management Journal, 6*(3), 257–272.

Morse, J.M., Penrod, J., & Hupcey, J.E. (2000). Qualitative outcome analysis: Evaluating nursing interventions for complex clinical phenomena. *Journal of Nursing Scholarship, 32*(2), 125–130.

Pal, L.A. (1992). *Public policy analysis: An introduction* (2nd ed.). Scarborough, ON: Nelson Canada.

Pal, L.A. (1997). *Beyond policy analysis: Public issue management in turbulent times.* Scarborough, ON: International Thomson Publishing.

Paras, A. (2004). *Administrative behavior in two cases of unexpected children's deaths.* Unpublished master's thesis, University of Alberta, Edmonton, Alberta, Canada.

Plumptre, T.W. (1990). *Beyond the bottom line: Management in government.* Halifax, NS: The Institute for Research on Public Policy.

Prescott, P.A. (1993). Nursing: An important component of hospital survival under a reformed health care system. *Nursing Economics, 11*(4), 192–199.

Quiney, R.G. (1991). How to create superior briefings. Ottawa, ON: Canadian Centre for Management Development.

Quinn, J.B., & Voyer, J. (1996). Logical incrementalism: Managing strategy formation. In H. Mintzberg & J.B. Quinn (Eds.), *The strategy process: Concepts, contexts, cases* (3rd ed., pp. 95–101). Upper Saddle River, NJ: Prentice Hall.

Rochefort, A.D., & Cobb, W.R. (1993). Problem definition, agenda access, and policy choice. *Policy Studies Journal, 21*(1), 56–71.

Ross Kerr, J.C., Warren, S., Schalm, C., Smith, D.L., & Godkin, M.D. (2003, December). Adult day programs: Who needs them? *Journal of Gerontological Nursing, 29*(12), 11–17.

Rowe, W.F., & Jacobs, N.F. (1998). Principles and practices of organizationally integrated evaluation. *The Canadian Journal of Program Evaluation, 13*(1), 115–138.

Rush. (1980). *Free will.* On Permanent waves [record]. Toronto, ON: Anthem Records.

Sabatier, P.A. (1986). Top-down and bottom-up approaches to implementation research: A critical analysis and suggested synthesis. *Journal of Public Policy, 6*(1), 21–48.

Sandelowski, M. (1996). Using qualitative methods in intervention studies. *Research in Nursing and Health, 19*(4), 359–364.

Schein, E.H. (1993). On dialogue, culture, and organizational learning. *Organizational Dynamics, 22*(2), 40–51.

Schon, D.A. (1971). *Beyond the stable state.* New York: W.W. Norton and Company.

Shamian, J., Skelton-Green, J., & Villeneuve, M. (2003). Policy is the lever for effecting change. In M. McIntyre & E. Thomlinson (Eds.), *Realities of Canadian nursing: Professional, practice and power issues* (pp. 83–104). Philadelphia: Lippincott Williams & Wilkins.

Sidani, S. (1996). Methodological issues in outcomes research. *Canadian Journal of Nursing Research, 28*(3), 87–94.

Skelton-Green, J.M. (1996). The perceived impact of committee participation on job satisfaction and retention of staff nurses. *Canadian Journal of Nursing Administration, 9*(2), 7–35.

Valentine, N.M. (2000). The evolving role of the chief nurse executive in the veterans health administration: policy and leadership lessons. *Policy, Politics, & Nursing Practice, 1*(1), 36–46.

Warren, S., Ross Kerr, J., Smith, D., Godkin, D., & Schalm, C. (2003). The impact of adult day programs on family caregivers of elderly relatives. *Journal of Community Health Nursing, 20*(4), 209–221.

Weller, G.R. (1980). The determinants of Canadian health policy. *Journal of Health Politics, Policy and Law, 5*(3), 405–418.

West, E., & Scott, C. (2000). Nursing in the public sphere: Breaching the boundary between research and policy. *Journal of Advanced Nursing, 32*(4), 817–824.

Wood, M. (1989). Evaluative designs. In P.J. Brink & M.J. Wood (Eds.), *Advanced design in nursing research* (pp. 223–237). Newbury Park, CA: Sage Publications.

Wrapp, H.E. (1979). Good managers don't make policy decisions. In Harvard Business Review (Ed.), *On human relations* (pp. 74–87). New York: Harper & Row.

Notes on Contributors

Anita Au, RN, BScN, MN is a graduate of the Faculty of Nursing at the University of Alberta. She has held a series of clinical positions in acute and long-term care. She is currently a clinical instructor in the Faculty of Nursing at the University of Alberta and a lab tutor for after-degree and undergraduate students.

Andrea Baumann, RN, PhD is Associate Vice-President, Faculty of Health Sciences International at McMaster University, a professor in the School of Nursing and Co-Principal Investigator in the Nursing Health Services Research Unit that studies health human resources and health services. This Ontario Ministry of Health and Long-Term Care nursing research unit coordinates many projects relevant to health human resources including economics, business, epidemiology, and industrial engineering. She has directed several international projects in relation to capacity building and higher education and is editor of the *Journal of Advanced Nursing* for the Americas. In 2004, she completed over 13 years as the Associate Dean of Health Sciences (Nursing) at McMaster University.

Jennifer Blythe, MLS, PhD is an Associate Professor at the School of Nursing, McMaster University and Senior Scientist at the Nursing Health Services Unit, formerly the Nursing Effectiveness, Utilization and Outcomes Research Unit (NEUORU). Her academic background includes degrees in anthropology, library and information science, and English language and literature. Her current research interests include nursing human resources and health care restructuring.

Vickie Boechler, RN, BScN, MN teaches Leadership and Current Issues in Nursing at the University of Alberta, Faculty of Nursing, Edmonton, Alberta. She is an experienced health professional in community/public health and home care, project management, program planning, evaluation, risk management, and quality assurance. She has been extensively involved in research with the Swift Efficient Application of Research in Community Health (SEARCH) Program at the Alberta Heritage Foundation for Medical Research.

John Church, BA (Hons), MA, PhD has spent the past two decades conducting research on health policy and politics, with a specific emphasis on the development of regional and community-based models for the management and delivery of health services. He is currently Associate Professor in the Centre for Health Promotion Studies and the Department of Political Science at the University of Alberta.

Lana Clark, RN, BScN, MN has served as General Manager, Women's Reproductive Services and Children's Health, Saskatoon and District Health. She is a former Assistant Executive Director, Patient Care at the Royal University Hospital, Saskatoon. She has several years experience as a front-line manager and in senior nursing administration.

Greta Cummings, RN, PhD is Assistant Professor in the Faculty of Nursing, University of Alberta. In her doctoral research completed in 2003, she examined the effects of hospital restructuring on nurses and how leadership styles intensify or mitigate these effects. She has served for 15 years in senior nursing leadership positions at local, regional, and provincial levels, and has been actively involved in health services policy development. She was co-chair of the Alberta Expert

Advisory Panel to Review Publicly Funded Services and is a member of the Access Standards Committee for Breast Cancer Services. She is currently President-Elect of the Canadian Association of Nurses in Oncology which will be hosting the 2006 International Cancer Care Nursing Conference in Toronto.

Germaine M. Dechant, RN, BScN, MHSA is the Executive Director of Child and Adolescent Services Association, an organization that provides community-based mental health services to infants, children, adolescents, and their families. She brings to this position a background rich in clinical work, teaching, research, management, and senior administration, including a position as Chief Executive Officer of an urban community hospital. In 2004, she received the Alberta Association of Registered Nurses Award for Excellence in Nursing Administration.

Linda M. Doody, RN, MEd is the Manager of Senior's Programs with the Division of Aging and Seniors at the Department of Health and Community Services, St. John's, Newfoundland. She has over 30 years of experience in the health care sector and has held a number of management positions both at the institutional and governmental level. She currently plays a leadership role in the development of standards and guidelines for a broad spectrum of services encompassing institutional and residential care as well as continuing care and home support.

Jennifer Dziuba-Ellis, RN is a PhD candidate in the McMaster University Clinical Health Sciences (Nursing) program, and a student of the Ontario Training Centre's Health Services and Policy Research Diploma program. Her areas of interest include nursing work design, employment strategies, and resource teams.

Joy Edwards, RN, BScN, MSN, PhD has worked as a public health nurse in a variety of settings including generalized public health in the Northwest Territories and Ontario as well as specialized public health with physically handicapped children. She has worked as a researcher in Public Health in the Edmonton area for over 24 years. She is currently Manager, Population Health Assessment with the Population Health and Research Department, Public Health, Capital Health, Alberta.

Richard Fraser, QC has practiced law for 34 years in Alberta. He has a BA (1968) and LLB (1969) from the University of Alberta and a Masters of Law Degree (1972) from the London School of Economics. He provides legal services to health care clients including the Caritas Health Group, operator of the Grey Nuns Community Hospital, Misericordia Community Hospital, and Edmonton General Continuing Care Centre. He is also an Adjunct Assistant Professor at the John Dossetor Health Ethics Centre at the University of Alberta. He was the Chair of the Canadian Bar Association Health Law Section and was Chair of the Canadian Bar Association Task Force on Health Care Reform.

Nonie Fraser-Lee, BComm, MHSA is a population health researcher (health status) with the Department of Population Health and Research in the Public Health Division, Capital Health, Alberta. She has worked for 16 years in the field of health status, epidemiology, and population health under the public health domain with a particular interest in infant health.

Sheila Gallagher, RN, (EP), PhD has worked as a nurse practitioner in community-based settings in New York City and Edmonton, Alberta. She works with local, provincial, and national nursing organizations on policy development in primary health care and also advanced nursing practice. Currently, she is Health Leader in the Child and Adolescent Health Service, Children's Asthma Clinic, and a nurse practitioner in the High Risk Growth and Development Clinic in the Northeast Community Health Centre in Edmonton.

Grant Gillis, BSc Advanced (Immunology), BComm (Health Services Administration) is currently the Manager, Standards Liaison at the Canadian Institute for Health Information (CIHI), leading a team that is responsible for HL7 Canada, the Partnership for Health Information Standards, and the Canadian Advisory Committee to ISO/TC 215 Health Informatics. Previously, he served as Secretary, ISO/TC 176 Quality Management and Quality Assurance. He played a major role in recent international applications of the ISO (International Organization for Standardization) 9000 standards in the field of health care, in particular for laboratory medicine. Grant also has held corporate management positions with the University Health Network and the Saskatoon Regional Health Board.

Phyllis Giovannetti, RN, BN, ScD is Professor Emerita, University of Alberta where she held the position of Associate Dean of the Graduate Program in the Faculty of Nursing. She was involved in some of the earliest North American efforts to develop nursing information, particularly in the area of nursing-workload measurement, nursing-resource utilization, and costs. A former President of the Alberta Association of Registered Nurses, she chaired the Canadian Nurses Association Planning Committee for the First Canadian Nursing Minimum Data Set Conference.

Moira Hennessey, BComm is Assistant Deputy Minister—Board Services, Department of Health and Community Services, in St. John's, Newfoundland. In this capacity, she has executive responsibilities for the regional health boards and emergency health services. She has 30 years of experience in the health sector and has been extensively involved in health care reform in Newfoundland and Labrador. Her previous work experience includes progressive senior administrative responsibilities in community-based agencies and private consulting work in health administration.

Alan Heyhurst, CA is currently Director of Corporate Services, St. Mary's Hospital, Camrose, Alberta. He previously served as Director of Business Support with the Community Care and Public Health Division of Capital Health in Edmonton, Alberta, and as an Auditor with the Office of the Auditor General of Alberta.

Judith M. Hibberd, BScN, MHSA, PhD is Professor Emerita, University of Alberta where she taught leadership and management courses to graduate and undergraduate students in the Faculty of Nursing. A graduate of the Nightingale School of Nursing, St. Thomas' Hospital, London, England, she practiced as a midwife before emigrating to Canada. In Toronto, she practiced in the field of home care with the Victorian Order of Nurses, and held positions in teaching and front-line management at the Toronto General Hospital. Following completion of her master's degree in health services administration she was appointed Assistant Executive Director—Nursing at the Glenrose Rehabilitation Hospital in Edmonton, Alberta. Her doctoral research on the labour disputes of Alberta nurses remains a classic in this field of study, and she pursued this and related interests in nursing worklife in subsequent research. Dr. Hibberd has served as chair of the Professional Conduct Committee of the Alberta Association of Registered Nurses and as a board member of the Canadian Association for the History of Nursing and the Alberta Registered Nurses Educational Trust. As first author/editor of the original edition of this book, *Nursing Management in Canada* (1994) and subsequent editions, Hibberd has made a distinguished contribution to education and scholarship in the field of nursing leadership in Canada.

Bernadette Hobson, RN, BScN is a student in the MN program, Faculty of Nursing, University of Alberta pursuing studies in leadership, teaching, and learning. Her areas of clinical interest are in transplantation and patient education strategies.

Noela Inions, ORPG, BScN, LLB, LLM, CHE is Legal Counsel—Health Information for the Information and Privacy Commissioner of Alberta. She is a nurse and lawyer with diverse experience in health and privacy law in the private and public sector. Inions is co-author of the book, *Canadian Health Information* (3rd ed.), and the author of the book *Quality Assurance and Privilege in Canadian Hospitals*.

Philip Jacobs, DPhil (Economics), CMA is a professor in the Department of Public Health Sciences, University of Alberta and is an affiliate professor with the Institute of PharmacoEconomics, Edmonton, Alberta. His research is in the areas of health-care funding and economic evaluation of health-care interventions.

Angela Kaida, MSc, BSc is a public health researcher trained in epidemiology and population health. She has experience working on public health issues both locally and internationally, primarily in eastern Africa and India. Currently, she works as an infectious disease epidemiologist with Alberta Health and Wellness in Edmonton, Alberta. Her previous employment was as a population health researcher with Public Health, Capital Health, Alberta.

Hester E. Klopper, RN, PhD has held leadership roles in nursing education in her native country of South Africa. She was Associate Professor in the Faculty of Nursing, University of Alberta when she contributed to this book.

Bonnie Lendrum, RN, BScN, MScN has held both line and staff positions during her career including Director of Education and Professional Development, Chedoke-McMaster Hospitals, Hamilton, Ontario; Director of Surgical Nursing, Royal Victoria Hospital, Montreal; Clinical Nurse Specialist, Sunnybrook Hospital, Toronto; and Planning Specialist, Hamilton Health Sciences Corporation.

Penelope Lightfoot, BSc(PT), MHSA is Director of Population Health and Research within the Capital Health Region in Alberta. She is responsible for assessment of the population's health and selected policy development, which focuses on prevention. She has 20 years of experience in the health field, including clinical practice and research, with a focus on pubic health, knowledge mobilization, and policy development.

Marianne McLennan, RN, PhD, CHE is Manager for Quality Improvement of the Vancouver Island Health Authority, one of six health authorities in British Columbia. She brings a rich understanding of the health care system based on her work experiences in community, acute, and rehabilitation settings from a variety of clinical, educational, and senior leadership roles. Her current research interests relate to quality work settings for nurses and knowledge translation in practice.

Carl A. Meilicke, BComm, DHA, PhD is Professor Emeritus, University of Alberta. He was founder and first Director of the Program in Health Services Administration, University of Alberta (1968–1980). He was then seconded to the Alberta Department of Health as the first Associate Deputy Minister, Policy Development. He returned to the University of Alberta from 1982–1993 and taught in the Department of Health Services Administration and Community Medicine. Throughout his career in health services administration, he maintained a special interest in the management of nursing services.

Shirley Meyer, RN, BN, MN is Director of Integrated Nursing Systems in the Calgary Health Region. Her 32-year career has spanned clinical, management, and informatic sectors in health care. She is presently responsible for the operation of the regional staff scheduling services, nursing workload measurement systems as well as nursing involvement with the electronic health record.

Margaret Mrazek, QC, BSN, MHSA, LLB is a partner with the law firm of Reynolds, Mirth, Richards & Farmer in Edmonton, Alberta. Her emphasis of practice is in the areas of health (including corporate and commercial transactions related to the health area), labour law, professional discipline work, and the facilitation of disputes. A registered nurse who has worked as a general duty nurse, she also taught in a hospital-based school of nursing and later became the director of that school. She held several senior administrative positions in a large active treatment hospital before beginning to practise law. She was appointed a Queen's Counsel in January 2004.

Cora Newhook, RN, BScN, MN (EP) has served in the Canadian Forces Medical Services since 1986 in Canada, Germany, and Bosnia. Her extensive clinical practice has included specialization in operating room nursing. Captain Newhook completed the Graduate Level Diploma Program for Advanced Nursing Practice at Athabasca University, qualifying as a nurse practitioner, and has been involved in implementing the innovative Primary Health Care initiative operationalized by the Canadian Forces over the past several years. While completing her MN degree in the Faculty of Nursing at the University of Alberta, she was a Student Research Partner in the LINCS Research Program funded by the Canadian Health Services Research Foundation, the Alberta Heritage Foundation for Medical Research and organizational partners in Alberta and Saskatchewan to study continuity of care.

Anita Paras, RN, BN, MN is a program consultant in the Quality and Accountability Branch of the Alberta Ministry of Health. She has extensive clinical experience in rural hospital settings and in perioperative and post-anaesthesia recovery room nursing. Her areas of interest are patient safety, accountability, and policy development. Her MN thesis, *Administrative Behaviour in Two Cases of Children's Deaths*, received the Ginette Lemire Rodger Award for Nursing Administration from the Canadian Nurses Foundation in 2002.

Leah Evans Parisi, RN, BScN, CRNA, MA, EdD, JD is Division Dean, Business Technologies, Technical College of the Lowcountry, Beaufort, South Carolina. She was formerly Professor, School of Nursing, McMaster University in Hamilton, Ontario, and Coordinator of the Leadership/Management Distance Education Program. Her career has included medical malpractice and medical staff privileges defense law in California, clinical practice as a nurse anaesthetist, and teaching in the areas of management, law, and ethics.

Carolyn J. Pepler, RN, BScN, MScN, PhD was Consultant for Nursing Research at the Royal Victoria Hospital of the McGill University Health Centre, Montreal, and is Associate Professor (retired), School of Nursing, McGill University. In 1992, she was awarded the prestigious Canadian Nurses Foundation/Ross Laboratories Award for Nursing Leadership, and in 2000, she received the Insigne de Mérite from the Ordre des infirmiers et infirmières du Québec for outstanding contribution to the profession.

Gerald Predy, MD, FRCPC is Medical Officer of Health for Capital Health in Edmonton and Associate Clinical Professor, Faculty of Medicine in the Department of Public Health Sciences at the University of Alberta. Dr. Predy holds a Fellowship in the Royal College of Physicians and Surgeons with a specialty in Community Medicine and has over 25 years experience in Family Medicine and Public Health in both rural and urban settings. His major responsibilities include managing health protection programs and monitoring and reporting on the health status of the population.

Ginette Lemire Rodger, RN, BScN, MAdmN, PhD is Vice President, Professional Practice and Chief Nursing Executive, Ottawa Hospital, and President of Lemire Rodger and Associates. She was awarded Canada's highest nursing honour, the Jeanne Mance Award in 2004, for her contributions to the profession. She served as Executive Director, Canadian Nurses Association, the Canadian Nurses Foundation, and the Canadian Nurses Protective Society from 1981 to 1989. She has held positions in clinical nursing, management, education, and research.

Michelle Salesse, RN, BScN, MN, OHNC is Program Leader of two 34-bed sub-acute care units at the Glenmore Park site of Carewest, a leading continuing care organization based in Calgary, Alberta. She is a certified Occupational Health Nurse whose professional interests include strategic health systems program and project planning, development, implementation, and evaluation.

Judith Skelton-Green, RN, BScN, MScN, PhD has extensive experience as a senior nurse executive in both educational and service settings. Since the fall of 1995, she has been President of TRANSITIONS, a consulting firm specializing in facilitating human and organizational change. During this period she also has held associate appointments with both Ernst & Young and Deloitte & Touche's health consulting practices. She has consulted to over 80 different clients in more than 120 engagements, mostly in the areas of corporate integration, organizational redesign, leadership development, strategic planning, and operational review.

Donna Lynn Smith, RN, BScN, MEd, CPsych, CHE is currently Associate Professor in the Faculty of Nursing, University of Alberta where she teaches courses in nursing leadership and coordinates the Leadership Stream in the Masters of Nursing Program. Between 1973 and 1988, she held senior nursing leadership positions in teaching and rehabilitation hospitals with responsibility for acute, long-term care, mental health, and home care programs. Between 1988 and

1995, she served as Manager of Program Development and Special Programs, and Manager of Strategic Development in the Long Term Care and Community Care Branches of the Alberta Ministry of Health. Throughout her leadership career, Professor Smith has been a champion of evidence-based practice and innovation. In 1979, she initiated the Nursing Research and Scholarly Activities Committee in the Nursing Division of the University of Alberta Hospitals that served as a focus for research development and knowledge transfer for a 10-year period. She played a leadership role in the development of the John Dossetor Centre for Health Ethics on the University of Alberta campus and was the first Executive Director of the Coordinating Council of Health Sciences, an innovative partnership of the Deans of all health science faculties at the University of Alberta. Professor Smith has research expertise in policy analysis and research, policy and program evaluation, and case study methods. She currently leads a nationally funded, interdisciplinary research program focused on continuity of care. Other research interests include safety quality and accountability in health services, policy, and programs for older people and vulnerable populations, and the scholarship of collaboration.

Jane E. Smith, RN, BScN, MN is a graduate of the Vancouver General Hospital School of Nursing and has held nursing positions in rural and urban acute-care settings. Her career also includes working as a police constable in the Vancouver City Police Department. Later, she served as coordinator of a project to develop interdisciplinary case management education at the University of Alberta. She recently worked as a program manager in geriatric rehabilitation and currently is pursuing advanced nurse practitioner studies.

Heather K. Spence Laschinger, RN, PhD is Professor and Associate Director, Nursing Research in the School of Nursing at the University of Western Ontario. Since 1992, Dr. Laschinger has been Principal Investigator in a program of research designed to investigate nursing work environments. She is the recipient of many awards including Best Paper in the Health Care Management Division of the American Academy of Management in 2002 and the Sigma Theta Tau International Elizabeth McWilliams Miller Award for Excellence in Nursing Research. Dr. Laschinger and her colleague Carol Wong are Co-Principal Investigators in the Canadian Nursing Leadership Study funded by the Canadian Health Services Research Foundation and supported by a number of organizational sponsors from across Canada. The study is designed to inform decision-making for effective nursing leadership role configuration and organizational structure in hospitals.

Janet L. Storch, RN, BScN, MHSA, PhD is Professor and former Director, School of Nursing, University of Victoria. She was previously Dean, Faculty of Nursing, University of Calgary and Program Director of the Health Services Administration Program at the University of Alberta. A noted teacher and author, she has written numerous articles on health-care policy and on ethical issues in health care and nursing. She continues teaching and research in health policy, health ethics, research ethics, and nursing ethics.

Ann E. Tourangeau, RN, BScN, PhD is Assistant Professor at the Faculty of Nursing, University of Toronto and Adjunct Scientist with the Institute for Clinical Evaluative Sciences in Ontario. Ann holds a Career Scientist award (2003–2008) with the Ontario Ministry of Health and Long-Term Care. Previous to her academic career commencing in 2001, she was a nurse administrator in several Alberta and Ontario acute care hospitals. Her program of research is in the area of understanding the determinants of clinical and organizational outcomes such as mortality and unplanned readmission to hospital. She uses large administrative data sets and primary data in her research.

Patricia E.B. Valentine, RN, PhD is Associate Professor, Faculty of Nursing, University of Alberta, where she has worked since 1987. She is Director of the International Nursing Centre. Her research is focused on gender (feminism) and nursing. Her work on culture of women-dominated organizations is featured in nursing and educational administration texts. She has written several articles on conflict management strategies used by various levels of women nurses and the impact that gender has on the types of strategies used by nurses.

Ardene Robinson Vollman, RN, BSN, MA, PhD is Adjunct Associate Professor in the Faculties of Nursing, Medicine (Community Health Sciences) and Kinesiology, University of Calgary. She is also a health and evaluation consultant. Her interests are public health and health promotion of vulnerable populations.

P. Susan Wagner, RN, MSc (Nsg) is Professor at the College of Nursing, University of Saskatchewan. She served two terms as a member of the Saskatoon Regional Health Board, including one elected by the public and two and a half years as the Board chair. She has extensive background on other health agency boards, and her professional practice and research is in the evaluation of community-based programs.

Dorothy M. Wylie, RN, BScN, MA, MSc (HRD) held many senior management positions including that of Vice President of Nursing at the Toronto General Hospital. More recently, she was a consultant in organizational and management development and Associate Professor (part-time), Faculty of Nursing, University of Toronto. She was Editor of the *Canadian Journal of Nursing Administration*, now known as the *Canadian Journal of Nursing Leadership*.

Leona Zboril-Benson, RN, BSN, MN is a doctoral candidate in the Faculty of Nursing, University of Alberta. She currently is employed as a Quality Consultant in the Capital Health Region, Edmonton, Alberta, where she formerly held the position of Unit Manager for Adult Operative Services at the University of Alberta Hospital. Her areas of interest include nursing leadership, patient safety, nursing practice environments, and continuity of care.

Index